Management of Diabetes Mellitus

Diana W. Guthrie, PhD, ARNP, FAAN, BC-ADM, CDE, NCC, AHN-BC, CHTP, FAADE She received an associate arts degree from Graceland College in Iowa; a bachelor of science in nursing, and a master's of science in public health from the University of Missouri–Columbia; an education specialist in counseling and development at the Wichita State University; and a doctorate from Walden University, St. Paul, Minnesota. She is now Professor Emeritus, Department of Pediatrics, University of Kansas School of Medicine–Wichita. She holds an adjunct professor appointment with the School of Nursing at the Wichita State University. She has been involved in the field of diabetes since 1969 as a diabetes educator, consultant, specialist, and nurse practitioner. She is certified in counseling, community health, stress management education, holistic nursing, healing touch, as a diabetes educator, and holds advanced status as a diabetes nurse practitioner and as a holistic nurse. She holds diplomate status in clinical biofeedback and is a fellow of the American Board of Medical Psychotherapy and the National Board for Certified Clinical Hypnotherapists. Dr. Guthrie is a clinical member of the American Association of Marriage and Family Therapists, is a fellow of the American Academy of Nursing and the American Association of Diabetes Education. In Kansas, she is also licensed in clinical marriage and family therapy and clinical professional counseling. Dr. Guthrie received the Outstanding Educator Award from the American Diabetes Association and the Distinguished Service Award from the American Association of Diabetes Educators. She has also received the Exemplar Award from the Epsilon chapter of Sigma Theta Tau and Kansas Counselor of the Year from the State Counseling Association.

Richard A. Guthrie, MD, FAAP, FACE He is a clinical professor of the Department of Pediatrics and Family & Community Medicine, University of Kansas School of Medicine–Wichita, medical director of the Robert L. Jackson Diabetes Research Institute, president and medical director of Mid-America Diabetes Associates, president of Great Plains Diabetes Research, Inc., and fellow of the American Academy of Pediatrics and the American College of Endocrinologists. He has been in the field of diabetes since 1966 and has served on various committees and chaired or been a member of the local and national Board of Directors of the American Diabetes Association and the American Association of Diabetes Educators. He is boarded in Pediatric Endocrinology and, because of the increasing number of nonpediatric patients referred to him, opened his practice to adults in 1979. He was given the award for Camping and Youth and was also recognized as the Outstanding Physician Clinician of the year in 2004 by the American Diabetes Association. He has held membership and worked in various roles supporting the International Diabetes Federation, the International Society of Pediatric and Adolescent Diabetes, the Diabetes Education and Camping Association, and the American College of Endocrinology for more than 30 years.

6
EDITION

Management of Diabetes Mellitus

A Guide to the Pattern Approach

Diana W. Guthrie, PhD, BC-ADM, CDE, FAADE
Richard A. Guthrie, MD, FACE

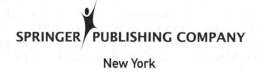

SPRINGER PUBLISHING COMPANY

New York

Springer Publishing Company, LLC
11 West 42nd Street
New York, NY 10036
www.springerpub.com

Acquisitions Editor: Allan Graubard
Production Editor: Julia Rosen
Cover Design: David Levy
Composition: Apex CoVantage, LLC

09 10 11 12/ 5 4 3 2 1

Library of Congress Cataloging-in-Publication Data

Guthrie, Diana W.
  Management of diabetes mellitus : a guide to the pattern approach / Diana W. Guthrie, Richard A. Guthrie.—6th ed.
    p. ; cm.
  Rev. ed. of: Nursing management of diabetes / [edited by] Diane W. Guthrie, Richard A. Guthrie. 5th ed. c2002.
  Includes bibliographical references and index.
  ISBN 978-0-8261-1909-4 (alk. paper)
  1. Diabetes—Nursing. I. Guthrie, Richard A., 1935- II. Nursing management of diabetes mellitus. III. Title.
  [DNLM: 1. Diabetes Mellitus—therapy. WK 815 G984m 2008]
  RC660.N83 2008
  616.4'62—dc22

                              2008024571

Printed in the United States of America by Hamilton Printing

The author and the publisher of this Work have made every effort to use sources believed to be reliable to provide information that is accurate and compatible with the standards generally accepted at the time of publication. Because medical science is continually advancing, our knowledge base continues to expand. Therefore, as new information becomes available, changes in procedures become necessary. We recommend that the reader always consult current research and specific institutional policies before performing any clinical procedure. The author and publisher shall not be liable for any special, consequential, or exemplary damages resulting, in whole or in part, from the readers' use of, or reliance on, the information contained in this book. The publisher has no responsibility for the persistence or accuracy of URLs for external or third-party Internet Web sites referred to in this publication and does not guarantee that any content on such Web sites is, or will remain, accurate or appropriate.

We dedicate this book to our mentor, Dr. Robert Jackson, to our three daughters (Laura, Joyce, and Tammy), and to our parents for what they have sacrificed to support us in this work.

Contents

Contributors

Belinda Pruitt Childs, RN, MN, ARNP, BC-ADM, CDE has been a clinic and research coordinator since 1978 and has served as editor or author of many articles and books. As an adjunct faculty member at the Wichita State University School of Nursing (WSU-SON), she coteaches an online graduate diabetes course with Deborah Hinnen. Her involvement as past President of the Health Care & Education of the American Diabetes Association (ADA), Sigma Theta Tau, and the Nursing Director of Camp Discovery earned her the Rachmeil Levine Award for Outstanding Service and the ADA's Outstanding Educator Award. She is known for the quality of research she coordinates and the multiple speaking assignments in which she engages.

Judy Friesen, RD, LD, MEd, FADA, CDE contributed to chapters on nutrition. She is a clinical dietitian specializing in diabetes since the late 1970s. She also holds a graduate degree in counseling from Wichita State University. As a member of the American Association of Diabetes Educators (AADE), the American Dietetic Association, and the American Diabetes Association, she has been recognized for her fine participation through the awarding of Fellow status by the American Dietetic Association. She has written articles and books related to diabetes, and is especially well known for *The Points Book,* which has been an important resource to patients and professionals alike.

Deborah Hinnen, RN, MN, ARNP, FAAN, BC-ADM, CDE is author of Appendix K. She has been a Diabetes Education Manager since 1976 and holds academic appointments as Clinical Assistant Professor at the University of Kansas School of Medicine-Wichita, adjunct faculty at the WSU-SON, and adjunct faculty at Butler County Community College Department of Nursing. She has been a past president of AADE and served on the Board of Directors for both AADE and ADA. She is recipient of the Outstanding Educator Award from the ADA and the Distinguished Service Award from AADE. A frequent speaker both nationally and internationally, Hinnen has been awarded Fellow status in the American Academy of Nursing in recognition of the high quality of her work.

Diana Rhiley, EdS, LCMFT, CDE contributed to the chapter on the psychologic effects of diabetes in people with Type 2 diabetes. She is a marriage and family therapist and approved supervisor for students in this field for Friends University. She has passionately worked with people who have diabetes, since the 1980s, both in private practice and with Mid-America Diabetes Associates.

Foreword

Practice-changing events are rare in diabetes, but the Guthries have often been the forerunners in education, research, and practice of diabetes over the past 40 years.

Having the opportunity to learn diabetes and practice with Drs. Richard and Diana Guthrie is one of those rare events. Richard and Diana have dedicated their lives to people with diabetes. They are passionate about good diabetes control and independence through self-management.

The Guthries' careers in health care began nearly a half-century ago. Their diabetes work began almost immediately thereafter. Both began their training at the University of Missouri–Columbia.

Richard Guthrie was recruited to Wichita to Chair the Department of Pediatrics for the University of Kansas School of Medicine–Wichita Branch. He has been driven to do diabetes work. Long before the Diabetes Control and Complications Trial (DCCT) results verified it, he believed good glycemic control was imperative. Being a fourth generation preacher, Dr. Guthrie has always been articulate and persuasive about sharing his convictions about good control. He and Diana built a diabetes team of which I am proud to be the first to join. The University supported their efforts in research. Early muscle biopsies documented normal blood glucose levels reversed early basement membrane thickening, a precursor to microvascular disease.

The first injection in the world of rDNA Lilly insulin was given to a person with diabetes in Wichita by Dr. Richard Guthrie. Publications, state, local, and international lectures, burgeoning clinical practice, and professional education created a reputation for both Dr. Richard and Diana Guthrie.

Diana's additional work on the Nursing Faculty at Wichita State University was the launching pad for the development of the first graduate program in diabetes. She later consulted with Yale to help them develop their program. Diana took the lead in creating group patient education programs that taught self-management and insulin adjustments to patients in the days when urine testing was the only method for self-monitoring.

Both Dr. Guthrie and Diana have mentored literally thousands of students, many of them doctors, nurses, dietitians, physician assistants, and others. Dr. Guthrie has received lifetime achievement recognition by way of the American Diabetes Association's Outstanding Clinician Award and Diana by way of the Outstanding Non-physician Educator's Award. Diana is one of only a handful of Kansans admitted as a Fellow of the American Academy of Nursing.

This book is an example of their labor of love to ensure that people are well educated to take better care of people with diabetes. Now in their 70s, they show no signs of slowing down. Rather than retire and do international medical mission work, they have declared their diabetes work in Kansas to be their mission. Truly that is the case. Thousands of people with diabetes and health professionals are grateful for that commitment as they travel to the far corners of the state every month to see patients in outreach clinics.

This book, now in its 6th edition, reflects the current practice of diabetes and the diabetes management philosophies of many in the heartland. I know you will find it enlightening.

Enjoy!

Deborah Hinnen, RN, MN, ARNP, FAAN, BC-ADM, CDE

Preface

Our mentor, the late Dr. Robert L. Jackson, felt that the treatment of diabetes should be as physiologic as possible, matching the treatment to the actual functioning of the pancreas. He determined that patterns, even those obtained with the archaic use of urine tests, were useful in determining the correct dose of medication to cover the food and activity of the active child (and adult). As machines are now made available to match the body's functioning release of insulin in real time, and the blood glucose levels after a period of time, knowledge of these values will be useful in directing the algorithms used in the pump, the artificial pancreas, or the injected or oral diabetes medications. A rapid, reactive response is needed when the person is in diabetic ketoacidosis (DKA), in hyperglycemic hyperosmolar nonketotic syndrome (HHNS), or having a severe hypoglycemic reaction. Daily use of diabetes medications to maintain a hemoglobin A1c lower than 6.5% (American Diabetes Association, 7%) does not need to be as dramatic, especially when the decision making is done by the patient or family member. The physiologic or pattern approach to management not only gives a safety factor, but also has proven quite useful in maintaining a high degree of control over long periods of time (evidence by the average, from the worst to the best hemoglobin A1c in our tertiary care diabetes clinic, is 7.4%). As a tertiary care clinic, we get individuals with newly diagnosed diabetes, people who are failing on oral agents, people who have already developed complications, and others that are difficult to control. We therefore have had extensive experience with numerous patients for more than 40 years.

We have attempted to put our years of experience in this book and to make this book user friendly for a variety of health professionals. Although the first edition was written as a guide for the working nurse who cared for a patient with diabetes, we recognized, over the years, that the book has become a working reference for all health professionals, including those professionals specializing in the field, and as a textbook for professionals wanting to know more about the disease and how to manage it by using the pattern approach.

I am reminded of an airplane ride in which I became involved in a conversation with a physician seated close by. During the course of the conversation I found that she was using our book as a guide for managing patients with diabetes. When I disclosed that I was one of the authors, tears welled up in her eyes and she thanked me for the help it had given her and her patient population.

When Richard and I discovered that some physicians, in addition to nurses and other health professionals, were using this book, we decided to develop the edition for broader use and for better ease of use. What you will find in the proceeding pages is the result.

The introduction takes you from the beginning to the present, including history, statistics, criteria for diagnosis, etiology, and physiology of the disease itself. Although acute care treatment (Chapter 6: In-Hospital Management of Diabetes Mellitus) perhaps should have been placed first, for handy reference, we decided to include some background to aid the reader in recognizing why a particular treatment is espoused. Treatment of diabetes when one has an infection and the effect of sleep apnea related to diabetes management (Management in the Clinic), along with treatment of hypoglycemia and school issues (In-Home Management), are also included. In this light, a reader interested in aspects of acute care or general diabetes treatment could read only the first two parts (Part I Introduction and Part II Management) or just Part II and obtain the immediate information desired.

The decision to separate Type 1 (Part III Ongoing Treatment and Care in Type 1 Diabetes) and Type 2 management (Part IV Type 2 Diabetes in Children and Adults), despite some controversy that one type is an extension of the other type, highlights major concerns and interventions associated with each of these conditions. If some of the information is a bit repetitive here, which we hope it is not, we trust it will be useful in the learning process.

A key addition to Part III is the particular focus on the needs and responses of children through adulthood; for example, the response of one unit of insulin to a 40-pound child is different than one unit of insulin to a 140-pound adult. Children with Type 2 diabetes, included in Part IV, remind us of the epidemic proportions of diabetes occurring in persons who are not yet adult.

We have coined the term "intermediate complications" to represent those conditions of a limited duration (refer to Part V). Pregnancy goes from preconception counseling through to labor and delivery and follow-up. Sexual dysfunction might be "cured" with today's medications or might require some surgical intervention. Surgery needs some prior considerations with blood glucose control before, during, and after the procedure. Pain management interventions are essential to maintain more normal blood glucose levels and for the healing to best take place. Poor control may lead to gingivitis and other dental problems that, with adequate interventions, may be resolved.

Part VI emphasizes chronic complications and is intended as an overview of the four specific classifications. Books are written on each topic for in-depth coverage of the pathophysiology and treatments involved. Cardiovascular disease includes the large-vessel problems and is placed first in relation to its impact on society and the need to keep blood glucose levels, cholesterol, and triglyceride levels in check to prevent damage from occurring. The retinopathy chapter includes more than just the problems related to the retina of the eye, but also related to those other conditions that might occur in a more frequent manner in someone who has diabetes. The nephropathy chapter was conveniently placed after the retinopathy chapter. If you have small-vessel disease in the eye, you are more apt to have small-vessel disease in the kidneys. Neuropathy not only includes the various types of neuropathy, but also the discomfort or pain management that may be needed to accompany the "healing" condition.

There is so much to cover in relation to diabetes that a special subjects section (Part VII) was a must. Self-management education tops the list as do barriers to care. Reference to standards of care and the two most useful journals to have on hand are recommended here. Interaction of social drugs and alcohol, including smoking, is also in need of attention. Complementary and alternative therapies are of importance and, although this chapter is not intended to be exhaustive, it will form a basis from which to gain further insight and knowledge to use when counseling patients. In addition, being prepared and knowing what to do in a disaster may save lives.

Finally, the promise of breaking developments and potential of those soon to come give hope to professionals and to the "whole person" who has diabetes (Part VIII). This, in a sense, is the most important section of all. At the same time, what is it like to be a parent of a child (or an older person) with diabetes? We trust that this section will continue to provide insight into what occurs when a person is diagnosed with a potentially life-threatening disease.

The Appendices should bring you fingertip information that we trust will be of ready assistance, especially the various protocols and listing of diabetes-related websites.

Diabetes is not the patient—the *person* with diabetes is the patient. Diabetes is a disease that affects every organ and organ system of the body; moreover, it affects and is affected by the emotions. This requires a cadre of professionals: a team effort (the individual with diabetes, the family and significant friends, and the family physician, the diabetes specialist, the acute care nurse, the nurse educator, the dietitian, the psychologist, counselor, social worker, podiatrist, physical therapist, or exercise specialists). This book is dedicated to the proposition that diabetes can and should be controlled through the coordinated interdependency of the health care professionals and the person with diabetes.

All of us join together in wishing that diabetes may soon be cured and, even better, prevented, so that one day this book will become unnecessary. Until that time, we hope that the book will assist those who are afflicted with this chronic problem, those who care for them professionally, and those they are close to, family and friends alike.

Acknowledgments

Appreciation is expressed to numerous people that have contributed to various chapters found in the five previous editions of this book. They are Elizabeth L. Burke on assessment; Betsy S. Desimone and Diana Rhiley on psychologic implications; Liddy Dye and Belinda Childs on surgery; Dr. Ronald James and Colleen Sheets on the older adult; Judy Jordan on complications and hygiene; Ben Leedle and Jayne McDaniels on exercise; Maria Smith on diagnosis and intermediary metabolism; Rita Nemchick and B. J. Maschak-Carey on the development of an education program; Donna Nickerson on urine testing, hygiene, and oral hypoglycemic agents; Virginia Stucky and Judy Friesen on meal planning; Deborah Hinnen on pregnancy, with Dr. Joseph Hume, and self-monitoring of blood glucose levels; and Ida Unsain, Michael Goodwin, and Marvel Logan on the effect of diabetes on sexual functioning. We also thank those that have challenged us to accomplish more, and most importantly, we thank the patients and their families from whom we have learned so much.

A special note of thanks goes to Joan Hoover, president of Diabetes Consultants, Inc., and mother of a daughter with diabetes, on "The Parents' and Patients' Perspectives," a chapter included in each edition of this book, and to Dr. Carle Lee and her fine contributions to a better understanding of the physiology of glucose metabolism.

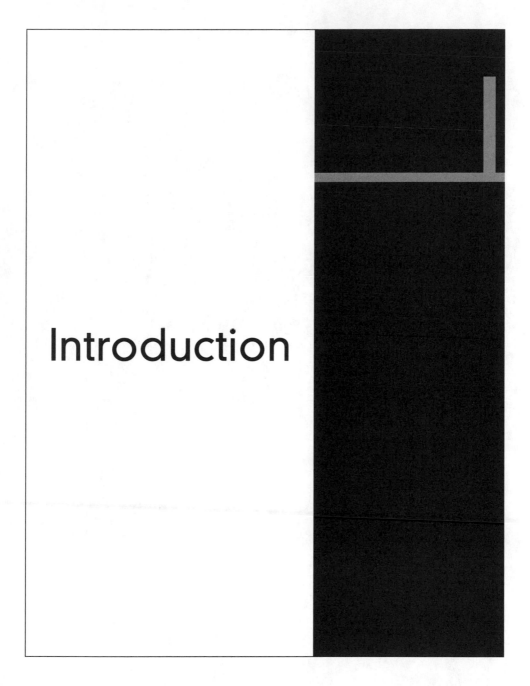

Introduction

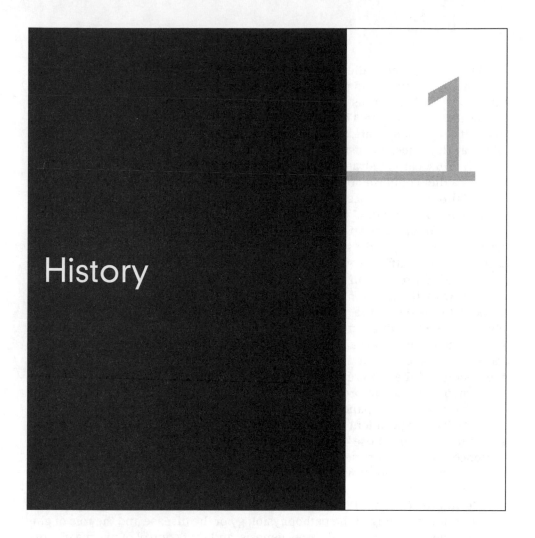

History

Diabetes is a metabolic disease or group of diseases of unknown cause resulting from an alteration in the availability and use of the pancreatic hormone insulin and irregularities in the endocrine system that may involve other hormones and the body's ability to use insulin. The disease has been known for centuries, and although research has elucidated many of the mysteries and resulted in the design of lifesaving treatments, the cause and the prevention of diabetes has remained elusive. The word *diabetes* is derived from the Greek word meaning *to siphon* and refers to the most obvious sign of the disease—marked loss of water by urination, or polyuria. The word *mellitus* comes from the Latin word for *sweet* or *honey* and thus differentiates diabetes mellitus (sweet urine disease) from diabetes insipidus (bland urine disease), a disease associated with the posterior pituitary gland (see Appendix A). In 1490, Paracelsus was the first to record that when a container of urine from a person with diabetes was allowed to evaporate it changed from a syrupy consistency to one that appeared to be a salt (the term for solids). He noted that it attracted flies. By allowing the urine to ferment, Thomas Willis, born in 1621, proved that its taste was sweet, because of sugar rather than salt.

From early times, dietary intake was viewed as a treatment. If a person did not eat as much, the person did not urinate as much. If a person ate certain foods, such as lentils or meats, they did not urinate as much as when they ate sweets. Around the 1790s, it was determined that foods contained certain amounts of carbohydrate, and they were organized into 3%, 6%, and 12% groups. Diets, at that time, consisted of guidelines to eat animal foods (proteins) and just 3% or 6% carbohydrate foods. Out of this type of thinking came other diets such as a diet composed of rancid meat or just composed of eggs, or vegetables cooked three times, or rice cooked, drained, and recooked several times to "cook all the carbohydrate out." Other programs included a week of fasting (no foods, just water) followed by an alternate week of feeding. One diabetes center on the East Coast actually had a small hut with bars on the windows for patients to stay when they had difficulty with the fasting week.

Scientific progress in our knowledge of diabetes began in the eighteenth century with the development of the microscope and Langerhans's descriptions of the islets in the pancreas that contain the beta cells. The "most celebrated diabetes clinician in the world," at that time, was Bouchardat of France (1806–1886). He is perhaps the first to associate the pancreas with diabetes. Pathologists such as Virchow (1821–1902) and others subsequently described the lesions of the pancreas, leading Minkowski (1858–1931) and von Mering in Germany in 1889 to prove that diabetes was caused by this gland. They did this by removing the pancreas from a dog and observing the resulting severe diabetes. This experiment led to the speculation that the pancreas contained an internal secretion whose deficiency was responsible for the disease. Many experienced investigators searched in vain for the internal secretion of the pancreas. All efforts were thwarted because the enzymes of the exocrine pancreas digested the beta cells.

Bernhard Naunyn (1839–1925) is one of the early scientists to report on a clearer understanding of the pathophysiology of the disease and the role of glucose "derived from protein, gluconeogenesis, and that control of plasma glucose levels in diabetic children required dietary limitations on both carbohydrates, and protein" (Loriaux, 2006). Dr. Naunyn published some of the first works on diabetes, promoting the treatment of "near starvation" to control blood sugars. One of his students (Hallevorden) noted in the urine large amounts of ammonia, which was later determined to be an acid (which Minkowski found to be butyric acid)—or the first understanding of ketone bodies.

In the dramatic summer of 1921, Dr. Frederick Banting devised a way of ridding the body of the exocrine pancreas while preserving functioning beta cells. Charles Best, a young graduate student working with Dr. Banting that summer, developed the alcohol techniques for extracting the hormone from the remaining pancreatic tissue and for measuring blood glucose. In August 1921, after several failures, Banting found that an extract of pancreas produced a dramatic drop in the blood glucose level of a dog that they had made diabetic by removing its pancreas. Thus, the internal secretion of the pancreas was isolated. This secretion, named insulin, was soon purified and concentrated, and a new era dawned for the unfortunate victims of diabetes.

Hagedorn, in Copenhagen, Denmark, noted that the insulin developed only lasted a few hours, so he sought to remedy this defect. He did so by using protamine, which had been discovered in 1868 (by Miescher in Germany) in fish sperm. Dr. Hagedorn experimented with many protamines and found the one that would cause a precipitation of insulin, resulting in a compound that absorbed so slowly that it acted twice as long as the initial insulin (neutral protamine Hagedorn, or NPH). Later, Scott and Fisher, in Canada, found they could prolong the action of insulin for more than a day by adding a very small amount of zinc (protamine zinc insulin, or PZI).

Insulin has since been further refined, concentrated (from U10 to U20 to U40 to U80 to present day use of U100; and also available directly from the companies in concentrations of U400 or U500), and humanized (to alter the chain of amino acids from beef [eight amino acids different from humans] or pigs [one amino acid different from humans] to human insulin with a same sequence in the chain of amino acids). It has been modified to alter the duration of action and designed to change its rate of absorbability (by altering and/or adding to the sequence and addition of another amino acid). The continuing discovery of various oral agents, the further alterations of insulin, and the discoveries of the kinds and causes of diabetes have all opened new avenues of research.

Throughout this period, a variety of approaches to the dietary management of persons who had diabetes developed. Already noted are the types and amounts of foods (the near starvation) used in treatment. One of these later programs was the point system, which was developed by Dr. Roland T. Woodyatt, who became involved with diabetes in the early years after insulin was discovered. His method of calculating the teaching diet involved the use of points and colored symbols and was originally developed for a non-English-speaking population in Chicago. This program was further defined by Virginia Stucky, the author of this chapter as it appeared in the first and second editions of this book. Judy Friesen, who studied with Dr. Stucky, has continued to refine and update this material. The exchange program of the American Diabetes and American Dietetic Associations has been the commonly used method of diet calculation and patient education. The exchange system often places foods of diverse content into an arbitrary category. For instance, peanut butter would be placed in the meat list, with some notice of its fat content. The point system overcomes some of the problems of the exchange system by assigning carbohydrate points for its carbohydrate content, fat points for its fat content, and protein points for its protein content or calorie points for the total caloric content. Carbohydrate counting is another major program. It is a variation of the point system without counting the fat and giving protein recognition when the advanced level of this program is taught. The point system, like the exchange system and carbohydrate counting, is not perfect but does represent an alternative method of meal planning, which should be carefully considered by the health care team. The pros and cons of various programs are discussed.

With the discovery of insulin in 1921, certain complacency settled over the diabetes world—diabetes was "cured." After a few years, however, it became evident that insulin treatment was not the final answer. Insulin extended the life span, but within a few years, people with diabetes began to go blind and die of vascular disease. Thus began the most important of the many controversies concerning diabetes, one that continued until the report of the Diabetes Control and Complications Trial study (DCCT, 1993).

The previous controversy was briefly stated as follows. Is the vascular and neuropathic disease that results in most of the morbidity and mortality when diabetes mellitus is diagnosed a genetic concomitant of diabetes or of the control of blood sugars? Or, is the vascular disease and neuropathy a complication of diabetes, somehow related to insulin deficiency and hyperglycemia, and thus preventable by control? If the first position were correct, diabetes control would be of little importance because the vascular disease was inevitable and unalterable. Little effort should be made to achieve control and diabetes education would be unnecessary. If the latter position were correct, as found to be true by many scientists and health care professionals, every effort should be made to effect control. Then, the burden is put on the diabetes specialists to educate the person who has diabetes, his or her family, the public, and other health care professionals who care for patients with diabetes in order to accomplish the goal of normalizing blood glucose levels as much as safely tolerated. This controversy, thought to have been settled by the DCCT study, has now been reactivated by the findings of the recently released ACCORD study, which shows that persons with preexisting cardiac disease have a higher mortality rate when the diabetes is very tightly controlled (A1c < 6%) than do people whose blood glucose levels are less tightly controlled. Further research is being carried out to finally settle this issue.

In 1946, the U.S. Public Health Service was developed. This unit of the government expanded to all states and internally developed sections, such as the Centers for Disease Control and Prevention (CDC). The CDC then developed a subsection devoted to diabetes mellitus.

The American Diabetes Association was founded in 1940 and also expanded to be the large, influential organization that it is today. Other significant organizations also developed programs, influenced legislation, and supported research such as the Juvenile Diabetes Foundation and the International Diabetes Federation (1952; the first congress was held in Holland with 15 countries represented) and the International Society for Pediatric and Adolescent Diabetes (started in 1973). What followed was input, coordinated research, and education to lessen the impact of this disease on individuals and society and to improve the treatment, care, and education of professionals and the people with diabetes and their families and significant friends. This is why the brief discussion of some of the controversies in diabetes was included—to put this book in proper perspective.

A Historical Review of the Pattern Approach

The three-meal, three-snack eating pattern with four doses of regular insulin was devised more than 60 years ago (Jackson & Guthrie, 1986). It was a time when a number of physicians, especially in Europe, recognized that the results of a blood glucose test represented what had passed rather than just what was occurring.

Jackson, as a pediatric resident at the University of Iowa, noted that children, despite receiving insulin, were not growing well and continued to have high blood sugars. He logically assumed that if children were given the nutritious foods for appropriate growth and development and adequate insulin to "cover" the food in relation to the child's activity level, they would maintain weight for height as the children who did not have diabetes. With this logic in mind, he then set about to observe more than 200 children who did not have diabetes. He noted what they ate, how often they ate, and when they ate.

What he observed was the three-meal, three-snack eating pattern. This same meal pattern was applied to children with diabetes, and insulin doses were administered in such a way that externally administered insulin levels would cause the child's blood glucose levels to be within the normal range as much as safely possible for 24 hours a day without the child experiencing any significant hypoglycemia. The percentages of 35%, 22%, 28%, and 15% of the total daily insulin or regular insulin with meals and at midnight were initially determined—from bedside research on children eating three meals and three snacks and controlled by four doses per day of short-acting insulin.

When intermediate insulin became available, Dr. Jackson completed the same meticulous, around-the-clock testing and developed the program to have a mixture of 2 parts intermediate-acting insulin and 1 part regular insulin before breakfast (globin was the only intermediate-acting insulin available then) and one part each short-acting (crystalline) insulin, and intermediate-acting insulin before supper (at that time and with that population, the largest meal was at noon). The evening meal was small, so intermediate insulin alone 2 hours before the meal without the use of short-acting insulin could be used to result in acceptable blood glucose levels at bedtime and before the morning meal the next day.

In the 1960s and with a different population of families that ate their larger meal at supper time, Dr. Guthrie (Jackson & Guthrie, 1986) added regular insulin to the supper-time intermediate-acting insulin (now NPH insulin, because globin insulin had been removed from the market). Premixing of the insulins had been started for the purpose of safety and stability of the dosing. Globin, an early intermediate-acting insulin, and regular were compatible. Later when NPH and regular had the same pH and globin insulin was subsequently taken off the market, the mixing of insulin continued. Eventually, with the recognition that when the insulin was purified it seemed to have a shorter duration of action, the short-acting insulin was "broken out" and administered before supper and the intermediate-acting insulin was used at bedtime.

Changes continued over time as insulin was humanized and attained an even shorter duration of action. So, a mixture before breakfast, a short- or rapid-acting insulin before supper, and an intermediate-acting insulin at bedtime became popular. One thing was still noted, even with the advent of long-acting insulin (which appeared to work better with adults than children—Ultralente and PZI or protamine zinc insulin): the use of multiple doses of insulin increased the flexibility of the lifestyle and decreased the possibility of hypoglycemia because smaller amounts of insulin were needed at each dosing.

When insulin analogs became available, not only was increased blood glucose level control possible, but insulin was made available to the body in a way similar to the physical response of the release of insulin when a person without diabetes ingests food. The addition of continuous subcutaneous insulin infusion (CSII), blood glucose sensing, etc., has led to safer and more effective management of the disease.

The three-meal, three-snack program for children has become a popular phenomenon. Small children gravitate to such an eating pattern because of their small glycogen stores. Adults have found that the body handles food better when given in small, frequent feedings (especially helpful for weight loss). Numerous studies have noted that 87% of teenagers eat in a three-meal, three-snack pattern, although the composition of the snacks may not be as nutritious as might be desired. Some states have instituted a midmorning nutrition break in the public schools, and teachers and parents have reported to us, by observation, a marked increase in effective teaching time.

Children are not able to hold as much food because of the small size of their stomachs; yet their caloric needs for activity and growth are larger than those of adults. Adults have coffee breaks, which often include caloric intake. Why then restrict the child with greater needs and decreased stomach capacity to fewer meals and snacks than are taken by adults? As children become adults, their lifestyles may change and variations may be needed. Medication is then adjusted to cover the needs of the food intake in relation to the activity to follow.

The increased incidence of Type 2 diabetes (T2DM) in children is especially noteworthy. Obesity and a sedentary lifestyle go hand in hand with the potential for an increasing number of children to be diagnosed with diabetes. Good nutrition and exercise are essential to having healthy children, and their being healthy requires the input of a variety of health professionals whether or not they have a chronic disease. The team approach (the multidisciplinary approach) is a need as much as for those youngsters with T2DM as for the youth with Type 1 diabetes (T1DM; Hall & Jacques, 2007). Hall and Jacques state, "Health care providers must understand this disease to insure proper management. A multidisciplinary approach is advocated . . . to help prevent the disabling and often incapacitating complications associated with T2DM."

The Goal

The goal of diabetes therapy should be to safely achieve normal blood glucose levels around the clock. This should take into account school, physical activity (such as gym or play), sleep and rest times, and stage in development (initial treatment, metabolic recovery, middle childhood, pubescent growth spurt, post puberty, and early, middle, and late adulthood). This objective may only be achieved with adequate education. The parents and adults as well as the youth must learn to adjust diabetes medication and/or insulin dosages and food intake to control glucose on a 24-hour basis. The child, the adolescent, and the adult must also be able to participate in activities with friends and at school or work without fear of hypoglycemia. As the family adjusts to the fact that the one who has diabetes mellitus has a chronic condition and as the individual adjusts to the same fact, methods must be devised to support continued understanding, good judgment, self-discipline, and motivation in order to obtain optimum health.

The principles are based on the following:

1. Food intake should be adjusted with exercise.
2. Insulin dose and/or oral agents should be adjusted and individualized as needed to match food intake and activity/exercise.
3. Food intake should conform to the needs of each individual and should be in relationship to the medication and blood glucose values noted in regard to the patterning of that person.

It is of utmost importance, therefore, to use the correct blood glucose values to adjust the insulin, oral agents, and food. Utilization of the wrong blood glucose values for adjustment of insulin (e.g., sliding scales) appears to be the most common error in diabetes management today and often leads to erratic blood glucose level control.

Summary

We have always believed that control of diabetes has been and is important in the prevention of both acute and chronic complications. Data from the DCCT and studies carried out in other countries have confirmed this belief. They also have found that education of the person with diabetes is a vital part of the control program.

It is also our belief that people with diabetes and/or their significant others should understand their disease so well that they can make their own individual adjustments (self-management) in their program. Health professionals should assist these individuals when necessary in altering their program to meet changing needs, but basically if diabetes is to be well controlled, it should be self-managed.

Knowledge and motivation are needed if such a self-management program is to be effective. Motivation must come from within the person, but self-motivation is facilitated by knowledge. Rarely will individuals do what they should unless they understand why they are being asked to do it. Thus, emotional support and ongoing educational programs are clearly needed to assist in attaining both the motivational force necessary to control the diabetes and the information needed to carry out the prescribed program safely.

Diabetes is not the patient—the person with diabetes is the patient. Diabetes is a disease that affects every organ and organ system of the body; moreover, it affects and is affected by the emotions. Diabetes can be difficult to control under the best of circumstances, but in the presence of emotional disturbance, home instability, or lack of a will to try, it is impossible. Control of diabetes requires a team effort, involving the cooperation of individuals with diabetes, the family and significant friends, physicians, nurses, dietitians, pharmacists, podiatrists, psychologists and/or counselors, and often social workers, exercise specialists, and physical therapists. The team must be alert to prevent or handle problems as they arise or, more importantly, to prevent problems.

This book is dedicated to the proposition that diabetes can and should be controlled through the coordinated interdependency of the health care professionals and persons with diabetes and their families.

References

Diabetes Control and Complications Trial Research Group. (1993). The effect of intensive treatment of diabetes on the development and progression of long-term complications in insulin dependent diabetes mellitus. *New England Journal of Medicine, 329*(14), 957–985.

Hall, C. A., & Jacques, P. F. (2007). Weighing in on the issues of type 2 diabetes in children: A review. *Pediatric Physical Therapy, 19*(3), 211–216.

Jackson R. L., & Guthrie, R. A. (1986). *The physiologic management of diabetes in children.* New York: Medical Examination Publishers (out of print).

Loriaux, D. L. (2006). Bernhard Naunyn (1839–1925). *The Endocrinologist, 19*(5), 239–240.

2

Facts and Statistics

Diabetes mellitus encompasses a heterogeneous group of diseases with various etiologies. All of these diseases affect the ability of the endocrine pancreas to produce, or the body to use, the hormone insulin. All of the diseases of the diabetes mellitus syndrome are characterized by variable and chronic hyperglycemia and other disturbances of carbohydrate, lipid, and protein metabolism. Diabetes mellitus is also associated chronically with a variety of vascular and neurologic changes that result in considerable morbidity and mortality as well as economic loss.

Because of the variety of diabetes syndromes and the varying definitions of what constitutes diabetes, authorities have disagreed not only on the incidence or prevalence of diabetes mellitus, but also on the terminology. To bring some order to the ambiguous terminology of diabetes syndromes, such as borderline diabetes, asymptomatic diabetes, chemical diabetes, latent diabetes, and prediabetes, the National Institutes of Health (NIH) appointed a select international committee on definition and terminology, the National Diabetes Data Group.

Classification

The various forms of diabetes, by present terminology, are divided into diabetes mellitus, gestational diabetes, other types of diabetes, and the various early or asymptomatic states of abnormal carbohydrate metabolism.

Diabetes mellitus is defined as a symptomatic or asymptomatic state of altered carbohydrate metabolism characterized by two or more fasting plasma glucose levels of 126 mg/dl (7.0 mmol/L) or greater or a value of 200 mg/dl (11.1 mmol/L), or greater, at 2 hr, on an oral glucose tolerance test. A diagnosis of diabetes can also be made with a random blood glucose value of 200 mg/dl (11.1 mmol/L) or greater, if it is associated with symptoms (polydipsia, polyuria, polyphagia, and unexplained weight loss). If the fasting plasma glucose is above normal (100 mg/dl or 5.6 mmol/L), but less than 126 mg/dl (7.0 mmol/L), the diagnosis is impaired fasting glucose, or IFG. If an oral glucose tolerance test is performed (and it is rarely needed) and the 2-hr value is greater than normal (140 mg/dl or 7.9 mmol/L), but less than 200 mg/dl (11.1 mmol/L), the diagnosis is impaired glucose tolerance, or IGT. IFG and IGT are now called prediabetes. The term borderline diabetes is obsolete and should never be used. (See Appendix B for etiological classification.)

Type 1 Diabetes Mellitus

What we once called juvenile or insulin-dependent diabetes mellitus is now simply called *Type 1 diabetes mellitus*, or T1DM. This is an insulinopenic state of the disease usually seen in young people, but it can occur at any age. Individuals with T1DM depend on exogenous insulin for life and become ketotic when insulin is removed, and most of these individuals have classic symptoms and certain human leukocyte antigen (HLA) haplotypes. They may also have islet cell antibodies early in their disease. Subgroups of T1DM include autoimmune and nonautoimmune forms (Imagawa, Hanafusa, Miyagawa, & Matsuzawa, 2000). Anything that can produce absolute insulin deficiency can be classed as T1DM. This form of diabetes accounts for about 5%–10% of the people with the disease in the United States.

Type 2 Diabetes Mellitus

What we used to call non-insulin-dependent diabetes mellitus, or NIDDM, is now simply referred to as *Type 2 diabetes mellitus*, or T2DM. This form of the disease occurs predominantly in adults, especially in persons older than 30 years of age, but it may occur at any age. In the past 10 years there has been a dramatic upsurge of T2DM in children, some younger than 4 years of age. The disease was formerly called adult or maturity-onset diabetes, but with the increasing prevalence of the disease in children, we can no longer use age-related terminology. Use of the term NIDDM was also awkward because many of the individuals with NIDDM required insulin for control. With these problems in mind, the 1997 committee decided to simplify the terminology by adopting the acronym T2DM and the etiological classification of diabetes (Report, 1997).

These individuals are not initially insulin deficient but are insulin resistant and hyperinsulinemic. With time, they will usually develop a relative insulin deficiency and require insulin, especially during periods of stress (e.g., during infection or surgery). T2DM is a genetic disease and the gene or genes are prevalent in all societies, but the disease becomes manifest primarily as societies industrialize (i.e., as calorie intake increases and calorie expenditure decreases) (Harris, 1995).

Other Types of Diabetes Mellitus

Other types of diabetes mellitus were formerly referred to as secondary diabetes as opposed to the familial or genetic forms of the disease. There are several subgroups of the class:

1. Pancreatic causes—pancreatectomy, pancreatitis, cystic fibrosis, hemochromatosis, and others.
2. Hormonal causes—acromegaly, Cushing's syndrome, etc.
3. Drug-induced causes—phenytoin (Dilantin), steroids, birth control pills, and others.
4. Receptor site abnormalities—acanthosis nigricans, congenital lipodystrophy.
5. Other causes—Turner's syndrome, Prader-Willi syndrome, progeria.

Some of these individuals are insulin dependent and occasionally massively dependent (i.e., receptor site abnormalities). Insulin dependency may be temporary, however. In drug-induced syndromes, the diabetes may remit if the drugs are discontinued. This category of diabetes causes accounts for less than 1% of all diabetes.

Gestational Diabetes

Gestational diabetes is diabetes in pregnant women who were previously healthy. This classification does not refer to the woman with T1DM or T2DM who becomes pregnant, but to the individual whose diabetes becomes known during pregnancy. Women with gestational diabetes were called Class A diabetics in the old White classification. Many are obese and, in the past, were managed by diet alone. The disease may be mild and even asymptomatic, but the incidence of fetal and perinatal complications is increased. Diagnosis of this condition is based on the criteria of O'Sullivan, Mahan, Charles, and Dandrov (1973). After pregnancy, the disease of these individuals must be reclassified as T1DM or T2DM, impaired glucose tolerance or prediabetes, or previous abnormality of glucose tolerance as determined by postpartum testing.

Asymptomatic States of Carbohydrate Intolerance

Impaired Glucose Tolerance

The term impaired glucose tolerance (IGT), now called prediabetes, applies to persons with abnormal results on a glucose tolerance test who have a fasting plasma glucose level that is normal or only slightly elevated (less than 126 mg/dl [7.0 mmol/L]). Glucose tolerance testing and the criteria for interpretation will be dealt with later. Most individuals with prediabetes are asymptomatic. This condition has been called by many names: asymptomatic diabetes, chemical diabetes, borderline diabetes, latent diabetes, and other ambiguous names. All of these incorporate the word diabetes. When that term is used, insurance companies and some employers do not differentiate these mild forms of carbohydrate intolerance from full-blown diabetes mellitus. Because many of these individuals do not progress to diabetes mellitus and many revert to normal glucose tolerance, especially if they lose weight, and because most do not seem to develop the microvascular complications of diabetes mellitus, it is unfair to classify them with the word diabetes. Because diabetes is occurring in epidemic proportions, it is now considered best to identify such individuals as having prediabetes, a codeable diagnosis. These patients have a very great risk of macrovascular disease when they do not receive a diagnosis or remain untreated. In August 2001, data from the Diabetes Prevention Program, reported by the *New England Journal of Medicine* (Fodor & Adamo, 2001), confirmed that lifestyle changes and weight loss can prevent full diabetes in many of these individuals and thus prevent or delay macrovascular disease.

On July 21–22, 2008, a conference was held in Washington, DC. This was a consensus conference involving the American Association of Clinical Endocrinologists, the American College of Endocrinology, the American Diabetes Association, the Centers for Disease Control, and a representative for the Food and Drug Administration. The purpose of the conference was to develop a consensus on whether prediabetes was a problem that should be recognized and treated. Several questions were asked, including: Did prediabetes lead to diabetes? Did people with prediabetes have a higher likelihood of developing micro- or macrovascular disease? If so, should people with prediabetes be diagnosed earlier and should they be treated? And finally, would treatment of people with prediabetes be cost-effective? The final report from this conference will not be available until fall 2008, but the preliminary report was released July 23, 2008. This preliminary report answered all of the questions above as "yes" and recommended guidelines for diagnosis and treatment. In essence the discussion at this conference leads to the conclusion that prediabetes really does not exist. Prediabetes, IGT, and IFG are just stages of diabetes, and we should probably just call it diabetes any time the blood glucose level is above normal. The problem is determining what exactly normal is. An analogy would be blood pressure. If blood pressure is above normal, we do not say the person has prehypertension, we say they have hypertension. Again, the problem is: What is a normal blood pressure? Most values considered normal are norms, that is, an average of a population. This does not mean this is truly normal, as another population might be different. An analogy here might be cholesterol. We call less than 200 normal but is it normal? It is the average + 2 standard deviations above the mean for the American population, but is that normal? We don't have the answers to these questions yet, but work will continue to find the proper values. Until then we need to do the best we can to keep blood glucose levels as low as possible without harming the patient. The final report of the consensus committee will be awaited with great interest.

Classifications Recognized in Other Parts of the World

Protein-Deficient Pancreatic Diabetes

Individuals with protein-deficient pancreatic diabetes (PDPD) have fasting blood glucose levels at or greater than 126 mg/dl (7.0 mmol/L), or a 2-hr glucose tolerance test value at or greater than 200 mg/dl (11.1 mmol/L). They are usually very thin (cachexia), and they might be insulin dependent at some times and not at others. PDPD was once known, by some, as Jamaican diabetes.

Fibrocalculus Pancreatic Diabetes

The characteristics of individuals with fibrocalculus pancreatic diabetes fit the description of PDPD, but they have pancreatic calcification. The only other diagnostic criterion is having a fasting blood glucose level at or above 126 mg/dl (7.0 mmol/L). In Africa and the Mediterranean region, this is often referred to as Type 3 diabetes.

Facts and Figures

The facts and figures regarding diabetes are constantly changing and those presented here may be obsolete by the time this book is published. The data we present here was up to date at the time the manuscript was submitted to the publisher. Data were obtained from the American Diabetes Association (ADA), the National Institutes of Health (NIH), the International Diabetes Federation (IDF), the Centers for Disease Control and Prevention (CDC), and numerous other sources.

It is difficult to estimate the prevalence of diabetes in the world. Many countries do not report diabetes data. In many underdeveloped countries people with diabetes die without a diagnosis being made. This is particularly true of T1DM in children who live in countries where early medical care for chronic disease is unavailable. It is also difficult to report world data because the data are changing rapidly in many countries. In countries such as China, India, and others where the standard of living is changing rapidly, so is the prevalence of diabetes, particularly T2DM. The IDF has estimated that there are more than 200 million people in the world with diabetes. This is probably a low estimate. The World Health Organization (WHO) has estimated that there will be 350 million people with diabetes in the world by 2012. A United Nations resolution in November 2007 (Silink, 2007) acknowledged these facts and asked the WHO to develop a program for worldwide diabetes control. T2DM is increasing rapidly in China and India and other countries where the standard of living is increasing in association with their increase in obesity. T1DM is increasing not only in the Western world, as it has been for many years, but also in Middle Eastern countries for reasons that are unclear.

The highest prevalence of T1DM in the world is in Finland. In general, the prevalence of T1DM is lowest at the equator and increases as you go north. There are exceptions to this generalization, such as the island of Sardinia in the Mediterranean where the prevalence of T1DM is about the same as in Finland. This may represent a genetic input from old Viking seamen raiding and then settling in Sardinia in centuries past. It may also be due to a change in feeding that occurred about the time of the turn of the twentieth century. At that time, there was a change from using milk from Brahman cattle to northern European cattle. There is some evidence that a protein found in the milk of Northern European cattle may be diabetogenic, though this is far from proven.

The increase in the prevalence of T2DM in the world is understandable in light of the increased industrialization and more sedentary lifestyle occurring in much of the developing world. In China, bicycles are being replaced by cars. Food supply is increasing as is income, and exercise is decreasing. Obesity is on the increase as is T2DM. The increase of T1DM is harder to understand, especially in Middle Eastern countries where there has been little change in food supply or customs. The increase in T1DM is about 3.5% per year in the United States but it is greater than 7% per year in many countries. It is unfortunate that the increase in the United States is in the younger children, usually under school age. Studies are under way in Europe and through TrialNet in this country to find the causes of the increase in T1DM and various treatments are being tested.

The increase in diabetes in the United States has caused a marked increase in health care costs, but statistics on diabetes mellitus are difficult to acquire for many reasons. Questionnaires, for example, can be misleading because many persons with diabetes do not want the fact of their disease to be known and they will deny having it. In the past, criteria for diagnosis have been highly variable from one center to another. The new criteria, as explained earlier, will change the data in the future. Unless otherwise noted, the data reported here are from *National Diabetes Fact Sheet* (ADA, 2008; CDC, 2008), *Diabetes Facts and Figures* (IDF, 2008a, 2008b), and *Diabetes Public Health Resources* (National Institute of Diabetes and Digestive and Kidney Diseases, 2008).

Prevalence

The prevalence of a disease is defined as the frequency of the disease in the population at the time of the survey. In 1973, there were 4.2 million people with diagnosed diabetes in the United States—2% of the noninstitutionalized population. In 1987, there were 6.51 million known persons with diabetes in the United States for a prevalence of 2.8%. Based on the National Health Interview Survey (NHIS) from 1993, there were 7.8 million persons with a diagnosis of diabetes at that time. This is a rate of 3.1% of the population of the United States and is more than a threefold increase from the prevalence of 0.93% in 1958. Part of this increase is attributable to better diagnosis, but much of it results from an actual increase in the incidence and prevalence of this disease (Margolis & Saudek, 2001). The change in diagnostic criteria in 1997 resulted in a shift in classification with more people in the diagnosed class and fewer in the undiagnosed and IFG and IGT (prediabetes) classes, but the total numbers of people with diabetes did not change at that time. In 2002, the estimate was a total of 17 million people in the United States. The present estimate is 23.8 million (ADA, 2008) or 24 million (CDC, 2008a) diagnosed and undiagnosed. Of these, 5.7 million are undiagnosed. This total constituted 5.9% of the population in 2000 and increased to 8% in 2008. It has been estimated that there are another 57 million people in the United States with prediabetes and/or the metabolic syndrome. The following is a summary of the latest data from the ADA and CDC:

> TOTAL ADA 23.8 million (7.8%), CDC 24 million (8%).
> Undiagnosed—5.7 million.
> Prediabetes 57 million.
> New cases per year—1.6 million in persons over 20 years of age.
> Prevalence under 20 years of age—186,000 or 0.22%. This equals about 1 in every 400–600 children with T1DM.
> Prevalence in persons age 20 and older—23.5 million or 10.7% of all people in this age group.
> Prevalence in persons age 60 and older—12.2 million or 23.1% of all people in this age group.
> Prevalence in men age 20 and older—12 million or 11.2%.
> Prevalence in women age 20 and older—11.5 million or 10.2%.
> Non-Hispanic Whites—14.9 million or 9.8%.
> Non-Hispanic Blacks—3.7 million or 14% of this group.
> American Indians and Alaskan Natives—14.2%.
> Adjusted for age over 20 years for patients of the Indian Health service— 16.5% (total), 6.0% (Alaska), and 29.3% (Southern Arizona) of these populations have diabetes.
> Adjusting again for age 20 or above—6.6% of non-Hispanic Whites, 7.5% of Asian Americans, 10.4% of Hispanics, and 11.8% of non-Hispanic Blacks have diabetes mellitus.

Many people without diabetes now will develop diabetes sometime in their lives. In children born after the year 2000, 1 in 3 will develop diabetes. In some ethnic groups the number is 1 in 2 (Lee, Herman, McPheeters, & Gurney, 2006). The increase in the number of persons with diabetes in the United States and in the world seems to be accelerating. The number of people with diabetes in the United States will double every 9–11 years. This fact is of concern because of the high prevalence of vascular and neurologic complications, and the high cost of these complications. Of particular concern in the United States is the high prevalence of diabetes in certain racial and ethnic groups. The prevalence of diabetes in African Americans is nearly twice that of Whites and even higher in Latinos, Asians, Pacific Islanders, and Native Americans. The Latinos and Asians are the most rapidly growing groups in the United States today.

Incidence

Incidence of a disease is defined as the frequency of new cases of the disease developing during a specified time interval. The incidence of T1DM in the United States in persons younger than 20 years of age has been estimated to be 18.2/100,000/year, and for those older than 20 years of age, 9.2/100,000/year. This represents a total of 29,713 new cases per year. For T1DM the risk is twice as high for Whites as for Blacks. A useful comparison of the burden of diabetes is found in a comparison with childhood AIDS. The number of children who develop diabetes is 14 times higher than those who develop AIDS and the economic impact is large, with a cost to age 40 of nearly $40,000 per case. The incidence and prevalence of T1DM varies with race and geographic area, with the increasing incidence in Asians and the highest in people of northern European extraction.

For T2DM, the incidence varies with age, diagnostic criteria, and the sampling system. For all ages, the incidence was between 8.2 and 17.6/1,000 population/year in 1991. In the United States, the incidence and prevalence of diabetes is highest in the Pima Indians, slightly less in other Native Americans, next highest in Asians and Pacific Islanders, next in Mexican Americans, slightly less in Puerto Rican and Cuban Americans, next highest in Blacks, and lowest in Whites. Based on the 2008 data, there are about 1,600,000 people under age 20 years, with newly diagnosed diabetes in the United States each year. This represents about 4,384 people diagnosed with diabetes every day. This number was 2,500 persons/day or 912,500 people with a diagnosis of diabetes mellitus per year in 2005.

Undiagnosed Diabetes

The number of persons with undiagnosed diabetes in the United States cannot be determined with great accuracy. Various projections indicate that there are from 4 to 6 million persons with undiagnosed diabetes in the population at any given time. The number of 24 million people with diagnosed and undiagnosed diabetes indicates that this disease is one of the most common chronic diseases in American society today. In addition to the diagnosed and undiagnosed diabetes in the U.S. population, there may be as many as 48–57 million people in the population with prediabetes and/or dysmetabolic syndrome (hyperinsulinemic syndrome). Most of these people will go on to develop diabetes in the future. Since the complications of diabetes begin to develop in the prediabetic state and develop rapidly in the diabetic but undiagnosed state, it is imperative that the health care system develop methods to bring all these people into the system and under treatment. If this could be done the cost savings would be tremendous.

Diabetes Mortality

The exact mortality rate for diabetes is unknown because diabetes is infrequently listed as the cause of death even for those known to have the disease. Cardiovascular disease is the immediate cause of death in most cases, usually listed first on the death certificate, and usually recorded as the diagnosis for statistical purposes. Diabetes may or may not even be listed as a comorbidity. T2DM is thought to account for at least 17.2% of all deaths in the United States for persons over the age of 25. In 1987, there were 40,018 deaths attributed directly to diabetes (diabetic ketoacidosis, hypoglycemia, and so forth).

In 1986, estimates of the number of cardiovascular, cerebrovascular, and renal deaths in which diabetes was the underlying cause of the vascular disease that led to death indicated that there were probably some 342,000 deaths/year caused by diabetes mellitus and its associated complications. In 1993, about 385,000 deaths from diabetes and its complications were estimated. The official number of deaths attributable to diabetes listed in 1996 was 198,140, but this does not account for the associated deaths where diabetes was not listed on the death certificate but was the underlying cause of the mortality.

The number of deaths due to diabetes are increasing at an alarming rate and represent a major epidemic of disease in the United States and in the world. Diabetes is now the sixth leading cause of death by disease and accounts for more than 233,619 deaths per year based on death certificate data in 2005. It is estimated that diabetes is the underlying cause of death, or listed as a secondary or tertiary cause of death, on death certificates in more than 440,000 people.

Mortality from diabetes mellitus is primarily from cardiovascular and renal disease. Morbidity is also a result of vascular diseases, coronary artery disease, cerebral artery disease, arterial occlusion of the arteries of the lower extremities, small-vessel disease as evidenced by retinopathy and nephropathy, and of neuropathy. Both vascular disease and neuropathy contribute to ulcers and gangrene of the lower extremities. Diabetes mellitus is now the leading cause of new cases of adult blindness, renal disease with dialysis and transplant, and amputation of the lower extremities.

Diabetes Costs

All of the aforementioned problems contribute to the massive economic costs of diabetes. The economic loss to the nation in 1975 in direct medical care costs, direct costs from complications, and indirect costs from loss of productivity was estimated to be $56 billion. This $56 billion figure was surpassed in 1992, reaching $90 billion when the increased numbers and costs plus inflation were taken into consideration. In 1992, $37 billion was spent on hospital care. Indirect costs based on premature death cannot be estimated but would also be in the billions. Direct costs for medical care and supplies, in 1997, were estimated at $44 billion. Indirect costs for short-term morbidity, long-term disability, and premature mortality estimated at $54 billion make the total cost $98 billion. This estimate was published by the ADA (1997) and was probably a conservative estimate. Some estimates for 1999 ran as high as $140 billion. In 2002, the costs were still increasing (ADA, 2003).

Today, the cost exceeds $174 billion dollars (ADA, 2008). One of every 7 health care dollars in the United States is spent on diabetes. For Medicare, 1 of every 4 health care dollars is spent on diabetes. This economic loss is especially appalling because much of it is avoidable. Several studies have indicated that the economic loss from diabetes can be greatly reduced by careful medical control of the diabetes, careful continued medical surveillance, and patient education programs. In one of the first comparative reports, Miller and Goldstein (1972) in Los Angeles were able to save Los Angeles County $53 million/year in direct hospitalization costs by such a program. Diabetes Control and Complications Trial data (1993) confirm these savings by showing a reduction in microvascular disease of 50%–76%. A consensus conference on diabetes (1999) revealed similar savings and a marked reduction in amputations because of improved patient programs. In their update of the ADA report (2003) of the economic costs of diabetes in the United States, D'Souza and Padiyara (2008) revealed that diabetes costs have gone up 32% since 2002.

Projected nationally, interventions would result in savings and could reduce the national loss from diabetes by at least half. This projection makes it difficult to understand why the national government and third-party payers fail to cover some of the costs for patient education and follow-up programs, and, in some cases, to pay for glucose-monitoring equipment and supplies. This problem was being corrected by national and state legislation, some of which has been too easily negated by budgetary crunches.

Summary

The high incidence, prevalence, morbidity, and mortality of diabetes mellitus are a national tragedy that should be attacked immediately in a concerted effort. The only bright spot in these dreadful statistics is a reduction in emergency hospital admissions and hospital days per year of individuals with diabetes. Narayan, Boyle, Geiss, Saaddine, and Thompson (2006) estimated the increased prevalence of diabetes would be 48.3–51 million people by 2050. This would make the financial burden of the disease in the United States by 2050 $369,750,000 a year without including a correction for inflation. Intervention should occur now with the recognition that more research is needed to reduce these costs.

References

American Diabetes Association. (1997). Estimated direct and undirect cost. Alexandria, VA: American Diabetes Association.

American Diabetes Association. (2003). Economic costs of diabetes in the US in 2002. *Diabetes Care, 26,* 917–932.

American Diabetes Association. (2008). *Fact sheet and other information.* Retrieved April 7, 2008, from www.diabetes.org

Centers for Disease Control and Prevention. (2008). *National diabetes fact sheet.* Retrieved April 7, 2008, from http://www.cdc.gov/nccdphp//ddt/fact.htm

Centers for Disease Control and Prevention. (2008). *National diabetes surveillance system. Data and trends.* Retrieved July 11, 2008, from www.cdc.gov/diabetes/statistics

Diabetes Control and Complications Trial Research Group. (1993). The effect of intensive treatment of diabetes on the development and progression of long-term complications in insulin dependent diabetes mellitus. *New England Journal of Medicine, 329*(14), 957–985.

D'Souza, J. J., & Padiyara, R. S. (2008). Update on ADA clinical practice recommendations. *Review of Endocrinology, 2*(3), 40–43.

Fodor, J. G., & Adamo, K. B. (2001). Prevention of type 2 diabetes mellitus by changes in lifestyle. *New England Journal of Medicine, 345*(9), 696–697.

Harris, M. I. (1995). Prevalence of non-insulin dependent diabetes and impaired glucose tolerance. In *Diabetes in America* (2nd ed., NIH Publication No. 95-1468, pp. VI 1–31). Washington, DC: U.S. Department of Health and Human Services.

Imagawa, A., Hanafusa, T., Miyagawa, J., & Matsuzawa, Y. (2000). A proposal of three distinct subtypes of type 1 diabetes mellitus based on clinical and pathological evidence. *Annals of Medicine, 32*(8), 359–363.

International Diabetes Federation. (2008). *Diabetes facts and figures.* Retrieved April 7, 2008, from www.IDF.org

Lee, J. M., Herman, W. H., McPheeters, M. I., & Gurney, J. G. (2006). An epidemiologic profile of children with diabetes in the US. *Diabetes Care, 29,* 420–421.

Margolis, S., & Saudek, C. D. (2001). *Hopkins white paper: Diabetes mellitus.* Baltimore, MD: The Johns Hopkins Medical Institutions, 4–5.

Miller, L.V., & Goldstein, J. (1972). More efficient care of diabetic patients in a country hospital setting. *New England Journal of Medicine, 286,* 1388–1391.

Narayan, K. M., Boyle, J. P., Geiss, L. S., Saaddine, J. B., & Thompson, T. J. (2006). Impact of recent increase in incidence on future diabetes burden: U.S. 2005–2050. *Diabetes Care, 29*(9), 2114–2116.

National Institute of Diabetes and Digestive and Kidney Diseases (NIDDK). (2008). *Diabetes public health resources: Diabetes statistics from the NIDDK, Centers for Disease Control and Prevention, and the National Diabetes Information Clearinghouse.* Retrieved July 11, 2008, from www.niddk.nih.gov

O'Sullivan, J. B., Mahan, C. M., Charles, D., & Dandrov, R. V. (1973). Screening criteria for high-risk gestational diabetes patients. *American Journal of Obstetrics and Gynecology, 116,* 895.

Report of the expert committee on the diagnosis and classification of diabetes mellitus (1997). *Diabetes Care, 20*(7), 1183–1197.

Silink, M. (2007). United Nations resolution 61/225: What does it mean to the diabetes world? *International Journal of Clinical Practice Supplement, 157,* 5–8.

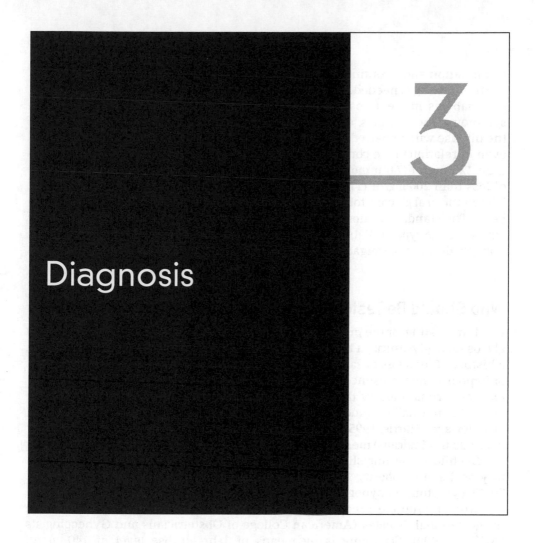

Diagnosis

The diagnosis of diabetes mellitus was simplified by the National Institutes of Health (NIH) consensus criteria of 1995 (Harris, 1995) and the select committee of 1997 (Diabetes Quality Improvement Project [DQIP] and Health Plan Employer Data and Information Set [HEDIS] Guidelines, 1999; Report of the Expert Committee, 1997). Other diagnostic criteria, such as the World Health Organization (WHO) criteria, are available and have been used in many studies. All data should always be scrutinized in light of the diagnostic criteria used.

Diabetes mellitus may be extremely easy to diagnose or extremely difficult. In the ketosis-prone individual (Type 1, T1DM), the onset of diabetes is usually sudden and fulminating. Signs and symptoms are usually present, and the fasting blood glucose level is usually elevated, but occasionally the onset can be insidious. Diagnosis can be made on the basis of a fasting plasma glucose of 126 mg/dl (7.0 mmol/L) or greater or a random plasma glucose level of 200 mg/dl (11.1 mmol/L) when symptoms are present. If, for example, the child has polydypsia, polyuria, polyphagia, weight loss, and a fasting blood glucose level of 600 mg/dL (33.3 mmol/L), no further testing is needed. Likewise, if the child presents in diabetic ketoacidosis and coma, no further testing is needed. Occasionally, however, a child may present for an annual school or athletic physical examination and a routine urinalysis may show mildly elevated glucose levels. Further testing is needed.

Diabetes in the ketosis-resistant person (Type 2, T2DM) may be without symptoms and, at times, difficult to diagnose. The earlier and milder forms of the disease with impaired glucose tolerance are often very difficult to diagnose, even in relation to the consensus criteria. A fasting plasma glucose level of less than 126 mg/dl (7.0 mmol/L) but more than 100 mg/dl (5.5 mmol/L), or value of less than 200 mg/dl (11.1 mmol/L) but more than 140 mg/dl (7.7 mmol/L) at 2 hr on the oral glucose tolerance test are the criteria for the diagnosis of prediabetes. The standard values previously mentioned lead to a diagnosis of diabetes whatever the type of diabetes mellitus, including those in the Spanish population (Valdes, Botas, Delgado, Alvarez, & Cadorniga, 2008).

Who Should Be Tested for Diabetes?

In adults, testing for the presence of diabetes should be carried out when there is glycosemia, glycosuria, a history of diabetes, a strong family history of diabetes, a history of fetal loss or large babies (babies more than 9 lb at birth), symptoms of hypoglycemia, presence of obesity, evidence of neuropathy, retinopathy, premature coronary artery disease, or early peripheral arteriosclerosis, evidence of lipid abnormalities (such as hypercholesterolemia or hypertriglyceridemia), or older age (Harris, 1995). There should also be a high index of suspicion for diabetes in Mexican Americans, Native Americans, or African Americans.

In children, testing should be carried out when there is a strong family history of diabetes, obesity, the presence of acanthosis nigricans (Jones & Ficca, 2007), symptoms of hypoglycemia, or glycosuria.

Women who are pregnant should be screened at 24–28 weeks' gestation for gestational diabetes (American College of Obstetricians and Gynecologists [ACOG], 2000). Screening is by means of 1-hr glucose level of 140 mg/dl (7.8 mmol/L) or higher after a 50-g glucose load. If the screening value is elevated, a 100-g glucose tolerance test is performed and interpreted according to the criteria of O'Sullivan (1967).

If children are obese, they should be suspected of having diabetes until proven otherwise (Franks et al., 2007; Jones, 2008). If the values fall within what used to be called the impaired glucose tolerance range (now, prediabetes), all risk factors should be addressed to aid in preventing the progression to frank T2DM, that is, instituting preventive interventions such as diet and exercise (Weiss, 2007). Gao, Dong, Nan, Tuomilehto, and Qiao (2008) were concerned with the "clinical and social implications of labeling," such as might influence marriage ability in some countries and employment and health insurance in others. Recent legislation in the United States is being proposed to address this type of discrimination.

Recommended Tests

A variety of tests are available for screening for diabetes. They are discussed here in the order of their effectiveness from least to most sensitive.

Urine Testing for Glucose Values

Testing of the urine for levels of glucose or reducing substances is one of the oldest and least effective methods of screening for diabetes. The urine glucose test has the advantage of being inexpensive, quick, and painless, and it is insensitive. The urine test will be positive for glucose only after the blood glucose values have become sufficiently elevated to allow glucose to spill into the urine, usually blood glucose values of 160–180 mg/dl (8.9–10 mmol/L) or more. Thus, the urine test will be positive, especially in adults, only in the advanced stages of the disease and has no value for detection of the early stages of the disease.

Blood Testing for Glucose Values

Random Blood Sampling

Random sampling (i.e., the taking of blood samples at any convenient time) is performed without standardization. Values obtained by random sampling are difficult to interpret because there are no norms with which to compare them. Again, if the values are grossly abnormal, they may be meaningful, but normal or mildly abnormal values are meaningless without standardization. Random blood sampling is being used extensively by public health departments, some diabetes associations, pharmacists, fairs, and so on for mass screening because of its simplicity, relative inexpensiveness, and convenience to the population being screened, but it is of limited sensitivity. Because the 2-hr postprandial glucose level goes up in T2DM before the fasting blood glucose level does, there is some support for developing standardized criteria for this value for diagnosis.

Fasting Blood Glucose Test

The fasting blood glucose test is the standard laboratory test for the diagnosis of diabetes mellitus. The fasting plasma glucose (FPG) value of 126 mg/dl (7.0 mmol/L) or greater is diagnostic for diabetes mellitus. An FPG of more than 100 mg/dl (5.5 mmol/L) is prediabetes. Values between 110 and 126 mg/dl (6.1 mmol/L and 7.0 mmol/L) may still be called impaired fasting glucose (IFG) along with impaired glucose tolerance but are now in the category of prediabetes. This category may assume more diagnostic significance in the future because people with prediabetes are more prone to macrovascular disease than the general population. FPG is a poor diagnostic tool for persons with impaired glucose tolerance (IGT); however, because the fasting blood glucose values usually remain relatively constant early in the course of the disease, the ability to handle a glucose load declines.

Oral Glucose Tolerance Test

The most sensitive method for detecting diabetes mellitus or impaired glucose tolerance is some modification of the oral glucose tolerance test. Properly standardized and performed, this test will detect early-impaired glucose tolerance and mild overt diabetes with great accuracy. There are many pitfalls, however, to accurate glucose tolerance testing. The individual to be tested should receive a high-carbohydrate diet for 3 days before the test. For adults, the diet should contain 80 g of protein, 150 g of carbohydrate, and the rest fat. For children, the diet should contain 60%–65% of carbohydrate and the appropriate amount of calories for size and age. A high-carbohydrate intake standardizes the glycogen reserves and sensitizes the beta cell to the glucose stimulus. Artificial diabetes can be created by starvation or carbohydrate deprivation because of a loss of beta cell sensitivity to the glucose stimulus.

After an overnight fast of 8–10 hr, the adult is given 75 g of glucose in a palatable base. For the child, the fasting period should be standardized to 10 hr; a snack is given at 10 p.m., and the test is started at 8 a.m. the next day. Failure to standardize the fasting period in children will result in an abnormal baseline (fasting) value. The child is given 1.75 g of glucose/kg ideal body weight for height, which is administered as a 30% solution in a palatable, carbonated base.

The glucose solution should be consumed within 5 min. Samples of blood and urine are obtained while the person is fasting and then 30, 60, 90, 120, and 180 min after oral glucose is administered. Some investigators extend the test to 4, 5, and even 6 hr. Standardization of the oral glucose tolerance test to the 2-hr test for the diagnosis of diabetes and the 5-hr test for confirmation of reactive hypoglycemia are now the established protocol. The criteria call for a 2-hr test with samples every 30 min using only the 2-hr value for diagnosis. A value of 200 mg/dl (11.1 mmol/L) or greater at 2 hr is diagnostic for diabetes mellitus and a value between 140 and 200 mg/dl (7.9–11.1 mmol/L) is diagnostic for impaired glucose tolerance. Medication should not be given during the test, and smoking or drinking anything (except water) should not be allowed. Simple, light activity is desirable.

Various drugs will affect the outcome of the oral glucose tolerance test. The following drugs elevate the blood glucose levels: glucocorticoids, which stimulate gluconeogenesis; thiazide diuretics, which diminish insulin secretion and total body potassium levels and aggravate existing diabetes; birth control pills containing mestranol, which impairs glucose metabolism; and nicotinic acid, which may damage liver cells. The following drugs decrease blood glucose levels: salicylates; alcohol, which inhibits the release of glucose by the liver; monoamine oxidase inhibitors (MAOs), which are "mood elevators" that stimulate insulin release; and propranolol.

Other Carbohydrate Tolerance Tests

Other diagnostic tests for carbohydrate tolerance are the cortisone-primed oral glucose tolerance test and the intravenous glucose tolerance test. Of these tests, the cortisone-primed oral glucose tolerance test is most useful for early diagnosis. This test is more sensitive than the standard test because it adds cortisone to glucose as an additional stress to the insulin-producing mechanism. It will diagnose impaired glucose tolerance in the earliest stages, but it has not been standardized for children and is most useful in a research setting. It is rarely used in the clinical setting.

The intravenous glucose tolerance test (IVGTT) is the most useful tool for studying persons with impaired glucose tolerance—especially for studying the insulin reserve; however, it is not as sensitive as the oral glucose tolerance test for diagnosis. This test was used in the National Diabetes Screening Program, known as DPT 1 and 2 (Diabetes Prevention Trial 1&2), for testing the insulin secretory capacity of the pancreas in persons who screen positive for islet-cell antibodies. IVGTT is now being used for the same purpose in TrialNet (an NIH-sponsored program to detect children with early diabetes or susceptibility to diabetes and test measures to prevent progression of the disease).

Testing for Serum Insulin Values

Since the advent of the radioimmunoassay for insulin in the early 1960s, it has been possible to measure the insulin-secreting ability of the pancreas during glucose tolerance testing. Testing for insulin-secreting ability increases the reliability of the oral glucose tolerance test. When the laboratory has the capability for measuring serum insulin values, this measurement should always be part of the oral glucose tolerance test for the diagnosis and definition of hypoglycemia but is rarely needed or useful for the diagnosis of diabetes mellitus. Fajans and Conn (1959) have published norms for serum insulin values for adults, and Pickens, Burkeholder, and Womack (1967) have published norms for children.

Screening Tests

Human leukocyte antigen (HLA) gene typing and anti-beta cell and anti-insulin antibodies are newer ways to screen for T1DM and impaired glucose tolerance (Eisenbarth, 1986). These tests are expensive if obtained commercially, and their use is usually confined to a research setting. They are more often used in research studies such as the Diabetes Prevention Trials and TrialNet.

Another consideration concerns the metabolic syndrome (dysmetabolic syndrome, cardiovascular risk syndrome, syndrome X), which, in the past, had only been noted when all of the following are found: hypertension, hypertriglyceridemia, obesity, impaired fasting glucose, and low high density lipoprotein (HDL). On further study, in a joint statement, the American Diabetes Association (ADA) and the European Association for the Study of Diabetes (EASD) found that the criteria used for defining the syndrome were not complete and somewhat ambiguous. They also found that the criteria differed between the National Cholesterol Education Program Adult Treatment Panel III (NCEP ATP III) and the World Health Organization (Kahn, Buse, Ferrinnini, & Stern, 2005). The major question was the inclusion of patients with cardiovascular disease (CVD), and they noted that other factors were involved such as C-reactive protein as an inflammatory marker. They concluded that more studies needed to be done regarding the criteria for a diagnosis of metabolic syndrome, the definition of the syndrome, the decision of whether to remove CVD factors or not, and the examination of underlying causes of such a grouping of risk factors.

The ADA is proposing the concept of "cardiometabolic risk" (as global diabetes/CVD risk) as an alternative name for metabolic syndrome and the inclusion of, besides obesity and hypertension, abnormal lipid metabolism, inflammation/hypercoagulation, smoking, age, race, sex, family history (genetics), and insulin resistance syndrome—insulin resistance/elevated cholesterol/hypertension/hyperglycemia (Bectly, 2006).

Summary

The oral glucose tolerance test is the most sensitive test for the diagnosis of diabetes mellitus—especially in the earlier and asymptomatic stages (i.e., impaired glucose tolerance). Properly standardized and interpreted, this test, combined with serum insulin determinations, is an extremely sensitive tool for the diagnosis and study of diabetes. Its only disadvantage to the patient is expense and inconvenience. When symptoms suggestive of diabetes are present, the fasting plasma glucose or 2-hr postprandial blood glucose determination may be all that is needed for diagnosis, as noted in Gavin's report of the "new" classification and diagnostic criteria for diabetes (1998), and in keeping with the clinical practice recommendations for the Diagnosis and Classification of Diabetes Mellitus (2008). When these are negative or when diabetes is suspected in an asymptomatic individual, an oral glucose tolerance test combined with serum insulin values, when available, should be performed under rigidly controlled conditions and the results compared with the carefully selected appropriate norms for age, especially in children.

Caution must be taken not to overdiagnose diabetes. It is important to detect diabetes as early as possible because treatment will prevent complications. A false diagnosis of diabetes though has serious implications in employment, insurability, and emotional impact. The standard oral glucose tolerance test properly performed and rigidly controlled and interpreted should lead neither to false-positive nor to false-negative tests, but to a proper diagnosis of diabetes mellitus or impaired glucose tolerance. It should be remembered, however, that the correct criteria for the diagnosis of actual diabetes mellitus are based on the fasting plasma glucose values, not on oral glucose tolerance testing, although oral glucose tolerance criteria can be included.

References

American College of Obstetrics and Gynecology. (2000). *Technical Bulletin, 92,* 1–5.

Beckley, E. T. (2006). *New ADA initiative moves beyond "Metabolic Syndrome."* Retrieved August 21, 2008, from www.diabetes.org/docnews

Diabetes Quality Improvement Project (DQIP) and Health Plan Employer Data and Information Set (HEDIS) guidelines. (1999). *Diabetes Care, 22*(Suppl. 1), S5–S19.

Diagnosis and classification of diabetes mellitus. (2008). *Diabetes Care, 31*(1, Suppl. 1), S55–S60.

Eisenbarth, G. S. (1986). Type I diabetes mellitus: A chronic autoimmune disease. *New England Journal of Medicine, 314,* 1360–1368.

Fajans, S., & Conn, J. (1959). The early recognition of diabetes mellitus. *Science, 82,* 208.

Franks, P. W., Hanson, R. L., Knowler, W. C., Moffett, C., Enos, G., Infante, A. M., et al. (2007). Childhood predictors of young-onset type 2 diabetes. *Diabetes, 56*(12), 2864–2972.

Gao, W., Dong, Y., Nan, H., Tuomilehto, J., & Qiao, Q. (2008). The likelihood of diabetes based on the proposed definitions for impaired fasting glucose. *Diabetes Research in Clinical Practice, 79*(1), 151–155.

Gavin, J. R. (1998). New classification and diagnostic criteria for diabetes mellitus. *Clinical Cornerstone, 1*(3), 1–12.

Harris, M. I. (1995). Classification, diagnostic criteria, and screening for diabetes. In National Diabetes Group, *Diabetes in America* (2nd ed., NIH Publication No. 95-1468, pp. 15–35). Washington, DC: U.S. Department of Health and Human Services.

Jones, K. L. (2008). Role of obesity in complicating and confusing the diagnosis and treatment of diabetes in children. *Pediatrics, 121*(2), 361–368.

Jones, L. H., & Ficca, M. (2007). Is acanthosis nigricans a reliable indicator for risk of type 2 diabetes? *Journal of School Nursing, 23*(5), 247–251.

Kahn, R., Buse, J., Ferrannini, E., & Stern, M. (2005). The metabolic syndrome: Time for a critical reappraisal. Joint statement from the ADA and the EASD. *Diabetes Care, 28,* 2289–2304.

O'Sullivan, J. B. (1967). Oral glucose tolerance tests. In G. J. Mammi & T. S. Danowski (Eds.), *Diabetes mellitus: Diagnosis and treatment* (Vol. 2, pp. 47–50). New York: American Diabetes Association.

Pickens, J. M., Burkeholder, J. N., & Womack, W. N. (1967). Oral glucose tolerance test in normal children. *Diabetes, 16,* 11–18.

Valdes, S., Botas, P., Delgado, E., Alvarez, F., & Cadorniga, F. D. (2008). Does the new American Diabetes Association definition for impaired fasting glucose improve its ability to predict type 2 diabetes mellitus in Spanish persons? The Asturias Study. *Metabolism, 57*(3), 399–403.

Weiss, R. (2007). Impaired glucose tolerance and risk factors for progression to type 2 diabetes in youth. *Pediatric Diabetes, 8*(Suppl. 9), 70–75.

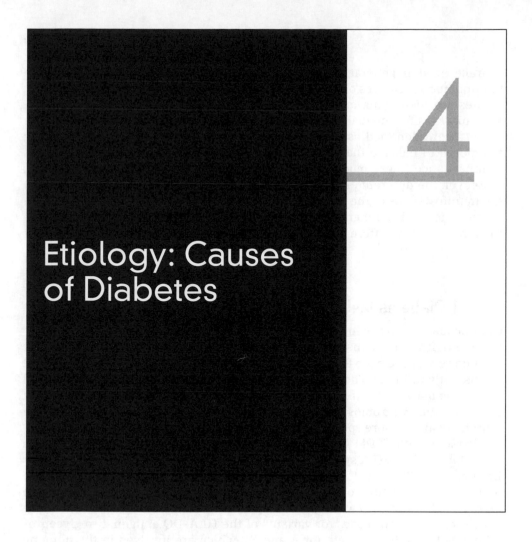

Etiology: Causes of Diabetes

The cause of diabetes mellitus remains unknown, but new research is leading us toward the concept that diabetes may have many causes. Indeed, diabetes is a syndrome, not a single disease, yet a few thinkers have recently suggested that the older concept of one disease may be right after all. Type 1 diabetes mellitus (T1DM) might be a telescoped form of diabetes manifesting somewhat differently between Type 1 and 2 because of age and environment on the genetic background. Age, body size, and other environmental factors affect the genetic background differently, causing the disease to be manifest differently in different people, as T1DM in younger patients and T2DM in older patients. This is called the acceleration theory (Wilkin, 2008). Epidemiologic studies are under way to prove or disprove this theory, but only one piece of supporting data is, as yet, available. At diagnosis, adolescents with T1DM appear to be heavier than expected even though they may have lost weight. Thus, body weight may be a factor in the etiology of T1DM as it is in Type 2 diabetes mellitus (T2DM) (Jones, 2008).

Diabetes is, then, one of many diseases that ultimately cause beta cell failure and/or peripheral insulin resistance. Diabetes has always been thought of as a genetic or inherited disease, although the mode of inheritance has not been characterized. In general, this is true because a genetic marker for the disease in nondiabetic relatives of persons with diabetes has not been found. Genomic studies are identifying many genes on many different chromosomes as possible markers for the diabetes diseases but no one gene or group of genes has as yet been identified as the cause of the diseases. Data are now beginning to emerge to indicate that diabetes is an inherited disease with many modes of inheritance. These modes of inheritance are different in different families; moreover, the different environmental factors that determine (at least in part) the manifestations of the inheritance may be different for the different inheritance patterns. The inheritance of T1DM and T2DM is probably different, and the inheritance of different types of T2DM and other types of diabetes are most likely also different.

Type 1 Diabetes Mellitus

Genetic markers are being developed for T1DM mostly in the human leukocyte antigen (HLA) system that controls immunity in humans. Though no consistent HLA patterns have been found in T2DM, several HLA antigens have been found consistently in T1DM. The HLA-B8 and HLA-B15 antigens were first identified as genetic markers for this type of diabetes. These genes are on the short arm of the number 6 chromosome. B-8 and B-15 antigens are not very specific, so a search began for more specific genes perhaps linked to B-8 and B-15.

Persons with T1DM have been found to also have at least 2 antigens in the D locus of the HLA system—DR3 and DR4 (Kolb, 1999). Data presented by Lernmark (1989) indicate that these genes are linked to alleles in the DQ band on the number 6 chromosome that encodes for Class II antigens, and may be more closely associated with the development of diabetes than the neighboring DR genes. This locus codes for variants of the HLA-DQ antigen, two glycoproteins labeled alpha and beta (or A and B), which are involved in the immune system's recognition of antigens and their presentation to macrophages. Antigen recognition and presentation is a vital step in immunity to foreign bodies such as bacteria and viruses. These alleles must also recognize self in order to differentiate self from foreign bodies. If an abnormality exists in these alleles, they may not be able to differentiate self, allowing the immune system to attack self, that is, an autoimmune process resulting in destruction of self-tissue such as the beta cells of the pancreas-T1DM.

Several abnormalities in the DQ band of the number 6 chromosome have been found that are related to the development of T1DM. One amino acid difference in the sequence of the glycoprotein can alter the ability of the locus to encode for recognition and presentation of foreign antigens and differentiation of self. Several such abnormalities have been found, in particular, deletion or substitution for aspartic acid at the number 57 position in several alleles. Such abnormalities have been found in loci labeled DQA1*0301, DQB1*0302, DQA1*0501, and DQB1*0201. Other amino acid deletions or substitutions have also been found, especially in other racial groups, in particular East Asians (Japanese and Chinese), so these abnormalities can be quite diverse. There are also some protective loci such as DQA1*0102 and DQB*0602. How all of these loci work to facilitate or protect against T1DM is unknown, but this opens possibilities for further research that may soon provide not only immune markers for the diagnosis of T1DM, but also immune system therapies that may cure or prevent this disease (Sperling, 2008). The form of diabetes now known as Type 1A is usually associated with islet cell antibodies (Juneja & Palmer, 1999).

Genetic Abnormalities

Genetic abnormalities in other genes on other chromosomes have also been identified in small populations of families with T1DM. Fifteen such forms of T1DM have been identified and are labeled IDDM1–15. Three of these (IDDM5, -9, and 15) are located on chromosome 6 like Type 1A, but at other loci. IDDM2 and -4 are located on chromosome 11. IDDM3 is on chromosome 15, IDDM6 is on 18, IDDM7, -12, and -13 are on 2; IDDM9 is on 3; IDDM10 is on 10; and IDDM11 is on 14. The locus for IDDM14 has as yet not been defined. These forms of T1DM are phenotypically similar to the classic form, but they are genetically different and are limited to a few families each. In some of them, there are chemical markers in the blood facilitating identification.

The abnormalities of the HLA system may cause several abnormalities of the immune system. Some of the abnormalities may cause an underreaction of the immune system so that an environmental antigen (such as a virus) can invade the beta cells of the pancreas and destroy them before the immune system can react. Another abnormality can cause overreaction of the immune system or interfere with the immune system's ability to recognize self, resulting in an autoimmune problem. With the latter problem, the onset of diabetes is slower than with the former and an association is often seen with other autoimmune diseases such as Hashimoto's thyroiditis, Addison's disease, pernicious anemia, alopecia areata, vitiligo, celiac disease, and, perhaps, autoimmune hepatitis, which are autoimmune diseases of the thyrogastric cluster. In all types of T1DM, there must be an environmental trigger before the immune system abnormality is activated. We know this because of twin studies. Identical twins have the same genetics but in a classic study, Tattersall, Pyke, Ranney, and Bruckheimer (1975) demonstrated that less than 50% of the second twins will develop the disease even after many years. These environmental triggers are discussed below.

Islet Cell Antibodies

In Type 1A diabetes, islet cell, insulin, and GAD 65 antibodies are present in the serum often for many years before the onset of the disease. Evidence from studies of siblings of people with diabetes suggests that early identification of these individuals could lead to prevention of this disease. Additional evidence for this is the remission or honeymoon phase of T1DM in which early treatment with insulin seems to arrest the beta cell destruction for a time and even promotes recovery of beta cell function. People with pancreatic antibodies and declining insulin secretory capacity have been given small doses of insulin and have slowed or stopped their beta cell destruction as measured by insulin requirement and C-peptide secretion. These provocative but limited observations have led to the development of a national prevention program known as Diabetes Prevention Trial (DPT 1 and 2).

In DPT 1, first-degree relatives of people with known T1DM were screened for islet cell and insulin antibodies. Those with a positive titer were then given an intravenous glucose tolerance to define their first-phase insulin-producing capacity. Those with a decreased insulin-producing capacity that had normal or only slightly abnormal oral glucose tolerance tests were entered into a treatment protocol for treatment with low doses of insulin. The purpose of this study was not to treat blood sugar with insulin but to administer small doses of insulin to immunize the person, thus creating antibodies that could block the immune system's attack on the beta cells and prevent the development of diabetes. Unfortunately, the procedure, at least in the insulin dosage and distribution used in the study, did not work and this portion of the DPT study was terminated in the spring of 2001 (Pozzilli, 2002). In DPT 2 similar screening procedures are carried out on second-degree relatives as well as first-degree relatives. In this study, the person with positive results was treated with an oral form of insulin (an insulin that is coated by a substance that will not break down until past the stomach and small intestine). Again, this insulin is not to control blood glucose but to immunize. This study was also unsuccessful but has led to a new trial with a different oral preparation. This study is a part of TrialNet, a network of groups across the country and in Europe testing various methods of solving the immune system problems and preventing diabetes.

Immune Mechanism of Diabetes

A simplified but unifying concept of the immune mechanism of diabetes is as follows. The immune system may be thought of as having an on and an off switch. When the DR4 and its associate DQ allele genes are present, there is a defect in the on switch in which the system does not properly turn on. It does not recognize the presence of the virus or other insult and so does not destroy it. The defect may be in cellular or humeral immunity or both ("Lazy T" cells is one hypothesis). In any event, the insulting force is not destroyed and is allowed to penetrate the beta cell and destroy it. This form of the disease, with an early and explosive onset and poor beta cell recovery with treatment, is increasing worldwide and in the United States mostly in children under the age of 6 years.

When the DR3 and its associate DQ allele genes are present, the defect is in the off switch. The environmental insulting agent such as a virus activates the on switch of the immune system and the virus is destroyed. The problem in these individuals is that the immune system is not turned off. The T-killer cells remain activated and attack the beta cells in an autoimmune type reaction. This form of the disease comes on later and is slower in onset. Islet cell, anti-insulin, and GAD 65 antibodies may be present for years before the actual onset of the disease. These people have a more profound remission phase of the disease indicative of less initial beta cell loss. Continued autoimmune assault and/or repeated assaults result in slow loss of beta cell function over several months or years. This form of the disease becomes manifest in later childhood usually during the preadolescent growth spurt or even later in life and has a better recovery or remission period. It is also associated with other autoimmune diseases. This has been a very simplified explanation of the process. Obviously, it is much more complex with many intervening steps and chemicals, including a variety of lymphocytes, cytokines, and other immune substances and cells. New research is clarifying these steps, identifying environmental triggers, and bringing new understandings that, in the future, may allow for interventions that will prevent T1DM.

Various treatment strategies are currently being developed to attack the immune system in new-onset T1DM and to preserve beta cell function. Immune therapy has had only marginal success so far, but much new knowledge is being gained and the immune theory of the etiology of T1DM is being proved. The first successful use of immunosuppressant was with cyclosporin A (Dupre et al., 1988). Extensive studies in Canada and Europe have shown the drug to be somewhat effective in preserving beta cell function, but cost and toxicity have been a problem. The effect is only temporary and when therapy is stopped, beta cell function is lost. Several other forms of immunotherapy such as the use of monoclonal antibodies to T cell proteins to deliver toxic enzymes specifically to the T cells and the use of monoclonal antibodies to block interleukin-2 receptors and other cytokines are being tried. All such therapies are experimental and should not be used except in carefully controlled research studies.

Other new approaches to the prevention or early treatment of diabetes are the administration of nicotinamide, restriction of cow's milk feeding in susceptible infants, heat-shock proteins, thalidomide derivatives, CD-3 or 4 monoclonal antibodies, and many others. Researchers are also looking for the genome for diabetes so that diabetes might be prevented (Pani & Badenhoop, 2000) or perhaps reversed, along with the early recognition of HLA typing (Morwessel, 1998). For treatment, researchers are trying almost every substance known in non-obese diabetes mice (NOD) mice, a species that develops an insulin-dependent diabetes very similar to that in humans, and the substances that show promise without severe toxicity are then proposed for human experimentation. Other than insulin and nicotinamide very few of these chemicals have as yet been cleared for trial in humans. Nicotinamide trials have been completed in Australia and New Zealand, and are under way in Europe, but nicotinamide, like many other chemicals, which have shown potential in NOD mice have not shown the same protective effects in humans.

Cow's Milk

Cow's milk has an interesting story in the understanding of the etiology of T1DM. It was reported several years ago from Scandinavia that breast-fed infants had a lower incidence of diabetes than those fed cow's milk (Dahl-Jorgensen, Joner, & Hanssen, 1991). It was proposed that human milk contained certain antibodies that protected the infant from the viruses that could initiate the immune problem, and that substance was not found in cow's milk or was destroyed by the preservation process in formula. Later research in Canada and New Zealand, however, showed that it was not a protective effect of human milk but an antigenic effect of cow's milk. Cow's milk seemed to contain something that triggered the immune attack on the beta cell. Further studies are under way to delineate that substance. Many researchers believe that it is bovine albumin and that this protein is incompletely digested in the infant's intestinal tract. The incomplete protein fragments are absorbed and trigger an immune response that is retained in the memory of the immune system. Later in life proteins form on the beta cells, which are similar to the cow protein fragments, and are then recognized by the immune system as foreign bodies. The immune system then attempts to eliminate these proteins and in the process kills the beta cells, causing diabetes. This same process is thought to be responsible for the increase of asthma in children where the foreign substance is the too early feeding of solid foods. An interesting sidelight of this issue is that milk from cows common to northern Europe (the milk used in Europe, United States, Canada, etc.) will cause the problem, but milk from Brahman cattle used commonly in Asia and Africa does not.

If the theory of a heat-resistant protein in cow's milk is true, then human infants, especially those who are genetically susceptible to diabetes, should not be exposed to cow's milk until they are at least one year of age. Further studies are needed to unravel this story, which may give us clues to other environmental triggers or insulting agents that may be involved with the etiology of T1DM. A study from Denver refutes the milk connection (Norris et al., 1996). The final story is not yet in.

Extensive studies are under way in Finland to delineate the role of cow's milk and other potential triggers in the etiology of diabetes. Viruses, especially the Coxsackie viruses and perhaps other intestinal viruses, have been implicated as etiologic agents, but other environmental factors such as other foods, methods of cooking, environmental contaminants, and so on, are likely in some cases as well (Knip & Akerbloom, 1999).

Additional Theories

Two additional theories for T1DM have been proposed. The first of these was mentioned earlier (the accelerator hypothesis). It was proposed by Wilkins, who is an immunologist who has worked on the immune theory of diabetes for more than 30 years, without success in unraveling it. He has proposed that T1DM and T2DM are the same disease. There are genetic differences in the 2 types of diabetes which impact the age of onset but environment triggers are the same. Some evidence for this is the observation that children who develop T1DM have previously been heavier than children who do not develop diabetes at comparable ages. Another bit of evidence is the observation that there is an impairment of beta cell mass and function early in T2DM and may be the primary defect rather than insulin resistance (Florez et al., 2007). If this is true, loss of beta cell mass and function is the initial common denominator in both types of diabetes, and they may be the same disease.

An additional theory has been labeled the *germ theory*. An observation during the polio era was that polio and certain other intestinal viruses were more common in cleaner people and societies than in poorer societies and the "slums." The idea was that in the less clean societies the infants were exposed to germs or viruses in infancy while they still had transplacental antibodies to protect them. They then developed immunity and had no disease. Infants in cleaner societies were not exposed while protected; thus, they had no immunity and when exposed later in life developed the disease. At the border between Finland and Russia, there is a population of Finns who are genetically the same but of higher socioeconomic status on the Finnish side. These two populations are being studied to see if there is a difference in the prevalence of diabetes between them that might be explained by environmental exposure early in life. Data from this study are not yet available. This study is part of extensive studies in Finland on the epidemiology of T1DM because this nation has the highest prevalence of T1DM in the world. We eagerly await the results of all of the studies on the cause of T1DM, so that we may more intelligently develop ways to prevent this disease.

Type 2 Diabetes Mellitus

The etiology of T2DM is even less well understood than the etiology of T1DM. It is genetic, but it has nothing to do with the immune system and the genes are not located on the same HLA locus on the number 6 chromosome. Indeed, there are probably many genes causing T2DM, located on several chromosomes. Some candidate genes have been identified but most have not. We also know that there is a strong environmental influence in the development of T2DM. The gene or genes seem to be widespread throughout the world and in every race and culture. But we see the disease manifest only in developed or developing countries where it is associated with increased caloric intake and decreased caloric expenditure (obesity). Underdeveloped countries have a very low incidence and prevalence of the disease and it occurs primarily in the elderly. When these countries begin to industrialize or the people immigrate to more developed countries, a virtual explosion of diabetes occurs. How this change in lifestyle interacts with the genetic precursor is not known.

Insulin Resistance and Obesity

We do know that obesity is involved in insulin resistance and hyperinsulinemia, yet not all obese people develop diabetes. Insulin resistance may therefore not be the primary, or at least the genetic, defect. As previously noted, there appears to be a loss of insulin secretory ability by the beta cells and a loss of beta cell mass (Florez et al., 2007). This is probably the main genetic defect. When insulin resistance develops, the person without the gene can increase insulin secretion and compensate. Those with the gene cannot compensate and develop a relative insulin deficiency and consequent elevated blood glucose levels. This scenario is fairly well understood. What is not understood is why. The gene or genes for T2DM are very widespread throughout the world and even occur in animals. If it is an undesirable gene, why has it been bred in instead of being bred out over time? Perhaps it had a function. Human history is one of recurrent famine, not the plenty we see today. The gene may have been evolved as a thrifty gene to improve energy utilization during times of famine. In other words, the gene allows us to get more miles to the gallon. During times of famine then, it was the people with the diabetic gene who survived, thus perpetuating the gene. Today, we still see little T2DM in countries with low caloric intake and high caloric expenditure. When those people increase caloric intake and decrease activity by improving economic conditions or moving to developed nations, diabetes develops, often at alarming rates. The key to prevention of T2DM, then, is to prevent obesity, a finding recently confirmed by the Diabetes Prevention Program (Fodor & Adamo, 2001).

The obesity associated with T2DM is not generalized, but centralized, obesity. It is not only central, it is also primarily intra-abdominal obesity. Fat tissue was once thought to be inactive tissue, but it is now known to be an active organ producing many hormones and cytokines. Some of these hormones, such as leptin, are beneficial. They reduce appetite and enhance metabolism and insulin utilization. Other substances produced by fat tissue are harmful especially in increasing food intake and causing insulin resistance. Subcutaneous fat tends to produce more of the good substances, and intra-abdominal fat the harmful substances. Much research remains to be done on fat hormones. This is a fruitful area of research that may lead to better treatments in the future. Genetic defects in diabetes may lead to the production of abdominal fat as well as decreased beta cell function and mass. The insulin resistance of diabetes may also be caused by genetic defects in insulin receptors on cells and/or the cascade of kinase reactions inside the cells. This remains to be established.

Metabolic Syndrome

Whatever the name given to this syndrome, the metabolic syndrome has taken a major role in association with diabetes mellitus. Pradhan (2007) relates this syndrome to an inflammatory basis of glucose disorders, whereas McGill, Molyneaux, Twigg, and Yue (2008) question whether the metabolic syndrome exists, even whether it matters when concerning T2DM. DeFerranti and Osganian (2007) discuss, in length, the epidemiology of pediatric metabolic syndrome and its relation to T2DM. They contend that the prevalence of this syndrome is increasing in children and especially adolescents. Their fear is if not caught early enough, the associated complications will occur in younger individuals, leading to an increase in morbidity and mortality in this age population. In any case, whether it is called syndrome X, or even the more recent name of cardiovascular syndrome, hypertension, hyperglycemia, hyperlipidemia, and obesity as such relate to potential problems that have an endpoint in disability or death whether controlled in part or in whole.

Maturity Onset of Diabetes in the Young

In the 1960s, Fajans and Conn (1960) studied some families in Michigan who had an unusual form of diabetes. In 1989, Fajans reviewed this field of study and reported on his findings accumulated over the years. These were non-insulin-dependent children with diabetes resembling T2DM. He called this maturity onset diabetes in the young (MODY). MODY has now been identified as a group of genetic diseases primarily involving enzyme defects in the liver. A number of diseases labeled MODY have been identified genetically, but the numbers are small and each form is usually confined to one family group.

Recently, another form of non-insulin-dependent diabetes has been reported. Occasionally there are newborn infants with diabetes. They have always been treated with insulin but may not need to be so treated. Research has shown that these babies have a gene that results in a defect in the potassium receptor on the beta cell that is involved in signaling of the beta cell to produce insulin. This is the receptor that is activated by sulfonylurea drugs. These infants can therefore be treated with oral drugs instead of insulin (Rafig et al., 2008).

Other Forms of Diabetes

Gestational diabetes will be discussed in Chapter 23 dealing with diabetes in pregnancy. Other forms of hyperglycemia (see Appendix B) may be caused by a variety of rare syndromes. They may also be associated with stress, steroid use, and ingestion of some drugs that are toxic to beta cells. This group of diseases, labeled *other*, accounts for less than 1% of the total number of people with diabetes.

Etiology of Complications

Basement Membrane Biochemistry

One of the primary lesions seen in the vasculature of people with poorly controlled diabetes is thickening of the capillary basement membrane. This membrane surrounds the blood vessels and serves as a filtration system. It contains slit pores that filter small molecules out of the vessels and into the interstitial tissue and prevent the loss of protein from the blood. When these membranes thicken, the slit pores increase in size and lose their electrical activity. The membranes then can leak protein into the tissue (as in the eyes) or in the urine (as in the kidney). Thickening of the membrane occurs because of glycation of the membrane proteins by glucose. This process may occur via enzymatic glycosylation (Spiro & Spiro, 1971) or by nonenzymatic glycosylation, a process widespread in nature. The blood glucose levels drive both these processes, that is, poor diabetes control.

Polyol Pathways of Glucose Metabolism

The polyol pathway of glucose metabolism leads to other changes in the body when kept metabolically imbalanced by high glucose levels that lead directly or indirectly to problems in oxygen availability to the cells. The polyols are sugar alcohols and represent an alternate pathway of glucose metabolism when insulin-dependent pathways are blocked. Winegrad, Morrison, & Clements (1973) have demonstrated the presence of enzymes of the polyol pathway (aldose reductase and sorbitol dehydrogenase) in various tissues of the body, including capillaries, large vessels, nerves, and the lens of the eye. When glucose levels are high and the normal insulin-dependent glycolytic pathways are blocked by low insulin levels (poor control), the polyol products are formed and accumulate in the respective tissues. The accumulation of polyols decreases the absorption into the cell as myoinositol, an important compound in oxidative metabolism. A myoinositol deficiency can develop and result in cellular death by oxidative stress in the vascular endothelium and nerve tissue.

The Process of Glycosylation

The use of the HgbA$_{1c}$ as a clinical tool in the assessment of diabetic control will be discussed in chapters 6, 7, and 8 in Part II regarding treatment. Here, we discuss this phenomenon as a model of tissue damage. HgbA$_{1c}$ is hemoglobin to which glucose has become attached at the terminal amino acid of the beta chain of the hemoglobin. The initial reaction is a loose bonding of the terminal nitrogen of the amino acid with the number one carbon of glucose to form a Schiff base. This reaction is reversible if glucose levels decline. However, if glucose levels are high, the law of mass action keeps the glucose in contact with the amino acid and an internal rearrangement of the double bond occurs (an Amadori rearrangement) resulting in a permanent bonding of the glucose to the amino acid (HgbA$_{1c}$). This process is called glycosylation and is widespread in nature. The toasting of bread and the browning of fruit are examples of glycosylation of proteins in nature.

In humans, glycosylation of tissue has now been described not only for hemoglobin but also in red blood cell membranes, serum albumin (fructosamine—another test of glucose control), serum globulins and other plasma proteins, lens tissue, and collagen and elastic tissue. Glycosylation of collagen and elastic tissue in blood vessel walls is responsible for the stiffening of the vessels that, along with glycosylation and stiffening of red blood cells, may be responsible for, or associated with, large vessel disease in diabetes. The glycosylation of tissue proteins is a non-enzymatic process that is directly related to the blood and tissue glucose levels and causes acceleration of the aging process. Because the process is non-enzymatic and is directly related to the glucose level, there is a direct need to keep blood and tissue glucose levels as low as possible to prevent this reaction.

The common denominator of the glycosylation and other reactions of tissue with glucose is the permeability of that tissue to glucose without the presence of insulin. Only in tissue into which glucose may enter without the presence of insulin (such as vascular tissue, lens tissue, and nerve tissue) does damage occur in diabetes mellitus. Apparently, in those tissues permeable to glucose without the presence of insulin, the glucose level inside the cell will be the same as the ambient or blood glucose level. The cell must dispose of this glucose in some way. The normal glycolytic pathway for glucose disposal through the Kreb's cycle is blocked, because the enzymes necessary for the chemical degradation of glucose are insulin dependent. The cell in some manner must dispose of the accumulating glucose by alternate pathways of metabolism. Spiro and Spiro (1971) described a pathway called enzymatic glycosylation. The polyol pathway was described by Morrison and Winegrad (1971) (operative in tissues that contain aldose reductase enzymes). The third pathway of glucose disposal is the glycosylation of tissue proteins, which is non-enzymatic and is directly proportional to blood glucose levels.

Recent Advances in Nonenzymatic Glycosylation

A recent addition to the non-enzymatic glycosylation story has been the discovery of advanced glycosylation end products (AGEs). The AGEs are the final stage in the glycosylation process after the formation of the Amadori product. These two stages of glycosylation are progressive spatial rearrangements of the amino acid-glucose-bonded molecule. The bonding is permanent and alters the properties of the protein. Indeed, the AGE is now in a configuration where it can bond to the same amino acids with which the glucose bound. This can result in cross-linkage of proteins such as collagen and elastic tissue that, when cross-linked, lose their elasticity and become rigid. Low density lipoprotein (LDL) cholesterol also contains the same amino acid complexes as collagen and can bond to the AGE, resulting in permanent infiltration of the tissue with lipid (an atheromatous plaque). Elevated blood glucose is the driving force in these reactions, which also happens in persons without diabetes, but to a much lesser extent because the glucose level is lower.

Summary

All of the mechanisms of glucose disposal are related either to elevated blood and tissue glucose levels or to deficiencies of tissue insulin. It therefore becomes apparent that it is vitally important to keep blood and tissue insulin and glucose levels normal or near normal to promote the normal disposal of glucose and to prevent tissue damage from the alternative methods of glucose disposal. This is called physiologic diabetes control and requires that insulin therapy in the insulin-dependent individual be carried out to simulate normal insulin secretion patterns, that is, to maintain a 24-hr basal tissue insulin level accompanied by a burst of insulin with each feeding. This is the rationale for the multiple-dose insulin administration regimens and for the use of insulin minipumps. As explained earlier, clinical data confirm the benefit of such forms of treatment. Biochemical, morphologic, and clinical data are consistent, indicating the need for a high degree of metabolic control of diabetes mellitus to prevent or at least slow and, in some cases, reverse microvascular and perhaps macrovascular and neurologic diseases in diabetes mellitus.

References

Dahl-Jorgensen, K., Joner, G., & Hanssen, K. F. (1991). Relationship between cow's milk consumption and incidence of IDDM in childhood. *Diabetes Care, 14*(11), 1081–1083.

DeFerranti, S. D., & Osganian, S. K. (2007). Epidemiology of paediatric metabolic syndrome and type 2 diabetes mellitus. *Diabetes Vascular Disease Research, 4*(4), 285–296.

Dupres, J., Stiller, C. R., Gent, M., Donner, A., VonGrafferied, B., Heinricks, D., et al. (1988). Clinical trials of cyclosporin in insulin-dependent diabetes mellitus. *Diabetes Care, 11*(Suppl. 1), 37–44.

Fajans, S. S. (1989). Maturity onset diabetes of the young. *Diabetes Metabolism Review, 5*(7), 579–606.

Fajans, S. S., & Conn, J. W. (1960). Tolbutamide-induced improvement in carbohydrate tolerance of young people with mild diabetes mellitus. *Diabetes, 9,* 83–88.

Florez, D. C., Gablonski, K. A., Cnop, M., Vidal, J., Hull, R. L., Utzchneider, K. M., et al. (2007). Progressive loss of beta cell function leads to worsening glucose tolerance in first degree relatives of subjects with type 2 diabetes. *Diabetes Care, 30*(3), 677–682.

Fodor, J. G., & Adamo, F. B. (2001). Prevention of type 2 diabetes mellitus by changes in lifestyle. *New England Journal of Medicine, 345*(9), 696–697.

Jones, E. L. (2008). Role of obesity complicating and confusing the diagnosis and treatment of diabetes in children. *Pediatrics, 121*(2), 362–368.

Juneja, R., & Palmer, J. P. (1999). Type 1 1/2 diabetes: Myth or reality? *Autoimmunity, 29*(1), 65–83.

Knip, M., & Akerbloom, H. K. (1999). Environmental factors in the pathology of type 1 diabetes mellitus. *Experimental and Clinical Endocrinology in Diabetes, 107*(Suppl. 3), S93–S100.

Kolb, H. (1999). Pathophysiology of Type 1 diabetes mellitus. *Experimental and Clinical Endocrinology and Diabetes, 107*(Suppl. 3), S88.

Lernmark, A. (1989, November). *Determination of IDDM.* Paper presented at the Annual Scientific Session of the Diabetes Treatment Center of American Foundation, Palm Desert, CA.

McGill, M., Molyneaux, L., Twigg, S. M., & Yue, D. K. (2008). The metabolic syndrome in type 1 diabetes: Does it exist and does it matter? *Journal of Diabetes Complications, 22*(1), 18–23.

Morwessel, N. J. (1998). The genetic basis of diabetes mellitus. *AACN Clinical Issues in Advanced Practice—Acute Clinical Care, 9*(4), 539–554.

Norris, M., Beaty, B., Klingensmith, R. K., Lipsing, Y., Hoffman, M., Chase, P., et al. (1996). Lack of association between early exposure to cow's milk protein in Bell Autoimmunity. *Journal of the American Medical Association, 276*(8), 609–614.

Pani, M. A., & Badenhoop, K. (2000). Digging the genome for diabetes mellitus: The 2nd ADA Research Symposium on the Genetics of Diabetes, San Jose, CA. *Diabetes, 40*(Suppl. 3), 17–19.

Pozzilli, P. (2002). The DPT-1 trial: A negative result with lessons for future type 1 diabetes prevention. *Diabetes/Metabolism Research and Reviews, 18*(4), 257–259.

Pradhan, A. (2007). Obesity, metabolic syndrome, and type 2 diabetes: Inflammatory basis of glucose metabolic disorders. *Nutrition Revolution, 65,* S152–S156.

Rafig, M., Flanagan, S. E., Patch, A. M., Shields, B. M., Ellard, S., & Hattersley, A. T.; Neonatal Diabetes International Collaboration Group. (2008). Effective treatment with oral sulfonylurea in patients with diabetes due to sulfonylurea receptor 1 (Sur 1) mutations. *Diabetes Care, 31*(2), 204–209.

Sperling, M. A. (2008). Light at the end of the tunnel? *Pediatric Diabetes, 9*(3, Pt. 2), 1–4.

Spiro, R. G., & Spiro, M. J. (1971). Effect of diabetes in the biosynthesis of the renal glomerular basement membranes. Studies on the glycosyltransferase. *Diabetes, 20,* 641.

Tattersall, R. M., Pyke, D. A., Ranney, H. M., & Bruckheimer, S. M. (1975). Hemoglobin components in diabetes mellitus: Studies in identical twins. *New England Journal of Medicine, 273*(23), 1171–1173.

Wilkin, T. J. (2008). Diabetes: 1 and 2, or the same? Progress with the accelerator hypothesis. *Pediatric Diabetes, 9*(3, Pt. 2), 23–33.

Winegrad, A. L., Morrison, A. D., & Clements, R. S., Jr. (1973). Polyol pathway activity in aorta. *Advances in Metabolism Disorders, 2*(Suppl. 2), 117–127.

5

Glucose Metabolism Physiology

Care of individuals with diabetes requires an understanding of metabolism. Metabolism is a complex process of interrelationships between multiple regulatory factors and receiving sites and tissues. This process is essential to life, as all systems and their constituent cells rely on the maintenance of a balance, which is often, in addition to being complex, a delicate mechanism in healthy states. Also, the metabolic process is built to respond to nonmaintenance conditions, such as starvation, stress, injury, and inflammation. This response is predicated on the understanding of the need for restitution and replacement therapy undergirded by an understanding of the adaptive mechanisms of the human organism (Guthrie & Guthrie, 2004).

Metabolism

Metabolism can be described as a combination of the anabolic and catabolic processes of metamorphic stages of cellular life. Anabolism is the process of cellular production and tissue building, which relies on many factors, including the intricacies of the glucose–insulin relationship. This relationship is paramount to supplying cells with energy resources. In a disorder such as diabetes mellitus, this derangement must be attended to carefully.

Catabolism, in contrast, refers to the breaking down processes of cellular metabolism. In normal situations, a balanced state exists between anabolism and catabolism. Imbalanced states, such as uncorrected diabetes states that are not managed carefully, result in multiple degenerative effects. The degenerative effects elicit negative nitrogen balance states and tissue destruction. Examples in persons with diabetes are microvascular disease, neuropathy, and muscle wasting. In recapitulation, metabolism and its concomitant stages are the essence of life.

The human body is built for the maintenance of functions based on a stable metabolic state. In contrast to stable states, the human body contains adaptive mechanisms that use various chemicals and other factors to adjust to conditions of starvation, stress, injury, and trauma. This chapter discusses the mechanisms of carbohydrate, protein, and fat metabolism as well as concepts of fluid, electrolyte, and acid–base balance as they relate to diabetes. The physiologic role of insulin, the consequences of insulin deprivation, and the special nutrient conditions related to diabetes are described.

Blood glucose is maintained in the human body in very narrow ranges (fasting blood glucose of 60–100 mg/dl [3.3–5.6 mmol/L] and post meal glucose of 80–125 mg/dl [4.4–6.94 mmol/L]) through a dynamic, delicate homeostatic mechanism. A delicate balance is necessary between the release of insulin by the beta cells of the pancreas, the secretion of catecholamines (epinephrine and norepinephrine) by the adrenal medulla, glucocorticoids by the adrenal cortex, glucagon by the alpha cells of the pancreas, and growth hormone by the pituitary as well as pancreatic polypeptide and somatostatin, hormones of the islets of Langerhans that mediate and balance the secretion and action of insulin and glucagon. Another hormone, amylin, is also secreted by the beta cells and functions to decrease glucagon secretion by the alpha cell of the pancreas to slow gastric emptying and depress appetite. With nutrient intake (i.e., in the postprandial condition), glucose load is increased; therefore, insulin is secreted by the beta cells of the islets of Langerhans. The net effect is to mediate the hormonal balance between insulin and glucagon secretion to decrease the serum blood glucose level, facilitate storage of excess glucose in liver, muscle, and lipid tissue, and encourage synthesis of muscle proteins. Thus, insulin has crucial effects on the metabolism of the three major nutrients: carbohydrates, fats, and proteins. In other words, insulin does not just affect sugar, but also fat and protein metabolism. When insulin secretion is compromised, and the body can no longer use glucose from carbohydrates, it then uses fat and protein by also converting some of the protein to glucose. This process is known as gluconeogenesis. A decline in insulin and the concomitant increased metabolic needs call for the release of fatty acids from fat storage depots (adipose tissues) and amino acids from muscles. Consequently, both fatty acids and amino acids are transported to the liver to be used for energy. Special conditions of starvation, stress, and trauma will also be discussed, enumerating the variations from the homeostatic mechanism.

Altered metabolism leads to and is threatened by obesity. With the current rise of obesity in children, an association of metabolic complications has occurred (Nathan & Moran, 2008). The metabolic syndrome clusters insulin resistance, hypertension, dyslipidemia, hyperglycemia, and obesity, and the cardiovascular disease found in childhood and adolescence is the outcome if homeostasis is not accomplished.

Pathogenesis of Diabetes Mellitus

Diabetes is a disease of the derangement of metabolism. It is now regarded as a syndrome of multiple diseases with common symptoms but different etiologies and pathogenesis. To date, the only common denominator used to define diabetes operationally is an abnormal blood glucose level.

Diabetes mellitus may be caused by defects of insulin secretion and/or insulin resistance. There are two major types. Type 1 (T1DM) is an absolute deficit of insulin with elevated fasting blood glucose levels and increased postprandial blood glucose levels. This lack of insulin causes depletion of lipid and protein stores. In Type 2 (T2DM), insulin receptors in the peripheral tissues, enzymatic reactions within the cell, and the insulin secretion from the pancreas are compromised. Both types, then, are defined based on the relationship to insulin, not to an age classification (i.e., juvenile onset or adult onset).

The third type of diabetes mellitus is referred to as other types of hyperglycemia and encompasses a wide variety of genetic syndromes, pancreatic diseases, hormonal abnormalities, chemical exposures, and insulin-receptor abnormalities.

Carbohydrate–Insulin Relationship

Glucose is the primary fuel for all body tissues. The brain uses 50% of the total body glucose—an especially high demand. Because brain energy stores are small, a constant supply of glucose must always be available to maintain adequate brain function. It is therefore imperative that the blood glucose level be maintained in the 60–120 mg/dl (3.3–6.6 mmol/L) range to prevent central nervous system compromise.

Insulin is the primary hormone for regulating blood glucose levels and does so by controlling the rate at which blood glucose is taken up by muscle, fat, and liver cells. Each of these three types of cells uses glucose in a different way, as determined by specific enzyme systems and glucose uptake proteins on the cell membrane. Many of the principles of diabetic management and control are based on the intricate interaction of insulin and other hormones with these three cellular processes.

Fat Cell–Lipid Metabolism

The primary function of the fat cell is to provide energy storage. It contains unique enzymes that convert glucose into triglycerides as well as enzymes that convert triglycerides to fatty acids, which are released as needed and converted to ketones in the liver.

The conversion of glucose to triglycerides and the breakdown of triglycerides to free fatty acids occur continuously and simultaneously within the same fat cell, and both processes are regulated by insulin. High blood insulin levels stimulate the uptake of glucose by fat cells to form triglycerides; thus, there is a net gain of storage fat. During low blood insulin levels, glucose uptake into the fat cell is poor; thus, fewer triglycerides are formed. Triglyceride breakdown, then, exceeds formation, resulting in a net loss of the storage fat. Thus, by regulating glucose uptake into fat cells, insulin influences net fat metabolism.

Insulin also inhibits the enzyme, lipase, which breaks down storage fat into fatty acids and glycerol. When insulin is high and lipase is inhibited, there is a net increase in storage fat. A net decrease in storage fat occurs when insulin is low, because lipase becomes activated and fat is then broken down.

Muscle Cell

The muscle cell has two primary functions. It converts glucose into the energy needed for muscle function, and it serves as a reservoir for protein and glycogen. When a person starves, the protein of the contractile apparatus itself can be made available in the form of amino acids, which can then be converted into glucose in the liver to maintain blood glucose at an adequate concentration for brain function (gluconeogenesis).

In the muscle cell, as in the fat cell, insulin promotes the uptake of glucose. The muscle cell, however, has different enzymes that control two metabolic pathways for glucose. First, glucose can be converted into *contractile energy*. Second, glucose can be converted to glycogen, a storage form of glucose that is more readily available than triglycerides in times of glucose insufficiency. When blood glucose levels are normal, insulin also assists muscle cell enzymes to maintain muscle mass by promoting the uptake of amino acids and preventing the breakdown of protein.

Liver Cell

Liver glycogen is another storage form of glucose. As mentioned earlier, glycogen is more readily available for use than are triglycerides, which first have to be converted to free fatty acids and then converted to ketones. The liver monitors these conversions and also converts amino acids to glucose when necessary. The latter process is called *gluconeogenesis* (new glucose formation). Although insulin is not required for the transport of glucose into the liver, insulin directly influences the liver to promote the uptake of glucose by reducing the rate of glycogenolysis (glycogen breakdown), increasing glycogen synthesis, and decreasing the rate of gluconeogenesis.

Beta Cell

Insulin is secreted by the beta cells of the islets of Langerhans in the pancreas, which continually monitor glucose levels. The beta cells function first as a sensor of blood glucose levels, then they secrete enough insulin to regulate the carbohydrate load, maintaining the blood glucose level within a narrow range. A feedback system exists whereby a small amount of carbohydrate stimulates a small amount of insulin release. The liver responds to increased insulin secretion by stimulating glycogen synthesis (glycogenesis) and suppressing glycogen release (glycogenolysis). The formation of new glucose (gluconeogenesis) is likewise suppressed. A large carbohydrate intake stimulates a greater insulin response, and the peripheral and liver cells take up glucose. When glucose levels are low, insulin release is suppressed and glycogenolysis and gluconeogenesis occur to feed glucose into the system and maintain the blood glucose levels.

Although the process of beta cell stimulation and insulin release is not entirely understood, it is recognized that glucose metabolism signals the synthesis of the precursor of insulin called proinsulin. Proinsulin is transformed into insulin within the beta cell, and the insulin is then stored in granules and released in response to several stimuli. Glucose is the most profound stimulus to insulin release. Other stimuli include amino acids, hormones, vagal stimulation, sulfonylureas, and ketones. Those substances diminishing insulin secretion are epinephrine, norepinephrine, thiazide diuretics, starvation, and hypoxia. Pancreatic insulin is secreted directly into the portal circulation to the liver, the central organ of glucose homeostasis, where 50% of the insulin is degraded. The peripheral circulation then transports insulin to body cells and to the kidney, where 25% is degraded, and excretion occurs.

Intracellular Functioning Through Second Messengers

Insulin affects glucose, lipid, and protein metabolism in all tissues, as discussed earlier. In fat cells, insulin promotes the uptake and enhances triglyceride stores. In muscle cells, glucose enters via the cell membrane made permeable by insulin, and is converted to glycogen stores or used for energy. In liver cells, glucose is stored as glycogen. The intracellular effects of hormones are accomplished by *second messengers*, which are activated by receptors on cell membranes that determine whether or not the cell responds to the hormones. Specific enzymes then allow the cell to perform its functions in response to hormones and second messengers. The second messenger for most hormones is cyclic adenosine monophosphate (cAMP), which is activated by the enzyme adenyl cyclase in the cell membrane. Insulin suppresses adenyl cyclase and cAMP and activates other second messengers. These messenger enzymes are activated by closure of the potassium channels and opening of the calcium channels so that calcium can flow into the cell and activate formation of cAMP.

One enzymatic mechanism that insulin-responsive cells have is the phosphorylase–kinase system. Insulin stimulates the cells by interaction with a specific receptor on the cell surface, and this stimulates a series of enzymatic phosphorylation reactions within the cell. Finally, this phosphorylase cascade activates the PPar gamma enzyme in the cell nucleus. This enzyme activates the gene for the formation of the RNA, which synthesizes a protein called a glucose transporter to facilitate the uptake of glucose by the cell. Glucose transporter proteins modify the cell membrane to absorb the glucose into the interior of the cell for utilization. These transporters are manufactured inside the cell and carried to the cell membrane under the control of insulin and the subsequent enzyme reactions within the cell. Insulin also controls the reabsorption and degradation of the transporters that are numbered to differentiate the proteins of different cells—GLUT 4 (Glucose Transporter 4 is found within muscle cells). A hexokinase enzyme inside the cell is also stimulated to facilitate the glycolytic process for the metabolism of glucose to CO_2, water, and energy (the Kreb's cycle). This hexokinase enzyme is the only enzyme of the glycolytic pathway activated by insulin. It catalyzes the initial step of this process that is the phosphorylation of glucose to form glucose 6-phosphate.

This catalysis is a vital step in the metabolism of glucose for energy, and insulin deficiency will result in blockage of the entire glycolytic pathway for energy production. The enzymatic system for lipogenesis (to fats) is specific to the fat cell, whereas the enzymatic system for conversion of glucose to energy occurs in all cells. By a separate set of enzymes, the fat can, of course, also convert glucose to energy for its own metabolic processes, because the conversion of glucose to fat is an energy-requiring process. All of these specifics are probably mediated by a second messenger through an activation of the sodium potassium pump and by the calcium flux.

Hormones Relative to Metabolism

Epinephrine

Epinephrine works to prepare the body for many different kinds of stress. Its effect on glucose is rapid and can produce continuous changes in blood glucose levels. Stress stimulates epinephrine release, and the hormone then serves to mobilize glycogen to yield a higher blood glucose level. This part of the fight-or-flight mechanism supplies the energy needed by the body to meet emergencies.

Corticosteroids

Corticosteroids increase gluconeogenesis (new glucose) from protein (amino acids) by the liver. Glucocorticoids can respond to acute stress but are more generally associated with chronic stress. Treatment with high-dose steroids is a potential trigger to the development of hyperglycemia and diabetes especially if the genetic component is already present.

Growth Hormone

Growth hormone, together with insulin, promotes body growth. Its effect on blood glucose levels is much slower than epinephrine or glucocorticoid hormones. Epinephrine acts in seconds, glucocorticoids in minutes, and growth hormone in hours. Growth hormone elevates blood glucose, making it available for the growth process, but its physiologic role in glucose control is unknown. Although growth hormone elevates blood glucose levels and hypoglycemia will increase growth hormone levels, it is now doubtful that growth hormone plays any meaningful role in continuous regulation of blood glucose levels.

Metabolism in Starvation, Stress, and Injury

Normal metabolism within the context of homeostasis occurs as described earlier. In starvation, stress, and injury states, however, the mechanisms can alter, escalate, or compensate in various ways. Each of these states is discussed, as they are germane to the maintenance of a balanced or steady state in the person with diabetes.

Insulin Deficiency

The abnormal state of insulin deprivation as observed in individuals with unknown or uncontrolled diabetes is similar to a state of severe starvation. The degree of lack of insulin will influence the extent of this process. If untreated, complete insulin deprivation, as often observed in the young child with diabetes, will terminate in ketoacidosis and coma. The adult with diabetes with a minimal lack of insulin may not even experience symptoms of the disease.

An immediate consequence of insulin deficiency is the lack of glucose uptake by cells. In fat cells, triglyceride stores are liberated in the absence of insulin, yielding free fatty acids that are ultimately converted into ketones and glycerol. In muscle cells, glycogen stores are activated and protein is degraded to amino acids that are then converted into glucose in the liver.

Diabetes mellitus may be defined as an absolute or relative lack of insulin that results in aberrations of fat, protein, and carbohydrate metabolism. Absence of insulin production initially affects the uptake of glucose in muscle and fat cells. As glucose's entry into cells diminishes, the body signals for fuel, and glycogen is released from the liver. The blood glucose level is thereby further elevated. As the glucose levels approach 180 mg/dl (10 mmol/L) of blood, the capacity of the renal tubules to reabsorb glucose (renal threshold) is exceeded, and glucose is excreted into the urine (glucosuria). The renal threshold is known to be lower in women during pregnancy and in children. It may be elevated in the older patient or in persons with a long history of diabetes. Because glucose is an osmotic diuretic, water and salts are also excreted in large quantities, and cellular dehydration occurs. Prolonged, excessive diuresis (polyuria) combined with caloric loss causes polydipsia (increased thirst), polyphagia (increased hunger), and fatigue, the classic symptoms of diabetes mellitus. Despite polyphagia, there may be weight loss because the food ingested cannot be used in the absence of insulin.

In addition to the classic symptoms mentioned, others may also be present. Weight loss, commonly seen in the child with diabetes, is uncommon in the adult, who is often obese. Fluctuation in blood glucose levels with changes of osmotic pressures may change the shape of the lens of the eye and the content of the vitreous humor, resulting in refractive changes manifested by blurred vision. Headache is often a major complaint and may be related to the vision problems. Faintness, nervousness, and hunger, experienced chiefly by adults, occur 1 or 2 hr after a meal; these problems are caused by rapid gastric emptying in the absence of the hormone amylin and the intestinal hormones GIP and GLP1 with a delayed insulin release, resulting in immediate hyperglycemia and later hypoglycemia. Weight gain, skin infection, and recurrent vulvovaginitis are fairly common complaints in the adult with diabetes.

Individuals with stable T2DM are often asymptomatic, and the diagnosis is made incidentally by routine blood or urine laboratory tests. These individuals frequently have the chronic complications of diabetes, such as recurrent infection, atherosclerosis, peripheral vascular disease, neuropathy, and ocular complications, at diagnosis because the diagnosis is delayed.

When the onset of diabetes continues unchecked, especially in younger, ketosis-prone individuals, cells attempt to respond to glucose deprivation initially by metabolizing protein, resulting in the liberation of amino acids in large quantities. Some of these amino acids are converted into urea in the liver and are excreted, which results in a negative nitrogen balance. Other amino acids are converted to glucose, further enhancing the hyperglycemic state.

In the absence of insulin, fat cells attempt to provide fuel by mobilizing fat stores. The free fatty acids are initially used for energy production, but the majority reach the liver in which three organic acids are formed: acetoacetic acid, beta hydroxybutyric acid, and acetone. The keto acids are ultimately excreted by the kidney along with sodium bicarbonate. The combination of keto acid accumulation and bicarbonate excretion causes a fall in plasma pH, resulting in acidosis. The body attempts to correct the acidosis by the characteristic Kussmaul's respiration, which is deep, labored respiration caused by the body's effort to convert carbonic acid (H_2CO_3) to carbon dioxide and water, and to excrete the carbon dioxide via the lungs. In an unchecked state, acidosis, dehydration, and electrolyte imbalance ultimately affect brain function, and coma results. Death may occur if insulin deficiency remains untreated.

Total body potassium may be decreased because of cellular breakdown and excretion. Dehydration, however, may cause the serum potassium to be concentrated in less body fluid, resulting in low, normal, or elevated serum potassium levels. Potassium may also show a false positive because of pH-buffering mechanisms. Sodium is lost along with water in the urine, and serum sodium is almost always severely depleted, indicating a water (cellular) deficit.

Insulin treatment reverses the catabolic state created by insulin deficiency. Blood glucose levels fall, fats cease to break down, ketones are no longer produced, serum bicarbonate and pH levels rise, and potassium shifts intracellular as anabolism (tissue rebuilding) begins.

Incretins (GLP-1 and GIP) are hormones secreted by the gut that mediate insulin release and glucagon suppression (Fujioka, 2007). Glucagon suppression is most noticeable in individuals with T2DM, although it is present in various forms in T1DM. Glucagon-like peptide-1 (GLP-1) has an insulinotropic effect, and appears to preserve this ability when enhanced by medication. Glucose-dependent insulinotropic polypeptide (GIP) is inactivated in persons with T2DM. Both GLP-1 and GIP are inactivated by dipeptidyl peptidase 4 (DPP-4). The use of DPP-4 inhibitors and GLP-1 and GIP analogs have aided in glucose processing in the presence of adequate insulin.

Starvation

Insulin deficiency in the pathogenesis of diabetes mellitus was initially reported by many people in the 19th century from studies in pancreatectomized animals. The hormone itself was not discovered until long after it had been named. The name of the hormone insulin comes from the discovery by such men as Bernard, Vircow, Minkowski, and others that it came from the islets of Langerhans in the pancreas (*islands* in Latin is *insular,* thus the name *insuline* initially).

Historically, Banting and Best (Banting, 1925), more than 80 years ago (1921), are credited with the epoch-making discovery of insulin. Further investigation by many other investigators showed the relationship of pituitary and adrenal hormones interfering with insulin action and contributing to hyperglycemia. This latter finding relates to the stress mechanism, a discussion to follow. In the 1960s hormonal analysis through radioimmunoassay studies to measure polypeptide type hormones was developed. This technique has further confirmed that insulin deficiency characterizes T1DM and some people with T2DM.

In general, the body's basic response to starvation is to lose nitrogen compounds in the urine. The person with diabetes and without appropriate treatment is in a state of metabolic response to starvation, because glucose and other nutrients are not properly transported to cells and metabolized. Calories to sustain life in a starvation state are derived from fat stores (80%–90%) and the remaining calories are taken from protein catabolism. Survival is related to the body's ability to enhance oxidation of lipids and reduce breakdown of proteins.

The usual hallmark of starvation is progressive weight loss, seen as flaccid skin, lean body mass, poor skin turgor, and flaking skin. Initial weight loss reflects a disproportionate loss of water. A healthy individual can lose 5%–10% of normal body weight in water without loss of function; 40% loss is incompatible with life. After initial water loss, overall tissue loss occurs in the visceral organs (i.e., liver, pancreas, and gut). Studies of prolonged starvation show that the greatest weight loss is in visceral organs with least loss occurring in skeletal and orbital tissue. Additionally, increased glucagon and protein catabolism increases sodium, potassium, and magnesium losses. In later stages, urinary loss of sodium and potassium may buffer increased urinary ketone levels. The excretion of sodium and potassium in early starvation is decreased by administering glucose and insulin.

Changes in body composition from starvation include increased extracellular fluid (saline), loss of intracellular fluid (water), disproportionate loss of fat, and lesser losses of lean body tissue. Bone minerals are usually maintained. The tissue lost in early starvation is thus a mixture of fat, protein, and water, a caloric equivalent of 2,000 kcal/kg. Untreated or prolonged starvation could result in losses of up to 8,000 kcal/kg. The metabolic response is to use any available glucose (provided insulin is available), then fat stores, then proteins. With the exception of nervous tissue, body organs lose fat in proportion to their original lipid content (from fat stores). Protein loss follows, and it is important to note that there is no protein depot or stored protein as such. Every protein molecule serves a vital function. Thus, the use of protein (even 5%–10%) for energy results in loss of protein molecules essential to enzymatic and cellular functions. Skeletal muscle is first catabolized raising the blood urea nitrogen and urinary nitrogenous compound excretions, in a mean output of 12 g/day during 3–5 days. If this initial rate continued, death would quickly ensue. So the adaptive responses in long-term starvation result in the sparing of body proteins. Urinary losses decrease to 3–4 g/day.

Further, starvation reduces energy expenditure by neuroendocrine responses discussed in the stress section. Cardiac load is reduced, noted by bradycardia and decreased triiodothyronine (T_3). Skeletal energy needs are decreased with decreased glycogen, resulting in decreased muscle tone. Examination shows loss of more red muscles than white muscle (Levenson & Seifter, 1983).

In summary, the overall effect of starvation is as follows:

1. Initial rise of urinary nitrogenous excretion.
2. Increase in blood fatty acids, keto acids, and ketones, producing metabolic acidosis and ketonuria.
3. Increased blood glucose levels in persons with diabetes (lowered in persons without diabetes).
4. Increased urinary excretion of sodium, potassium, and other minerals.

Thus, persons with untreated diabetes experience a complicated starvation state and are particularly vulnerable, because compensatory mechanisms are often compromised in the absence of insulin and its multiple effects.

Stress

Stress states are ubiquitous with life. Persons with diabetes are additionally challenged, however, because much of the stress response mechanism is geared toward hyperglycemia to provide energy for the fight-or-flight syndrome (Cannon, 1953). The stress mechanism is a complex quality control system, in general, a negative feedback system that is directed to respond to increased body demands. It is a complicated neuroendocrine-mediated response to a trigger event. A discussion of the intermediary relationships between various neurologic and endocrine enzymes follows.

The stress response functions through intermediaries called hormones. The master hormones are secreted by the pituitary gland and the hypothalamus, which stimulate specific target glands throughout the body. Because diabetes is a metabolic disorder and because the insulin–nutrient relationships are impaired, stress phenomena make the person with diabetes additionally vulnerable. Consequently, stress (such as surgery, infection, or major psychosocial events) must be acknowledged in the medical management regimen. Most of the neuroendocrine hormones are involved in the stress mechanism, but some are more specifically involved.

The stress mechanism, a normal metabolic reaction, regularly triggers the hypothalamus area of the brain that in turn stimulates the anterior pituitary gland to produce the following hormones: growth hormone (HGH) also known as somatotropin (STH), thyrotropin (TSH), adrenocorticotropin (ACTH), the gonadotrophic hormones (follicle-stimulating [FSH] and luteinizing hormone [LH]), and prolactin. The posterior pituitary secretes two additional hormones for stress, antidiuretic hormone (ADH) and oxytocin, involved in blood pressure control and childbirth. All of these master gland hormones are facilitated for secretion by intermediaries released in the hypothalamus called releasing hormones. After release by the pituitary, the hormones are transported via the bloodstream to stimulate target receptor sites in biologically programmed glands. The target glands (e.g., the adrenal cortex, thyroid gland, gonads, kidney, and so on) respond by secreting additional hormones, such as steroids, thyroxin, cortisol, and so on.

Hormones mediate the metabolism of nutrients. Persons with diabetes are affected not only regarding the insulin (a hormone) and glucose relationship previously discussed, but also in other hormone–nutrient relationships: growth hormone-protein synthesis and cellular factors; thyrotropin-thyroxin-cellular metabolic rate; adrenocortical hormones, glucose, and fluid and electrolyte metabolism (primarily salt balance); and antidiuretic hormones and water balance. Gonadotrophic hormones and the stress of pregnancy in the person with diabetes must be closely managed.

Stress, as a normal metabolic process, as well as increased stress, is important to the metabolic management of people with diabetes. Increased stress, or distress as defined by Selye (1976), prepares the body for fight or flight by release of adrenal medullary hormones, catecholamines, specifically epinephrine and norepinephrine. Each of these hormones facilitates specific effects. The hypothalamus is also stimulated by stress, causing the release of the pituitary hormones. In persons with diabetes, balance is particularly precarious, as multiple nutrient relationships are affected, especially glucose, sodium-potassium, and water balance. Glucose metabolism is affected by ACTH release (glucocorticoids and mineralocorticoids), thyroxin, and growth hormone. Glucocorticoids increase release of proteins and stimulate their conversion to glucose by the liver (gluconeogenesis), increasing blood glucose levels. Additionally, the release of epinephrine for additional stress mobilizes glycogen (glycogenolysis) to yield higher blood glucose levels. Thus, all hormones except insulin contribute to an increased blood glucose level, which requires more insulin production to facilitate transport of glucose into the cell; without sufficient insulin, hyperglycemia results. Additionally, the catecholamines suppress insulin release as does the stress of starvation and hypoxia.

Thus, the general effects of stress are a response to *hormonal metabolism*. Concurrently, the responses of the autonomic nervous system are elicited. Further information on this response follows in the discussion on injury and inflammation.

Injury and Inflammation

Adaptations to body changes caused by injury and inflammation elicit a set of characteristic responses. This challenge is particularly arduous for the person with diabetes. Thus, all goals in diabetic management are directed toward prevention of injury, trauma, surgical and critical illness, and infection.

The neuroendocrine mechanisms undergirding the human body's response to injury and inflammation are altered, causing a profound effect on the person with diabetes. Injury elicits an autonomic nervous system response escalating to a central nervous system response, thus connecting with the pituitary for mediation. The autonomic nervous system mediates internal homeostasis, with the sympathetic branch being the chief effector in stress, injury, and inflammation. This response accentuates release of catecholamines, which, in turn, increase glucose and free fatty acids *and* suppress the expected elevation in insulin.

In injury, the characteristic shifts of fluids and electrolytes are directed at fluid and electrolyte balance (preservation of intravascular fluid and therefore tissue perfusion). Obligatory retention of sodium and water is mediated by ACTH and ADH, respectively. Initially, this results in saline excess (lowered hematocrit) *and* water excess (lowered serum sodium). If shock or hypoxia occurs, metabolic acidosis ensues (pH lowered and serum carbon dioxide lowered because of lactic acidosis). The stress raises the blood glucose, and catecholamines suppress insulin release, resulting in hyperglycemia. Normally, wound healing depends on aerobic energy. The person without diabetes has a strong response to stress; a person with diabetes has an aggravated stress response, resulting in the use of lipids and protein for cellular energy, leading to ketoacidosis and delayed wound healing. Profound effects (severe metabolic acidosis) of combined lactic and metabolic acidosis can occur.

In the postinjury and postinflammatory phases, adequate energy is required to maintain bodily functions, to free reparative processes, and to respond to pathologic energy demands. Sources of energy are either exogenous or endogenous, and the caloric, fluid, and electrolyte needs in the individual with diabetes must be closely monitored. Typically, as is the case of *uncomplicated* starvation, lipid stores will supply approximately 80%–85% of energy needs. Long-term protein stores will be challenged to provide the remaining 20%. Protein use for energy can result in as much as a 10% weight loss. Thus, the potential for muscle wasting is metabolically increased in the person with diabetes.

In injury, *without shock,* proteins from lean tissue are mobilized, which is reflected in increased urinary nitrogen. It is unclear if proteins are mobilized because of increased muscular protein catabolism or reduced protein synthesis; this may depend on the severity of injury. In severe injury, sulfur-containing amino acids are elevated, indicating increased protein breakdown. Exogenous glucose can reduce loss of nitrogen. Therefore, treatment of hyperglycemia and supplying glucose is important in decreasing nitrogen loss. Additionally, decreased insulin levels inappropriate to plasma glucose levels favor lipolysis and release of fatty acids—again, emphasizing the propensity for ketoacidosis of the person with diabetes.

In comparison, the metabolic response to starvation, in general, differs from the metabolic response to injury in relation to nitrogenous losses, gluconeogenesis, and resting energy expenditure. In general, responses are *augmented* in injury and are *diminished* in starvation. The starvation response is directed to conserve tissue to prolong life, whereas injury accentuates tissue loss. The person with diabetes is particularly vulnerable to both.

Altered States: Acidosis and Hyperglycemia

Acidosis, a serious and critical state in diabetes, is a result of the primary pathogenesis of diabetes—insulin deficiency. The inability to transport glucose to cells and to metabolize cellular glucose leads the body to burn fats (lipids) for energy. The stored lipids are split into free fatty acids, then to ketone derivatives. Thus, this disorder is named *ketoacidosis*. Lipids are split to acetoacetic acid, beta hydroxybutyric acid, and acetone that rise in the extracellular fluid. Consequently large quantities of ketones are excreted in the urine, sometimes as much as 500–1,000 mmol/day. Diabetes acidosis results, then, primarily from the presence of keto acids (measured as ketones in blood and urine). This high acidic state (high hydrogen ion concentration) causes chemoreceptors to increase respiratory rate and depth; a key diagnostic sign is called Kussmaul's respiration. Diabetes acidosis also results from the loss of large amounts of sodium bicarbonate, the alkaline half of the bicarbonate–carbonic acid buffer system (measured as a low serum carbon dioxide level, less than 22 mEq/L, and a large anion gap). Metabolic acidosis often results in profound reduction of serum carbon dioxide in contrast to respiratory acidosis. The major effect, which is death producing if unattended, is depression of the central nervous system, ranging from lethargy, dulled sensorium, disorientation, to coma. In persons with diabetes, the central nervous system depression and shock caused by metabolic acidosis progresses to a comatose state (McCance & Huether, 1998).

This hyperosmolar state created by high levels of glucose, free fatty acids, and ketones also results in excessive urinary excretion of saline fluids, thus leading to a saline depletion state, a type of hematogenic shock. The concomitant altered metabolic state can be prevented by adequate ammonia secretion by renal tubules, as hydrogen ions combine with ammonia and thereby release sodium for tubular reabsorption. When the total amount of acids (i.e., keto acids) entering the tubules *exceed* the rate of ammonia secretion, the excess acid transports sodium with it into the urine rather than allowing it to reenter the extracellular fluids as sodium bicarbonate.

Additionally, levels of potassium must be concurrently evaluated as the acidotic state increases. Cells, the third of the four-part buffering system (plasma, lungs, cells, and kidneys), will absorb hydrogen (acids) from the extracellular fluids to decrease the acidity of the plasma and therefore decrease the severity of the acidosis. This reaction results in the release of potassium from the cell to the plasma, however, resulting in a redistribution hyperkalemia. If the extracellular levels rise above 6.0 mEq/L, a toxic state is created and must be treated accordingly. Key diagnostic signs of potassium alteration are specific configurations in electrocardiogram tracings, such as high tented T waves in hyperkalemia, widening of the QRS complex, lowering and flattening of P waves leading to bradycardia and atrial arrest and flattened T waves, and the appearance of U waves in hypokalemia.

Buffering Mechanisms

Because the maintenance of acid–base balance is crucial to equilibrium, the body has several levels of defense or compensatory mechanisms against changes in pH. Physiologic compensatory mechanisms or *compensation* enables the adjustment by the organs to stress or physiologic disruption. These mechanisms can be total, partial, or noncompensatory in action, and they include the action of four regulatory systems: chemical serum buffers, lungs, cells, and kidneys.

The four mechanisms are triggered by a stressor, an event leading initially to physiologic imbalance, such as the excess of hydrogen ions (acids), which might result from ketoacidosis in uncontrolled diabetes (metabolic condition) or hypoventilation (respiratory condition). This state of excess of hydrogen ions (acidemia-acidosis) subsequently triggers the buffering mechanisms to respond. The response is time sequenced as follows: serum chemicals (seconds to minutes), lungs (10–30 min), cells (2–4 hr), and kidneys (hours to days).

Serum Chemical Buffers

A buffer is a certain combination of chemicals contained in the fluids of the extracellular compartment that act as a deterrent against spontaneous and critical changes in the hydrogen ion concentration. A buffer is sometimes conceptually likened to a "chemical sponge," because it can "soak" up surplus hydrogen ions or release or donate them to calibrate or balance the fluctuations in pH. A buffer is composed of a "weak" acid combined with one of the salts of that acid. Although there are several buffering mechanisms in the human body, the most important one is the carbonic acid–sodium bicarbonate system in the serum.

The chemical serum buffers are the first level of defense against changes in the body's acid–base balance. They begin to react immediately to counteract the slightest change in pH balance. Chemical buffers are *paired* compounds—a weak acid is paired with a weak base or salt. The weak acid separates to neutralize strong bases. The weak base separates to neutralize strong acids. Once the chemicals have reacted, they are consumed and cannot be used again as a defense until the body has had time to replenish them. Three primary (serum) chemical buffers function in the donor–acceptor pattern: bicarbonate, hemoglobin, and plasma proteins. The bicarbonate buffer is the key compensating mechanism in diabetes.

Bicarbonate Subsystem

One part of carbonic acid exists in relationship to 20 parts of bicarbonate. The base bicarbonate system must maintain this ratio of 20 parts bicarbonate to 1 part carbonic acid in the blood to keep a slightly alkaline pH (normally pH 7.4). Bicarbonate is produced when carbonic acid dissociates into hydrogen and bicarbonate. For example, if a strong acid like hydrochloric acid enters the bloodstream, the weak base sodium bicarbonate combines with it to form the weak carbonic acid and salt, sodium chloride. The salt does not affect the pH level, and the weak acid only slightly reduces the pH.

Hemoglobin Subsystem

When the bicarbonate or carbonic acid is consumed, the bicarbonate buffers can no longer react, and the next level of the blood chemical buffer regulatory system, hemoglobin, is challenged. The chloride in hemoglobin shifts in and out of the red blood cells as the level of oxygen changes in the blood. Chloride also leaves the cell in relation to pH changes. As the plasma becomes more alkaline, chloride shifts out of the cell. As a result, bicarbonate moves in. Conversely, if chloride moves into the red blood cells, bicarbonate moves out. In this way the body has another level of chemical control. The chloride shift corrects acidosis, or alkalosis, by varying the level of bicarbonate available to handle the stress. In acidosis, chloride may also combine directly with hydrogen. For example, a person whose system has become acidic from a starvation diet or a fad high-protein, low-carbohydrate diet may develop mild acidosis. This mild state of acidosis usually ranges from pH 7.34 to pH 7.30 and can be corrected by the chemical buffer bicarbonate. If slightly more bicarbonate is needed than is available in the bloodstream, the oxygen level decreases. The reduced oxygen causes chloride to shift into the red blood cells and the bicarbonate to move into the bloodstream to buffer the excess acid that is not neutralized by bicarbonate. Chloride shifts occur in acute diabetic coma.

Protein Subsystem

The third chemical buffer is plasma protein, primarily albumin and globulin. Plasma protein, functioning in conjunction with the liver, has the ability to attract or release hydrogen ions. For example, alkalosis is diagnosed in a person having gallbladder problems with a pH range of 7.47 to 7.55 because of the loss of hydrochloric acid resulting from vomiting. In this case, the liver reacts to a decrease of acid by breaking down the plasma protein, thereby releasing more hydrogen ions that add acid to the blood and neutralize excess base. If the alkalosis or acidosis is too severe, the chemical buffers can reduce it only slightly.

Lungs

If serum chemical buffering systems are not able to correct the pH change, the second buffering mechanism is stimulated (i.e., the lungs). The lungs are unique in that they can regulate only the problems caused by metabolic acid–base imbalances. They cannot compensate for respiratory acid–base problems because the lungs themselves are part of the problem. The lungs initially assist the chemical buffers to maintain the correct metabolic base balance and act directly as a regulator system after the chemical serum buffers are consumed. During acidosis, the lungs aid the base bicarbonate and chloride chemical buffers. Bicarbonate neutralizes the excess strong acid into the weaker acid (i.e., carbonic acid). The lungs then break the carbonic acid, a volatile acid, into carbon dioxide and water, which is exhaled as a gaseous substance. In this way, the lungs act as a facilitator to the bicarbonate buffer system.

When the chemical buffers are consumed, the lungs react either to the excess or deficit in the ratio of bicarbonate to carbonic acid in the bloodstream by changing breathing patterns. With normal body pH, respiratory depth and speed are constant. When there is too much base or too little acid in the blood, resulting in a pH greater than 7.45, the lungs automatically *reduce* depth and speed of respiration to compensate for metabolic alkalosis. This slowing action (hypoventilation) causes carbonic acid to build up in the bloodstream. The retained carbonic acid neutralizes the excess base in the blood, thus reducing the metabolic alkalosis. If there is too much acid or too little base in the bloodstream and the pH drops below 7.35, the lungs *increase* the depth and speed of respiration, exhaling (hyperventilation) the excess acid in the form of carbon dioxide and water. This compensates for metabolic acidosis. An example of acidosis regulation is seen in patients who are hyperventilating as a result of diabetic acidosis. The lungs respond in 10–30 min to decrease the amount of acid in the bloodstream. Because the lungs can only exhale or retain carbon dioxide and water, they are only able to neutralize the hydrogen ions of carbonic acid. Fixed acid imbalances must be corrected by other regulatory systems, the cells and kidneys, especially in diabetic acidosis.

Cells

The cells regulate acid and base imbalances by exchanging potassium ions for hydrogen ions. Normally, 98% of the potassium is located inside the cell with only 2% in the serum. During acidosis, however, hydrogen ions move into the cell to reduce the acid in the serum. Potassium ions move out of the cell into the interstitial fluid and eventually into the serum to allow room for the hydrogen ions.

Although this hydrogen potassium exchange temporarily relieves the acidosis, it has the potential of creating a toxic state. As the quantity of potassium outside the cell increases, it rapidly becomes toxic causing a potassium excess called *hyperkalemia*. The hydrogen potassium exchange causes the level of potassium in the serum to increase six tenths for each one-tenth decrease in the pH reading. At this rate, the potassium rapidly reaches the toxic level (especially on the heart) of 6.0 mEq/L; consequently acidotic persons may evidence hyperkalemia or a "false" normal, with excessive gastrointestinal losses in diabetic acidosis. The excess serum potassium may be reduced by renal excretion causing a total body potassium deficit.

Kidneys

The kidneys are the last level of defense the body has against acid–base imbalances. The kidneys control the acid–base balance by regulating bicarbonate, converting phosphate to phosphoric acid, and changing ammonia to ammonium. The kidneys can control the amount of bicarbonate in the body by selectively secreting hydrogen ions into the urine and retaining bicarbonate ions, *or* excreting bicarbonate and retaining hydrogen. In the normally functioning kidneys with a normal serum pH, proportional amounts of hydrogen and bicarbonate are secreted into the kidney tubules. The tubules select whether to retain bicarbonate or hydrogen. The electrolytes not retained are excreted in the urine. Normal urine pH is 5.5 to 6.5. If the extracellular fluid becomes acidic, bicarbonate is used in the extracellular fluid to reduce acidosis, resulting in more hydrogen ions in the kidney tubules than bicarbonate. These excess ions, combined with the tubular fluid, are then excreted in the urine. In this way, hydrogen ions are removed from the body, and acidosis is reduced. This is primarily a kidney compensation for respiratory acidosis. Although it takes hours to days, this process can also help reduce severe metabolic acidosis. Bicarbonate is also used if the extracellular fluid becomes alkaline. The excess bicarbonate in the kidney tubules combines with sodium and is secreted in the urine in the form of sodium bicarbonate. This process is primarily a correction for severe metabolic alkalosis.

A buildup of phosphoric acid (H_2PO_4) from a kidney dysfunction can also create an acid–base imbalance. A chemical reaction, phosphate and hydrogen, in the kidney tubules allows both to be excreted in the urine as H_2PO_4, which reduces the acid in the serum.

Another mechanism by which the kidneys control the amount of acid in the extracellular fluid is a combined function with the liver called the *ammonium mechanism*. When the acidotic state becomes so severe that the kidneys cannot control the acidosis with buffers in the kidney tubules, the distal tubules begin to secrete ammonia. Ammonia combines with hydrogen ions to form ammonium. This combination hooks to chloride and is excreted in the form of a salt. Both phosphoric acid and ammonium are fixed acids and are only excreted through the kidneys. The kidneys are slower to react than any of the other defenses against acid–base imbalances, but they are also more thorough. The kidneys take from several hours to several days to respond. The pH level of the serum is controlled by the regulatory systems in both health and disease states. During a disease state, the regulatory systems are less effective and medical intervention is usually needed. Observation of urinary responses to metabolic imbalanced states in diabetes is important. Attention to renal responses in acute diabetes shock and coma is paramount.

Summary

Metabolic balance is the challenge that all persons face. This is particularly crucial to the patient with diabetes, however, and therapeutic regimens may be necessary to achieve this balance. The body works to maintain a balanced state (pH 7.35 to 7.45 arterial blood gases) by use of the buffering mechanisms just described. Thus, stages of buffering in acidotic and ketoacidotic states follow a usual pattern, assisting in the assessment of worsening or improving states. The therapeutic regime is predicated on the knowledge of these buffering mechanisms in metabolic balance.

The diagnosis of acidosis is made from physical findings and laboratory assessment. Major clinical findings center on the following metabolic conditions present (new or concurrent) or escalated because of stress: hyperventilation (a compensatory mechanism), stupor leading to coma, neurologic hyperirritability with twitching and convulsion in uremia, and stupor and acetone breath in ketoacidosis. Laboratory findings show plasma bicarbonate less than 22 mEq/L, arterial blood gases show lowered pH (<7.35, more reduced than with respiratory acidosis), bases lowered, and elevated or false normal potassium (cellular compensatory mechanism). Note that persons with diabetes mellitus are primarily vulnerable but may also have other conditions concomitantly with diabetes. Fluids such as normal saline are used to correct the fluid and sodium losses and potassium is added when renal blood flow is established. Other fluids can be administered depending on the etiology of the imbalance. Fluid and electrolyte administration will be further discussed with the discussion of DKA in Chapter 6. Metabolic acidosis is a major derangement of metabolism. Attention to early recognition, return to balance, and prevention of complications is paramount for the person with diabetes. Diabetes mellitus is a complex disease based on the pathogenesis or the creation of a catabolic state caused by a deficiency (absolute, T1DM, or relative, T2DM) of insulin. Deficiency of insulin leads to inhibition of normal body functions, improper cellular metabolism, and tissue degeneration leading to a ketoacidotic state. Fluid, electrolyte, and keto acid balances are critical to blocking serious metabolic derangements affecting almost every body organ and its constituent functioning (Kee, Paulanka, & Purnell, 2004 [a programmed instruction manual]; Lee, Barrett, & Ignatavius, 1996; Reusens, Host, & Remacheo, 2001). The metabolic processes, including the altered states of starvation, stress, and injury, have been described. Administration of proper care to prevent further deterioration is paramount to management of the person with diabetes (see the American Association of Diabetes Educators' chapter on pathophysiology [Bardsley & Ratner, 2006] in *The Art and Science of Diabetes Self-Management Education* and American Diabetes Association's [Hirsch, 2005] *Complete Nurse's Guide to Diabetes Care*).

Giugliano, Ceriello, and Esposito (2008) note that not one, but all three measures of glycemic control (HbA1c, fasting glucose levels, and postmeal glucose peak), must be taken into account to achieve normal blood sugars the majority of the time and as safely as possible. If an imbalance occurs in the body, there are likely to be complications associated with that imbalance. The sooner this "rebalancing" is achieved, the sooner homeostasis delays or prevents complications.

References

American Association of Diabetes Educators. (2001). Diabetes and complications. In M. Franz (Ed.), *A core curriculum for diabetes educators* (4th ed.). Chicago: American Association of Diabetes Educators.

Banting, F. (1925). *Diabetes and insulin.* Nobel lecture. September 15, Stockholm, Sweden.

Bardsley, J. K. & Ratner, R. E. (2006). Pathophysiology of the metabolic disorder. In C. Mensing (Ed.), *The art and science of diabetes self-management education* (pp. 143–161). Chicago: American Association of Diabetes Educators.

Cannon, W. B. (1953). *Bodily changes in pain, hunger, fear and rage* (2nd ed.). Boston: Bradford.

Fujioka, K. (2007, December). Pathophysiology of type 2 diabetes and the role of incretin hormones and beta-cell dysfunction. *Journal of the American Association of Physician Assistants,* (Suppl.), 3–8.

Giugliano, D., Ceriello, A., & Esposito, K. (2008). Glucose metabolism and hyperglycemia. *American Journal of Clinical Nutrition, 87*(1), 217S–222S.

Guthrie, R. A., & Guthrie, D. W. (2004). The pathophysiology of diabetes mellitus. *Critical Care Nursing Quarterly, 27*(2), 113–125.

Hirsch, I. B. (2005). Acute complications of diabetes. In B. P. Childs (Ed.), *Complete nurse's guide to diabetes care* (pp. 76–91). Alexandria, VA: American Diabetes Association.

Kee, J. L., Paulanka, B. J., & Purnell, L. D. (2004). *Fluids and electrolytes with clinical applications: A programmed approach.* New York: Thompson Publisher.

Lee, C. A., Barrett, C. A., & Ignatavius, D. (1996). *Fluids and electrolytes: A practical approach* (4th ed.). Philadelphia: F. A. Davis.

McCance, K. L., & Huether, S. E. (1998). *Pathophysiology: The biologic basis of disease in adults and children* (3rd ed., pp. 686–687). St. Louis: Mosby.

Nathan, B. M., & Moran, A. (2008). Metabolic complications of obesity in childhood and adolescence: More than just diabetes. *Current Opinions in Endocrinology, Diabetes and Obesity, 15*(1), 21–29.

Reusens, B., Host, J. J., & Remacheo, C. (2001). Anatomy, developmental biology and pathology of the pancreatic islets. In L. J. DeGroot & J. L. Jameson (Eds.), *Endocrinology* (4th ed., pp. 654–666). New York: W. B. Saunders Co.

Selye, H. (1976). *The stress of life* (Rev. ed.). New York: McGraw-Hill.

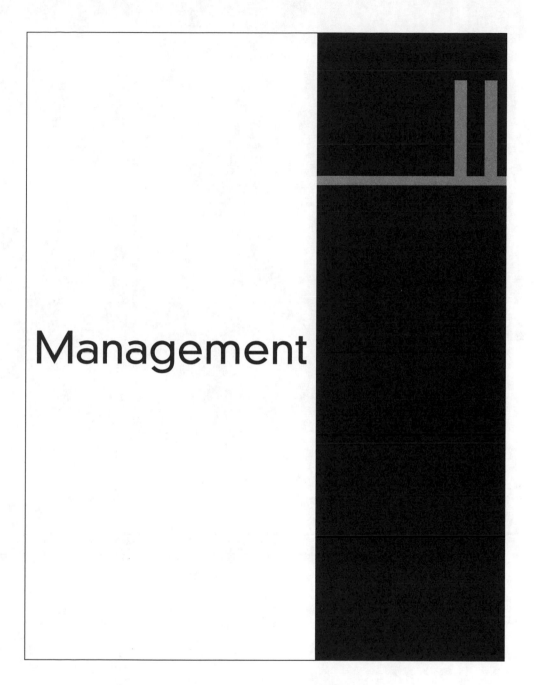

Management

6

In-Hospital Management of Diabetes Mellitus

Management of people with diabetes in the hospital is often difficult because of co-morbidities. Rarely are people with diabetes hospitalized just for their diabetes except for people with newly diagnosed Type 1 diabetes mellitus (T1DM) or diabetic ketoacidosis (DKA). Adults are usually hospitalized because of heart disease, surgery, pneumonia, chronic obstructive pulmonary disease (COPD), pregnancy, and so on, all of which will frequently complicate diabetes treatment. Patients with diabetes who have pneumonia or COPD treated with steroids will usually need to be changed from oral agents to insulin. Protocols should be established for hospital treatment, especially for IV insulin, transition to subcutaneous insulin, daily insulin management, and hypoglycemia. Examples of protocols are given in the appendices C, D, E, and F.

Although many people have advocated for better control of blood glucose levels in hospitals for many years, the statistics for diabetes care in hospitals have not been good. Krinsley (2003); Van den Berghe et al. (2001); Funary, Zerr, Grunkeineier, and Starr (1999); Pomposelli et al. (1998); and Zerr et al. (1997) all agree that glucose control lowers the risk of morbidity. Organizations such as the American Diabetes Association, the American Association of Clinical Endocrinologists, and many surgical societies have stressed the need for better hospital control of blood glucose. The concern of these societies led to a consensus conference in 2002 that produced a list of goals for improvement. A second conference was held in Washington, DC, in January 2006 to see why these goals had not been achieved and what could be done to accomplish them. Although much has been done to improve in-hospital diabetes control, much remains. This chapter includes discussion of acute care management, as in the care of patients with DKA, and the care of patients with more chronic conditions, who may be admitted because of diabetes, or of patients who may have diabetes but are admitted because of other comorbidities.

Recent studies have shown that diabetes constitutes 38% of all hospital admissions as a primary diagnosis or as comorbidity. When diabetes or hyperglycemia is listed as a problem in the hospital the mortality increases. Quite surprisingly, the mortality is higher for people admitted to the hospital who are found to have an elevated blood glucose level but without known diabetes, than for people with known diabetes (Umpierrez et al., 2002). The mortality rate in the hospital for patients without diabetes, or elevated blood glucose levels, is 1.7%. The mortality rate for people with known diabetes is 3%, and for people with elevated blood glucose levels, but who are not known to have diabetes, 16%. The higher mortality in patients without diabetes but with elevated blood glucose levels probably occurs because the elevated blood glucose levels are either not recognized and treated or are inadequately treated because primary attention is given to problems other than blood glucose. These findings suggest strongly that all patients entering the hospital should be screened for elevated blood glucose levels and diabetes and that blood glucose levels should be normalized as nearly as possible in all patients (Funary et al., 1999; Krinsley, 2003; Van den Berghe et al., 2001).

Hyperglycemia

Hyperglycemia results when there is too much glucose and not enough insulin present. The causes of hyperglycemia are numerous, but the major difficulty is a lack of available insulin either because of a lack of insulin-making capability or resistance to insulin use. The deficiency may be relative or absolute.

A lack of insulin may result when an insulin injection or the oral hypoglycemic (secretagogue) agent is forgotten or purposefully omitted. Hyperglycemia may also develop when the person with diabetes deviates from the diet by ingesting large quantities of carbohydrate (such as sweet desserts or starches, or increased calories over and above the meal plan or desired intake), especially when this extra intake is not compensated by exercise or medication. When an individual's occupation necessitates heavy labor and the laborer is off work and no longer doing heavy labor, increased blood glucose levels may be seen if food intake is not decreased. For example, if the laborer does heavy labor 5 days a week and then is off work for 2 days, his or her blood glucose levels will increase during the 2 days that he or she does not do heavy labor. Persons with diabetes should try to get the same amount of exercise daily or vary their food intake or insulin or oral agent on days of changed activity.

One of the primary causes of severe hyperglycemia is infection, which almost always causes an elevation in blood glucose levels. Infection and fever also increase blood glucose levels by activating the adrenal medulla and cortex, which produce epinephrine and cortisol, respectively. When a person with diabetes has an infection that elevates blood glucose levels, diabetes medications may need to be increased to control such exacerbations (Clement et al., 2004). Elevated blood glucose levels support the infectious process. The more normal the blood glucose levels, the less the diabetes state will influence the process of the disease, that is, the healing process will be slowed with higher blood glucose levels.

Stress (physical or psychological), treatment with certain drugs such as steroids, surgery, myocardial infarction (MI), and stroke (cerebrovascular accident, or CVA) may also result in a hyperglycemic state. Hyperglycemia resulting from emotional stress is often underestimated. The mechanism resulting in increased blood glucose levels during stress is hormonally related. When individuals with diabetes are upset, epinephrine from the adrenal medulla is released into the blood, increasing the rate of glycogenolysis and lipolysis, and hence the discharge of glucose and free fatty acids from the liver. Also, the adenocorticotropic hormone (ACTH) causes a release of glucocorticoids from the adrenal cortex, promoting gluconeogenesis. Emotional reactions appear to influence individuals with Type 2 diabetes (T2DM) as much as it does individuals with T1DM, but those with T1DM may have a blunted response because of a longer history of counterregulatory challenges.

Symptoms

Symptoms of hyperglycemia in the earlier stages include polyuria (frequent urination), polydipsia (frequent thirst, dry mouth), and polyphagia (increased appetite). Questioning an individual about the number of urinations during the night (nocturia) is often a method for gross screening for hyperglycemia. Remember that diabetic ketoacidosis can mimic the flu, stomach upset, appendicitis, and, less frequently, a heart attack.

When a person has insulin deficiency and glucose is unable to enter the cells, fat in the fat cells is broken down into fatty acids, the fatty acids travel to the liver to become ketone bodies (acetone, acetoacetic acid, and beta hydroxybutyric acid) and, as a result, ketones appear in the blood and urine. As the body becomes more hyperglycemic, ketones, sodium, and glucose are released into the urine. Carbonic acid is formed and released as its component parts in the lungs (into carbon dioxide and water) by Kussmaul's respiration. As the cycle continues, the physiology becomes more imbalanced until the intervention of fluids, insulin, and electrolytes occurs.

Laboratory Tests

As the situation deteriorates, the urine reveals positive glucose and ketone values. Blood tests at home or in the laboratory will reveal blood glucose levels at usually more than 250 mg/dl (14 mmol/L) and usually with positive serum ketone levels. A carbon dioxide content of less than 20 vol% is termed ketosis, and a carbon dioxide content of less than 15 vol% is termed acidosis. A person can be in diabetic ketosis, but not in diabetic ketoacidosis. Because leukocytosis is present in nearly all cases of diabetic ketoacidosis, physicians should not depend on white blood cell counts in distinguishing infection from other causes of diabetic ketoacidosis.

The differential diagnosis may involve ruling out DKA, diabetic ketosis (DK), hyperglycemic hyperosmolar nonketotic syndrome (HHNS), lactic acidosis (LA), alcoholic ketoacidosis, pregnancy-associated ketoacidosis, and some organic poisonings. Extremely elevated blood glucose levels without the presence of ketones or the presence of only trace or more amounts of ketones in the urine and blood, plus a presence of an elevated blood urea nitrogen (BUN) and creatinine, easily identifies HHNS (the anion gap is usually normal, i.e., the sodium and potassium are both elevated). Elevated lactic acid levels identified with the lack of glucose in the presence of elevated ketones in the urine assist in identifying lactic acidosis. The history or observation of alcoholic intake or of the intake of an abusive substance, or presence of pregnancy, leads to the diagnoses of other conditions.

Treatment

Treatment involves four major steps:

1. Restoration of normal carbohydrate, fat, and protein metabolism;
2. Restoration of fluid balance;
3. Prompt recognition and treatment of circulatory complications; and
4. A focus on an underlying cause, that is, infection.

As hyperglycemia progresses to ketonuria and ketoacidosis, there will be a feeling of tiredness, nausea, abdominal cramps, decreased appetite, and, in more advanced stages, Kussmaul's respiration (labored breathing). With the depression of the central nervous system, there is headache, drowsiness, stupor, and decreased muscle tone and reflexes. The breath will smell of overripe bananas (acetone breath).

Ideally, the person with diabetes should not progress beyond hyperglycemia with mild ketonuria. Instructed properly, the person with diabetes can recognize signs and symptoms of hyperglycemia, call the health professional, and receive treatment before the progression to diabetic ketoacidosis.

The members of the health care team should be careful to identify the underlying cause of the hyperglycemia. If the person does not get proper attention, it will become more difficult to control the blood glucose levels. In the acute state of diabetic ketoacidosis, fluids and insulin must be administered to restore the body's fluid balance and the normal metabolism of carbohydrate, fat, and protein. Regular insulin is the insulin of choice because, intravenously, it has an immediate action and a short duration. The IV profile of regular and the newer analog rapid-acting insulins is the same, but regular insulin is much less costly than the analogs.

Management of Diabetic Ketoacidosis

DKA is a common complication of T1DM and is occasionally seen in people with T2DM who have lost all or most of their insulin-secreting ability. This is most often seen in patients with newly diagnosed T2DM who have had unknown disease for a long period of time. In T1DM, DKA is common in patients with newly diagnosed diabetes, but it is not common when the diabetes is well controlled. It can occur with infection, steroid treatment, and other similar stresses, but recurrent DKA is most often the result of omitted insulin doses. Such patients should always be monitored for their ability to follow the treatment regimen or for their ability to obtain the insulin.

The classic symptoms are polyuria, polydipsia, and polyphagia with weight loss. The classic signs of DKA are Kussmaul's respiration and dehydration. A list of signs and symptoms of DKA compared with hypoglycemia can be found in Table 6.1. The diagnosis of diabetes and DKA are confirmed with an elevated blood glucose level. Initial lab screens should include electrolytes (BMP or CMP) and perhaps an arterial blood gas (ABG). The blood glucose level can vary from minimal elevation (>126 mg/dl or 7 mmol/L) to more than 3,000 mg/dl or more than 166 mmol/L. The actual blood glucose level (unless it is grossly elevated) is of less importance than the state of the acidosis and hydration. Therefore, the sodium and potassium levels and the pH, bicarbonate level and anion gap, and serum creatinine levels are of greatest significance. Arterial pH will be below 7.35 and may be as low as 6.8. Serum sodium levels are usually low but must be corrected for the osmolarity of the serum. Serum potassium levels may be normal or elevated or decreased. Total body potassium is always depleted and potassium must be added to the fluids as soon as renal function is established. The initial serum level, though, is a function of cellular breakdown with loss of potassium into the blood, the state of hydration, and the rate of clearance of potassium by the kidney.

Standing Orders for the Treatment of DKA

Refer to Appendix C for suggested standing orders for the treatment of diabetic ketoacidosis. Reviewing such a list can assist in the preparation for an emergency. Blanks are provided for individualized amounts related to patients' personal needs.

Starting IV Insulin

Many IV insulin therapy protocols are currently available from various institutions and on the Internet. One problem with most protocols is that the starting dose of IV insulin is based on the blood glucose level at initiation. The problem with basing the starting IV insulin dose on the blood glucose level is that people who are thin are insulin sensitive and may present with high blood glucose levels. A starting insulin dose based on these high blood glucose levels may be too high and could cause hypoglycemia. By contrast, people who are obese are insulin resistant, usually have T2DM, and present with only modestly elevated blood glucose levels. A low starting insulin dose based on a low blood glucose level in a person who is insulin resistant may be much too low and delay getting the blood glucose level to normal. A better way to start insulin is to base the starting insulin dose on body weight. IV insulin in DKA is usually started at 0.1 unit·kg^{-1}·hr^{-1}. Half that dose (0.05 unit·kg^{-1}·hr^{-1}) is a safe starting

6.1 Hyperglycemia Versus Hypoglycemia

Signs and Symptoms

Similar

Hyperglycemia	Hypoglycemia
Irritability	Irritability
Headache	Headache
Hunger	Hunger
Nausea	Nausea
Vomiting	Vomiting
Coma	Coma
Convulsion (blood sugar, >1,800 mg/dl)	Convulsion

Different

Polyuria	Nervous
Polydipsia	Trembly
Polyphagia	Change in personality
Double vision	Blurred vision
Dry skin	Cold, clammy sweat
Soft pupils	Dilated or constricted
Chest pain	pupils
Blood pressure down	Blood pressure up 30 min+
Autonomic	*Neuroglycopenic*
Anxious	Confusion
Strong pulse	Cognitive dysfunction
Tingling	Faintness
Trembling	Blurred vision
Hunger	Weakness
Sweating	Drowsiness
	Loss of consciousness

dose regardless of body weight and negates the problem of insulin resistance or sensitivity. Once the insulin is started, the IV insulin dose can be titrated by the blood glucose value measured hourly to maintain the blood glucose level wherever it is ordered. Van den Berghe et al. (2001) recommends maintaining the blood glucose level at below 110 mg/dl. Other levels are used in other institutions. I believe that maintaining a blood glucose level between 70 and 140 mg/dl (3.9–7.8 mmol/L) is safe and effective and relatively easy for the nurse to maintain. Continuous blood glucose monitoring for patients receiving IV insulin is being developed and will ease the workload of nurses in the future.

IV insulin therapy is usually carried out in intensive care units. Patients who are stable can be treated on hospital floors if the nurses are trained to handle IV insulin therapy and if the floor is equipped for cardiac monitoring.

Several good discussions and protocols are available for treatment of DKA in adults and in children. The Consensus Guidelines for Treatment of Diabetes in Children published by the International Society for Pediatric and Adolescent Diabetes (ISPAD) in 2008 is the best discussion of the treatment of DKA in children.

Dr. George Cahill of the Joslin Clinic once said, "There are two things to do in the management of DKA-HURRY UP AND WAIT." By this he meant that it was imperative to hurry up and start IV fluids and rehydrate the patient, but it was not critical to start the insulin. Often when physicians see an elevated blood glucose level, they are tempted to immediately give insulin, usually as an IV bolus. Treating with insulin is not urgent in these patients because IV fluids will often bring down the blood glucose level by several hundred milligrams per deciliter. The most important aspect of therapy is to start IV fluids and reestablish renal blood flow. The kidney is an amazing physician and will correct a lot of problems (and even mistakes), if it is in play. The level of dehydration should be established and maintenance and depletion amounts calculated. An initial bolus of 10–20 cc of normal saline per kg of body weight is usually given over the first hour, and then the flow rate calculated for the next 23 hours for maintenance and for correction of the calculated deficiency. An initial insulin bolus of 0.1 Unit/kg body weight can be given by IV push but is usually not needed. An IV insulin drip is established at a rate of 0.1 Unit of regular insulin per kilogram per hour as soon as the solution can be made by the pharmacy or when the patient reaches the intensive care unit. The initial fluid should be normal saline. Ringer's lactate is sometimes used, but the consensus today is that normal saline is the fluid of choice. Ringer's lactate contains lactate that can be detrimental if the patient has lactic acidosis, which is hard to differentiate from DKA or may be concurrent with it. Fluids are changed to D5 0.45 normal saline (NS) when the blood glucose level falls below 250 mg/dl (13.9 mmol/L). The addition of glucose to the fluids allows for an increase in the insulin flow rate with faster correction of the acidosis.

Insulin

There are many ways to give insulin. It can be given subcutaneously, intramuscularly, or intravenously. All of these work, but the current consensus is that the intravenous route is the easiest to control, the most efficient use of personnel time, and the safest with less danger of hypoglycemia. The IV insulin solution is best made by the pharmacy and is usually made as a solution of regular insulin and normal saline in a concentration of 1 unit of insulin to 1 cc of NS. The drip is started at a rate of 0.1 Unit of insulin per kilogram of body weight per hour. The drip rate is modified to obtain a reduction in blood glucose levels of 50–100 mg/hr (2.8–5.6 mmol/L). Too slow a correction leaves the patient in acidosis longer and may be detrimental to renal, hepatic, and cardiac function. Too rapid a drop in blood glucose levels may precipitate cerebral edema. A method of adjusting the insulin drip rate is found in the protocol in Appendix D. Appendix D may also be referred to for the non-DKA initiation of insulin.

Electrolytes

Sodium

Sodium replacement is usually not controversial. Maintenance sodium is calculated, and the deficit is calculated and added to correct the sodium level to 140 mEq/L. The most important aspect of sodium correction is determining the correct sodium level, and the laboratory value must be corrected for the blood glucose level. A very high blood glucose level will give a spuriously low serum sodium value. Correction should be based on the corrected value, not on the laboratory value. The formula for correction is as follows: add 1.6 mEq/L to the lab sodium value for every 100 mg/dl (5.56 mmol/L) the blood glucose is above 180 mg/dl (10 mmol/L), or in formula for correct Na = 1.6 × (glucose − 100)/100.

Potassium

As stated earlier, initial serum potassium measurements may not be of much value because they vary with the rate of cellular breakdown, renal excretion, and degree of dehydration. Of more importance is the rate of fall of the serum potassium. All patients with DKA have depletion of total body potassium and it must be replaced. I have been an expert witness in many legal cases of deaths from DKA, and 90% of the time the cause of death is either inappropriate IV fluids or hypokalemia. In most cases of hypokalemia, the problem has been insufficient monitoring. Potassium should be added to the IV fluids as soon as renal blood flow and urinary output have been established. Electrolytes should initially be monitored at least every 2 hr by laboratory value and the patient's electrocardiogram (ECG) should be continuously monitored for the effect of hyper- or hypokalemia on T waves. This means that most patients with DKA should be in an intensive care unit or on a floor with cardiac monitoring. Maintenance potassium is 1 mEq·kg^{-1}·day^{-1} and deficiencies should be calculated to correct the potassium level to 5 mEq/L. Traditionally, potassium is replaced as chloride. If this is done, a hyperchloremic alkalosis will usually occur by the end of treatment. This is not a serious problem unless the patient has renal disease because the kidney will sort out and correct the problem. I prefer, however, to correct the potassium with phosphate rather than chloride. This prevents the problem of hyperchloremia and replaces the phosphate, which is deficient in most patients. Giving half of the potassium as chloride and half as phosphate is also acceptable. Remember that potassium chloride is dispensed as milliequivalents and phosphate as millimoles. The two are not equivalent, but a concentration of 20/L of fluids of either will usually be safe, unless the fluid rate needs to be extremely high to correct dehydration.

Bicarbonate

The use of bicarbonate to correct acidosis is one of the most controversial issues in DKA therapy. The problem is this: If the pH is very low, there is poor function of many organs with continued tissue breakdown, tissue hypoxia, potassium loss, and continued ketone production. The temptation then is to give bicarbonate and correct the acidosis quickly. Bicarbonate and carbonic acid exist in a fixed ratio of 17–20 mmol of CO_2 to 1 mmol of carbonic acid (depending on temperature, P_{CO_2}, and other variables) in the blood according to the Henderson–Hesselbach equation. If the bicarbonate level is increased, the carbonic acid level is raised as well. In the blood, this is not a problem because the ratio favors bicarbonate and the carbonic acid is broken down to carbon dioxide and water, and the CO_2 is excreted by the lungs. The problem is in the brain. Carbonic acid passes the blood–brain barrier but bicarbonate does not. When bicarbonate is given, the serum pH rises but the central nervous system pH falls and the cerebral spinal fluid becomes more acid, which may precipitate increased coma and/or cerebral edema. Except in very severe acidosis (pH < 6.9) or in severe hyperkalemia (pH > 10), bicarbonate is not indicated in the treatment of DKA. With severe hyperkalemia or cardiac arrest, the bicarbonate may be given by bolus, but otherwise should be given as part of the IV fluids over 24–48 hr. There is no maintenance dose of bicarbonate, and correction doses should be given to correct to a bicarbonate level of 12 mEq/L of the bicarbonate space, which is about 60% of the total body weight. Example: weight 50 kg × 0.6 = 35 kg or liters, the bicarbonate space. The serum bicarbonate level is 2 mEq/L so 12 − 2 = 10 mEq × 35 kg = 350 mEq every 24 hr. The fluid flow rate can be calculated and the bicarbonate then calculated per liter of fluid.

Monitoring

As stated earlier, I have been involved as an expert witness in many malpractice cases involving deaths from DKA. In almost all instances, the cause of death could be traced to inadequate monitoring of the patient. In some cases, patients were treated on floors without cardiac monitoring and with inadequate laboratory monitoring. In other cases, there was inadequate laboratory monitoring even though the patient was in intensive care. A preprinted set of orders with the minimal laboratory monitoring will correct these problems. The patient should always have cardiac monitoring and nurses who are trained in reading the ECG tracings for T wave abnormalities. Minimal laboratory monitoring should include a basic metabolic profile containing sodium, potassium, and bicarbonate levels and a serum creatinine level to monitor the state of hydration. These levels should be checked at least every 2 hr two times, then every 4 hr four times, and then every 8 hr until values are in the normal range. There can *never* be too much monitoring. There is often too little. The first rule of DKA management is *hurry up and wait*. The second rule is *monitor, monitor, and monitor*.

Cerebral Edema

Cerebral edema is an uncommon complication of DKA, but when it occurs, it is a serious problem. Most cases of cerebral edema are fatal or leave the patient with significant brain damage. The cause of the brain swelling is unknown. Many theories have been proposed but none proven. Theories of causation include too rapid a fall in blood glucose levels, administration of the wrong IV fluids, the use of bicarbonate by IV push, and others. I have treated several thousand patients with DKA over 40 years, in all age groups, and have never managed a case of cerebral edema. I have seen several instances of cerebral edema in other physician's patients and have testified in several malpractice cases as an expert witness. Analysis of these cases has led to the conclusion that there is no single cause of this condition. The most common underlying cause has been administration of inappropriate IV fluids. The use of fluids without electrolyte (D5W) is rarely appropriate and is certainly not appropriate for children. Even children with hypernatremia should receive some sodium chloride in the IV fluids. Bolus bicarbonate has also been a common finding, although no real evidence exists that this causes the problem. The common denominator in all of the suggested causes of cerebral edema is the vulnerability of the child's brain subjected to rapid changes in fluid, glucose, or electrolyte levels. Although cerebral edema is primarily a problem in children, it can occur, though rarely, in adolescents and adults. Preprinted DKA orders should include an order for frequent monitoring of the neurologic status. If there is any hope of saving these patients or preventing brain damage, the problem must be detected early and treated vigorously. Treatment is with IV mannitol and monitoring of intracranial pressure.

Transition From IV to Subcutaneous Insulin

Transition from IV to subcutaneous insulin is relatively simple if certain principles are followed. It is important that basal insulin be given before the IV insulin is discontinued. The half-life of IV insulin is about 4 min, so the blood insulin level will be zero very quickly. Blood glucose levels will then rise very quickly and will require large correction doses of insulin. Long-acting basal insulin (Glargine or Detemir) should be given the night before the IV insulin is discontinued for optimal therapy. The basal 24-hr insulin will be in place when the IV insulin is stopped, which can occur at a meal time so that rapid-acting insulin can be given with the next meal. If the long-acting insulin is not given the night before IV insulin is stopped, then IV insulin should not be discontinued until the long-acting insulin takes effect, which is about 2 hr. If this is not done, there will be gaps in the insulin given at mealtime, because most rapid-acting insulins have an effective duration of action of only 3–4 hr. A transition protocol can be found in Appendix E.

Monitoring

During the process of giving insulin and replacing fluid, the patient must be carefully observed for circulatory complications. Hypotension, which is caused by contracted vascular volume from dehydration and decreased blood flow peripherally and to the kidneys, is often a problem. Particular attention should be given to the heart, lungs, and kidneys. Temperature, pulse rate, blood pressure, respirations, and urinary output, as well as the general level of consciousness, should be charted often. Increased temperature, which may indicate an infection, should be noted so that treatment can be started immediately.

The health professional has an important role in caring for the individual with diabetic ketoacidosis. An accurate flow sheet indicating the amount and time of insulin administration, electrolyte, and fluid therapy, temperature, respirations, pulse rate, level of consciousness, intake and output, urine glucose, urine ketone, and blood glucose should be kept. The success of treatment may very well depend on the ability to obtain and accurately record these items in the flow sheet. The patient with diabetes in a severe stage of diabetic ketoacidosis or coma should be in an intensive care unit and carefully monitored. Cardiac monitoring helps in adjusting potassium therapy, and blood glucose levels can be monitored at the bedside with the use of the blood glucose meter.

Other Types of Coma

A person with diabetes is subject to any type of coma that the general population is subject to, but two types of coma are seen most often in association with diabetes. These are hyperosmolar nonketotic syndrome and lactic acidosis.

Hyperglycemic Hyperosmolar Nonketotic Syndrome (HHNS)

Hyperglycemic hyperosmolar nonketotic syndrome (HHNS or HHNK) is most often seen in individuals with T2DM diabetes or in those people who have no previous diagnosis of diabetes. It is most commonly seen in people older than 60 years, but may also be found in children. The cause of this condition is a relative insulin deficiency sufficient to produce hyperglycemia but not sufficiently severe to allow ketonemia (Delaney, Zisman, & Kettyle, 2000). The person may have the classic signs of diabetes, that is, polyuria, polydipsia, and weight loss, but no or little ketonemia or ketonuria.

This syndrome has most often been identified as hyperglycemic hyperosmolar nonketotic coma. Because most of these individuals do not present in coma, the term syndrome has been suggested as the more appropriate diagnosis for this occurrence.

The distinguishing features of this condition are:

a. Marked serum hyperosmolarity,
b. Very high blood glucose levels (900–3,000 mg/dl [50–166.6 mmol/L]),
c. Frequent hypernatremia,
d. Severe dehydration and hypokalemia, and
e. Coma not associated with ketosis or acidosis.

Treatment consists of replacement of fluids and electrolytes, especially potassium, and administration of insulin. Less insulin is required with HHNS than with diabetic ketoacidosis because the patient is not ketotic, but fluid requirements are higher because of the extreme hyperosmolality. Many of these people are very dry and require massive amounts of fluid. They usually are older, though, and may have renal insufficiency and/or congestive heart failure. Fluid administration must be done carefully to prevent fluid overload. The help of the nephrology service or the cardiology service may be needed.

Lactic Acidosis

Lactic acidosis—a condition of increased levels of lactic acid in the blood—carries with it a high incidence of death. It occurs in individuals without diabetes as well as those with diabetes. The major concern is not the increased lactic acid but the grave underlying problems producing the abnormality. Lactic acidosis occurs in advanced stages of diabetes—especially in individuals who have uremia, arteriosclerotic heart disease, pneumonia, acute pancreatitis, chronic alcoholism, and bacterial infection. Treatment of the individual with lactic acidosis consists of applying the principles described previously for the treatment of diabetic ketoacidosis, namely, the administration of insulin, fluids, and electrolyte replacement as needed. Intravenous administration of solutions containing lactate must be avoided.

Hypoglycemia

Hypoglycemia is considered an acute complication that occurs when the opposite imbalance to hyperglycemia is present (too much insulin in relation to blood glucose levels). Besides leading to cognitive dysfunction, it can lead to fear or embarrassment (some of the actions of persons with hypoglycemia can be weird—eating a bar of butter, appearing naked in public, having seizures and/or coma) and thereby can become an obstacle to intensive insulin therapy. In all cases, it must be respected, and is to be avoided whenever possible. In the hospital, hypoglycemia is usually due to physician or staff error. The physician may order the wrong insulin or the nurse may give the wrong dose. A common cause of hypoglycemia in the hospital is poor coordination of nursing (insulin administration) and food service (service time for the meal). All such errors are avoidable with proper planning and supervision.

In-Hospital Management of Diabetes Other Than DKA

Outcomes data from various studies (Umpierrez et al., 2002) have led to recommendations that all patients admitted to hospitals be screened for diabetes and those with diabetes or elevated blood glucose levels have blood glucose levels kept as near to normal as possible throughout the hospitalization. For people with known diabetes this may mean an increase in insulin requirements, conversion from older diabetes regimens to IV or basal-bolus therapy, or conversion from oral antidiabetic agents to insulin. For those who were not known to have diabetes, inauguration of therapy with insulin is superior to oral hypoglycemic agents in the hospital. For patients with or without known diabetes, who on admission have significant comorbidities such as an MI, CVA, serious surgery, steroid therapy, serious infection, and so on, IV insulin therapy may be appropriate.

Maintenance of Glucose Control in the Hospitalized Patient

Oral antidiabetic agents are of little use in the hospital because of the comorbidities of most hospitalized patients. Patients who were on insulin prior to hospitalization, especially when on basal-bolus therapy, can be started on their old insulin dose and regulated as needed. If patients are using insulin but not basal-bolus, they should be changed to basal-bolus insulin. If they are not receiving insulin prior to hospitalization, basal-bolus insulin can be started at a dose of 0.5 unit per kg body weight per day, divided up as 20% of the total insulin as rapid-acting insulin (Lispro, Asparte, or Glulisine) for breakfast, 13% of total daily insulin as rapid-acting insulin for lunch, 17% of total daily insulin as rapid-acting insulin for the evening meal, and 50% of the total daily insulin as long-acting insulin (Glargine or Detemir) at bedtime.

Blood glucose is monitored by bedside monitoring and the insulin adjusted by patterns as explained in detail in Chapter 15 on pattern control. The goal in hospitalized patients should be to keep fasting blood sugar (FBS) at 70–120 mg/dl (3.89–6.67 mmol/L) and the postprandial blood glucose level at less than 140 mg/dl (7.78 mmol/L).

Enteral or Parenteral (TPN) Feedings

Special consideration must be given for patients receiving enteral or parenteral feedings. Enteral feedings must be handled differently depending on whether the feeding is continuous or by bolus. Continuous enteral feeding can often be handled by adequate administering doses of basal long-acting insulin or basal insulin and every 6 hrs regular insulin. When enteral feeding is by bolus then basal insulin once or twice daily plus rapid-acting insulin with each bolus works well.

Parenteral feeding (TPN) is best handled by IV insulin but can be handled by basal insulin once daily and regular insulin every 6 hr. Insulin in the TPN bag is not recommended because insulin sticks to the bag and the dose reaching the patient cannot be calculated and will vary from day to day. The rate of flow of the insulin is determined by the rate of flow of the TPN fluid and thus is not determined by the patient's need. Control will be variable with insulin in the TPN bag. Blood glucose is better controlled by the physician directly rather than by indirectly by the IV fluid flow. A protocol for insulin therapy in enteral and parenteral therapy may be found in Appendix F.

Summary

The diagnoses just described are emergencies, and each should be treated promptly (American Diabetes Association [ADA], 2004a; Kitabchi & Nyenwe, 2006), especially in children (Wolfsdorf, Glaser, & Sperling, 2006). Diabetes emergencies should be closely monitored (ADA, 2004b), and guidelines for admission are needed for each hospital (ADA, 2004c).

Encouraging people with diabetes to wear proper identification aids in giving assistance more quickly, especially if a person is found in a hotel room, in an accident, or at other times when unaccompanied by a knowledgeable person.

Because the most common causes of hyper- or hypoglycemia in hospitals, in general, were found to be related to inadequate prescribing (with use of sliding scales), decreased nutrition without the counterbalance of decreased insulin infusion or injection, lack of appropriate monitoring, and poor communication practices (Smith, Winterstein, Johns, Rosenberg, & Sauer, 2005; Vriesendorp et al., 2006), there is a problem. Recognizing that diabetes is a very logical disease (in most instances), that the blood glucose reading is a reflection of what has previously been done (food, medication, and procedures), and that people heal faster when blood glucose levels are kept in the normal range as much as possible—more logical decisions could be made with the potential for more favorable outcomes.

References

American Diabetes Association. (2004a). Hyperglycemic crisis in diabetes (position statement). *Diabetes Care, 27*(Suppl. 1), S94–S102.

American Diabetes Association. (2004b). Bedside blood glucose monitoring in hospitals. *Diabetes Care, 27*(Suppl.1), S104.

American Diabetes Association. (2004c). Hospital admission guidelines for diabetes. *Diabetes Care, 27*(Suppl. 1), S103.

Clement, S., Braithwaite, S. S., Magee, M. F., Ahmann, A., Smith, E. P., Schafer, R.G., et al. (2004). Management of diabetes and hyperglycemia in hospitals (technical review). *Diabetes Care, 27,* 553–591.

Delaney, M. F., Zisman, A., & Kettyle, W. M. (2000). Diabetic ketoacidosis and hyperglycemic hyperosmolar nonketotic syndrome. *Endocrinology and Metabolism Clinics of North America, 29*(4), 683–705.

Funary, A. P., Zerr, K. J., Grunkeineier, G. L., & Starr, A. (1999). Continuous intravenous insulin infusion reduces the incidence of deep sternal wound infection in diabetic patients after cardiac surgery procedure. *Annals of Thoracic Surgery, 67*(2), 352–362.

International Society of Pediatric and Adolescent Diabetes. (2008). *Guidelines for the treatment of children with diabetes.* Retrieved March 31, 2008, from www.ISPAD.org

Kitabchi, A. E., & Nyenwe, E. A. (2006). Hyperglycemic crises in diabetes mellitus: Diabetic ketoacidosis and hyperglycemic hyperosmolar state. *Endocrinology and Metabolism Clinics of North America, 35*(4), 725–751.

Krinsley, J. S. (2003). Association between hyperglycemia and increased hospital mortality in a heterogeneous population of critically ill patients. *Mayo Clinic Proceedings, 78*(12), 1471–1478.

Pomposelli, J. J., Baxter, J. K., III, Babineau, L., Pomfret, E. A., Driscoll, D. F., Forse, R. A., et al. (1998). Early post operative glucose control predicts nosocomial infection rate in diabetic patients. *Journal of Parenteral and Enteral Nutrition, 22*(2), 77–81.

Smith, W. M., Winterstein, A. G., Johns, T., Rosenberg, E., & Sauer, B. C. (2005). Causes of hyperglycemia and hypoglycemia in adult inpatients. *American Journal of Health-System Pharmacy, 62*(7), 714–719.

Umpierrez, G. E., Isaacs, S. D., Bazargan, N., You, X., Thaler, L. M., & Kitabchi, A. E. (2002). Hyperglycemia: An independent marker of in-hospital mortality in patients with undiagnosed diabetes. *Journal of Clinical Endocrinology and Metabolism, 87*(3), 978–982.

Van den Berghe, G., Wouters, P., Weekers, F., Verwaest, C., Bruyninckx, F., Schetz, M., et al. (2001). Intensive insulin therapy in the critically ill patient. *New England Journal of Medicine, 345*(19), 1359–1367.

Vriesendorp, T. M., Van Santen, S., DeVries, J. H., de Jonge, E., Rosendaal, F. R., Schultz, M. J., et al. (2006). Predisposing factors for hypoglycemia in the intensive care unit. *Critical Care Medicine, 34*(1), 96–101.

Wolfsdorf, J., Glaser, N., & Sperling, M. A. (2006). Diabetic ketoacidosis in infants, children, and adolescents: A consensus statement from the American Diabetes Association. *Diabetes Care, 29*(5), 1150–1159.

Zerr, K. J., Funary, A. P., Grunkemeier, G. L., Bookin, S., Kanhere, V., & Starr, A. (1997). Glucose control lowers the risk of wound infection in diabetics after open heart operations. *Annals of Thoracic Surgery, 63*(2), 356–361.

7

Management in the Clinic

The clinic or physician's office is the crossroads of care of anyone having diabetes mellitus. The clinic or office should be considered the medical home for the care of diabetes and should be delivered by a knowledgeable and caring team. People can be cared for or diagnosed in the clinic or office. Both team and group therapy can be carried out in an office setting. Cost for patient care was appreciably lowered by successfully using "group visits" (Clancy, Dismuke, Magruder, Simpson, & Bradford, 2008). Yearly physical and laboratory screens, as recommended in the American Diabetes Association (ADA) (2008) standards of care, aid in the diagnosis, early intervention, and treatment of diabetes as well as other disorders, especially of other autoimmune and lipid disorders. This information also leads to the prediction of cardiovascular risk as reported by Colhoun (2007), and office-based screening of the feet is a facet of clinic care that decreases the possibility of a future amputation (Farber & Farber, 2007).

These are just a few aspects of clinic care that are evidence-based with the outcome of enhancing the life span and the quality of life for the person with diabetes. The key goal is the normalization of all biochemical parameters in a safe and efficacious manner. The ADA (2008) recommends that the level of hemoglobin A1c should be 7% or less and, in some individuals, 6% or less.

American Association of Clinical Endocrinologists (AACE) (2007) guidelines recommend that the goal be 6.5% or less. Both the ADA and AACE note that the goals should be individualized depending on personal situations and age. The best recommendation as a goal for the control of diabetes is "work to achieve the best A1c and blood glucose levels that can be achieved without significant hypoglycemia in each individual" (Cefalu, 2004).

If more hypoglycemia occurs than can be handled by management practices or by referral to a specialist, then less stringent criteria must be set. If preprandial goals cannot be met, then there must be a focus on postprandial goals. In our practice, postprandial goals will, the majority of the time, meet the target set for preprandial goals.

Weight loss or weight maintenance, plus adequate attention to calorie and nutritional needs, should be the goal for each patient. Insulin's major purpose is to act as a storage hormone. Too much food in the face of internal or external available insulin leads to weight gain. Intensified blood glucose control should not be traded for weight gain due to the management of medication alone. Weight control is about portion control and the composition of food intake. High-fat meal plans with the same total calories as a low-fat meal plan may also lead to weight gain despite portion size (this has been documented only in animal studies—Surwit et al., 1995).

Adolescents need a transition of care, especially if their diabetes is not monitored in a diabetes center. Lane et al. (2007) found that a diabetes clinic for young adults that focuses on the specific needs of older adolescents promotes better diabetes control than the general endocrine clinic does. They concluded that a specialized clinic and the earlier introduction of pump therapy results in the best outcome.

The Clinic Visit

There are a variety of aspects of care that must be assessed at each clinic visit. Not only must blood glucose control, food intake (amounts, kinds, and patterns of eating), and exercise or activity level be assessed, but also the quality of sleep, the levels of stressors (at home and/or at work or school), and the use of supplements and other aspects of alternative and complementary self-care (see Appendix G).

First and foremost, the patient must feel comfortable in stating particular needs. The usual 20-min visit with the health professional cannot achieve what is needed. For the routine visit: check vital signs including blood pressure, the parameters of height (every 3–4 months for children 18 years of age and under; once a year for 55 years of age and older), weight, laboratory tests (HbA1c every routine visit; thyroid-stimulating hormone [TSH] and/or lipid profile, if on medication, every 6 months; and once a year a complete metabolic profile with estimated GFR [Glomerular Filtration], a thorough foot exam, and off-loading blood glucose meters (if they have such a meter) or averaging blood glucose levels per time of day with the use of a handheld calculator (see Table 7.1 for blood glucose level averages compared with HbA1c).

Note: Glycated hemoglobin just indicates average blood glucose levels over a 2–3 month period of time. It does not tell where the problem might be

7.1	Comparison of HbA1c to Whole Blood and Plasma Mean Blood Glucose Levels[a]		
HbA1c	Whole Blood in mg/dl	Plasma in mg/dl	mmol
6.0%	115	135	7.5
6.5%	132	152.5	8.5
7.0%	150	170	9.5
7.5%	165	187.5	10.4
8.0%	183	205	11.5
8.5%	199	223.5	12.5
9.0%	217	240	13.5
9.5%	232	257.5	14.5
10.0%	253	275	15.5
11.0%	281	310	17.5
11.5%	298	327.5	18.5
12.0%	315	345	19.5
12.5%	330	362.5	20.0
13.0%	342	380	21.0
14.0%	369	405	22.5

[a]Adapted from ADA Standards of Medical Care in Diabetes, *Diabetes Care*, 2008, S18.

on a daily basis. Also, in interpreting this assay, results can be altered by the extrabiochemical stress responses in the body and the abnormal synthesis of hemoglobin (Roszyk, Faye, Sapin, Somda, & Tavern, 2007). For example, persons with iron deficiency anemia can have a falsely high reading or a falsely low reading (HbA1c) if they have a variety of other anemias, such as hemolytic anemia or sickle cell disease. This became very apparent to us when, during one clinic visit, a previously reliable person had an HbA1c of 11.4%. Her complete blood count revealed iron deficiency anemia. The second person had an HbA1c of 4.5% and his wife reported her annoyance when he chewed so much ice. He was found to have hemolytic anemia. The first patient had an HbA1c corresponding to his average blood glucose level once the anemia was corrected. In the second patient, glycated albumen (fructosamine) was used to measure overall control. This test is useful in all patients with hemoglobinopathies such as sickle cell disease, thalassemia, and others.

Asking what the person would like to achieve during the visit can often be an opening question. Be sure to include, before the end of the clinic visit, what the person states that is very important to him or to her or to the family as a whole. Intake history should then include the history of blood glucose averages; ketone testing, if needed; hypoglycemic episodes; medication changes; interval events, that is, surgery or illness, or hospitalization, and so on; examination of the feet (thoroughly once a year; every three months if feet are found to be insensate with the 5.07 [10 g] filament; and any time changes are noted); meter problems; nutrition concerns; injection site assessment; problem solving and discussion on lowering risks through a decrease or stopping in smoking, frequency of drinking, weight gain or loss; and total physical assessment.

In our clinic, our physical assessment sheet is filled out at the time of each visit and positive findings are discussed in depth. We do not complete a full physical because we wish patients to identify a family physician that co-ordinates their total care with a full history and physical at least once a year (see Appendix H). Once this information is gathered, appropriate education is given for specific needs or for a general review of a topic—now the patient is ready for the specialist. The specialist's task is to identify changes in manage-ment, reinforce key aspects of care, and identify further education needed by that individual and ensure that all the questions are answered. A special ad-dition to care is the sharing of new research findings related to diabetes. The pattern of return clinic visits is 2 weeks after hospitalization, then 1 month, to 2 months, and finally every 3 months if the patient is receiving insulin. If the indi-vidual is on diet alone and blood glucose levels are well controlled, it is possible that the person will be scheduled every 4 to 6 months (see Patient Recommen-dations [Take Home Sheet]—Appendix I). Note: all information in our clinic is now obtained and stored in a paperless form at the time of each visit.

Blood glucose measurements at home should be 4–6 times a day every day if the patient is on a pump; 4 times a day, fasting; and 2 hr after a meal and/or bedtime if the patient is on insulin, or for a specified period if a medication change has been made; 4 times (or equivalent) a day for 3 days a week if on oral agents; or 4 times (equivalent) a day, twice a week, if on diet alone. For patients who refuse to test several times a day the "equivalent" might be to obtain a fasting one day, 2 hr after breakfast another day; 2 hr after lunch the third day, and so on.

Postprandial Blood Glucose Level Testing

Postprandial blood glucose level testing is needed in the hospital—it is also needed for clinic visits, according to the Insulin Congress (Schaefer, 2007) and is recommended in the ADA Standards of Medical Care (2008). "Clinicians should consider incorporating agents that lower postprandial hyperglycemia in their treatment of patients with diabetes mellitus" (Perkins & Davis, 2007). Perkins and Davis sited five studies that associated postprandial hyperglycemia with cardiovascular disease and mortality from 1979 to 1996. The use of postprandial blood glucose testing should then come as no surprise. Even though it is sometimes more difficult to remember, it leads to an ability to make better recommendations, especially in using the pattern approach to therapy.

Preprandial Testing

Some blood sugar reports are better than none at all, however. If the person can't remember the 2 hr after meal blood sugars, we ask them to concentrate one day a week to obtain them—and at least do this the 3–5 days before the clinic visit. If this is still a problem, we will work with the premeal and bedtime blood sugars the best way we can.

Continuous Glucose Monitoring

For "real" problems and a look into the future, continuous glucose monitoring is best, especially if the machine can let the individual know if changes need to be made in the daily management in a timely manner. The readings on a 7-day monitor correlated significantly with hemoglobin A1c values and resulted in improved daily blood sugars with medical intervention (Garg & Jovanovic, 2006).

In General

Averaging these results to look for patterns, taking into account the ranges of blood glucose level readings, leads to the decision-making process in relation to any changes in the person's lifestyle (refer to Chapters 9 and 17 for more details).

Referrals to other specialists are made on the basis of laboratory findings and history—to the cardiovascular specialist; to the nephrologist; to the neurologist; once a year (or, as needed, sooner) to the ophthalmologist or retinologist; to the urologist; to the dermatologist; and, as needed, to the certified sex therapist, and so forth. We ask patients if they have seen their family physician, physician assistant, or nurse practitioner at least once during the year for a full history and physical examination.

Sleep Apnea and Depression

Within the past few years, it has become apparent in the diabetes field that quality of sleep and depression are associated with diabetes more than recognized earlier (Chaput, Depres, Bouchard, & Tremblay, 2007). Sleep apnea is discussed here. Depression will be handled in depth by referring to information found in Chapter 13 for those with Type 1 diabetes mellitus (T1DM) and Chapter 21 for those with Type 2 diabetes mellitus (T2DM).

Sleep Apnea Problems and Treatment

Quality of sleep can be assessed by asking if a person wakes up with a headache or wakes up during the night to go to the bathroom or to get a drink of water. The risk for sleep apnea is greater if persons are obese. Do they wake up with a dry mouth or they have problems with esophageal reflux? Do they feel rested after a night's sleep? Do they have a hard time staying awake during the daytime? Two major factors, the snoring and the report from another that he or she had stopped breathing for a short while, are indications of sleep apnea. A sleep center (go to www.sleepcenters.org for the nearest one) would record this breathing process with the use of electroencephalography, electrooculography, electrocardiography, chest impedance, airflow monitoring, carbon dioxide monitoring, pulse oximetry, sound sensors, and audio and video recordings.

If the person has demonstrated obstructive sleep apnea, then assessment is done to determine whether continuous positive airway pressure (CPAP) is in order.

Body positioning is the first resort, for example, the use of pillows to elevate the head and sleeping on the side. Sprays are the second resort. CPAP may be needed for moderate to severe apnea. Surgery is the last resort.

Individuals with T2DM appear to be more at risk (more likely than other patients) for sleep disorders. Sleep deprivation is a stressor to the body. The stress response increases cortisol levels that, in turn, indirectly raise blood glucose levels. The dryness, related to the snoring and/or open mouth, may trigger an inflammatory response. Repeated episodes during the night lead to oxygen deprivation which affects the person's immune response. Getting up at night to go to the bathroom and excessive need to drink water are certainly signs that a person needs to be screened for diabetes. Obesity is most often concurrent with the occurrence of sleep apnea. These individuals are not aware of the problem most of the time. They may assume that snoring is normal. Stressors at work may be blamed for the desire to sleep during the day and be responsible for not sleeping at night. A useful tool used to screen for diabetes is the Berlin Questionnaire, which is a 10-point sleep evaluation assessment that covers gender, age, weight, the frequency of breathing and snoring, tiredness, and high blood pressure. A copy may be obtained from the American College of Physicians.

Individuals may be educated to try having a routine before going to sleep and to not use any stimulants 2–3 hr before bedtime (e.g., caffeine, smoking, exercise, hot shower, spicy foods). They should also be told that they would sleep better in a cool room; not to sleep during the daytime; and go to sleep and get up at the same time each day whenever possible. The outcomes of interventions to control weight, body positioning, and, if needed, CPAP, are improved blood glucose levels, improved blood pressure, and a reduction in the inflammatory response, thereby reducing the risk of cardiovascular events.

Summary

The team approach to patient management and education is the best method of diabetes care. Abrahamson and Aronson, American College of Physicians (2007), have developed a CME/CEU programmed manual to assist in improving and updating knowledge in the diabetes field. It includes screening and prevention, controlling blood glucose, and comorbidities and complications. Guidance for emergencies in diabetes care of the hospitalized patient and for special populations is included.

Full screens are ordered once a year, every six months if the person is receiving a lipid and/or thyroid medication. Hemoglobin A1c levels are tested every 3–4 months. Glucose levels are averaged at the time of each visit, and patients are taught to review their own records once a week and make changes as necessary.

On our team, we have an endocrinologist, pediatrician, nurses, dietitian, and two marriage and family therapists. Health professionals who are certified diabetes educators and/or board certified in advanced diabetes management are invaluable in our office for taking patient calls and managing diabetes care by phone, after office hours and on weekends. Physician specialists take hospital calls unless routine surgical and obstetrical orders are faxed to the individual's hospital. Referrals are made as needed by any practitioner on the team.

Unless the person with diabetes is a member of the American Diabetes Association and attends support group sessions or available workshops, two years is the recommended reeducation time. Education for patients is just as simple as the Conversation Maps on diabetes management available through Healthy Interactions, Inc. Special topics encourage questions to be answered or the discussion to follow is led by a health professional. Learning in this way may be informative and also fun. So much is going on in this field and changes are happening so quickly that updated information is needed. Clinic or office visits are also useful for involving other family members and for renewing general information related both to self-care and to self-management.

There is a saying that it takes a village to raise a child. In the diabetes field, it takes a team to make a difference. The "coordinator" of the team is the patient. The focus is his or her present and future needs.

References

Abrahamson, M. J., & Aronson, M. (Eds.) (2007). *ACP diabetes care guide: A team-based practice manual and self-assessment program.* Philadelphia, PA: American College of Physicians.

American Association of Clinical Endocrinologists. (2007). Medical guidelines for clinical practice for the management of diabetes mellitus. *Endocrine Practice, 13*(Suppl.1), S3–S68.

American Diabetes Association. (2008). Standards of medical care in diabetes. *Diabetes Care, 31*(Suppl.1), S12–S55.

Cefalu, W. T. (Ed.) (2004). *The CADRE handbook of diabetes management* (pp. 145–168). New York: Medical Information Press.

Chaput, J. P., Despres, J. P., Bouchard, C., & Tremblay, A. (2007). Association of sleep duration with type 2 diabetes and impaired glucose tolerance. *Diabetologia, 50*(11), 2298–2304.

Clancy, D. E., Dismuke, C. E., Magruder, K. M., Simpson, K. N., & Bradford, D. (2008). Do diabetes group visits lead to lower medical care charges? *American Journal of Managed Care, 14*(1), 39–44.

Colhoun, H. M. (2007). Lipid goals in metabolic syndrome and diabetes. *Current Atherosclerosis Report, 9*(4), 286–295.

Farber, D. C., & Farber, J. S. (2007). Office-based screening, prevention, and management of diabetic foot disorders. *Primary Care, 34*(4), 873–885.

Garg, S., & Jovanovic, L. (2006). Relationship of fasting and hourly blood glucose levels to HbA1c values. *Diabetes Care, 29*(12), 2644–2649.

Lane, J. T., Ferguson, A., Hall, J., McElligott, M., Miller, M., Lane, P. H., et al. (2007). Glycemic control over 3 years in a young adult clinic for patients with type 1 diabetes. *Diabetes Research and Clinical Practice, 78*(3), 385–391.

Perkins, J. M., & Davis, S. N. (2007). The rationale for prandial glycemic control in diabetes mellitus. *Insulin, 2*(2), 52–60.

Roszyk, L., Faye, B., Sapin, V., Somda, F., & Tauveron, I. (2007). Glycated haemoglobin (HbA1c): Today and tomorrow. *Annals of Endocrinology, 68*(5), 357–365.

Schaefer, C. F., Jr. (Ed.) (2007). Proceedings of the Insulin Congress: The evolving science and practice of insulin therapy. *Insulin, 2*(Suppl. A), S1–A28.

Surwit, R. S., Feinglos, M. N., Rodin, J., Sutherland, A., Petro, A. E., Opara, E. C., et al. (1995). Differential effects of fat and sucrose on the development of obesity and diabetes in C57BL/GJ and A/S mice. *Metabolism, 44*(5), 645–651.

Yaggi, H. K., Araujo, A. B., & McKinley, J. B. (2006). Sleep duration as a risk factor for the development of type 2 diabetes. *Diabetes Care, 29*(3), 657–661.

In-Home Management

8

Diabetes mellitus is the only disease in which an individual or other family member is taught how to regulate a medication, sometimes on a dose-to-dose basis. Education and supportive guidance is necessary, and recognition of a person's capability to do this is an important consideration. Reinforcement of skills, knowledge, and accuracy are all a part of the safety needed for the administration of potentially dangerous medications, especially insulin (Bodenheimer, Lorig, Holman, & Grumbach, 2002).

The care of even one person who has diabetes in the family involves all members of the family in one way or another. Whether other members of the family might be the cook, the "bottle washer," or the emotional supporter, they are involved and, therefore, must have the education to become involved in the best ways possible. Besides the ways in which to support the person in the most effective way, whether an individual with diabetes or other family member, a number of things must be considered and, in some way, assessed at the time of each clinic visit.

Education is most important to learn self-management practices, to carry them out, and to report those aspects of self-care (i.e., blood glucose monitoring), that can aid the diabetes specialist and other health professionals to best meet the needs of that person. Problems were prevented or ameliorated by such interventions along with telephone- and cell-phone–based self-management support (Sakar et al., 2008).

Supplies on Hand

Glucagon When on Insulin and/or Hypoglycemic Treatment

The treatment of hypoglycemia is an emergency. If the person is taking insulin, glucagon kits are a must. A glucagon kit should be available in the home, in the school (as this applies), and/or in the work setting—and another person, other than the one who has diabetes, should be trained in its use. The kit supplies it all—the diluent is in the syringe and the vial of the lyophilized glucagon tablet. There is even a reminder on how to use the contents of the syringe once the diluent has been placed into the vial.

Other treatments for low blood sugars must also be on hand. Whether in a tablet or gel form, a juice form, or another form of easily digestible carbohydrate food, these treatments must be available 24 hr, 7 days a week. At one time, a friend said, on the phone, "There is no orange juice available." It may seem trite, but educating a person that any juice will do or even some table sugar in a small amount of water. These are simple things, but at the time of need, very important.

Medication(s): Delivery and Monitoring

Obviously, the medication to be administered and, in the case of insulin, supplies for administration will be needed. Insulin administration may include a choice of pen devices with various length needles, various size syringes, or supplies used in the attachment and delivery of insulin by a pump. Continuous glucose monitoring machines will more frequently be found in the list of supplies to have in the home. Alcohol wipes are handy, but any cleaning agent or just clean skin is considered appropriate at the time of injection.

Oral agents are not frequently changed by the person involved, but it is possible that they might be. The individual might be instructed to decrease a previous dose of one or more oral agents if the after-meal or pre-meal blood glucose levels get to a certain point (this is the same for insulin—if blood glucose levels are less than 70 mg/dl [3.8 mmol/L] then a change needs to be made in the dosage administered prior to the time of that finding, unless the person can explain it away by less food or greater activity).

A glucose monitor and appropriate strips must be available, and the patient taught to use the equipment. The strips must be kept fresh and dry and the date and time set properly on the meter. Schoolchildren should also have a meter at school and someone there trained to use it if the child cannot.

For patients with needle phobias, or even for those that wish such a convenience, injection ports might be useful adjuncts to aid in the frequency of actual injections. These in-site devices allow for multiple injections through a diaphragm or preset device resulting in the less invasive multiple-site injection areas.

These in-site placements are changed every 72 hr (or less) and are restricted to a 28 gauge ⁵⁄₁₆ in. (8 mm) needle.

During times of crises in the family or illness, larger doses of medication (or added medication, in the case of the person on oral medications) may be needed. Supplemental doses of insulin may be given hourly, intramuscularly (when using short-acting insulin) or subcutaneously (when using rapid-acting insulin). Other supplements over and above the usual dosage amounts might be needed at the usual time of administration during severe infections or emotional crises. Children and some adults will become hyperglycemic more rapidly than others, but they are also more sensitive to insulin treatment (White, 2000) so great care must be taken to not give too much insulin (refer to Chapters 9 and 17 for further guidance).

Some medications needed for the treatment of the emotional crises or infection may raise blood glucose levels. The use of prednisone or other adrenocorticosteroids are frequently prescribed drugs used at home and will raise blood glucose levels. When medications that raise blood glucose levels are given, concomitant increases in insulin (or oral agents) are expected. It is possible that someone taking steroids will need 2–3 times the total insulin dose or that someone on oral agents will need to go on insulin. The administration of greater amounts of insulin will prevent serious hyperglycemia from occurring. The ability to make contact by phone 24 hours a day is necessary under these circumstances.

Monitoring Blood and Urine

For monitoring, the variety of available meters is expanding. Tunis and Minshall (2008) demonstrated that monitoring blood glucose levels at home was found to be cost effective. When testing 3 times per day, the savings is $518 per quality-adjusted life-years over a 10-year period. If testing 4 times per day, the savings would be less, but still a savings.

A meter may be purchased, sent home from the hospital, or given out in the clinic or education program along with a prescription for strips and lancets. If that particular meter does not meet with the person's satisfaction, there are many other meters to try (see Chapters 12 and 20 for further information). The strips and lancets might be obtained through a local store or through a mail order service. A clean hand, clean arm, or clean ear lobe is then all that is needed. Alcohol wipes are, again, not needed when the part of the body to be lanced is clean.

Ketone test strips for testing urine are available in a bottle or in individually foil-wrapped units. These are needed for ketosis-prone individuals, but usually not for those with T2DM unless the person has been ill or highly stressed for a period of time. Decompensation can occur from an insulin-requiring state to an insulin-dependent state.

Careful monitoring of urine ketone and blood glucose levels during an infection or prolonged emotional stress aids in directing the amount of supplemental insulin to be given or oral agent. It also guides the person or professional as to when such supplements may be discontinued or altered in the amount of the dosage to be administered.

Food and Hygiene

Nutritious food and products for good hygiene practice should already be available, but for some families this might mean a change in lifestyle—and quite difficult for them to have or to do. In these cases, increased support and guidance are needed by the health professionals and others in the community until new habits are formed and feelings of self-efficacy are achieved.

Dawn Phenomenon

Hyperglycemia may result from improper insulin administration or it might be due to the *therapeutic* or *pharmacodynamic* duration of action of the medication, which is usually less than the *pharmacokinetic* action. More medication, such as sulfonylureas or insulin, may result in hypoglycemia or possibly hypoglycemic-hyperglycemia (rebound). Another such hyperglycemic excursion type is called the dawn phenomenon.

In an early paper, Milligan and Torrance (1986) noted that the *dawn phenomenon* is revealed by blood glucose monitoring. With this problem, the fasting blood glucose level is persistently elevated even on adequate doses of presupper or bedtime insulin or oral agents. Theory suggests that such a response from 4–7 a.m. is a delayed, physiologic reaction to the nighttime secretion of growth hormone and/or corticosteroids. An attempt to increase the evening or bedtime diabetes medication can lead to nocturnal hypoglycemia, and yet the increased fasting blood sugar persists. The use of metformin at bedtime in individuals with T2DM or bedtime long-acting basal insulin will usually solve this problem. Pump use (or administration of the awkward 3–4 a.m. dose of insulin) with an alternate basal insulin setting from 3 or 4 a.m. until 7 or 8 a.m. can cover this normal phenomenon.

Somogyi or Rebound Effect

Another problem is the rebound phenomenon, referred to as the *Somogyi phenomenon* (Bolli, Perriello, Fanelli, & DeFeo, 1993). The term *rebound* derives from the belief that hypoglycemia begets hyperglycemia. Some have questioned whether this really does occur (Raskin, 1984). The Somogyi phenomenon usually occurs when the action of the insulin causes the blood glucose levels to dip below normal or to drop rapidly, releasing a counterregulatory response. If this happens during the night, it results in elevated blood glucose levels in the morning or during the day. This phenomenon may easily be ruled out by increasing the previous snack or meal or decreasing the previous insulin or oral agent. The individual or family may observe a lowering of the blood glucose levels with the lowering of food intake, the increase of medication, or the increase in activity. If the opposite occurs, then suspect a rebound.

Hypoglycemia Occurring in the Home

Newer medications, especially insulins, have been made available so that there are fewer occurrences of hypoglycemia than in the past. Ratner et al. (2000) documented less peaking of long-acting insulin and, therefore, fewer problems with hypoglycemia (especially at night) than when using intermediate-acting insulin.

Patients and family members are taught that there are some similarities and some differences in symptoms and signs when hyper- or hypoglycemia occurs (see Table 8.1). For a mild hypoglycemia (40–60 mg/dl or 2.2–3.3 mmol), ½ to 1 calorie point (37–75 calories), such as a half glass of any juice, is recommended. If a moderate hypoglycemic reaction occurs (20–40 mg/dl or 1–2 mmol/L), simple sugar such as honey (1–2 tsp) or glucose tablets (1–3 depending on the child's size) or 1–2 tsp of glucose gel is used. Once the blood glucose levels exceed 60 mg/dl (3.3 mmol/L), a small snack is given or the meal is eaten with the insulin given after the meal.

If the person is unconscious or unable in any way to swallow efficiently (blood glucose levels may be 20 mg/dl or below [1 mmol]), glucagon is given with a one-quarter dose for a child younger than 3; a half dose for the child from 3–5 years of age; and the full dose (1 mg) if the child is 6 or older

8.1 Hyperglycemia Versus Hypoglycemia

Signs and Symptoms	
Similar	
Hyperglycemia	*Hypoglycemia*
Irritability	Irritability
Headache	Headache
Hunger (polyphagia)	Hunger
Nausea	Nausea
Vomiting	Vomiting
Coma	Coma
Convulsion (blood sugar >1,800 mg/dl)	Convulsion
Different	
Polyuria	Nervous
Polydipsia	Trembly
Double vision	Blurred vision
Abdominal pain	Sweaty
Soft pupils	Dilated or constricted pupils
Chest pain	Change in personality
Blood pressure down	Blood pressure up[a]
Dry skin	Cold, clammy skin

[a]Blood pressure may initially elevate (adrenaline response) for up to approximately 30 minutes and then decrease.

(or to an adult). Once the glucagon is given and the caregivers still feel insecure in their judgment, the emergency service should be called. It will take 15–20 minutes after the glucagon is given for the blood glucose to rise to a safe level or for the individual to awaken. In every case, if a severe insulin reaction occurs, and once blood sugars are under control, they are to call the nurse-on-call to report the incident and to follow the guidance given.

Everyone taking insulin should have glucagon available. There should be a glucagon kit in the home and more than one person should be trained on when and how to use it. The main side effect is transient nausea in some people. Pearson (2008) found that glucagon was not used as much as it could be. The author pointed out that if people understood and used glucagon, if needed, it might be helpful in alleviating some fears about hypoglycemia and obviating expensive trips to the emergency room.

Other innovations, especially for those patients who have more difficulty in controlling their blood glucose levels, were the use of the Web (McMahon et al., 2005). Web programs allowed for more frequent contact with health professionals, both from the education and the management standpoint. In this randomized controlled study, not only were blood glucose levels lowered and more stable, but also blood pressure levels were lowered and more stable.

Many parents have a fear of hypoglycemia in their child. This fear is also present with insulin-dependent adolescents and adults. Continuous subcutaneous insulin infusion (CSII) has alleviated much of this fear for some, and the newer long-acting "peakless" insulins has for others. Patton, Dolan, Henry, and Powers (2007) found that this fear is still present for some parents. The presence of this fear in parents or in individuals who have Type 1 diabetes mellitus (T1DM) can be a barrier to maintaining the best glycemic control possible. Continuous glucose sensors that alarm when sensing too low or too high blood sugars, or within a period of time going in that direction, may finally solve this problem.

Blood glucose monitoring has made fear of hypoglycemia less of a problem than in times past, but if individuals are unaware that their blood glucose levels are too low, then another problem exists. Note the information presented in Chapter 13 on Blood Glucose Awareness Training (BGAT) (Cox et al., 2001). There is recognition that the body can adjust and feel better at higher blood glucose levels, not respond to blood glucose changes (or respond, and the person ignores or misinterprets the symptoms), or adjust and feel better at blood glucose levels that are too low. Continuous monitoring is the answer for these individuals, enabling them to be more sensitive to counterregulatory hormones and blood glucose level changes. If hypoglycemia unawareness is present, then BGAT training is recommended which, in the study by Cox et al., demonstrated a reduction in the occurrence of diabetic ketoacidosis (DKA) and severe hypoglycemia.

Illness in the Home

Illness should occur less frequently if blood glucose levels are well managed. If any illness should occur, early initiation of treatment prevents more acute problems, such as DKA. Illnesses that involve vomiting and diarrhea are usually accompanied by lower blood glucose levels. All other illnesses appear to elevate glucose levels.

Fluid increase is the first line of therapy. In the case of nausea and vomiting, small amounts of regular sugar-containing fluids are given by teaspoon to tablespoon or sips. Once the nausea subsides, soft foods, crackers, and soups are usually tolerated.

If insulin supplements are needed the guidance is as follows: when blood sugar is 250 (13.8 mmol) or higher, 10% of the total daily insulin dose is given as rapid-acting insulin at the time of the usual dose; when blood sugar is 250 (13.8 mmol) or higher and ketones are present in the urine (or blood), 20% of the total daily dose is given as rapid-acting insulin at the time of the usual dose. If blood glucose levels are really challenged, supplemental doses may be given on an hour-by-hour or every-2-hr basis (see Chapter 9 for details).

Sleep Apnea

A problem that is often first noticed in the home is sleep apnea. Sleep apnea occurs more frequently in individuals who are obese, and when it occurs, there may be a change in glucose metabolism or general body functioning (Boyer & Kapur, 2002; Punjabi & Polotsky, 2005). Spouses report more snoring or more times when there is a short absence of noticeable breathing. Poor quality of sleep may lead to sleep deprivation and other problems related to deficits in cognitive and physiologic functioning. The person with sleep apnea might report using more than one pillow or finding it difficult to get a "good night's sleep." It is possible that hypoglycemic episodes during the night might be triggered by the lack of sleeping ability. In most cases, there is more of a problem in controlling blood glucose levels, which therefore needs to be addressed.

"Triggers" for Diagnosis or Missed Diagnosis

Other members of the family may develop diabetes. In one family, diabetes was diagnosed in one daughter, then a second, then in one parent, and then the other parent. Relatives become sensitized and more knowledgeable about the signs and symptoms and they report to the health professional those aspects that might lead to the diagnosis of diabetes. Diabetes mellitus is a great mimicker. It can be found to mimic the flu, gastroenteritis, appendicitis, and even a heart attack.

In a recent instance in our clinic, a person called and noted the symptoms of chest pain accompanied by high blood glucose levels and ketone production. His C-reactive protein levels had been normal as had his electrocardiogram (ECG) results. To be sure, he was advised to go to the Emergency Room, and after fluids, electrolyte adjustment, and insulin (plus another ECG), his chest pain went away and, to this day, he has had not further signs or symptoms of cardiovascular disease.

With children, and some adults, the gastrointestinal disturbances are overlooked more frequently. Multiple times, we have learned that a child or adult had been treated or told it was nothing to worry about and sent home from the doctor's or other health professional's office. Within hours, if not a few days, they were really sick and some were even in a coma with diabetic ketoacidosis.

It is easy to get a urine or finger stick to rule out such an occurrence and yet too many health professionals do not take the time or think of doing this. The advice is, if there is anything that is suspect in a patient's condition, at least rule out diabetes by such simple testing.

Summary

Management of diabetes in the home faces many obstacles, but with the intervention of newer innovations and empowering education, family-based therapy is an option to be considered. Wysocki et al. (2008) found that, for adolescents, family therapy could be better tailored to the family and the individual when the person with diabetes was seen in familiar surroundings. This is not always possible, but a home health nurse or a diabetes center's nurse practitioner (if a psychologist was not available) could be educated to do some home- or community-based therapy and mutually devise ways that an adolescent (or adult) could better manage their life and their blood sugars. Senior, MacNair, and Jindal (2008) found that such a community-based multifactorial intervention not only achieved better diabetes control, but also, with their nurse–dietitian teams, improved blood pressure and lipid levels. Wangberg (2008) successfully worked with an Internet-based intervention to improve self-efficacy. New ways and newer gadgets (such as cell phones, especially those with Web capabilities) are allowing the treatment and monitoring of diabetes to be much more feasible.

Self-management education makes the difference. Two references for self-management education are the national standards (Funnell et al., 2008) and third-party reimbursement (American Diabetes Association, 2008) for diabetes self-management education. The individual and/or family must be able to safely use the guidance of self-management education to reach the ultimate goal of more normalized blood glucose levels more of the time. Ways of connecting by phone, cell phone, e-mail, and Web sites, along with cost containment, third-party coverage, and ongoing "proactive" education, even for patients with Type 2 diabetes mellitus, and care combine to promote the best possible outcomes for all ages of people who have this potentially disastrous condition. Barriers to care are decreasing. Early intervention is helping to prevent or alleviate potential future problems.

References

American Diabetes Association. (2008). Third-party reimbursement for diabetes care, self-management education, and supplies. *Diabetes Care, 31* (Suppl. 1), S95–S96.

Bodenheimer, T., Lorig, K., Holman, H., & Grumbach, K. (2002). Patient self-management of chronic disease in primary care. *Journal of the American Medical Association, 288,* 2469–2475.

Bolli, G. B., Perriello, G., Fanelli, C. G., & DeFeo, P. (1993). Nocturnal blood glucose control in type I diabetes mellitus. *Diabetes Care, 16* (Suppl. 3), 71–89.

Boyer, S., & Kapur, V. (2002). Obstructive sleep apnea: Its relevance in the care of diabetic patients. *Clinical Diabetes, 20,* 126–132.

Cox, D. J., Gopnder-Frederick, L., Bolonsky, W., Schlundt, D., Kovatchev, B., & Clarke, W. (2001). Blood glucose awareness training (BGAT-2): Long-term benefits. *Diabetes Care, 24*(4), 637–642.

Funnell, M. M., Brown, T. L., Childs, B. P., Haas, L. B., Hosey, G. M., Jensen, B., et al. (2008). National standards for diabetes self-management education. *Diabetes Care, 31*(Suppl. 1), S97–S104.

McMahon, G. T., Gomes, H. E., Hohne, S. H., Hu, T. M. J., Levine, B. A., & Conlin, P. R. (2005). Web-based care management in patients with poorly controlled diabetes. *Diabetes Care, 28*(7), 1624–1629.

Patton, S. R., Dolan, L. M., Henry, R., & Powers, S. W. (2007). Parental fear of hypoglycemia: Young children treated with continuous subcutaneous insulin infusion. *Pediatric Diabetes, 8*(6), 363–368.

Pearson, T. (2008). Glucagon as a treatment of severe hypoglycemia; safe and efficacious but underutilized. *The Diabetes Educator, 34*(1), 128–134.

Punjabi, M. S., & Polotsky, V. Y. (2005). Disorders of glucose metabolism in sleep apnea. *Journal of Applied Physiology, 99,* 1998–2007.

Raskin, P. (1984). The Somogyi phenomenon. Sacred cow or bull? *Archives of Internal Medicine, 144*(4), 781–787.

Ratner, R. E., Hirsch, I. B., Neifing, J. L., Garg, S. K., Mecca, T. E., & Wilson, C. A. (2000). Less hypoglycemia with insulin glargine in intensive insulin therapy for type 1 diabetes. U.S. Study Group of Insulin Glargine in Type 1 Diabetes. *Diabetes Care, 23,* 639–643.

Sakar, U., Handley, M. A., Gupta, R., Tang, A., Murphy, E., Seligman, H. K., et al. (2008). Use of an interactive, telephone-based self-management support program to identify adverse events among ambulatory diabetes patients. *Journal of General Internal Medicine, 23*(4), 459–465.

Senior, P. A., MacNair, L., & Jindal, K. (2008). Delivery of multi-factorial interventions by nurse and dietitian teams in a community setting to prevent diabetic complications: A quality-improvement report. *American Journal of Kidney Diseases, 51*(3), 425–434.

Tunis, S. L., & Minshall, M. E. (2008). Self-monitoring of blood glucose in type 2 diabetes: Cost-effectiveness in the United States. *American Journal of Managed Care, 14*(3), 131–140.

Wangberg, S. C. (2008). An internet-based diabetes self-care intervention tailored to self-efficacy. *Health Education Research, 23*(1), 170–179.

White, N. H. (2000). Diabetic ketoacidosis in children. *Endocrinology and Metabolism Clinics of North America, 29*(4), 657–682.

Wysocki, T., Harris, M. A., Buckloh, L. M., Mertlich, D., Lochrie, A. S., Taylor, A., et al. (2008). Randomized, controlled trial of behavioral family systems therapy for diabetes: Maintenance and generalization of effects on parent-adolescent communication. *Behavior Therapy, 39*(1), 33–46.

Note. The ADAG (Alc Derived Average Glucose) study group conducted extensive research to more accurately associate the estimated average glucose (eAG) to hemoglobin Alc (Nathan et al., released June 2008). Kahn, of the ADA, and Fonseca, of Tulane University School of Medicine, stated that the language eAG will be an added aid in patients' (and professionals') understanding while "...current units and normal range will not vanish or change."

Kahn, R., & Fonseca, V. (2008). Translating the Alc assay. *Diabetes Care, 31,* 1704–1707 (published online June 7, 2008).

Nathan, D., Kuenen, J., Borg, R., Zheng, H., Schoenfeld, D., & Heine, R.J., for the ADAG study group. Translating the Alc assay into estimated average glucose values. *Diabetes Care, 31,* 1473–1478 (published online June 7, 2008).

Ongoing Treatment and Care in Type 1 Diabetes

9

Hormone Therapy for Type 1 Diabetes

For the individual with Type 1 diabetes (T1DM), the replacement of insulin is paramount in achieving optimal glucose control. In the individual without diabetes, normal physiology keeps the blood glucose in a very narrow range through the complex interplay of glucagon, insulin, amylin, and gastrointestinal peptides, including glucagon-like peptide-1 (GLP-1) and glucose-dependent insulinotropic polypeptide (GIP). GLP-1 suppresses glucagon secretion, and together GLP-1 and GIP increase insulin secretion. Both of these gut hormones are inactivated by dipeptidyl peptidase 4 (DPP-4) (Ahern, 2005). Insulin and glucagon have long been recognized as pivotal hormones that contribute to the regulation of glucose. Insulin and amylin are produced by the islet of Langerhans beta cells and glucagon is produced by the alpha cells.

Small physiologic amounts of insulin are released to maintain the blood glucose at a constant level; this is considered the *basal* insulin. There is never a peak. When a meal or other glucose load occurs, insulin is released as a *bolus,* to prevent the rise in the blood glucose following the glucose load. Insulin also acts to suppress the release of glucose from the liver during this "feeding" period by suppressing glucagon production and stimulating glycogen production. It is now recognized that another hormone, amylin, which is cosecreted with insulin by the beta cells, also plays a role in glucose homeostasis. Amylin inhibits postprandial glucagon secretion and slows gastric emptying and the resulting uptake of glucose into the bloodstream (Edelman, 2008).

Today, it is possible to closely mimic the normal physiology of glucose homeostasis with exogenous insulin by using the basal–bolus approach to therapy. A continuous subcutaneous insulin infusion (CSII) device or a multiple daily insulin injection regimen can be used. The amylin analog, Pramlintide, can be administered premeal with insulin to further enhance postprandial glucose control.

This chapter reviews the currently available insulin products, regimen options including CSII therapy, insulin storage and administration, and the use of Pramlintide (Symlin) in practice.

Insulin

Insulin pharmacokinetics is the description of how fast insulin appears in the blood after an injection. This is the most common insulin curve and is what appears in the package insert. It does not take into account the individual absorption factors of the injected insulin. Insulin pharmacodynamics, however, describes how long the insulin is active in lowering the blood glucose and is usually shorter than the more commonly used pharmacokinetic values. Insulin timing and action are measured in four general categories of insulin based on action times. The four categories are rapid acting, short acting, intermediate acting, and long acting.

Before 1983, the source of manufactured insulin was the pancreas of cattle and hogs. Human insulin, made by modification of pork insulin, that is, transaminated alanine to threonine (Novo and Nordisk, then separate companies), then by recombinant deoxyribonucleic acid (DNA) technology from *Escherichia coli* cells (Lilly), was made available. A few years later, Novo-Nordisk marketed recombinant DNA insulin made from yeast cells.

In 1996, Lispro (Lys-pro), the first "designer" insulin, was released by Eli Lilly and Company under the name of Humalog. This is insulin that has been biochemically altered to absorb more rapidly through the process of switching the lysine and proline amino acids on the beta chain of insulin (Glazer, Zalani, Anderson, and Bastyr, 1999). In 2001, Novo-Nordisk released Aspart insulin (Novolog), a rapid-acting insulin, made by substituting asparagine (aspartic acid) for proline at the 28 position of the beta chain (Mudaliar et al., 1999). In 2006, Glulisine (Apidra, Sanofi-Aventis) was produced by recombinant DNA technology utilizing a nonpathogenic laboratory strain of *E. coli* (K12). Insulin Glulisine differs from human insulin in that the amino acid asparagine at position B3 is replaced by lysine and the lysine in position B29 is replaced by glutamic acid. These insulins are considered rapid-acting insulins.

Long-acting insulins have also evolved to include Lantus (Glargine Sanofi-Aventis) and Levemir (Detemir Novo Nordisk) in the past several years. Lantus is relatively peakless insulin that lasts 24 hr ± 2 hr. Its slowed action is made by the replacement of aspargine with glycine as the terminal amino acid of the alpha chain and the addition of two amino acids, arginines, on the beta chain of insulin (Berger, 2000). Levemir (insulin detemir [rDNA origin] injection) is a peakless insulin with up to 24 hr duration produced by a process that includes expression of recombinant DNA in *Saccharomyces cerevisiae* (a yeast) followed by chemical modification. Insulin detemir differs from human insulin in that the amino acid threonine in position B30 has been omitted, and a C14 fatty acid chain (myristic acid) has been attached to the amino acid B29. These insulins are long acting and considered basal insulins. The other basal insulin that had been available in the United States, Ultralente, was removed from the market in the early 2000s.

The only intermediate-acting insulin available in the United States is NPH (neutral protamine Hagedorn). This insulin has been available for more than 50 years. It is used less today than in the past because it has a slow onset and a peak. It is difficult to use in a basal–bolus regimen but still has uses today because it is much cheaper that the "designer" or analog insulins. It is therefore useful for people with limited financial resources, especially older people with Type 2 diabetes mellitus (T2DM).

The only short-acting insulin available in the United States is regular insulin. This is the original insulin developed by Banting and Best in 1921 from animal sources. It became available in 1983 as recombinant DNA human insulin and is identical to the insulin produced by the human pancreas. This insulin is used less now than in the past because of the delay in onset in association with food intake, but it is still used for intravenous therapy and for people with limited finances.

Insulin Regimens

When developing an insulin regimen for an individual, the primary goal is to mimic normal physiology as much as possible. One must also consider the individual's lifestyle, physical, mental, and psychosocial capabilities, and financial resources. The usual total daily dose for starting insulin in the patient with T1DM is 1–2 Units·kg^{-1}·day^{-1}. For T2DM the starting insulin dose is 0.5–1.5 Units·kg^{-1}·day^{-1}. The dose is usually the highest in a child during growth periods or with insulin resistance because of ketosis. The initial dose ranges are determined by the degree of ketosis, not by the initial blood glucose level. Individuals with ketoacidosis have less endogenous insulin-producing ability left in the pancreas and therefore require a high starting dose. Individuals with T2DM who have been on oral agent therapy and are being converted to insulin, though insulin resistant, usually require lower doses per unit body weight than do individuals with T1DM.

The best insulin regimen to mimic normal insulin secretion is the basal-bolus regimen. This regimen uses a rapid- or short-acting insulin before meals as the bolus insulin and a long-acting insulin like Levemir or Lantus once or twice daily as the basal insulin. Basal insulin secretion normally is 40%–50% of the total daily insulin dose. Approximately 50%–60% is then given as bolus insulin divided between two or three meals based on the calorie or carbohydrate intake. The basal insulin rate of an insulin pump can be adjusted during the day and night and, more easily, can be programmed to cover the dawn phenomenon. A typical starting dose for injected insulin would be 50% of the total dose as basal insulin given in the evening, and the rapid-acting insulin would be divided into 20% before breakfast, 13% before lunch, and 17% before supper. Ideally the meals remain fixed as the insulin dose is adjusted. One can then determine the insulin-to-calories or insulin-to-carbohydrates ratio so that patients can make their own adjustments as their meals change.

In the individual with newly diagnosed T1DM, it is important to establish an adequate insulin dose to correct the glucose toxicity that is often present after running high blood glucose levels for a time. After the initial period of glucotoxicity and nutritional repletion, a period of partial remission of the diabetes may follow (often called The Honeymoon Period). During these two periods rapid changes occur in insulin requirements, often by as much as 10% a day. Rapidly changing insulin sensitivity makes nutritional-to-insulin ratios impractical at this point. It is important to use a pattern management approach for the adjustment of insulin and calories.

A four-shot regimen of regular insulin is an option for the initial management for newly diagnosed T1DM, the hospitalized patient, or for sick-day self-management. Using the current total daily insulin dose or 0.5–2 Units·kg^{-1}·day^{-1}, the dosage is divided into four doses by using the distribution of 35% before breakfast, 22% before lunch, 28% before the evening meal, and 15% of the total daily insulin dose at midnight with a small snack. The insulin would be administered injected 30 min before the meal and bedtime snack. This option could be used for someone without insurance for sick-day management. If the patient is to receive nothing by mouth, as in the hospital or on a sick day, the regular insulin can be given every 6 hr as 25% of the total daily dose. Regular insulin offers a lower-cost alternative to insulin analog therapy and the insulin can be obtained without a prescription. Delayed and peak action effects, however, make regular insulin, as well as neutral protamine Hagedorn (NPH) insulin, difficult to use. Analog insulins are simpler to use and more physiologic.

Another alternative therapy would be to use a *split-mix* regimen with two or three daily insulin doses. A mix of the intermediate-acting insulin, NPH, with a short-acting insulin (Humulin 70/30 or Novolin 70/30) or with one of the analog insulins (Humalog 75/25 or Novolog 70/30) could be administered in the morning; a second dose could be given before the evening meal. This regimen also requires that the individual eat meals and snacks at regular times. See Table 9.1 for the number of premix insulins available including Novolog 70/30, Novolin 70/30, Humalog 75/25, Humalin 70/30, and Humalog 50/50. An initial starting dose for this regimen would be to administer two-thirds of the total insulin dose before the breakfast meal and one-third before the evening meal.

The risk of the split-mix regimen is nocturnal hypoglycemia from the evening NPH. To minimize this risk, an insulin mix may be administered in the morning before breakfast, a dose of rapid- or short-acting insulin can be given with the evening meal, and NPH can be given at bedtime. This reduces the risk of nocturnal hypoglycemia and helps prevent the predawn glucose rise by more closely matching the insulin action to the occurrence of predawn hyperglycemia. The percentage split for this regimen would be approximately 60% prior to the breakfast meal, 18% before the evening meal, and 22% at bedtime.

Conversion from one regimen to another is relatively easy, especially when converting from regimens involving older insulins (regular and NPH) to analog insulins. The total daily insulin dose of the old regimen is calculated then redistributed to the new insulins. For example, for a person taking 70/30 twice a day, add up the total daily dose and redistribute as long-acting insulin (glargine or detemir), giving 50% of the daily total at bedtime; rapid-acting insulin (Lispro, Asparte, or Glulisine), giving 20% of the total daily insulin for breakfast, 13% for lunch, and 17% for the evening meal. Blood glucose levels should be checked fasting and 1–2 hr after the beginning of each meal. The optimal approach is to look at a pattern over a 3-day period. If the fasting blood glucose level is not in the right range, adjust the bedtime long-acting insulin. If the after-breakfast blood glucose level is not in the right range, then adjust the breakfast rapid-acting insulin. Adjust the lunch and supper rapid-acting insulin in the same way. Once base insulin doses are established, then the patient should be taught the adjustment of the mealtime insulin according to the amount of food eaten.

Insulin Administration and Delivery Devices

Many factors influence the absorption of insulin and thus how effective insulin is, day to day, for the individual with diabetes. How insulin is handled and administered can have a significant impact on the consistency of blood glucose levels day to day. How and where the insulin is administered and how it is stored can alter the time action of the insulin and thus the stability of the blood glucose levels.

Storage

In general, insulin that is being used, whether via a vial or an insulin pen, can be stored at room temperature or at a temperature between 46 and 86°F per the package inserts. Novo Nordisk has tested Novolog at up to 96°F. Extra insulin supplies should be kept refrigerated until used. Predrawing Lantus insulin is not advised (Grajower et al., 2003). Studies indicate that depending on the brand of syringe used, the Lantus may become cloudy within 20 min (Becton-Dickinson company, personal communication, 2008). Based on clinical experience, Lantus vials may be more stable if refrigerated between uses. This is not necessary or advised with the Opticlick pen and cartridges or the Solostar Lantus pen now in use. Levemir also does not need refrigeration, but vials of any insulin not in use should be refrigerated to prolong shelf life. Lantus and Levemir insulin should never be mixed in the same syringe with any other insulin.

People with diabetes should always have on hand at least one extra bottle (or pen) of each type of insulin they are using. When traveling, patients may use a simple wide-mouth plastic vacuum bottle that can hold several bottles of insulin or pens and keep the temperature stable. Several travel packs, such as the Frio products, are currently available that require only water to provide an acceptable storage temperature. It is wise for persons who have diabetes to carry insulin and other medical supplies in carry-on luggage when they are traveling via public transportation. The baggage compartment of an airplane is too cold for storage of diabetes supplies including insulin, Pramlintide, and glucose-testing supplies, and their supplies will then be at hand when they are needed.

Insulin carries an expiration date on the label. As a general guideline, outdated insulin should not be used. The potency of insulin used after the expiration date cannot be guaranteed by the manufacturer. It is important to advise patients to check the date on the bottle before leaving the pharmacy.

Supplies

Disposable syringes and insulin pens are the primary method for intermittent insulin delivery. Many sizes of syringes, needles, and pen needles are available. The needle lengths are 12.7, 8, and 5 mm. The gauge of the needle is from 28 to 32, that is, 32 g (just available June 2008) is the finest gauged needle. Syringes are available as ¼ cc, ⅓ cc, ½ cc, and 1 cc. There are ¼ cc and ⅓ cc insulin syringes that are marked with half-unit markings.

Pens, with or without removable cartridges, and infusion pumps are also available for the administration of insulin (to be discussed later in this chapter). Not all pen needles are interchangeable on the available insulin pens. Insulin will leak around the pen needle if the appropriate brand of needle is not used. The manufacturer's instructions should be followed.

Care of Supplies; Disposal of Syringes

Disposable syringes need no care before their use. They are designed to be used once and then thrown away. Care does need to be taken in the disposal of these syringes. The needle can be broken off from the hub through the use of a needle-clipping device or, preferably, the total syringe with the needle can be placed in a hard plastic container. Safe disposal of needles helps to prevent unauthorized persons from using the equipment and reduces the risk of blood-borne pathogens.

The classic study of 30 patients who reused disposable syringes from 1 week to 2 months showed only 1 syringe of 60 with a bacterial growth (Greenough, Cockcroft, & Bloom, 1979). These syringes had a removable needle that was changed after 3 or 4 days. Studies have measured the incidence of infection in individuals using the same syringe for widely varying periods. There appears to be little untoward effect from these practices (Aziz, 1984; Turner & Lancaster, 1984; Bosquet, Grimaldi, & Thervel, 1986). These studies were done by using larger gauge needles before the advent of newer, smaller (30, 31, and possibly a 32 g) needles. Even with one injection, the needle tip of a disposable needle can become bent to form a hook that may lacerate tissue or break off to leave needle fragments within the skin. The medical consequences of these findings are unknown but may increase lipodystrophy or have other adverse effects (American Diabetes Association [ADA], 2004b).

The most widely available syringes in this country have needles that cannot be removed; therefore, it is recommended that the syringe not be used for more than 2 or 3 days because of the needle becoming dull and the resulting tissue trauma. If one is using a basal–bolus regimen it is advisable to use one syringe for the basal insulin and one syringe for the bolus insulin to prevent contamination. Lantus and Levemir cannot be mixed with any other insulin. If these modifications in syringe reuse are indeed safe for most individuals, a dollar savings of major importance for certain groups of people could result. Although it goes against the recommendation by the manufacturers for a syringe to be used more than one time, social circumstances may warrant a need for reusing a syringe more than once. It is critical that the syringes be used by only one person. Unless there is a significant absence of personal hygiene, the probability of infection from self-injection is small with syringe reuse.

Injection through clothing is a frequent action by many patients with diabetes. Fleming, Jacober, Vandenberg, Fitzgerald, and Grunberger (1997) showed that this practice did not result in infection or deterioration in diabetes control. The study has not been replicated using the finer 30–31 gauge needles or the shorter length needles, that is, 8 mm or 5 mm. Careful glucose monitoring should be undertaken and if blood glucose levels are higher than goal, reviewing injection practices is warranted before altering insulin doses.

Length of needle could have an effect on the action of the insulin injection. If the point of the needle is to reach the subcutaneous fat, it must be of the appropriate length to do so. The 5-mm needle is most appropriate for children and lean adults. The original length needle is better for obese or overweight individuals. If or when a patient changes the length of needle for administration, careful glucose monitoring should be practiced to determine whether glucose control is altered with the change in needle length.

Accuracy of the Amount of the Insulin

The accurate measurement of the insulin dose is a critical part of insulin therapy. The person doing the measuring must be fully instructed and have adequate time to practice before being permitted to do so unsupervised. A calm, positive attitude on the part of the instructor will enhance the learning experience.

First, the user and a significant other person in the family should be allowed to become familiar with the equipment. They should handle the syringe or pen, get used to the feel, push the plunger in and out, and be shown the various ways they might hold it. Initially individuals with diabetes may feel self-conscious about the equipment and fearful about the upcoming injection. Offering an opportunity to explore the equipment prior to the administration of the injection may help them to gain confidence.

When the person (or family) is ready to learn how to measure and give the insulin, all supplies should be available. Encouraging parents, a family member, or the individual's significant other to also experience an injection helps the individual to feel less fearful and the family member or significant other to better understand what the individual with diabetes is feeling and to realize that the injection is not painful. In fact, we encourage all health professionals who may prescribe insulin therapy to also take a saline injection to have the opportunity to self-inject.

Measurement Procedure

Teach the patient to measure one type of insulin first. The procedure is as follows:

1. Roll the bottle of insulin between the hands (*only if using NPH,* i.e., mixing NPH is necessary to return any particles to suspension. Do not shake vigorously because this creates many bubbles, which are difficult to remove. This procedure is not needed for the clear insulins).
2. Wipe the top of the bottle with an alcohol sponge.
3. Inject air into the insulin bottle equal to the dosage of insulin to be taken out. (This step equalizes the pressure in the bottle to make it easier to withdraw the insulin.)
4. Withdraw the insulin into the syringe. (Using insulin that is at room temperature reduces the bubbles that may be seen in the insulin bottle and syringe.)
5. Withdraw the insulin into the syringe, adjusting to the required dosage.

Mixing Two Types of Insulin or Diluting Insulin

When a person is receiving both modified (i.e., intermediate-acting) and unmodified (i.e., short- and rapid-acting) insulin, the two types can be mixed in the same syringe, thus saving the patient extra injections. (Precaution: Do not mix glargine with any other insulin because glargine is an acid insulin, but other insulins are neutral pH). When one is measuring two types of insulin, care must be taken not to contaminate one insulin with the other. Follow this procedure:

1. Roll the bottle of modified insulin (i.e., intermediate).
2. Wipe the tops of both bottles.
3. Inject air equal to the insulin dosage into the bottle of modified insulin (or into the diluent). Do not withdraw this insulin (diluent).
4. Inject air into the bottle of unmodified (short- or rapid-acting) insulin equal to the insulin dosage and withdraw this insulin, being certain to remove all air bubbles.
5. Return to the bottle of modified insulin and withdraw the insulin (or diluent) to equal the total amount desired. Take care to have the insulin bubble-free before adding the second insulin (or the diluent). If an error in measurement is made, redraw the insulin.

Some patients, because of various limitations, cannot be taught to measure two kinds of insulin accurately. For increased safety and ease of use, it is best to use premixed insulin, that is, 70/30, 50/50, or 75/25. Today, insulin mixing or diluting is seldom done. If it is needed, having a visiting nurse or family member assist might be helpful if the patient has a problem in mixing or diluting insulin.

Pulling up insulin in disposable syringes for a couple of weeks at a time is discouraged, but, again, if necessary it may be done. Predrawing cannot be done with glargine because of the acid pH. The premixed insulins are stable until the expiration date or until mishandled (i.e., too hot or too cold). Glargine

9.1 Insulins

Manufacturer	Type/Name	Onset	Peak	Effective Duration
Eli Lilly & Co.	Humalog–Lispro	5<15 min	1.5 hr	3 ½ hr
	Humulin R	30–60 min	2 to 3 hr	6+/– hr
	Humulin N	2 hr	6–8 hr	10–12 hr
	Humalog Mix 75/25	75% lispro protamine/25% lispro		
	Humalog Mix 50/50	50% lispro protamine/50% lispro		
	Humulin 70/30	70% NPH/30% regular		
Novo Nordisk	Novolog–Aspart	5–10 min	40–50 min	4+ hr
	Novolin	R 30 min	2–4 hr	6+/– hr
	Novolin N	2 hr	6–8 hr	10–12 hr
	Novolin L	2 hr	8+ hr	14–16 hr
	Levemir/Detemer	2+ hr	nearly flat	14–24 hr
	Novolog Mix 70/30	70% aspart protamine/30% aspart		
	Novolin 70/30	70% NPH/30% regular		
Sanofi-Aventis	Apidra–Glulisine	2–3 hr	nearly flat	22+/– hr
	Lantus/Glargine	2+ hr	nearly flat	24+/– hr

and detemir insulin can be administered at any time of day to cover the 24-hr period. Family may be able to assist with administration at another time of day other than bedtime.

Mixing instructions are needed less now than in the past because of the availability of premixed insulins and the use of basal-bolus therapy with rapid- and long-acting insulins. The instructions have been included here because mixing is still done by some patients.

All of the currently available premixed insulins and their times of action are noted in Table 9.1.

Injection Sites

Throughout the years of insulin therapy, many sites have been used for insulin injection. The most frequently used areas have been the thighs, upper arms, abdomen, and buttocks. The backs of the forearms have also been used. The calves of the legs are not recommended because of the toughness of the skin and low subcutaneous fat content, which leads to a more painful injection, and a decreased blood supply, which leads to poorer absorption. With the modern insulin analogs, insulin is absorbed almost equally at all available injection sites.

Rotation of Sites

Adequate rotation of injection sites is probably the single most important factor in minimizing problems at the site of injection, despite the availability of purified insulins. As stated previously, some people have developed lipodystrophy, particularly lipohypertrophy, even with the purified human insulins when using poor rotation or superficial injection techniques. Not only should the anatomical region be rotated, but also even the site within the region. Individuals tend to use a small area of the abdomen repeatedly out of habit and eventually, with repeated use, that area has fewer nerve sensations. Lipohypertrophy will result from this practice.

Studies using regular insulin indicate that regular insulin is absorbed at different rates in various areas of the body at rest. The abdomen absorbs 86% faster than the legs, and the arms absorb 41% faster than the legs, in the classic study by Galloway (1980). This study identifies the disadvantages of rotating injection sites in a hit-or-miss pattern, such as abdomen one day, leg the next, and so forth. Rather, one should stay with one general area for 1 week or more at a time before moving on to the next site. Zehrer, Hansen, and Bantle (1991) even suggest only rotating in the abdominal area because of greater consistency in absorption rate. With many individuals now administering four injections daily, they may choose to give all the morning injections in one site, lunch in another, supper in another, and the bedtime dose in another. Insulin analogs have more consistent absorption than the older insulins. Even with the analog insulins, lipohypertrophy can occur if injections are given consistently in the same location.

Exercise also can affect the rate of absorption. Insulin should therefore not be injected into an extremity just before the exercise period. When a person is to exercise soon after injection or within a few hours after injection, the abdomen is the best site for injection.

When the abdomen is being used, injection sites should be below the rib cage above the waistline or below the waistline on either side of the middle. This area is relatively easy to pinch up and pull (giving the injection in the tight, pulled site) and is relatively free from any discomfort. The skin at the waistline itself is usually tough in adults and makes the injection more uncomfortable. The lower area of the abdomen is usually fatter, which makes the technique more difficult for obese adults. This area is acceptable for children who have thinner skin and fat layers.

Use of the arms and the back needs to be taught to those who are assisting the insulin-dependent person. Some people, especially adolescents, do give their own injections in the arms; however, self-injection into the arms is not as preferable for older, less dexterous people.

Most people initially feel that the back is taboo. Such is not the case. The back is a relatively painless site, is usually easy to pinch up, and has a wide surface area. Two or three rows of injections can be given on each side of the back. Injection sites are spaced to receive 1 week of insulin in each row. The individual to be injected may stand, sit, or lie down for the injection. The shoulders need to be in a relaxed position.

The important points to remember in the use and rotation of injection sites are:

1. Use as many of the available areas as possible.
2. Use a system that is easy to remember.
3. Do not use the inside of the thighs, the calves of the leg, the middle of the upper arms, or within 1.5 inches of the umbilicus.

Methods of Injection

Over the years, several insulin injection techniques have been used. One technique has been injection at a 45° or 90° angle directly into the subcutaneous fat layer. The skin and fat are pinched up, and the needle inserted at a 45° angle into the stretched skin adjacent to the pinched up area. Another technique is to inject into a deeper subcutaneous layer by injecting at a 90° angle and either stretching the skin taut or *pinching it up* (very short needles: inject straight in at 90°). Explain to the patient that injecting the needle through stretched skin and/or use of the dart, or quick, method of penetration will result in the least discomfort if any at all.

Although these techniques may be fine for some people, no single method works for all. The educator needs to determine individual needs carefully based on the thickness of skin and fat layers and manual dexterity.

Injection Procedure

1. Pinch up the skin, unless a 5-mm needle is used, and wipe the site with an alcohol sponge. (There has been some question about the practice of special skin cleansing. Although this is not overstressed, it is recommended that persons wash their hands and use an alcohol wipe or have recently cleaned skin. Infections are rarely seen when simple cleanliness is observed.)
2. Hold the syringe at the appropriate angle, with the thumb on one side and a few other fingers on the other side.
3. Trace the needle from the top of the hill to the bottom, keeping the syringe at the recommended angle without touching the skin. This exercise prevents guesswork by assuring that the needle is in the right place.
4. With the needle directly over the site to be injected, push the needle quickly through the skin, all the way to the hub.
5. Inject the insulin by pushing the plunger with the second fingertip, and release the pinch.
6. Keep the needle in place for 5–6 seconds for rapid- (or short-) acting insulin; for 10 seconds for long- (or intermediate-) acting insulins.
7. Place the cotton ball over the site and pull the needle straight out. (If the patient has a problem with bruising or insulin leaking, hold a cotton ball or finger firmly on the site for one full minute. This usually prevents bleeding just under the skin surface or leaking of the insulin directly out the same hole in which it was injected.)

Do not rub the injection site unless a more rapid absorption of insulin is desired.

Inspection of Injection Sites

Injection sites must be inspected periodically. The injection sites need to be checked for lumps or hollows or any evidence of infection. The individual, family member, or health professional should not only look at the areas of injection, but also should feel them. The best way to do this is by running the flat of the palm down the thighs, across the abdomen, and down the arms. Someone else will have to feel the back. The palm is more sensitive to variations in texture of the underlying tissues than the fingertips alone. If lumpy areas, thickening, or hollows are felt, the area should be allowed to rest for a time. These areas will soften and return to normal, usually within a few weeks, although occasionally it may take 6 months to 1 year or more.

Lipoatrophy is possible, even with the use of the "humanized" insulins. Ka-ordonouri, Lauterborn, and Deiss reported such a case in 2002. Al-Khenaizan, Al-Thubaiti, and Al-Alwan (2007) also observed the case of a 4-year-old developing lipoatrophy because of insulin injections. Lipoatrophy with CSII has also been seen, though it is rare. The only treatment for lipoatrophy is to create lipohypertrophy by the injection of insulin into the edge of the atrophied area at a 20-degree angle in a decreasing circular pattern (Wentworth et al., 1973). Injecting into the same small areas over and over may result in lipohypertrophy, although this is seen less frequently today than in previous years when nonhuman insulin was used. Lipohypertrophy can only be treated by letting the lump rest for 6–12 months.

Timing of the Insulin Dose

The timing of the injection should be based on food consumption, the type of insulin used, planned physical activity, and meal type. The insulin action (e.g., onset, peak, and duration) should also be considered when administering the insulin dose.

Rapid-acting insulin analogs should be injected 5-15 min before a meal or immediately after a meal. Typically the blood glucose rises immediately on food ingestion. The time that it takes an individual to consume a meal varies greatly. Administering insulin after the meal is only recommended if one does not know how much of the meal they will consume or if a parent is administering insulin to a small child who may or may not eat all (or any) of the meal. This is a problem mainly with preschool children. Apidra is promoted as being as effective as premeal and postmeal insulin, but the study comparison was to regular insulin (Novo Nordisk, 2008b). To be most effective, regular insulin is recommended to be given 30 min prior to the meal. Only rapid-acting analog insulins should be used for postmeal injection, except in some cases of delayed gastric emptying.

Special Injection Products

Injectors

For multiple injections, the Insulfon (Diabetes Onter, Inc., Wayzata, MN) or I-port might be helpful. The injection is given through the site connected to a tube inserted with a needle and replaced about once a week (to date, these have not been as popular in the United States as they have been in Europe).

Insulin Pens

Insulin pens are available for most insulin formulations (see Table 9.2). The benefit of using an insulin pen is that accuracy and consistency in dosing are improved when patients use insulin pens. The use of insulin pens should be promoted. Their use is increasing in the United States as people are learning

9.2 Insulin Pens

Manufacturer	Pen(s)	Features
Eli Lilly & Co.	Humalog Mix 75/25 Humalog Mix 50/50 Humulin Mix 70/30 Humalog and Humulin N	Prefilled, disposable, 3.0 ml, and reusable (cartridge)
	HumaPen Memoir	Reusable pen with memory for date/time of 16 past boluses
	HumaPen Luxura HD	Reusable, delivers in ½ units
Novo Nordisk	Novolog 70/30 Flexpen Novolog Flexpen Levemir Flexpen	Disposable, 3.0 ml
	NovoPen 3	Reusable pen (cartridge)
	NovoPen Jr	Reusable; delivers in ½ units
Owen Mumford, Inc.	Autopen AN3800 & AN3810	Automatic reusable cartridge, 3.0 ml
Sanofi-Aventis	Opticlick	Reusable for Apidra and Lantus, 3.0-ml cartridges
	SoloStar	Disposable, Lantus

Note. From *American Diabetes Association Resource Guide* (p. RG22), 2008. Copyright 2008 by American Diabetes Association. Adapted with permission.

about the convenience of using a pen, and there is more insurance coverage than in the past.

Patient satisfaction has been demonstrated once a pen is introduced and the patient educated in its use (Thurman, 2007). Increased compliance with therapy was also found.

Automatic Injectors

The automatic injector works by a push-button spring release of the needle that automatically gives the injection with little participation by the patient. Persons who have used injectors have done so because they could not learn to give themselves an injection. Most, if not all, people who have fears or other emotional adjustments to diabetes can give their own injections in time and the use of other devices may assist them in coping until they can be more comfortable doing otherwise. It is recommended that the person who has a physical handicap, such as cerebral palsy, use the automatic injector as an aid.

Continuous Subcutaneous Insulin Infusion (CSII)—Pumps

A subcutaneous insulin infusion pump may offer a more precise way of mimicking normal insulin delivery (see Table 9.3). In one of many studies, long-term use

9.3 Insulin Pumps

Manufacturer	Pump	Features
Animas Corporation	Animas IR 1250	Uses AA lithium or AA alkaline battery; 12 basal rates; 4 patterns; temporary rate Smallest bolus, 0.05 Units; 3 alarms; uses insulin-to-CHO ratio, insulin on board, correction factor; Weight, 3.13 oz full. http://www.animascorp.com
Insulet Corporation	OmniPod Insulin	Integrated battery; no tubing; temporary rate 7 basals (0.05–30.0 Units/hr); 3 alarms Weight, 1.2 oz full. http:www.MyOmniPod.com
Medtronic Diabetes	MiniMed Paradigm 722	Uses AAA battery; 3 basal patterns with up to 48 rates per pattern (0.05–35.0 U/hr); Smallest bolus, 1.0 Units; 3 alarms Displays glucose reading every 5 min. Uses insulin-to-CHO ratio; insulin sensitivity; correction factor; Weight, 3.8 oz 300-Unit reservoir.
	522	Uses AAA battery; 3 basal patterns with up to 48 rates per pattern (0.05–35.0 Units/hr); Smallest bolus, 1.0 Units; 3 alarms Uses insulin-to-CHO ratio; insulin sensitivity; correction factor; Weight, 3.5 oz 176-Unit reservoir. http://www.MiniMed.com
Smiths Medical	CosMore Insulin Technology System	Uses AAA battery; 4 basal patterns (0.05–35 Units/hr); temporary rate; 3 alarms; all-correction factor; uses standard infusion sets; Weight, 3.3 oz full. http://www.CozMore.com
Sooil USA	Diabe care II	Uses 3-volt DC battery; 24 basal rates (0.0–16 Units/hr); temporary rate; 3 alarms Smallest bolus, 0.1 Unit; Weight, 1.8 oz; 12 languages; can preset boluses. http://www.sooil.com

Note. From *American Diabetes Association Resource Guide* (pp. RG24–RG25), 2008. Copyright 2008 by American Diabetes Association. Adapted with permission.

of the pump (CSII) has been found to have benefits in lowering mean HbA1c and decreasing the occurrence of severe hypoglycemia (Scrimgeour et al., 2007). Despite these positive findings, Scrimgeour et al. also reported an increase in the number of diabetic ketoacidosis (DKA) episodes (because of the lack of delivery of insulin often related to the kinking of tubing). Even with normal

HbA1c values, they found that *blocking* of the insulin's ability to reach the patient only required an average of 6 hr until DKA or diabetic ketosis was identified.

The insulin pump provides the potential of a variable basal insulin rate throughout a 24-hr period. Any of the rapid-acting insulins or regular insulin can be administered continuously through a patient-placed subcutaneous needle. Bolus insulin is then administered with meals and snacks as needed. The newer model insulin pumps, some with glucose sensor augmentation, allow the patient and provider to establish preprogrammed correction factors, insulin-to-carbohydrate or insulin-to-exchange ratios, and insulin sensitivity parameters. For example, Joe has a blood glucose level of 200 mg/dl (11.1 mmol) before lunch. If his exchange ratio is 1 Unit per exchange, his correction factor is 1 Unit to drop the blood glucose by 25 mg (1.4 mmol) and his target glucose is 100 mg/dl (5.5 mmol), he would enter into his pump the blood glucose of 200 mg/dl (11.1 mmol). He would enter into the pump that he was going to eat 8 exchanges. The insulin pump would calculate automatically that he needed 12 Units of insulin as a bolus. He could activate this dose or he could choose to decrease the dose because he knows that he is going to play 45 min of racketball after lunch and those 12 Units would be too much.

With the sensor-augmented pump, like the MiniMed 722 (Paradigm Real Time Sensor, see the Web site http://www.MiniMed.com), the patient also can see what the blood glucose is continuously and use the data from the continuous sensor to determine the premeal doses and correction doses, should blood glucose be out of the target range. For a glucose sensor-augmented insulin pump, a second needlelike sensor is inserted in addition to the insulin pump infusion needle. The glucose reading is sent to the insulin pump by infrared or radio-frequency (RF) technology.

Subcutaneous insulin infusion pumps can be used with individuals with T1DM and T2DM, but Medicare does not cover insulin pumps for individuals with T2DM and requires c-peptides on all patients with T1DM. Many state-funded plans and private insurance plans follow the same reimbursement guidelines.

Indications for CSII include:

- A1C greater than target with maximized current regimen
- Marked daily variability
- History of severe hypoglycemia
- Dawn phenomena
- Need for flexibility such as shift work or working night shift

When assessing a patient for insulin pump therapy, one must consider the patient's motivation to undertake insulin pump therapy. They must be willing and able to self-test their blood glucose at least four times daily. They must have realistic expectations for insulin pump therapy. A diabetes management team that is experienced in managing CSII and is available 24/7 is necessary to ensure the safe utilization of pump therapy patients and their families. Patients must be willing to undertake the education process to learn the self-management skills necessary to successfully manage CSII.

A CSII education program includes counseling regarding:

- Accurate glucose monitoring and appropriate timing.
- Needle insertion, with change every 2–3 days, for prevention of abscess formation.

- Management of hyperglycemia including troubleshooting the technical cause of hyperglycemia.
- Management of hypoglycemia including not suspending the pump for prolonged periods of time.
- Knowing glucose targets.
- Sick day management.
- Knowing how and when to contact pump-experienced personnel 24 hr a day, 7 days a week.

Hypoglycemia, even though seen less frequently in pump use, has been observed. Franklin et al. (2007) reported that a 10-year-old was using the prime function (rather than the bolus—that didn't quite control the glucose excursions) to cover the ingestion of candy. This is an excellent example of the resourcefulness and the ability of today's children in using various technologies and the need of appropriate supervision by the parent(s).

Overall, when compared with multiple injections, CSII has been found to achieve the same degree of blood glucose level control but with the occurrence of fewer hypoglycemic episodes (Hirsch et al., 2005).

Incretin Hormones

In 1986, amylin was recognized as a hormone that was cosecreted with insulin from the β-cell (Nauck et al., 1986). Amylin along with insulin is instrumental in the regulation of postprandial glucose. Although insulin regulates the disappearance of glucose from the bloodstream, amylin helps to regulate the appearance of glucose in the bloodstream from the stomach and the liver.

Amylin and insulin have complementary actions in regulating glucose homeostasis. The key functions of amylin are to inhibit postprandial glucagon secretion, regulate food intake, and slow gastric emptying. Amylin suppresses glucose production during the postprandial period, when endogenous glucose is not necessary to maintain glucose concentrations. However, in persons who are insulin and amylin deficient (anyone who has T1DM or has insulin-requiring T2DM), the deficiency of amylin causes inadequate glucagon suppression after meals, excessive glucose production, and resultant hyperglycemia in the postprandial period. Through a centrally mediated modulation of appetite, food intake is decreased and, for many individuals, this decrease in food intake results in weight loss. Finally, amylin regulates the inflow of glucose from the gut after meals by restraining the rate of gastric emptying. The deficiency of amylin leads to accelerated gastric emptying. This accelerated gastric emptying also contributes to postprandial hyperglycemia (Kruger, Aronoff, & Edelman, 2007).

Because native amylin tends to self-aggregate and is insoluble in pharmaceutical diluents, a human amylin analog was developed by researchers at Amylin Pharmaceuticals and is called Pramlintide (Symlin). Pramlintide has pharmacokinetic and pharmacodynamic properties similar to human amylin. If individuals are insulin deficient, they are amylin deficient. Therefore, anyone who is on insulin is potentially a candidate for Pramlintide. A candidate for Pramlintide is someone who is not achieving adequate postprandial glucose control and is willing and able to aggressively self-monitor the blood glucose.

The willingness to test the blood glucose up to six times daily and to add three injections daily is paramount to success in using Pramlintide. However, not all patients on insulin will choose to take Pramlintide because it is given by subcutaneous injection prior to each meal and up to one snack daily. The primary side effects of taking Pramlintide are nausea and the risk for hypoglycemia, especially if the insulin dose is not titrated appropriately.

Another side effect is weight loss, which is often an added benefit to the improvement of the blood glucose levels and subsequent lowering of the A1C.

Pramlintide is given subcutaneously with an insulin syringe. For individuals with T1DM, the dose is initiated at 2½ Units (15 µg) and is increased after 3 days if the patient experiences no nausea in that 3-day period. The dose is then increased to 5 Units (30 µg), 7½ Units (45 µg), and finally to 10 Units (60 µg). For individuals with T2DM the dose is initiated at 10 Units (60 µg) and increased to 20 Units (120 µg). The dose is increased every 3 to 5 days depending on the level of nausea one may experience. Not all patients experience nausea. But if nausea is experienced, the dose should not be increased until the nausea has subsided. Some patients have chosen to stay at a lower-than-maximum dose, especially those with T1DM who only need postprandial glucose control, but do not need to lose weight.

Patients are instructed to take the Pramlintide with the first bite of food and their insulin with the last bite of food. In general, the insulin doses need to be decreased by one-third to one-half of their usual meal bolus dose. This reduction is due to physiologic changes that occur with Pramlintide and the reduction in calories. For the individual on an insulin infusion pump use of the dual-wave or extended bolus may enhance coverage of the meal. To start, one-third to one-half of the bolus may be given as a bolus and the remainder of the bolus may be given over 60–90 min to accommodate the delay in gastric uptake of the glucose from the gut. The long-acting insulin dose or basal insulin dose may or may not need to be changed. If the individual tends to "graze" on calories during the day, this may be decreased by the Pramlintide and, thus, a lower basal dose may be required. If patients tend to not eat between meals, they will likely not need to alter the basal insulin dose.

Insulin doses should be titrated carefully to prevent hypoglycemia. Individuals should test their blood glucose at fasting, 2 hr postprandial, and premeal. Frequent communication with the health professional by e-mail or telephone is valuable during the initiation and titration of Pramlintide and insulin doses. Initially, frequent contact is important to minimize the effect of potential nausea and to reduce the risk of significant hypoglycemia.

The treatment of hypoglycemia should be reviewed to ensure that individuals are using the 15 gram–15 minute rule. With the delayed gastric uptake, one would not want to use a snack with fat or protein to treat hypoglycemia. Simple carbohydrates (15 g) should be used and repeated in 15 min if the blood glucose is not greater than 70 mg after treatment. A simple carbohydrate treatment should be repeated.

The potential for nausea is present with Pramlintide. Tips to minimize nausea include taking the injection with the meal rather than 10–15 min before the meal and instructing individuals to stop eating when they are full. Oftentimes the feeling of nausea is actually the feel of overeating. Encouraging individuals to use their appetite as a guide to fullness is important.

Pramlintide should be stored much like insulin at 77°F or less. The vial or pen that is being used can be stored at room temperature; otherwise, what is not being used currently can be refrigerated.

It is important to set realistic expectations with the initiation of Pramlintide. Many individuals have been told that this is a weight loss medication. However, research shows that the average patient loses only about 6 pounds in a year (Mack et al., 2007; Ratner et al., 2002) unless the 120-µg dose level is used in patients with T2DM (Aronne et al., 2007). Postprandial hyperglycemia control is the most important role of Pramlintide.

Teaching Others

Many health professionals feel uncomfortable when they have to teach patients or family members how to give insulin. Some do not like to teach at all. Some simply have not done it often enough to really become accustomed to teaching insulin injection, or they do not know enough about how to teach it. Actual teaching is probably the best way to learn.

The following guidelines should be helpful:

1. *Learn as much as possible.* This can be done by reading and talking to others about insulin injection practices.
2. *Have self-confidence.* Remember, the health professional knows more about insulin injection than the patient, and it does not take many instruction periods for educators to feel like they have been teaching insulin injection all their lives.
3. *Be positive.* Assure the individuals that they will be able to give the injections. They may tell you that they cannot do it, but be calmly firm and refuse to take no for an answer. Do not let them off the hook. Some people take longer than others to learn, but all will eventually learn. Self-injection is something they have to do and will face, but some people are more upset by self-injection than others. Accept that fact and help them with it. The person might practice on the health professional first if the professional feels comfortable in the practice. Most will be saying, "I can't do it," while they are being given directions each step of the way. As they stick in the needle, their faces will suddenly change from fear, to surprise, and then to acceptance, not from sticking themselves or the subject, but from having mastered a task they did not believe they could do. Self-injection is then just one step away. A bright 4-year-old boy had a mother who was terrified of the injection process. She decided she would have to give herself an injection to realize that it did not hurt, before attempting to give her child an injection. After 1 hr of tears and much self-denial, she was finally able to give herself an injection. She was so pleased that she asked her son if she could give him a shot even though it was not yet time for insulin and it would have to be a dry run. He pulled up his sleeve and pinched up his skin, saying, "Do it right there." He did not even flinch, and both of them felt quite pleased with themselves.
4. *Give directions each step of way.* Do not just hand syringes to the patients and expect them to use them. Show how to select the injection site, and help

them pinch up the skin and wipe it off. Show them how to hold the syringe and the angle of the needle. Continue detailed instruction until the injection is finished and the needle is out. This will give them assurance that they are not doing something wrong.

5. *Be calm and unhurried.* Assure your patients that they will be given support and education before doing it on their own.

6. *Use the same basic approach with everyone.* Simple language works well with all people. The technique is new to them; thus, it does not matter whether they are intelligent. The simple approach can be understood. Medical terms, such as injection, may be used. If your patient feels more comfortable with the term *shot,* then use that term.

7. *Teach patients to inject in the thigh first: unless that area is contraindicated.* Use of the thigh seems to be less emotionally charged than the abdomen. They can easily see what they are doing and manipulate the equipment. Have them use the abdomen once or twice before completing the teaching, however, so that they can become accustomed to the idea.

8. *Begin teaching early.* Begin teaching insulin injection as soon as it is known that the patients will be using insulin. Do not put off injection instruction because it only causes patients the needless anxiety of knowing they will have to learn self-injection but have not begun. In addition, it is helpful to have as much time as possible for practice; if instruction is delayed, the time will be limited.

9. *Do not try to teach the entire injection process at one time.* There is too much to learn, and your patients will become confused or tired. Do it in several short sessions: injection, measurement, and review of sites. Teach the injection procedure first. This may seem backward, but the injection is the cause of the greatest anxiety. If you begin there, the rest will be easier. Occasionally the health professional has slaved over teaching the measurement of insulin and has gotten nowhere because the patient was worrying about self-injection. When the injection was performed, the patient settled down and was able to practice and succeed with measurement. Sometimes the patient can succeed in performing the self-injection but cannot measure because of poor eyesight, shakiness, or related problems. In these instances, teach someone else to measure the insulin and allow the patient to give the injection. This plan certainly helps the patient maintain independence.

10. *Alert them about the untoward side effects in a nonthreatening manner.* Lipodystrophy, more likely hypertrophy, is possible if insulin is given constantly in the same location. Insulin allergy is possible (Heinzerling, Raile, Rochlitz, Zuberbier, & Worm, 2008). Immunotherapy and/or the desensitization process, or changing brands of insulin, have been successful in treatment. If a rash is localized at the injection site, a more in-depth injection usually results in its disappearance. Please do not give your patients an orange on which to practice injections. It is strongly believed that this allows the denial of the reality of injection. Moreover, it leads patients to believe that self-injection is no harder, which is not true. Giving oneself insulin and giving an orange insulin are really not the same. If patients need a crutch, let them give *you* an injection first. For young children, the use of a rag doll is suggested. This allows children to feel that they are participating in their care even though they may not be capable of managing self-injection on

their own. Use of the doll may also serve to encourage children to act out other feelings they may have about their diabetes.

11. *Allow children to give their own injections as soon as they show interest.* They may not be capable of doing the entire procedure at first. Start them off by letting them hold up the pinch, if a pinch is needed, and push in the insulin. Then let them go for a free ride by putting their hand on top of yours, on the syringe, while you give an injection. This helps them get the feel of the action. Next, you go for the free ride and let the children do the work. They will think you are helping when actually they may be doing most of it. Even very young children can do part of the injection with encouragement and praise. Ask them to help you. When they trust you, they will usually be cooperative.

Apply these same guidelines when you are teaching family members or others involved in the care of the patient. It is advisable to have the family member perform a self-injection before giving an injection to the spouse or child. This practice is the best reassurance for family members, to let them know that they are not hurting their loved ones, and it usually frees them from any negative feelings they may have had. In addition, try to involve the whole family in the care of the patient. In this way, one person will not feel that the patient depends only on a single family member who always has to be available. Care should be a shared responsibility.

Summary

Use a portion of every hospitalization or clinic visit as a time to review the use of insulin and the injection technique. Do not assume that, just because patients have had diabetes for a while, that they know everything or that they do what they should. Ask where they inject insulin and inspect the sites.

Review the importance of site rotation. If they have any site problems, make appropriate recommendations—that is, better rotation or different technique.

If there is a question of visual accuracy, ask them to measure their insulin doses for you. Many times these reviews help to identify a problem in control that had not been recognized previously.

If the person has difficulty drawing up an accurate dose, vision may be a problem. Several products assist the person in drawing up and getting an accurate dose (a catalog is available through the Department for the Blind and Vision Impaired [www.vdbvi.org] or the Center for Vision Impaired (www.cviatlanta.org), among others.

Develop an attitude of helpfulness, not of criticism. Assure the patients that you want what is best for them and their management of diabetes. Even hostile patients will often come around and recognize how well they feel when blood glucose levels are controlled by insulin and when they feel you are really concerned and interested in them.

References

Ahern, B. (2005). What mediates the benefits associated with dipeptidyl peptidase 4 (DPP-4 or IV) inhibition? *Diabetologia, 48*(4), 605–607.

Al-Khenaizan, S., Al-Thubaiti, M., & Al-Alwan, I. (2007). Lispro insulin-induced lipoatrophy: A new case. *Pediatric Diabetes, 8*(6), 393–396.

American Diabetes Association. (2004a). Continuous subcutaneous insulin infusion. *Diabetes Care, 27*(Suppl. 1), S110.

American Diabetes Association. (2004b). Insulin administration. *Diabetes Care, 27*(Suppl. 1), S106–S109.

American Diabetes Association Resource Guide. (2008). Retrieved on April 9, 2008 from www.diabetes.org/diabetesforecast/RG22/RG 24/RG25insulindelivery.pdf

Aronne, L., Fujioka, K., Aroda, V., Chen, K., Halseth, A., Kesty, N. C., et al. (2007). Progressive reduction in body weight after treatment with the amylin analogue Pramlintide in obese subjects: A phase 2, randomized, placebo-controlled dose escalation study. *Journal of Clinical Endocrinology and Metabolism, 92*(8), 2977–2983.

Aziz, S. (1984). Recurrent use of disposable syringe-needle units in diabetic children. *Diabetes Care, 7,* 118–120.

Banting, F. (1925). *Diabetes and insulin.* Nobel lecture. September 15, Stockholm, Sweden.

Berger, M. (2000). Safety of insulin glargine. *Lancet, 356*(9246), 2013–2014.

Bosquet, F., Grimaldi, A., & Thervel, F. (1986). Insulin syringe reuse (letter). *Diabetes Care, 9,* 31.

Edelman, S. W. (2008). Optimizing treatment success with an amylin analogue. *The Diabetes Educator, 34*(Suppl.1), 45–105.

Eli Lilly and Company. (2008a). Humalog package insert. Retrieved on April 9, 2008, from http://pi.lilly.com/us/humalog-pen-i.pdf

Eli Lilly and Company. (2008b). Humalog 75/25 package insert. Retrieved on April 8, 2008, from http://pi.lilly.com/us/humalog-pen-i.pdf

Fleming, D. R., Jacober, S. J., Vandenberg, M. A., Fitzgerald, J. T., & Grunberger, G. (1997). The safety of injecting insulin through clothing. *Diabetes, 20,* 244–247.

Franklin, V. L., Bluff, S., Ramsay, V., Stirrock, C., Greene, S. A., & Alexander, V. (2007). Unexplained hypoglycaemia on a pump. *Pediatric Diabetes, 8*(6), 391–392.

Galloway, J. A. (1980). Insulin treatment in the early 80's. *Diabetes Care, 3,* 615–622.

Galloway, J. A. (1993). New directions in drug development: Mixtures, analogues, and modeling. *Diabetes Care, 16*(Suppl. 3), 16–23.

Glazer, N. B., Zalani, S., Anderson, J. H., Jr., & Bastyr, E. J. (1999). Safety of insulin lispro: Pooled data from clinical trials. *American Journal of Health-System Pharmacy, 56*(6), 542–547.

Grajower, M. M., Fraser, J. H., Holcolme, J. H., Daugherty, W. C., De Flippis, M. R., Santiago, O. M., et al. (2003). How long should insulin be used once a vial is started? *Diabetes Care, 26,* 2665–2666.

Greenough, A., Cockcroft, P. M., & Bloom, A. (1979). Disposable syringes for insulin injection. *British Medical Journal, 2,* 1467–1468.

Heinzerling, L., Raile, K., Rochlitz, H., Zuberbier, T., & Worm, M. (2008). Insulin allergy: Clinical manifestations and management strategies. *Allergy, 63*(2), 148–155.

Hirsch, I. B., Bode, B. W., Garg, S., Lane, W. S., Sussman, A., Hu, P., et al., for the Insulin Aspart CSSI/MDI Comparison Study Group. (2005). Continuous subcutaneous insulin infusion (CSII) of insulin aspart versus multiple daily injections of insulin aspart/insulin glargine in type 1 diabetic patients previously treated with CSII. *Diabetes Care, 28,* 533–538.

Kaordonouri, O., Lauterborn, R., & Deiss, D. (2002). Lipohypertrophy in young patients with type 1 diabetes. *Diabetes Care, 25*(3), 634.

Kruger, D. F., Aronoff, S. L., & Edelman, S. V. (2007). Through the looking glass: Current and future perspectives on the role of hormonal interplay in glucose homeostasis. *The Diabetes Educator, 33,* s32–s46.

Mack, C., Wilson, J., Athanacio, J., Reynolds, J., Laugero, K., Guss, S., et al. (2007). Pharmacological actions of the peptide hormone amylin in the long term regulation of food intake, food preferences, and body weight. *American Journal of Pharmacologic Regulation, Integration, Composition Physiology, 293*(5), R1855–R1863.

Mudaliar, S., Lindberg, F., Joyce, M., Beerdsen, P., Strange, P., Lin, A., et al. (1999). Insulin aspart: A fast-acting analog of human insulin: Absorption kinetics and action profile compared with regular human insulin in healthy non-diabetic subjects. *Diabetes Care, 22*(9), 1501–1506.

Nauck, M. A., Homberger, E., Siegel, E. G., Allen, R. C., Eaton, R. P., Ebert, R., et al. (1986). Incretin effects of increasing glucose loads in man calculated from venous insulin and C-peptide responses. *Journal of Clinical Endocrinology and Metabolism, 63*(2), 492–498.

Novo Nordisk. (2008). Levemir package insert. Retrieved April 9, 2008, from www.levemirus. com/patient prescribing-information asp

Novo Nordisk. (2008). Novolog package insert. Retrieved April 9, 2008, from www.novolog.com/ Novol.or_Prescribing_Info.pdf

Ratner, R. E., Want, L. L., Fineman, M. S., Velte, M. J., Ruggles, J. A., Gottlieb, A., et al. (2002). Adjunctive therapy with the amylin analogue pramlintide leads to a combined improvement in glycemic and weight control in insulin-treated subjects with type 2 diabetes. *Diabetes Technology Therapy, 4*(1), 51–61.

Sanofi-Aventis. (2008). Apidra package insert. Retrieved April 9, 2008, from http://products. sanofi-aventis.us/apidra.html

Sanofi-Aventis. (2008). Lantus package insert. Retrieved April 9, 2008, from http://products. sanofi-aventis.us/lantus/lantus.html

Scrimgeour, L., Cobry, E., McFann, K., Burdick, P., Weimer, C., Slover, R., et al. (2007). Improved glycemic control after long-term insulin pump use in pediatric patients with type 1 diabetes. *Diabetes Technology & Therapy, 9*(5), 421–428.

Thurman, J. E. (2007). Insulin pen injection devices for management of patients with type 2 diabetes: Considerations based on an endocrinologist's practical experience in the United States. *Endocrinology Practice, 13*(6), 672–678.

Turner, J. G., & Lancaster, J. (1984). Multiple use of disposable syringes by 1000: Incidence of inflammation at injection sites. *The Diabetes Educator, 10,* 38–41.

Wentworth, S. M., Galloway, J. A., Haunz, E. A., Duncan, T. G., Klink, D. D., & Kirtley, W. R. (1973). The use of purified insulins in the treatment of patients with insulin lipoatrophy. *Diabetes, 22*(Suppl. 2), 290.

Zehrer, C., Hansen, R., & Bantle, J. (1991). Reducing blood glucose variability by the use of abdominal insulin injection sites. *The Diabetes Educator, 16,* 474–476.

10

Nutrition in Type 1 Diabetes Mellitus

Medical nutrition therapy (MNT) is a key component in diabetes management. Following nutrition and meal-planning recommendations can often be the most challenging part of diabetes care. The key to satisfactory management of diabetes lies in sound, realistic education and an individualized meal plan appropriate for the patient's treatment program and lifestyle. Frequently, the nutrition of the whole family improves when meals are planned around the eating recommendations given to the family member with diabetes. The nutritional guidelines for persons with diabetes are based on the recommendations of good nutrition for all Americans for overall health and optimal nutrition from the 2005 Dietary Guidelines (U.S. Department of Health and Human Services, 2005), and the recommended dietary allowances (Institute of Medicine, 2002). The Diabetes Control and Complications Trial (DCCT) also contributed to the importance of behaviors related to nutrition and achieving glycemic control (Delahanty & Halford, 1993).

In their position statement, the American Diabetes Association (ADA) (2008) describes science-based nutrition recommendations for the individual with diabetes. The goal of this report is to make people with diabetes and health care providers aware of beneficial nutrition interventions. Education should consist of basic nutrition plus a goal-oriented treatment plan and the individual must have a diet that supplies all the necessary calories and nutrients for normal growth, development, and activity. The key to achieving effective dietary control consists of an understanding of the nutrient composition of food, time actions of insulin, diabetes medications, exercise, monitoring, and diabetes management skills.

Referral to a registered dietitian for medical nutrition therapy is recommended (ADA, 2005). Studies of MNT provided by a registered dietitian have reported decreases of A1C of approximately 1% in Type 1 diabetes (T1DM; Pastors, Warshaw, Daly, Franz, & Kulkarni, 2002). There is no specific diabetic diet or ADA diet and the use of preprinted menus in place of nutrition counseling is strongly discouraged. An individualized, flexible plan that allows for a variety of food choices and input on food preferences is far more likely to be implemented and may result in healthy food habits and long-range diabetes control. Furthermore, the term diet often has the negative connotation of starvation and denial; therefore, meal planning may be preferable to use in counseling. As opposed to diet advice in the past, sugar and sweets are not the focus of diabetes nutrition care and a general admonition at diagnosis to avoid sugar is misleading. All members of the diabetes team should be knowledgeable about MNT and continually assess food, insulin, and activity for optimal diabetes management.

Specific Goals

The following are specific ADA Nutrition Recommendations and Interventions for Diabetes (2007):

1. Achieve and maintain:

   ■ Blood glucose levels in the normal range or as close to normal as is safely possible.
   ■ A lipid and lipoprotein profile that reduces the risk for vascular disease.
   ■ Blood pressure levels in the normal range or as close to normal as is safely possible.

2. Prevent, or at least slow, the rate of development of the chronic complications of diabetes by modifying nutrient intake and lifestyle.
3. Address individual nutrition needs, taking into account personal and cultural preferences and willingness to change.
4. Maintain the pleasure of eating by only limiting food choices when indicated by scientific evidence.

   Goals of MNT that apply to specific situations:

1. For youth with T1DM (ADA, 2005), meet the nutritional needs of the unique times in the life cycle.
2. For individuals treated with insulin, provide self-management training for safe conduct of exercise, including the prevention and treatment of hypoglycemia and diabetes treatment during acute illness.

MNT, including assessment, goals, intervention, monitoring, and evaluation, is necessary immediately after the diagnosis of diabetes. The goal is to educate and support the person with diabetes in becoming an independent decision maker. It is essential to consider the person with diabetes as the center of the diabetes team. When the health professional respects the individual's lifestyle and food issues, the professional will make only the dietary changes that are absolutely necessary. Fortunately, MNT has evolved from rigid, difficult diets to flexible, patient-centered strategies. As our concern for the individual becomes more evident in medical nutrition therapy, we will see greater responsibility taken by the person who has diabetes and more successful self-management.

Nutrition Assessment

Nutritional needs can be determined through interviews including the client and family, medical records, consultant evaluations, and dietary history. Assessment requires a thorough analysis of the following factors:

- Physiologic data, such as laboratory data and clinical data, that reveal height, weight, growth charts if applicable, body mass index, blood pressure, pulse rate, skin color and texture, vision and hearing, dental and oral hygiene, and medications.
- Environmental data, such as ethnic and cultural orientation, education, religion, economic situation, living conditions, recreation, hobbies, exercise or physical activity, and family health.
- Behavioral data, such as readiness to learn, eating habits, and the usual schedule related to eating.
- Food intake data, such as diet history that reveals food preferences, food rejections, meals eaten per day and week, regularity of meals, eating out, supplemental vitamins and minerals, current meal plan, and general knowledge of nutrition.

Many forms are available to obtain food histories (refer to Appendix J: Nutrition Assessment). The 24-hr food intake record may report the food and drink intake of 1 or more days. A 3- to 5-day food and drink record is preferred for assessment, including a weekend day, if possible. Assessments are needed, as demonstrated by Ford and Mokdad (2001) in their work on fruits and vegetable consumption by people in the United States who had diabetes. Because the most accurate method for evaluating the adequacy of food intake uses the computer, numerous computer programs are available for analysis of food intake. MyPyramid (U.S. Department of Agriculture [USDA], 2005) illustrates nutritional recommendations for all healthy Americans, including people with diabetes and their families. The pyramid can be used as an assessment tool. *Points in Your Favor* (Friesen, 2000) includes a variety of resources, useful for both the professional and the lay person in understanding and planning food intake. *Dietary Reference Intakes* (Institute of Medicine, 2002) is a useful tool indicating a number of nutrients and the recommended values that should be included in meal planning.

Nutrition Intervention

Intervention strategy depends on the assessment of dietary history and on individual needs. A patient-centered or empowerment approach including problem solving and adjustments can improve compliance. Dietitians plan goals to prioritize nutrition implementation and education with the patient and family. The goals established should help the patient with diabetes to make positive changes that will result in improvements in blood glucose levels, lipid levels, and nutrient intake. The meal-planning objective is to coordinate food intake, insulin action, and exercise to achieve glucose goals. This approach must assist the patient and family in learning the effect of food on blood glucose levels. Including the family, especially those family members involved in meal planning, is most important. Goals should be reasonable and negotiable.

Approaches to Meal Planning

Carbohydrate Counting

Carbohydrate is a major factor in insulin requirements, so carbohydrate counting has become a prevalent meal-planning approach. Resources for patients to use in carbohydrate counting are available from the American Dietetic Association (2001) and the American Dietetic Association (Daly, Bolderman, Franz, & Kulkarni, 2003a, 2003b). Food labels list the grams of carbohydrates in each food, and books that list the grams of carbohydrate in food are readily available. Carbohydrate counting is used by many people on insulin pumps.

A meal plan can be developed based on grams of carbohydrate to be eaten at each meal (and snacks, when needed). Or, 15-g carbohydrate portions can be counted at each meal and snack. This follows the exchange portions for starch, fruit, and milk groups. In its simplest form, carbohydrate counting is used to focus on consistency in food intake. The next level of education focuses on adjustment of food, medication, and activity based on patterns of daily records. Advanced carbohydrate counting is determining ratios of insulin units to carbohydrate grams by using blood glucose results for intensive insulin therapy and insulin pump therapy. The dietitian is a good resource for initial and follow-up education and support, that is, a dietitian, after initial education, should be seen at least once a year.

When carbohydrate counting is used, the protein and fat content of food must be considered because of the calories they add, the potential for weight gain, and the effect on blood glucose, especially in large portion sizes.

Exchange Lists

The *Choose Your Foods: Exchange Lists for Diabetes* (2008) by the ADA and the American Dietetic Association is based on food groups. The list of foods in one group contains somewhat similar amounts of carbohydrate, protein, fat, and nutrients. Individuals are to choose a food from an exchange list as indicated in their meal plan. They may exchange one food for another within the same allowed group. Exchange lists have been published since 1950 and were revised in 1976, 1986, 1995, 2003, and 2007. Since the 1995 revision, the lists reflect the emphasis on the amount of carbohydrates consumed rather than the type of carbohydrate. An additional list, Sweets, Desserts, and Other Carbohydrates, was added, incorporating more foods into the exchange lists. A very-lean-meat group was added for fat-free protein choices. Any food within a list can be substituted or exchanged for any other food in that list. For example, in list 1, the starch exchange contains one slice of bread, ½ cup of cooked cereal, ⅓ cup of rice, and many other foods that would contain 15 g of carbohydrate or approximately 80 calories. A patient told to eat two exchanges from the starch list could choose any two foods in the amounts listed or two portions of one food. Two slices of bread would be the equivalent of two starch exchanges as would one slice of bread and a ⅓ cup of rice. This same procedure is followed for the fruit list, which is equivalent to 15 g of carbohydrate or 60 calories. Of course, choosing a nutritious meal plan is important for good health, so knowing protein and fat recommendations is necessary.

Total daily exchanges of each food group are determined, then the exchanges are distributed into meals (and snacks as needed). A meal plan may be developed from the assessment and diet history. The best approach to distributing food is based on the individual's typical eating pattern tailored to a medication regime.

The First Step in Diabetes Meal Planning (ADA and ADA, 2003) presents very basic nutrition education as the introduction to meal planning. In-depth counseling should follow as part of the total program and the use of the *Choose Your Foods* (2008), along with or in place of the 2003 booklet.

Calorie Point System

The calorie points system is based on the principle that one calorie point equals 75 calories (Friesen, 2000). All calories count in the management of blood glucose, blood pressure, lipids, and body weight. Food can easily be assigned a calorie point value based on the calorie content (divided by 75). Many common portions such as 1 egg, 1 slice of bread, 1 orange, 1 cup of skim milk, 1 ounce of hamburger, or 1 apple are equal to 1 calorie point. The daily calorie allowance is divided by 75. Counting 20 calorie points is easier than counting 1,500 calories. The total daily points are distributed into meals and snacks according to individual needs and the medication regime. Table 10.1 compares food groups with calories and calorie points. Table 10.2 shares a 1-day sample menu using calorie points. Refer to Table 10.3 for calorie points related to various plans for meals and snacks of various calorie levels.

Points can be used to calculate insulin doses based on intake in exactly the same way it is done in carbohydrate counting for intensive insulin therapy and insulin pump therapy. In fact, carbohydrate counting is basically a version of earlier point systems.

Meal Planning Application

Effective use of any meal planning approach depends on accurately measuring food. When persons are first learning, weighing or measuring assists them in recognizing the size of servings and in realizing the importance of accuracy.

10.1 Comparing Food Groups With Calories and Calorie Points

	Carbohydrate	Protein	Fat	Calories	Cal. Points
Starch/bread/cereals/ vegetables		15	3	Trace–80	1
Meats					
Very lean meats	–	7	0–1	35	½
Lean meats	–	7	3	55	¾
Medium-fat meats	–	7	5	75	1
High-fat meats	–	7	8	100	1½
6% Vegetables	5	2	–	25	½
Fruits	15	–	–	60	1
Dairy/milk					
Skim	12	8	Trace	90	1
Low-fat	12	8	5	120	1½
Whole	12	8	8	150	2
Fats/nuts/dressings	–	–	5	45	½

The amount of food eaten makes such a major impact on blood glucose that a common term now is portion distortion. The portion of rice in a serving is ⅓ cup, but the usual portion of rice at an Asian restaurant is 2 cups. The discrepancy in portion size affects insulin adjustments and the postprandial glucose significantly. It takes time and practice to learn the portions for insulin adjustments (one carbohydrate portion, one calorie point, or one exchange portion). Once the patient has learned accurate portions, estimations can be made, then occasional reevaluation of estimated serving sizes may be needed. It is especially necessary to begin measuring food again if blood glucose levels rise, or if the A1C increases.

Patients using intensive insulin management consisting of basal insulin and bolus insulin doses or insulin pumps have flexibility in the timing of meals, the frequency of meals, the amount eaten at meals, and the timing of physical activity. Self-management education is the foundation of glycemic control. Patients learn to use blood glucose monitoring results to evaluate the balance of food, exercise, insulin, and the effectiveness of food and exercise changes to meet glucose goals. MNT discussions with caregivers and children with T1DM may include nutrition issues for school and day care, flexible schedules, sports, peer influence, hormonal effects on blood glucose, growth, and development (American Association of Diabetes Educators [AADE], 2006).

10.2 Possible *Individualized* Meal Pattern (About 1,700 Calories)

Amount in Food Group	75 Cal.=1 Point	15 g CHO= 1 Carb	Example
Breakfast			
1 c. skim milk	1 Point	1 Carb	1 c nonfat
1 piece of fruit	1 Point	1 Carb	1 orange
2 grain-based foods	2 Points	2 Carb	½ c cereal and 1 slice wg bread
1 meat serving	1 Point	0 CHO	1 oz ham
1 tsp fat	½ Point	0 Carb	1 tsp margarine
Coffee or tea (any amount)	—	—	N/A
Subtotal	5 ½ Points	4 Carbs	
Midmorning snack			
1 piece of fruit	1 Point	1 Point	1 apple, small
Subtotal	1 Point	1 Carb	
Lunch or supper			
1 c skim milk	1 Point	1 Carb	1 c nonfat milk
1 serving of fruit	1 Point	1 Carb	2 small plums
2 grain-based foods	2 Points	2 Carbs	2 slices bread
2 meat servings	2 Points	0–1 CHO*	2 oz of low-fat lunch meat
1 serving of fat	½ Point	0 Carb	1 tsp mayonnaise
__ Coffee or tea (any amount)	—	—	N/A
Subtotal	7 Points	5–5 ½ Carbs	
Afternoon snack			
½ c skim milk	½ Point	½ Carb	½ c nonfat milk
Subtotal	½ Point	½ Carb	
Dinner or main meal			
½ c skim milk	½ Point	½ Carb	½ c nonfat milk
1 c 3%–6% vegetables	½ Point	0–½ CHO	½ c beets
½ c 12% vegetables	1 Point	1 Carb	½ c mashed potatoes
1 piece of fruit	1 Point	1 Carb	1 medium peach
1 grain-based food	1 Points	1 Carb	1 slice wg bread
2 meat servings	2 Points	0–1 CHO*	2 oz roast beef
1 serving of fat	½ Point	0 Carb	1 tbsp gravy

(continued)

		Possible *Individualized* Meal Pattern (About 1,700 Calories) (*continued*)	

Amount in Food Group	75 Cal.=1 Point	15 g CHO= 1 Carb	Example
__ Coffee or tea (any amount)	—	—	N/A
Subtotal	6 ½ Points	4–5 Carbs	
Bedtime snack			
1 serving of grain	1 Point	½ Carb	4 wg crackers
1 meat serving	1 Point	0–½ Carb	1 oz low-fat cheese
Subtotal	2 Points	½–1 Carb	
Total	1,700 Cal	22½ Points	14½–16½ Carbs

CHO* = Carb equivalent or 1 protein = ½ CHO. wg = whole grain. ªFor detailed information, see *Points in Your Favor* by J. Friesen, contact at 1-316-689-6050, or *Calorie-Carbohydrate Controlled Diet* (2005). C. L. Gerwick & Assoc., at www.clgerwick.com.

Nutrition Recommendations

Medical nutrition therapy for T1DM is prescribed to meet the treatment goals and desired outcomes. In youth, nutrient recommendations are based on requirements for all healthy children and adolescents because there is no research on the nutrient requirements specifically in diabetes. In general, U.S. children are not eating recommended amounts of fruit, vegetables, and fiber and are consuming saturated fat well above the National Cholesterol Education Program (NCEP) (Expert Panel Committee, 2001) recommendations.

Some form of regularity of food intake appears to promote diabetes control, in particular, in those persons receiving insulin therapy. Most important is that the meal plan matches the action time of the individual's insulin. Medical nutrition therapy for T1DM includes adequate calories for growth and development needs and timing to match insulin's time action. Distributing calories into meals and snacks for young children has been used effectively by Jackson and Guthrie (1986). In patients using rapid-acting insulin in basal-bolus insulin therapy, snacks are not needed but should still be considered for bedtime, for growth, and for extra activity if the previous dose of insulin has not been decreased to meet the demands of the duration and intensity of the activity. Rapid-acting insulin or a pump bolus will be needed for snacks that are not required for extra exercise. A general guideline (Childs & Cypress, 2005) is that additional insulin is not necessary if the snack is less than 120 calories or 20 g of carbohydrates, but snacks with more than 120 calories or 20 g of carbohydrate may require extra rapid-acting insulin. Children under the age of 6 years typically prefer three meals and three snacks daily. Older children may want three meals plus afternoon (after school) and bedtime snacks. Snacks can be adjusted to

10.3 Suitable for Children—Add Snacks to Meals for Adults

		Breakfast	Morning	Lunch	Afternoon	Evening	Bedtime
	Cal	Meal	Snack	Meal	Snack	Meal	Snack
Cal[a]	Points	$\frac{4}{18}$	$\frac{1}{18}$	$\frac{5}{18}$	$\frac{2}{18}$	$\frac{5}{18}$	$\frac{1}{18}$
500	7	2	Free food	2	Free food	2	1
800	11	2.5	0.5	3	1	3	1
900	12	2.5	1	3	1.5	3	1
1,000	13.5	3	1	3.5	1.5	3.5	1
1,100	14.5	3	1	4	1.5	4	1
1,200	16	3.5	1	4.5	1.5	4.5	1
1,300	17.5	4	1	5	2	5.5	1
1,400	18.5	4	1	5	2	5.5	1
1,500	20	4.5	1	5.5	2	5.5	1.5
1,600	21.5	5	1	6	2	6	1.5
1,700	22.5	5	1	6	2.5	6.5	1.5
1,800	24	5.5	1.5	6.5	2.5	6.5	1.5
1,900	25.5	5.5	1.5	7	3	7	1.5
2,000	26.5	6	1.5	7	3	7	2
2,100	28	6	1.5	8	3	8	1.5
2,200	29.5	6.5	1.5	8	3.5	8.5	1.5
2,300	31	7	1.5	8.5	3.5	8.5	2

[a]75 cal = one calorie point.

individual preference. Caregivers of youth need to be carefully educated to not withhold food in an effort to control blood glucose because withholding food can result in inadequate calories for growth (AADE, 2006).

It is crucial that meals (and snacks, if needed) are distributed and insulin is adjusted to prevent hypoglycemia from occurring. The best program can be determined by observation and assessment during follow-up and adjustment based on glucose monitoring.

Nutrient Specific

Calories

The calorie recommendations for T1DM are the same as for persons who do not have diabetes. At diagnosis, patients with T1DM often present with weight loss that must be restored with insulin initiation, hydration, and adequate calories. As calorie requirements change with age, activity, and growth, evaluation of the nutrition plan is recommended at each diabetes checkup, but at a minimum of every year. Good metabolic control is essential for normal growth and development. Parents of children with diabetes should be educated to adjust the insulin dose (in consultation with their health care provider) rather than restrict food intake to control blood glucose levels. In children, adequacy of energy intake can be evaluated by weight gain and growth patterns and by asking the children whether they get enough to eat. Children and adolescents should be monitored on a weight and height growth grid every 3–6 months.

Adequate calories must be provided for growth and the maintenance of a healthy weight. It is essential that the person with T1DM always receive adequate calories. Too often the person who is not obese receives a prescription of reduced calories because the health professional is accustomed to restricting calories for the obese person. In the hospital, inactive individuals may say they are receiving adequate amounts of food. Because of their inactivity and the greater bulk in low-calorie foods, they may think their diet is adequate. After discharge from the hospital, they may find it necessary to cheat because their calorie intake is less than their body requires. They have inadequate adipose tissue to compensate for the deficiency in calorie consumption. They soon discover that they feel better when cheating or when those counting carbohydrates add excessive fat and protein calories to fill up. No one can tolerate calorie deficiencies unless they are overweight. Nonobese individuals have a protein deficiency if they have a calorie deficiency. With appropriate caloric intake and metabolic control, children and adolescents with diabetes will grow and mature at normal rates. Growth charts are vital to assess growth rate.

Carbohydrates

Carbohydrate foods are plant foods (i.e., fruits, vegetables, and grains), sweets, and the lactose in milk. The percentage of calories from carbohydrate will vary, based on the patient's eating habits and glucose and lipid levels. It has been assumed that complex carbohydrates are digested and absorbed more slowly than simple sugars, and therefore yield flatter blood glucose responses. This assumption has changed and, since 1994, ADA nutrition principles report that restriction of sucrose in the diabetic diet is not justified based on glycemic control (Franz et al., 2002). If consumed, it is recommended that sucrose-containing foods should be substituted for other foods in the meal plan. A dietary pattern including carbohydrate from fruit, vegetable, whole grains, legumes, and low fat milk is encouraged for good health. Low-carbohydrate diets restricting carbohydrate to less than 130 g daily was not recommended (ADA, 2007).

Fiber

Recommendations for fiber intake are the same for individuals with diabetes as for the general population: 14 g/1,000 calories (Institute of Medicine, 2002). Soluble fibers are found in legumes (dried beans), oats, barley, and some vegetables. Insoluble fibers are found in grains such as wheat and corn and in some vegetables. Fiber may improve glycemia, lipids, and gut motility, preventing gastrointestinal disorders, including colon cancer, and providing satiety in the diet. The effect of carbohydrate absorption, especially fiber, which may have beneficial metabolic effects in diabetes, continues to be studied.

Protein

The amount of protein recommended for adults is based on kilograms of ideal body weight. For adults, the recommendation is 0.8 g of protein per kilogram of ideal weight. Adequate amounts are necessary for growing children and pregnant women according to the recommended dietary allowances (Institute of Medicine, 2002). Too often patients try to minimize carbohydrate, which leads to an increase in the intake of protein and fat. Because of the higher intake of saturated fatty acids that may occur with increased meat and cheese, it may be prudent to use more vegetable proteins, such as beans and legumes. Research has been completed on the use of high-protein intake and weight loss (Clifton, Keough, & Noakes, 2008). Studies continue to be needed to determine whether the course of diabetic nephropathy can be altered by protein intake.

Fat

Research provides substantial evidence that fat modifications in the diet may improve plasma lipid levels and decrease cardiovascular disease. Several diet factors influence the incidence of developing macrovascular disease in diabetes. The primary goal is to decrease intake of saturated fat, trans fat, and cholesterol. Saturated fat intake should be less than 7% of total calories, trans fat should be minimal, and cholesterol intake is recommended to be less than 200 mg daily. Monounsaturated fats, which are peanut oil, olive oil, and canola oil, and omega 3 fatty acids, which are in fish, flax, canola oil, soybean oil, and nuts, are recommended for their cardioprotective benefits (ADA, 2007).

Micronutrients

There is no clear evidence of the benefit of vitamin, mineral, antioxidant, or herbal supplementation in diabetes for patients who do not have nutrient deficiencies. Exceptions are folate for the prevention of birth defects and calcium for bone health. The micronutrients most commonly mentioned in regard to diabetes are chromium, magnesium, folate, B vitamins, calcium, zinc, vanadium, and antioxidants. The response to supplements is mostly determined by nutritional status, so that only people with deficiencies are likely to respond favorably. Laboratory values may help to document deficiencies and provide evaluation of treatment. Regular assessment of supplement intake provides an opportunity to discuss with the patient fads that may affect diabetes and provide insight into the patient's health practices. Persons who may benefit from supplementation include pregnant and lactating women, older individuals, strict vegetarians, and patients on calorie-restricted diets (ADA, 2008). Persons with diabetes should receive education regarding the importance of a healthy diet and the potential toxicity of megadoses of supplements.

Alcohol

Precautions for alcohol use in persons with diabetes are basically the same as those that apply to the general public, with additional consideration for glycemic control, prevention of hypoglycemia, hyperlipidemia, and weight control. The evidence-based nutrition principles (ADA, 2008) recommend no more than two drinks per day for men and no more than one drink per day for women. One equivalent is equal to a 1.5-oz shot of distilled beverage, a 5-oz glass of wine, or 12 oz of beer. Alcoholic beverages should be consumed only with food. An alcohol equivalent may be taken in addition to the usual meal plan in individuals with T1DM, with no food omitted because alcohol is not converted to glucose and does not require insulin for metabolism (Franz, 2001).

Alcohol is best avoided for diabetes control. The effect of alcohol on glucose depends on the amount of alcohol ingested relative to food. Alcohol inhibits gluconeogenesis so that hypoglycemia can result if alcohol is consumed without food. The hypoglycemic effect may occur up to 12 hr after the last drink. Possible problems resulting from alcohol misuse include hypoglycemia, neuropathy, malnutrition, impaired glycemic control, hyperlipidemia, and alcohol abuse, and alcohol may interact with medications. Abstention from alcohol should be advised in cases of pancreatitis, neuropathy, hypertriglyceridemia, history of alcohol abuse, and pregnancy.

Sick Days

Illness requires individualized adjustment of food intake and insulin, but general guidelines can be recommended. Illness may cause days when the meal plan cannot be followed. Patients must be reminded of the necessity of always eating or drinking foods that supply calories. Sugar-containing fluids such as juice or regular soda will be necessary if the patient cannot eat, is vomiting, or has diarrhea. During illness, endogenous carbohydrate continues to be metabolized, and individuals should not omit their insulin or calories. The carbohydrate content of some sick-day foods is listed in Table 10.4.

Fluids are essential. Ideally, sips should be taken every 5–10 min or 1 cup/hr. In adults, drinking 45–50 g of carbohydrate every 3–4 hr should be sufficient to prevent starvation ketosis (ADA, 2007). Illness can lead to hyperglycemia and ketoacidosis, so testing plasma glucose and ketones is important. Guidelines should be available for when to call for professional assistance if glucose levels or hydration cannot be controlled.

Monitoring and Evaluation

A plan for ongoing nutrition care is essential to successful diabetes management. Adults should be seen every six months to one year or as changes occur in work schedule, activity, for MNT or health status, such as complications. Because of rapid

10.4 Sick-Day Carbohydrate Equivalents[a]	
Food	Amount
Gelatin dessert, sweetened	½ cup
Fruit juice	½ cup
Popsicle	1
Sherbet	¼ cup
Soft drinks, regular (preferably noncaffeinated)	½ cup
Sugar	4 tsp

[a]Approximately 15 g of carbohydrate = 60 cal or 1 point.

growth, young children with T1DM need close monitoring by registered dietitians to ensure that their individualized diet plans are modified appropriately as they grow (Patton, Lawrence, & Powers, 2007). Children should be seen at least every 6 months, preferably every 3 months, to assess growth and development.

The health professional can evaluate how well the individual has learned and applied diabetes education through review of the patient's food and blood glucose records, physical examination, and measurements of height, weight, growth, and laboratory values. Physical, psychologic, intellectual, social, and economic barriers that affect the individual's ability to implement a meal plan should be noted. Professionals must praise the positive, as well as revise, adjust, and educate as needed. It is important for them to emphasize that patients have not failed if the diabetes plan has not improved their blood glucose control. A change in food or medications is a natural progression in diabetes care, and whenever new plans are implemented, they must be evaluated. Coordination with diabetes team members is essential to diabetes management. As needs are identified, the patient may benefit from referrals to the dietitian, counselor, or exercise specialist. Follow-up is necessary for continuing education, updating the meal plan, and providing support.

Summary

The primary goal of nutrition in diabetes is to promote positive behavioral changes and optimal health. This requires an individualized meal plan and nutrition counseling appropriate for management goals and lifestyle. For individuals with T1DM, the primary considerations are adjusting food, insulin, and activity for glucose control. For some patients, appropriate traditional, ethnic, and cultural foods must be incorporated into meal planning. Nutrition education optimally progresses from initial teaching of survival skills through phases of increasing information acquisition, new skills, problem solving, identifying and overcoming barriers, continuing education, and reinforcement with the ultimate goal of positive behavioral changes and glycemic control. The best approach includes a multidisciplinary team using creative skills in education and counseling. Medical nutrition therapy (MNT) including individual planning with each patient is essential. No special dietetic or diabetic foods are required, and the meals should be no more expensive than meals for the general population. The guidelines can be incorporated for the entire family, and all family members may benefit from improved knowledge of nutrition.

References

American Association of Diabetes Educators. (2006). *The art and science of diabetes self-management education*. Chicago: Author.

American Diabetes Association. (2005). ADA Statement: Care of children and adolescents with Type 1 diabetes. *Diabetes Care, 28,* 186–212.

American Diabetes Association. (2007). Nutrition recommendations and interventions for diabetes. *Diabetes Care, 30*(Suppl. 1), S48–S65.

American Diabetes Association. (2008). Nutrition recommendations and interventions for diabetes. *Diabetes Care, 31*(Suppl. 1), S61–S78.

American Diabetes Association and American Dietetic Association. (2003). *Exchange lists for meal planning: The first step in diabetes meal planning.* Alexandria, VA: American Diabetes Association, and Chicago: American Dietetic Association.

American Diabetes Association and American Dietetic Association. (2008). *Choose your foods: Exchange lists for diabetes.* Alexandria, VA: American Diabetes Association, and Chicago: American Dietetic Association.

American Dietetic Association. (2001). *ADA medical nutrition therapy evidence based guidelines for practice for Type 1 and Type 2 diabetes.* Chicago: Author.

Childs, B. P., & Cypress, M. (Eds.) (2005). *Complete nurse's guide to diabetes care.* Alexandria, VA: American Diabetes Association.

Clifton, P. M., Keogh, J. B., & Noakes, M. (2008). Long-term effects of a high-protein weight-loss diet. *American Journal of Clinical Nutrition, 87*(1), 23–29.

Daly, A., Bolderman, K., Franz, M., & Kulkarni, K. (2003a). *Basic carbohydrate counting.* Alexandria, VA: American Diabetes Association, and Chicago: American Dietetic Association.

Daly, A., Bolderman, K., Franz, M., & Kulkarni, K. (2003b). *Advanced carbohydrate counting.* Alexandria VA: American Diabetes Association, and Chicago: American Dietetic Association.

Delahanty, L. M., & Halford, B. N. (1993). The role of diet behaviors in achieving improved glycemic control in intensively treated patients in the Diabetes Control and Complications Trial. *Diabetes Care, 16,* 1453–1458.

Expert Panel Committee on Detection, Evaluation, and Treatment of High Blood Cholesterol in Adults. (2001). Summary of the third report of the National Cholesterol Education Program (NCEP). *Journal of the American Medical Association, 285,* 2486–2497.

Ford, E. S., & Mokdad, A. H. (2001). Fruit and vegetable consumption and diabetes mellitus incidence among U.S. adults. *Preventive Medicine, 32*(1), 33–39.

Franz M. J. (Ed.) (2001). *A core curriculum for diabetes education diabetes management therapies.* Chicago: American Association of Diabetes Educators.

Franz, M. J., Bantle, J. P., Beebe, C. A., Brunzell, J. D., Chiasson, J. L., Garg, A., et al. (2002). Technical review: Evidence-based nutrition principles and recommendations for the treatment and prevention of diabetes and related complications. *Diabetes Care, 25,* 148–198.

Friesen, J. (2000). *Points in your favor.* Wichita, KS: Via Christi Regional Medical Center.

Institute of Medicine. (2002). *Dietary reference intakes: Energy, carbohydrate, fiber, fat, fatty acids, cholesterol, protein, and amino acids.* Washington, DC: National Academies Press.

Jackson, R. L., & Guthrie, R. A. (1986). *The physiologic management of diabetes in children.* New York: Medical Examination Publishers (out of print).

Pastors, J. G., Warshaw, H., Daly, A., Franz, M., & Kulkarni, K. (2002). The evidence for the effectiveness of medical nutrition therapy in diabetes management. *Diabetes Care, 25*(3), 608–613.

Patton, S. R., Lawrence, D. M., & Powers, S. W. (2007). Dietary adherence and associated glycemic control in families of young children with type 1 diabetes. *Journal of the American Dietetic Association, 107,* 46–52.

U.S. Department of Agriculture Center for Nutrition Policy and Promotion. (2008). Retrieved August 27, 2008, from www.MyPyramid.gov. Washington, DC: U.S. Department of Agriculture.

U.S. Department of Health and Human Services & U.S. Department of Agriculture. (2005). *Dietary guidelines for Americans.* Washington, DC: Author.

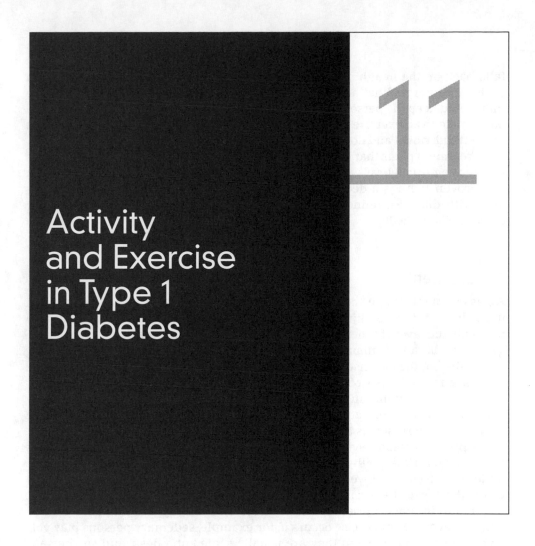

Activity and Exercise in Type 1 Diabetes

Exercise is important in maintaining fitness and good circulation and in aiding the person with diabetes to maintain health. In diabetes or even prediabetes, exercise is one of the best tools to attain and maintain weight loss or weight maintenance (Melkus, 2005). A person with Type 1 diabetes (T1DM) has the extra burden of needing to exercise or be more active and to avoid tipping the balance of blood glucose levels too high or too low. These people march to the same "drummer" heard in that old saying, "If you don't use it you will lose it."

Exercise is especially important in lowering blood glucose levels by utilizing glucose as an energy source during and after exercising (Daly, 2005). Exercise also plays a major role in decreasing cardiovascular disease by delaying or preventing damage to large blood vessels. Therefore, initiating an exercise program in the daily regimen is an opportunity to counteract the increased risk of cardiovascular disease and improve diabetes management.

Most people with diabetes do not know how to design a program to provide the proper amount of physical activity, aiming to obtain its benefits with the lowest risk. Exercise physiologists and personal trainers are helpful, but their services cost money and they are not always available. So, the responsibility falls back on the health care professional. Is the person *safe* to participate in such a program? What are the physical limitations, if any? What is available that would keep the person interested in increasing his or her activity level or to participate in an exercise program? What are the blood glucose level responses for that individual and do the blood sugars bounce too much?

Treatment plans that include exercise focus on keeping blood glucose levels within the normal levels as much of the time as possible. By doing so, research has proven there is a decreased risk of developing the complications associated with diabetes: retinopathy, neuropathy, nephropathy, and cardiovascular disease (Camp, 2006).

Assessment

An assessment must be completed before adding an exercise component to an individual's routine, not just to determine the status of the individual, but also to decide the level of functioning that is safe in relation to the exercise program. The maximal and minimal pulse rates (MPRs) per minute safe for each individual during the exercise period may be determined by the following formula: 220 – age multiplied by 65% and 85%. By using this information, the intensity of the exercise program can be adjusted periodically so that the person's capacity is challenged with the utmost safety. In other words, the threshold pulse rate needs to be increased as the exercise capacity increases.

A problem could develop whether the person with diabetes overexercises (going beyond the ability based on the physical status of the individual) or underexercises (what we most often do). Under- or overexercising, especially when the level of exercise varies from time to time in the same individual, may result in inappropriate levels of stress on the body and fluctuating blood glucose levels. Overexercise occurs if, for example, sedentary persons play volleyball all afternoon when they are usually seated at a desk, and so, the sensitivity to insulin is increased. This increase in insulin sensitivity may lead to prolonged hypoglycemia (i.e., for 12–24 hr) after the more intense exercise has occurred (Kranious, Cameron-Smith, Misso, Collier, & Hargreaves, 2000; Kristiansen, Gade, Wojtaszewski, Kiens, & Richter, 2000). Underexercise leads to more disuse.

According to Dr. Neil Gordon at Presbyterian Hospital in Dallas, Texas (1995), "To achieve a safer, more effective response when exercising, focus must be placed on safety aspects, modality of exercise, frequency, duration, and intensity of exercise, progress of exercise, and time of day to exercise. These are interrelated yet definitely connected to each individual purpose, intent, and need to exercise."

The health professional must consider the severity of any diabetes complications, which might necessitate participation in a more closely medically supervised program. If someone has had T1DM for a while, it is possible that silent ischemia could occur. Therefore, it is recommended that graded exercise testing be performed to determine the safest maximal pulse rate prior to the beginning of an exercise program. If the heart is found to be incapable of tolerating the level of aerobic activity that the skeletal muscles can tolerate (i.e., myocardial deficiency during the stress test), the level of exercise training should be gradually increased until the heart can tolerate more than the muscles. Cardiovascular monitoring should continue until the heart is strengthened.

Keeping this in mind, the National Institutes of Health (2006), the American College of Sports Medicine (ACSM) (1995; Kaufman, Berg, Noble, & Thomas, 2006; Morey, 1999), the American Diabetes Association (2004), and the American Heart Association (2006) recommend, after the preassessment, working up to exercising 20–30 min 3–5 times a week or preferably exercising daily at a moderate intensity. The question is, "What is moderate intensity?" In 1994, an ADA/ACSM joint statement on diabetes mellitus and exercise was published in *Diabetes Care* and *Health and Fitness Journal*.

Intensity

Intensity is described as the strength or degree of some action. In *diabetes language*, it could be described as the calories burned or the energy expended during or because of a particular activity (see Table 11.1). Various methods are available to monitor intensity. These include measurements such as percent maximal oxygen (V_{max}), percent maximum heart rate (HR_{max}), and rate of perceived exertion (RPE), usually on a scale of 5–20, 20 being the greatest exertion. Another test of tolerance to intensity is the Sing Talk Test, which tests the ability to sing or talk while exercising without getting out of breath.

Ideally, HR_{max} should be prescribed from data gathered after a graded exercise test. Individuals with cardiovascular complications or autonomic neuropathy or who are taking prescription drugs for coronary artery disease or high blood pressure usually find the RPE and Sing Talk Test the easiest

11.1	Activity Level Versus Calories Burned[a]
Activity	**Calories Burned**
Walking	
Strolling/1 mph	2.0–2.5 cal/min
Walking/2 mph	2.5–4.5 cal/min
Walking/3 mph	4.5–5.0 cal/min
Walking/3.5 mph	5.0–6.0 cal/min
Walking/ 4 mph	6.0–7.0 cal/min
Stationary cycling	5.0 cal/min
Stretching/range of motion	2.0 cal/min
Calisthenics (light)	6.0 cal/min

[a]Cal/min × time spent = total calories burned.

to understand, even though these are not the best indicators for therapeutic changes. These subjective personal assessment tests (RPE and Sing Talk Test) do not effectively support the person's optimum benefit possible from an ideal program. Sykes (2003) reported that the American College of Sports Medicine recommends that the heart rate reserve and percentage intake of oxygen uptake reserve (HR_{max}) are the best methods to be used even though the RPE is still considered appropriate.

Mode of Exercise

The greatest improvement in physical fitness through exercise results from using large muscle groups in a rhythmic pattern over a continuous amount of time. Because of the wide variety of exercises available, exercise can be tailored according to the individual's skill and enjoyment level, both of which affect exercise compliance. Whether walking, dancing, hiking, swimming, doing water aerobics or games, or performing machine-based exercises or nontraditional exercises (e.g., yoga, tai chi, qigong), individuals should exercise often.

Special caution needs to be taken if high-impact and/or high-intensity forms of exercise are being considered. Performing high-impact and/or high-intensity exercise increases the potential for injury if not properly supervised. It is appropriate to warm up by stretching and walking at a comfortable pace for 5–10 min. As the chosen exercise is performed, the heart rate should increase until the pulse rate is 75% of the previously determined MPR. This intensity should be maintained for about 20 min. The pace is too intense if it exceeds the 75% level by 5 beats per minutes.

The level of exercise might need to be kept at 70% if the pulse rate is more stable at this level. The intensity of the exercise may need to be increased or decreased before finding the stable pulse rate that can be held for 20 to 30 min. The pace should be adjusted until the pulse rate increases during the beginning moments and then can be maintained at the higher level for the entire exercise period. This is the maximum steady-state pulse rate (MSSPR).

At the end of the 20–30 min of exercise, there should be a cool-down period that includes a decreased exercise rate along with mild stretches.

Be aware! The placement and distribution of food and insulin prior to the exercise period may lead to hypoglycemia if not taken into consideration (Daly, 2005). This is of particular concern because exercise will increase insulin sensitivity.

Physiological Response to Exercise

Exercise requires both the availability of fuel and the handling of waste products. If there is not enough fuel, glucose, then muscle contractions will not be optimal. If fuel wastes are not removed, then the muscle may become ill (i.e., lactic acidosis). For this to happen, the body follows a specific chain of events involving responses of the cardiovascular, neurologic, and endocrine systems.

To have a sound fuel supply, the person must not only eat correctly, but also must use food appropriately (e.g., if the fuel is not used properly, from lack of insulin, the body responds in a negative fashion—hypoglycemia). To perform daily activities, a person must have a sound energy supply system. Energy comes from the nutrients obtained from the carbohydrates, fats, and proteins eaten. The body uses these nutrients for growth, tissue repair, and energy. Energy formation and use occurs through the formation of a chemical called adenosine triphosphate (ATP). This is the raw source of energy used by the cells. For the body to use the energy supplied by nutrients, the food must be digested and broken down into smaller particles: carbohydrates to glucose, fats to fatty acids and glycerol, and proteins to amino acids and glucose. Converted to these smaller forms, glucose, fatty acids, and amino acids travel through the bloodstream and arrive at the receptor sites on the cell walls. Once they get inside the cells, they are chemically changed into ATP.

Consider ATP as the actual fuel used for all types of activity (i.e., breathing, digestion, growing tissue, daily activity, glandular secretions, nerve transmissions, exercise, and so on). ATP is not stored in large amounts in the cells; consequently, the body must continually produce it. ATP provides the muscles power for contraction and movement. Energy is released when the high-energy phosphate bonds separate from the adenosine. Oxygen is the catalyst that makes this happen, is carried in the cells in the blood vessels, especially the small blood vessels. Exercise can open small blood vessels leading to better oxygen delivery. This, in turn, leads to increased ATP production.

On the other hand, if the exercise program is not handled appropriately, vasodilatation may lead to increased pulse pressure in people with vascular damage. This can lead to poorer oxygen delivery with lactic acid accumulation and a fall in the serum pH, which then can cause cardiovascular cell or renal cellular destruction.

The body constantly works to break down and replenish ATP, with replenishment accomplished through both the anaerobic and aerobic systems.

The anaerobic system occurs in the absence of oxygen. It has two pathways:

1. The ATP pathway where ATP is stored in the muscle in very small quantities (the response lasts for approximately 10 min),
2. The lactate pathway where ATP is produced at a relatively high rate from glycogen stores within the muscle tissue (lasts approximately 1–3 min). It is at this level that lactic acid is produced.

The system used to replenish ATP is the aerobic system that functions in the presence of oxygen. This system can use both glucose and fatty acids for ATP building and yields a higher amount of ATP at a slower rate when a person is exercising.

One must recognize that the body fights for a balance. If exercise is engaged in a way that causes imbalance, more harm is done than good. For the cells to function properly they need energy. If cells do not receive enough oxygen as well as fuel, their functioning is impaired. Limitations that can slow down the replenishment of ATP include the body's ability to (a) absorb oxygen, (b) transport oxygen, (c) deliver oxygen to the muscle blood vessels, (d) utilize oxygen at the muscle cell level, and (e) efficiently carry oxygen through the blood. Any one of these processes can have limitations, which can be magnified by complications related to diabetes.

Exercise Response Without Diabetes

When an individual begins to exercise, energy consumption by the muscle will very quickly increase to provide the high-energy ATP necessary for muscle contraction. The muscle's first source of energy comes from its glycogen stores because they are so readily available. The next source is the circulating glucose supplied by the liver. As the uptake of circulating glucose increases, so too will liver glucose production (gluconeogenesis and glycogenolysis). This is the body's avenue for maintaining blood glucose levels at a constant concentration even though the muscle's demand for energy when exercising is considerably greater than when at rest. It is vital to maintain a constant blood glucose level to deliver glucose to the brain at a constant rate.

As an individual begins to exercise for a prolonged period of time, the body will rely primarily on adipose tissue as its energy source. Fats are broken down into free fatty acids, bound to albumin, and transported in the blood to the active muscle. Mobilization of these fuels, whether glucose or free fatty acids, depends on the duration and intensity of the exercise, the fitness level of the individual, and the previous nutritional state. In essence, as long as the demand side of exercise does not exceed the supply capability of the body (fuel availability, oxygen capacity, circulation), exercise could be continued indefinitely when performed at a submaximal level.

The endocrine responses to exercise play a pivotal role in blood glucose control. Insulin secretion decreases at the onset of exercise, which initiates the process of liver glucose and free fatty acid production. Insulin supports the increase in muscle glucose uptake as it responds to exercise. Norepinephrine stimulates glycogen breakdown in both the liver and muscle cells and can also stimulate the breakdown of adipose tissue. Epinephrine assists in preserving the body's circulating glucose concentration and may also play a role in adipose tissue breakdown. This provides one more source for an alternative fuel for exercise. Glucagon, produced in the alpha cells in the islets of Langerhans in the pancreas, primarily stimulates and maintains liver glucose production while decreasing the risk of hypoglycemia due to muscle glucose uptake. Cortisol and growth hormones play a more dominant role when exercising for prolonged periods of time. They do this by assisting the body to increase adipose tissue breakdown, decrease insulin-stimulated glucose uptake in peripheral tissue, and increase liver glucose production. They have a lesser role when exercising for short durations of time.

Exercise Response With Type 1 Diabetes Mellitus

Individuals who have T1DM may not experience the same chain of events in the body's system as the individual who does not have diabetes. Why? Because the concentration of insulin and the presence of other counterregulatory hormones may be abnormal.

For the person with T1DM, the type of insulin, the injection site, the insulin's peak time, the time between injections, the onset of exercise, and the time between exercise and the last meal play a role in the body's response to exercise. The normal rate of insulin secretion from the pancreas is difficult to duplicate with subcutaneous injections. There will be a vacillating effect between deficiency and excess availability because of the erratic absorption and time action curves of the insulin. The pancreas of the individual who does not have diabetes runs on automatic pilot, making adjustments as needed. The person with T1DM is on manual control, making adjustments as can best be determined by using blood glucose monitoring results as the guide.

When a deficiency in insulin concentration exists, the blood glucose level increases and the formation of ketone bodies accelerates. An exercising muscle's ability to utilize glucose depends on insulin attaching it to the receptor site on the muscle cell. This then stimulates the process that allows glucose to enter the cell for its usage. If insulin is not present, muscle glucose uptake will not occur, causing a break in the normal chain of events. Hyperglycemia and increased ketone production are the direct result creating a negative environment for exercise. Further exercise would be detrimental and unsafe. Glucose would continue to be dumped into the circulating bloodstream for exercise fuel through glycogenolysis, but no insulin would be available to get it into the muscle cells. Unless externally injected and insulin is present, the concentration of glucose in the bloodstream would continue to increase. When insulin deficiency occurs, the fuel most available for use would be free fatty acids, but at the cost of a high concentration of ketones.

If the intake of insulin is greater than the calorie requirements for the exercise period, low blood glucose levels will be the outcome. Exercise should be discontinued until blood glucose levels are once again within proper management ranges and ketones are not present.

As indicated previously, glucose levels will decrease during exercise unless elevated at the start of the exercise period. If, at the same time, there is an excess concentration of insulin, a break in the chain of events will occur, resulting in a potentially drastic decrease in blood glucose levels. Liver glucose production would be inhibited, disrupting the release of glucose needed to replenish the glucose utilized from the circulation during exercise. This is a type of exercise environment that would create a higher risk for exercise-induced hypoglycemia.

Patients using an insulin pump (continuous subcutaneous insulin infusion [CSII]) must consider their basal insulin settings along with bolus injections prior to exercise or increased activity. Admon et al. (2005) studied children and adolescents with T1DM. They concluded that, although special attention was needed in the insulin management, exercise promoted more benefits than problems. Daly (2005) also supported the concept of good nutrition and the need for physical activity for the healthiest lifestyle possible. The total consensus was that children (and adults) benefit from exercise (Wolfsdorf, 2005).

Duration and Progression of Exercise

It is known that there is an inverse association between diabetes and exercise. Carnethon and Craft (2008) thought that this inverse association might be due to the autonomic function of the body and supported their hypothesis through their observations and their clinical studies.

Duration of each exercise session is inversely related to the intensity level desired. With individuals who are obese or severely deconditioned, a program of 5- to 10-min sessions of low to moderate intensity levels (i.e., as determined by a simple Sing Talk self-test), several times during the day, might initially be a better choice than prolonged or intense exercise, especially if an exercise specialist is not available to supervise and monitor the individual's progress.

The rate at which progression of exercise occurs depends on baseline cardiovascular fitness level, age, weight, health status, personal preference, and individual goals. A very conservative approach to progression would focus on duration instead of intensity. Instruct individuals to begin with what is a comfortable pace for them personally, that is, for 5 to 10 min, and to increase the time by 1–5 min per week until the desired duration is reached (i.e., 20–30 min 3–5 times a week). Increase intensity as cardiovascular adjustment dictates.

Frequency of Exercise

The ADA and ACSM recommend a frequency of 3–5 times per week for exercise, but remaining on a 5-times-a-week program is better. It fits into a personal pattern of management, that is, in most instances, it is easier to manage.

Types of Exercise

Various types of exercise have been promoted because of the different benefits derived from such participation. Research has revealed that many unusual types of exercise, in addition to those usually performed, are beneficial to people with diabetes. Kubota et al. (2006) found that horseback riding (the study used mechanical horses) enhances the insulin-induced glucose uptake in the subjects that participated in the study (older people with diabetes). Tai chi was found, in ethnic Chinese adults with cardiovascular risk factors, to improve flexibility, balance, and strength (Taylor-Piliae, Haskell, Stotts, & Froelicher, 2006). Although these two studies applied more to Type 2 diabetes mellitus (T2DM), interpolation for those with T1DM is possible, indicating that even when the patient is older, there are types of activity and/or exercise that can be of benefit.

With the advent of pump therapy, and according to studies that included children and adolescents, exercise appeared to be beneficial whether the person was receiving pump therapy or not. An important notation was the increase in delay in hypoglycemic events found in those individuals who had their pump on. This leads to the conclusion that the pump could be turned off or even removed during prolonged exercise periods. Associated with this conclusion was the expected recommendation for blood glucose monitoring before and for a number of hours after prolonged exercise (Admon et al., 2005).

Summary

The American College of Sports Medicine states, "The benefits of physical activity are well established and emerging studies continue to support the role for habitual exercise in maintaining overall health and well being" (ACSM, 1995). That exercise benefits cardiovascular health is still the consensus when exercising persons are appropriately preassessed, given evidence-based guidelines, and follow the guidance of health professionals in their exercise programs (National Institutes of Health, 2006).

In the late 1980s and early 1990s, there seemed to be a fear of injuring someone with exercise because of the potential for injury when exercises are performed incorrectly or with inadequate supervision. The goal is to "get more people more active more of the time." It is not to elevate everyone to an arbitrary fitness or activity level. Are health professionals doing a disservice to those who have diabetes and their families by not aiming for the healing abilities obtained in an optimum exercise program? Before developing an exercise prescription to obtain this optimum level, some special considerations must be noted: (a) the individual's health status and maximum safe exercise intensity, along with the pulse rate at that intensity; (b) determination of the individual's metabolic threshold or anaerobic threshold; (c) the potential side effects of any medications that the individual is presently taking; (d) the person's understanding and willingness to participate in such a program; and (e) the person's exercise preference(s).

The benefits of exercise training have a positive effect on the cardiovascular system when approached with guidance and caution. This has been found to be true in adolescent girls with T1DM (Heyman et al., 2007). The use of a personal trainer with youth has led to a lowering of HbA1c in this population, according to Nansel et al. (2007). As an aside, use of personal trainers also strengthened the safety factor of monitoring how much, how long, and how intense the exercise sessions were in relation to monitored blood glucose levels.

The actual first step in compiling an exercise prescription is medical screening and approval for exercise. Special attention needs to be implemented to minimize the potential adverse effects of exercise. The identification of possible macrovascular, microvascular, and neurologic complications that might be contraindications for exercise is essential (ADA, 2004).

Exercise is beneficial in both T1DM and T2DM diabetes and is necessary for the prevention of T2DM (American Association of Diabetes Educators, 2008). Exercise is helpful when appropriate precautions are taken whether the patient is an adult or, as more recently documented, a child (Wolfsdorf, 2005).

References

Admon, G., Weinstein, Y., Falk, B., Weintrob, N., Benzaquen, H., Ofan, R., et al. (2005). Exercise with and without an insulin pump among children and adolescents with type 1 diabetes mellitus. *Pediatrics, 116*(3), e348–e355.

American Association of Diabetes Educators. (2008). Position statement on diabetes and exercise. *The Diabetes Educator, 34*(1), 37–39.

American College of Sports Medicine. (1995). *Guidelines for exercise testing and prescription* (5th ed.). Media, PA: Williams and Wilkins.

American Diabetes Association. (2004). Physical activity/exercise and diabetes: Position statement. *Diabetes Care, 27*(Suppl. 1), S58–S62.

American Diabetes Association/American College of Sports Medicine. (1994). Joint statement: Diabetes mellitus and exercise. *Diabetes Care, 17,* 924–937.

American Heart Association. (2006). Exercise standards: A continuing statement for health professionals. *Circulation, 91,* 580–615.

Camp, K. K. (2006). Being active. In C. Mensing (Ed.), *The art and science of diabetes self-management education: A desk reference for healthcare professionals* (pp. 669–688). Chicago: American Association of Diabetes Educators.

Carnethon, M. R., & Craft, L. L. (2008). Autonomic regulation of the association between exercise and diabetes. *Exercise Sports Science Review, 36*(1), 12–18.

Daly, A. (2005). Healthy lifestyle changes: Food and physical activity. In B. P. Childs, M. Cypress, & G. Spollett (Eds.), *Complete nurse's guide to diabetes care* (pp. 20–32). Alexandria, VA: American Diabetes Association.

Gordon, N. F. (1995). The exercise prescription. In N. Ruderman & J. T. Devlin (Eds.), *The health professionals guide to diabetes and exercise* (pp. 71–82). Alexandria, VA: American Diabetes Association.

Heyman, E., Toutain, C., Delamarche, P., Berthon, P., Briard, D., Youssef, H., et al. (2007). Exercise training and cardiovascular risk factors in type 1 diabetes adolescent girls. *Pediatric Exercise Science, 19*(4), 408–419.

Kaufman, C., Berg, K., Noble, J., & Thomas, J. (2006). Ratings of perceived exertion of ACSM exercise guidelines in individuals varying in aerobic fitness. *Research Quality in Exercise and Sport, 77*(1), 122–130.

Kranious, Y., Cameron-Smith, D., Misso, M., Collier, G., & Hargreaves, M. (2000). Effects of exercise on GLUT-4 and glycogenic gene expression in human skeletal muscle. *Journal of Applied Physiology, 88,* 797–803.

Kristiansen, S., Gade, J., Wojtaszewski, J. F., Kiens, B., & Richter, E. A. (2000). Glucose uptake is increased in trained vs. untrained muscle during heavy exercise. *Journal of Applied Physiology, 89*(3), 1151–1158.

Kubota, M., Nagasaki, M., Tokudome, M. Shinomiya, Y., Ozawa, T., & Sato, Y. (2006). Mechanical horseback riding improves insulin sensitivity in elder diabetic patients. *Diabetes Research and Clinical Practice, 71*(2), 124–130.

Melkus, G. D. (2005). Review: Non-pharmacological interventions induce or maintain weight loss in adults with pre-diabetes. *Evidence-Based Nursing, 8*(4), 110–113.

Morey, S. S. (1999). ACSM revises guidelines for exercise to maintain fitness. *American Family Physician, 59*(2), 473.

Nansel, T. R., Iannotte, R. J., Simons-Morton, B. G., Cox, C., Plotnick, L. P., Clark, L. M., et al. (2007). Diabetes personal trainer outcomes: Short-term and 1-year outcomes of a diabetes personal trainer intervention among youth with type 1 diabetes. *Diabetes Care, 30*(10), 2471–2477.

National Institutes of Health. (2006). General recommendations as indicated in the Consensus Development Conference Statement, December 18–20, 1995 (originally published in *Physical Activity and Cardiovascular Health, 13*[3], 1–33).

Sykes, K. (2003). Promoting health through physical activity. *Journal of the Association of Chartered Physiotherapists in Women's Health, 94,* 35–38.

Taylor-Piliae, R. E., Haskell, W. L., Stotts, N. A., & Froelicher, E. S. (2006). Improvement in balance, strength, and flexibility after 12 weeks of tai chi exercise in ethnic Chinese adults with cardiovascular disease risk factors. *Alternative Therapies in Health and Medicine, 12*(2), 50–58.

Wolfsdorf, J. I.(2005). Children with diabetes benefit from exercise. *Archives of Diseases of Children, 90*(12), 1215–1217.

12

Monitoring Type 1 Diabetes Mellitus

The Diabetes Control and Complications Trial (DCCT) (1993) and the U.K. Prospective Diabetes Study (UKPDS) (1998) emphasized the need for normalization of blood glucose levels and for education and supervision to manage diabetes safely. Diabetes is unique in that it is a disease in which people must alter their own medication. It is a *self-managed disease*. How can self-management be done safely? Appropriate education and interpretation of blood glucose levels, with an eye on what has caused dramatic elevations and depressions, aid in determining how much medication is needed to cover how much food in relation to the activity that is to follow. In the fifth edition of this book, Hinnen (2002) said, "Self-monitoring of blood glucose (SMBG) is the road atlas used on the long and treacherous journey of diabetes." Therefore, if you do not know where you are going, you probably will not get there. There needs to be some guidance on making potentially dangerous decisions and SMBG is the way to get this guidance.

This chapter focuses on individuals with Type 1 diabetes and the decisions they must make. Type 2 diabetes is the subject of Chapter 20.

A person cannot safely participate in intensive control without blood glucose monitoring (Garg, Campbell, Delahanty, & Halvorson, 2000). Although urine testing has been used, it does not allow the safety that SMBG may give a person. Each urine specimen, whether a first or a second voiding, only gives information after the fact and only gave some idea of the renal threshold (which is lower for women who are pregnant, who have gestational diabetes, and for children). Renal thresholds have been monitored at 100–160 mg/dl (5.6 to 8.4 mmol/L) for children and pregnant women and at 180 mg/dl (10 mmol/L) or so for many adults (even 200 mg/dl [11 mmol/L] or higher).

Symptoms can occur if the blood glucose levels are below normal or if blood glucose levels are rapidly changing. Some individuals having symptoms of hypoglycemia indicated that their blood glucose levels were below 60 mg +/− (3.3 mmol/L), but rarely would someone experience symptoms of hyperglycemia until the blood glucose levels were well above 300 mg/dl (16.6 mmol/L). Self-efficacy literature has revealed that reports of symptoms are not consistently associated with estimations of high or low blood glucose levels (O'Connell, Hamera, Schorfheide, & Guthrie, 1990), and that postprandial blood glucose levels give better guidance related to overall control (Dungan et al., 2006; Slama, 2000). Standardization and guidelines are needed in diabetes care and prevention. Guidelines can be found in the first supplement of each year in *Diabetes Care* (ADA, 2008) (see Table 12.1 for recommended monitoring criteria). European health professionals have also developed such guidelines (Schwartz et al., 2007).

All medications have a time action. Blood glucose levels vary depending on the time action of the medication. They also depend on the level of emotional stress a person is experiencing, an illness or any level of pain, the types and amount of food eaten, and activity level. Absorption of medication will determine when and how much the blood glucose levels will be affected. Where an injection is given in relation to the absorptive factor, both at the site and in relation to food, fluid intake, and activity, also may be variable in glucose level outcome.

Choosing a Meter

A plethora of meters is now available to monitor blood glucose levels. A person, in choosing a meter, needs to be aware of readability, size, cost of strips (anywhere from 50 cents to over a dollar a strip), and insurance coverage. These meters can fit into the lifestyles of most busy people because the duration of testing has diminished from minutes to seconds. Accuracy has increased as the amount of blood needed to do the testing has decreased. Measurements had been calculated to plasma rather than whole blood (a 15% difference) in the past, but most meters today translate the value shown on the screen to whole blood. Smaller meters, shorter testing time, and smaller drops of blood are now accompanied by the varied sites from which blood specimens may be obtained. Sites of testing such as the arm are called off-site testing. Off-site testing is not recommended if blood glucose values are very high or very low because off-sites are less accurate than finger testing. Some machines are even calibrated to work hand-in-hand with insulin pumps so diabetes management decisions are easier. Devices for the visually impaired are also available. These latter machines are expensive. Now there is a machine for as low as $30 that audibly announces the results of the test.

Standardization of all of these machines allows the information made available to be reliable enough to make safe decisions as part of daily management of the disease (Rodgers & Wood, 2001). Cost of test strips is still a problem for people with low incomes, especially those without insurance coverage.

Blood glucose testing monitors work in a variety of ways. In the original meters, the blood was placed on a strip. The glucose oxidase enzyme reaction developed a color reaction in the strip. The blood was washed off and the color depth read in a colorimeter. Now, almost all strips and meters use an electrochemical process. The strip is placed in the meter, which turns it on. Blood is then placed on the strip and a glucose oxidase reaction occurs. Oxygen and water are generated in this reaction and electrons are transferred, by way of an electrochemical mediator (oxygen), to a silver-platinum electrode surface. This, in turn, generates a current that is measured by the meter. The size of the current generated is proportional to the amount of glucose present in the drop of blood. A computer chip compares this information with a standard in the meter and translates the value to milligrams per deciliter (or millimoles per liter) to read out on the meter's screen. The whole process of reaction and readout can be as short as 5 seconds and the amount of blood needed as little as 0.1 μl.

The package inserts include specifications and data obtained in the clinical trials of each of the meters. As is known, each manufacturer is obliged to list the details on their products and this information is subject to Food and Drug Administration (FDA) approval. Some variability occurs with each meter (not more than 10% variation from one meter to the other), but almost all portable meters have similar interferences. The National Steering Committee for Quality Assurance (NSCQA) has been the watchdog that promotes the guidance for the level of quality of reading and outcomes of each of the machines available.

There is less chemical or cellular interference that can affect glucose-testing results in today's meters than in the past. The hematocrit (in the oxygen-driven procedure) was one of the major factors that influenced the outcome of testing. Lowered hematocrits generally result in a false-negative hemoglobin A1c, but blood glucose monitors are configured, in plasma concentrations, so that there would be no problem in the newborn, in people who are fluid depleted, or in the patient with polycythemia. Conversely, the person with iron deficiency anemia may demonstrate a false-positive hemoglobin A1c but, again, this should not abnormally influence today's meters. Care must still be taken if the person is ingesting or being given large amounts of ascorbic acid (by mouth or by vein) or acetaminophen in toxic levels. If the lipid profile is grossly out of the normal range, it is still possible that results might also be altered—but the possibility of this happening is much less with the stabilized machines now available.

Another consideration is the range considered most accurate for each machine. This information may be found in the package insert or on the side of the bottle of strips. Some machines will include artificial blood or self-calibrated plastic inserts to conform to the range of acceptability when using the particular vial of strips.

The humidity range should be 20%–80% for best results, but this is not as much of a problem with modern meters as with the older machines. The same with temperature ranges. Ideally, the machine should be used at room temperature, but again, newer construction has allowed for more latitude for both humidity and temperature. Testing with a control solution should indicate if the machine if functioning correctly. If the strips have been exposed to extreme heat, it would be wise to throw them out. Be aware that high altitude may affect a meter's functioning, and is not always identified as a possible problem in package inserts. Despite all of the possible interferences, user error remains as the most common problem in glucose monitoring. A vial of strips (usually 10) is supplied with a new meter. The prescription will allow for further strips to be obtained. A change in meters will mean a change in strips. This change in meter might be because of user choice, suppliers, or third-party insurers. Manufacturers' rebates may make a particular meter essentially free if the person needs to purchase a machine, and most diabetes centers can supply free meters. The companies make their money from the strips, not from the sale of the meters. Most of today's strips have a capillary action to ensure that enough blood is available to correctly complete a test. One machine gives the user an opportunity to add blood if there has not been enough to complete the function on the original blood obtained. An error reading may be indicated if not enough blood is present. The sound of a bell or other auditory prompt may be available to also tell the user that enough blood is present.

All types of diabetes mellitus need blood glucose monitoring. The frequency of monitoring blood glucose levels usually depends on the type of diabetes a person has and whether changes have been made in medication requirements. Prescriptions usually require a diagnosis code, the frequency with which blood glucose levels are to be tested, the present dosage prescribed, if on insulin, and the number of strips desired. This specific documentation is requested when a person needs more than 100 strips at a time. The number of strips Medicare has *cleared* for coverage is not adequate for full coverage of the testing process especially when a person is testing four times a day, every day, is ill, or needs more documentation related to a change in medication.

Individual Features of Interest

The variety of sizes of glucose monitors gives the consumer more choices. Meters range from the smallest size (usually less than the size of the palm of the hand) to the largest units that might be found in a clinic, laboratory, or hospital. User errors, whether the person is testing at home or at another site, can be a problem especially if a patient is involved in self-management. These errors might be due to battery problems, inadequate sample size, dirt on or in the mechanism for display or function, loss of a lighting mechanism, or computer readout problems. The capability of machines to translate the readings into dosages of insulin to be administered is increasing. Some machines *speak*, or are combined with abilities to measure cholesterol or blood ketone or to monitor blood pressure.

It is also important to be aware of the range of blood glucose level readings that are characteristic of that machine. These readings may vary from 10 to 20 mg/dl (0.5–1.1 mmol/L) on the lower end to 500 to 600 mg/dl (27.7–33.3 mmol/L) on the upper end. The determination of the range for a particular machine gives the user information to complete a specific treatment protocol or to call for assistance. The indication of 240 mg/dl (13.3 mmol/L), 250 mg/dl (13.8 mmol/L), or even 300 mg/dl (16.7 mmol/L) also gives guidance, depending on the education direction as to when to check for ketones in the urine. One machine checks for blood ketones. In the future, this may be a more common feature. More machines should have an alarm system to be triggered when blood glucose levels reach a preset level so that the user will check for ketones in the urine and treat or report their findings as appropriate.

Timing of the test ranges from 3 seconds to 50 seconds; amount of blood needed ranges from 0.1 to 3.5 µl; the memory for home monitors may be from 1 to more than 1,000 tests; the testing range is from blood glucose levels of 10 mg/dl (0.5 mmol/L) to 600 mg/dl (33.3 mmol/L); the price range for a home meter may be from *free* to $200; the cost for strips is usually about $1 per strip. Data managers might include, besides date and time of the test (military or real time), such items as carbohydrate or calorie intake, unusual foods eaten, exercise or activity level, and perhaps a place to note emotional stressors. Some machines allow testing on alternate sites as well as fingertips. Many more of the machines are self-calibrating. Average blood glucose levels might be set for 7, 14, 21, 28, 30, 60, and/or 90 days. There are machines that average all the premeal and postmeal tests, whereas other machines average blood glucose levels before each meal and/or after each meal, plus the overall average.

The newest systems can collect and transfer data from a person's home to the health professional's office in seconds with or without the use of a computer. The user may purchase a linking device that allows the information to be transferred by telephone. A new device is a cell phone that also serves as a glucose meter, and can transmit the information to a similar device in the health care provider's office. Such devices will become much more popular in that future, especially with young people.

Results from the memory of the meters can be downloaded into computers, averaged, and graphed as pie charts, bar graphs, and so on. Another system takes into account variations that occur with differences in time, temperature, cleanliness, and ethnic groups as it analyzes blood samples in a way that leads to even more accurate results.

Lancing Devices

Lancing devices vary from the pen shape to the stubby to the round shape. Lances themselves are increasingly smaller in diameter, more defined (can be altered for depth of penetration), and less visible so that the users find that they can obtain a sample with less pain. Of course, people are still looking for noninvasive procedures that involve eye or mouth secretions or other noninvasive type testing. So far, all forms of noninvasive testing methods are too expensive and accuracy is still a problem.

Checking the Technique of Monitor Use

Overall, following manufacturer's recommendations for each lancing device and meter is a must. Meter accuracy and reliability cannot be obtained unless step-by-step procedures are followed. Calibrating is now done by many of the companies even before the machine reaches the user's hands. The blood glucose test strips should be checked for their expiration date. Using control solution and/or changing the control number to match that found on the bottle of strips, for those machines so needed, ensures an increase in both the reliability and accuracy of the monitor.

Each visit should include a time to observe the user's technique. If time does not permit such an observation, asking key questions about the location, care, and specific use of the identified machine may pick up some error. Observation of user technique is best. Because management decisions are based on reliable results, lack of skill in testing may prove a hazard in the wake of a self-management decision.

Whenever batteries are changed, remind the users to note if they need to reset the month, day, year, time, and/or other parameters of the machine. Many of these machines come with the day and date already set by the company. Some of the machines need the day, date, and time set when the machine is first used, but almost every machine needs some resetting when the battery is changed. The downloading capabilities of some of the machines will actually reset the day and time or will at least give some indication that such changes should be made.

A word on control solutions. Control solutions are sugar solutions that deteriorate within a few months after opening (observe the expiration date on the side of the bottle). New solutions must be obtained regularly from the pharmacists. Pharmacists should be advised to stock control solutions and ask their customers periodically if they need new control solutions. Ask if it is possible for these control solutions to work on all machines. If, when the control solution is used, results read outside of the range noted on the side of the vial, instruct the person to contact the company. It may be time for a new machine that the company usually sends by priority mail.

Using alternative sites for testing is possible with an increasing variety of meters. The first site to alternatively be cleared for use was the forearm, even though the outer aspect of the palm and the earlobe are also considered possible. A few considerations for using these alternative sites is whether or not the site is rubbed (McGarraugh, Schwartz, & Weinstein, 2001) and how the alternative site compares with a finger stick (Lee, Weinert, & Miller, 2001). The admonition is to test fingers when hypoglycemia is suspected. The second site found to be similar or statistically close enough to represent a finger stick has been the outer aspect of the palm of the hand (Kempe et al., 2005). Either this area of the palm of the hand or the fingers may be used for the testing sites when hypoglycemia is suspected.

One other point needs to be made. Even though there have been few if any reports related to infection because of blood glucose testing, careful handwashing can assist in keeping such reports to a minimum. The main principle to remember to use any meter is to follow the directions given by the manufacturer of the monitor to the letter.

Memory Capabilities of Meters

Blood glucose testing meters are getting more user friendly. These machines are increasingly capable of storing more information than before. Errors (mostly user errors) are noted. Beyond the storing of data in a memory bank are the indications for trends of increasing, lowering, or maintaining blood glucose levels. The use of alarm settings to remind the person to check a blood glucose level or to be aware of too high or too low a reading is increasing.

Data management is one of the most impressive advances available in glucose monitors. Almost all companies have some type of software package that is available free of charge or for a small fee. These data managers analyze and report the data by number, by graph, by pie charts, and by other methods. Multiple screens may even show bar graphs and even modal days so the individual might see how frequently they are outside or inside the goal areas. This is most useful for the hospital. The hospitals need systems that allow a method for quality assurance that relate to each meter, for each user, and, in some cases, patient billing. Individual billing may not require this specificity when the health care is given in a capitated system. In most hospitals, this type of documentation is most useful for the quality procedures for their individual laboratories.

Using the Monitor in the Clinic or Hospital

Today's monitoring of blood glucose levels is a long way from the laboratory-based analysis of the past. Stat blood glucose monitoring relies on bedside monitoring but laboratories still have a place in documenting glucose levels that are above (or, for some, below) the particular meter's capabilities. Additionally, obtaining a simple finger stick is easier than accessing the vein of a person who is dehydrated when in diabetic ketoacidosis or has hyperglycemic hyperosmolar nonketotic syndrome.

To maintain quality care, the laboratories have placed standards and developed guidelines to assure the public that accuracy and reliability are being maintained. The National Committee for Clinical Laboratory Standards (NCCLS) published rules (NCCLS, 1991) for laboratory practice that categorized glucose monitoring as a wavered test, requiring a certificate of waiver and biennial fee. This applies to bedside testing whether completed in a hospital, a clinic, a physician's office, or diabetes camp. Additional guidelines and regulations are published by state health departments, the Joint Commission for Accreditation of Health Care Organizations (JCAHCO), the College of American Pathologists (CAP), and NCCLS.

Development of a quality assurance (QA) program for a facility should be a collaborative process involving laboratory personnel and clinicians (National Steering Committee for Quality Assurance [NSCQA], 1993). Most meter companies have synthesized the many regulations and developed processes and forms to help meet the requirements. Whatever the facility, there is a need, if not already established, to implement written policies and procedures for all testing procedures, maintenance, daily quality control, proficiency testing, and troubleshooting. Most time-consuming, however, is the requirement for standard training and ongoing certification of all users whether in the hospital or clinic setting.

Careful attention to bloodborne pathogens and proper techniques to eliminate contamination are mandatory components of any system. In settings where multiple people are using the same meter, techniques of use, use of gloves, single-use lancets, and documentation of use if an accompanying data collector is not used are needed. These are but a few of the critical factors to consider when developing blood glucose testing policies and procedures for a specific site.

Use of Computer Meter Output

We have already alluded to the actual averaging capacity of many of the meters in use. This gives more guidance to the health professionals and, if used effectively, to the person who has diabetes. This assists the person with diabetes and the health professional to more actively participate in the pattern approach to management without having to write down the blood glucose levels or offload them from the machine. One problem occurs. This is related to the person who is using the meter. If the machine does not have a readily available way to readout or determine a pattern by visual or average blood glucose means, there is less possibility that the individual will participate in self-management. Too often, the machine is brought into the office and off-loaded at the time of the visit. It is also possible the blood glucose levels might be written in a notebook and not assessed until the time of the clinic visit.

The computerized programs for handheld or personal computers have aided many patients in questioning their body's response to insulin at an earlier stage than at the time of clinic visit. Sophisticated programs that take into account the food eaten, the activity, the exercise participation, and the type of insulin(s) allow for safer alterations in dosing when used in an educated manner. Some meters just provide the information so that the user might make the decisions for self-management at that time. They can question whether it is time to call for assistance or for follow-up with self-treatment. Others predict what dosage should be used depending on a precalculated ratio of carbohydrate or calorie points to insulin.

Care must be taken that these calculation programs are accompanied by a *bolus wizard* that can be used for children as well as adults. It must be remembered that a unit of insulin for a 40-lb child has a different effect than a unit of insulin for a 140-lb adult.

A number of continuous glucose monitoring systems (CGMS) are now available. These CGMS units monitor blood glucose levels over a 1- to 7-day period. Newer models of these monitoring devices should be able to monitor results for a longer and longer period of time. The cost of these devices is still high enough to keep them from being used on a routine basis. It should be possible in a few years to just hook one of these monitors/meters to a patient in an intensive care unit so that blood glucose levels can be assessed real time or in as little as 1 to 5 min.

General Procedures

The following is a procedural guide for blood glucose monitoring:

1. Blood glucose testing should be done four to six times a day until control is established or during a period of illness or prolonged emotional stress. Ideally, this should be after fasting and 2-hr postprandially (Goal: A reading of less

than 110 premeal and less than 140 mg/dl [6.1–7.7 mmol/L] postmeal by American Association of Clinical Endocrinologists [AACE] guidelines. Higher blood glucose levels may be considered for a child or an elderly person).

2. Once control is established, a daily blood glucose profile should be performed a minimum of four times a day; a minimum of three or more days each week (daily is recommended, especially if using a pump or if ill): fasting and 2 hr after each meal (first choice) or premeal and bedtime (second choice). Four times a day, once a week is acceptable for the person who is on diet alone.

3. A 24-hr profile (useful for determining overall levels of control) would include:
   a. Fasting (before morning insulin and breakfast)
   b. 2 hr after breakfast (or before lunch)
   c. 2 hr after lunch (or before supper)
   d. 2 hr after supper (or at bedtime before the bedtime snack if a bedtime snack is to be eaten)
   e. Occasionally at 2–3 a.m. (or midnight if neutral protamine Hagedorn [NPH] is given before supper, i.e., evening meal) or at bedtime.

4. If the Somogyi effect (or rebound effect) is suspected, the test for blood glucose levels could be done at 1 hr, 2 hr, and 3 hr after the previous dose of insulin (if the Somogyi response has occurred, the blood glucose level would seem to go up rather than down after insulin use—so long as total calories and carbohydrate content are at usual levels).

5. If the Dawn Phenomenon is suspected, a 2–4 a.m. blood glucose level would most likely be lower than a fasting blood glucose level.

See goals for blood glucose levels as shown in Table 12.1.

Other Monitoring Capabilities

Hemoglobin A1c

Using a hemoglobin A1c kit at home can be helpful if the results are correctly interpreted. These kits have been giving relatively stable, overall information since their introduction more than 10 years ago, though some questions have been raised regarding user reliability. Some professionals are concerned that the home kits do not have the oversight that is found in a clinic or hospital setting. There are similar but potentially more accurate machines for clinic use. Some of these machines can give results in as little as 10 min. The usual method of A1c determination in the office, clinic, or hospital uses high-performance liquid chromatography (HPLC) methodology and takes a longer time though it has been found to be more accurate than home kits and the rapid testing machines.

Methodologies for testing HbA1c do vary but are varying less from laboratory to laboratory. The gold standard for A1c has been, for many years, the HPLC method developed at the University of Missouri School of Medicine and used in the DCCT study. Further refinements of this methodology have been made and new standards of normal adopted in Europe and Australia (Goodall, Colman, Schneider, McLean, & Barker, 2007; Hoelzel et al., 2004). As noted previously, hemoglobinopathies can result in false-positive A1c values (iron deficiency

12.1 Recommended Monitoring Criteria

	ADA	AACE	IDF	WHO
In general:				
Fasting/premeal	90–130 (5–7.2 mmol)	<110 (6.1 mmol)	<110	<110
1 hr postmeal	<180 (10 mmol)			
2 hr postmeal		<140 (7.7 mmol)	<140	<140
Hemoglobin A1c	7.0% or less	6.5% or less	6.5% or less	6.5% or less
In pregnancy:				
Preexisting diabetes				
Fasting/premeal	<100 (5.5 mmol)			
1 hr postmeal	<120 (6.6 mmol)			
Gestational				
Fasting	<90 (5.0 mmol)			
2 hr postmeal	<110 (6.1 mmol)			
General medical and surgical				
	<126 (fasting) (7 mmol)			
	<200 (random) (11.1 mmol)			
	Preferably between 110 and 140 mg/dl			
Cardiac surgery	<150 (8.3 mmol)			
Critical care	<110 (6.1 mmol)			

Young children and elderly people should focus on the high side of normal. Blood glucose levels at bedtime should be approximately 100 mg/dl (5.6 mmol/L).

ADA, American Diabetes Association; AACE, American Association of Clinical Endocrinologists; IDF, International Diabetes Federation; WHO, World Health Organization.

anemia and Hb F) and false negatives (sickle cell disease, thalassemia, hemolytic anemia, etc.). When there is a distinct difference in average blood glucose levels and the hemoglobin A1c outcome, the patient should be checked for a hemoglobinopathy (Baynes, McIntosh, & Feher, 2001; Schnedl et al., 2000). Note that hemoglobin A1c only gives an overall report of blood glucose level averages rather than the need to alter treatment at a particular time of day.

Hemoglobin A1c has significantly predicted mortality in a prospective population study (Khaw, 2001). Barrett-Connor and Wingard (2001) also found an association between elevated glucose levels and coronary heart disease. These pieces of significant information reinforce the findings found in the DCCT (1993) and the UKPDS (1998). Therefore, careful documenting and comparison of the methodology of testing HbA$_{1c}$ is a must.

A National Glycohemoglobin Standardization Program (NGSP) was organized to implement and oversee the program established by the American Association for Clinical Chemistry (AACC) subcommittee. The laboratories that test for HbA$_{1c}$ are networked with the NGSP for checking their methodology against the standards established by the AACC subcommittee (Hoelzel et al., 2004; Little, 2000). Table 12.2, adapted from the LXN Corporation (San Diego, CA), gives comparisons between the whole-blood and plasma-calibrated average glucose levels, the glucoprotein (fructosamine: 10 days to 2 weeks overview), and the HbA1c (2–3 months overview).

Self-monitoring of blood glucose methods is presently the only way to determine the day-to-day or week-to-week management of diabetes. Averages from the individual samples of plasma blood glucose that meters are now set to report (ADA, 2008), taking into account the range of blood glucose levels being averaged, are recognized as a more significant guide from which to make decisions rather than HbA1c alone.

Presently, with the use of continuous monitoring devices, control of postprandial blood glucose levels is seen to be necessary for the overall management of diabetes (Monnier, Lapinski, & Colette, 2003). A marker (1,5-anhydroglucitol, or 1,5-AG) is believed to be another way to include and determine the extent of postprandial hyperglycemia in the continuous glucose-monitoring system (Dungan et al., 2006). This is a system that should be tested further, but its

12.2 Whole Blood/Plasma[a] Related to Fructosamine and HbA1c

Averages Whole Blood, mg/dl	Averages Whole Blood, mmol/L	Averages Plasma, mg/ml	Averages Plasma, mmol/L	Fructosamine, µmol/L	HbA1c, %
330	18.3	380	21.1	513	13
300	16.7	345	19.1	475	12
270	15.0	310	17.2	438	11
240	13.3	275	15.2	400	10
210	11.6	240	13.2	363	9
180	10.0	205	11.3	325	8
150	8.3	170	9.4	288	7
120	6.7	135	7.5	250	6
90	5.0	105	5.8	213	5

[a]Whole blood and plasma averages are rounded.

benefit may be in demonstrating further need to check out postprandial blood glucose levels, especially if the HbA1c is elevated and the 1,5-AG is low.

Summary

Monitoring blood glucose levels is a must. Whether this monitoring is done by the person who has diabetes or it is done by a responsible adult, determining who should do this and how it should be accomplished is part of the process. Automatic coding features of the meters erase further problems associated with coping errors (Baum, Monhaut, Parker, & Price, 2006). Education and reeducation with the support of a health care professional have been found to be the key to safely attaining and maintaining normal blood glucose levels most of the time. As a person learns his or her individual response to insulin, they are better able to predict what amount of insulin is needed to cover what food is eaten in relation to the activity to follow.

During usual daily activity and illness, blood glucose monitoring will guide self-management in the use of insulin to keep the diabetes controlled (McAndrew, Schneider, Burns, & Leventhal, 2007). As technology increases, the ability to control blood glucose levels becomes easier and easier as reported by the Centers for Disease Control and Prevention (2007). The result? An even healthier population, despite having diabetes.

References

American Diabetes Association. (2008). Standards of medical care in diabetes. *Diabetes Care, 31*(Suppl. 1), S5–S11.

Barrett-Connor, E., & Wingard, D. L. (2001). "Normal" blood glucose and complications risk. *British Medical Journal, 322*(7277), 5–6.

Baum, J. M., Monhaut, N. M., Parker, D. R., & Price, C. (2006). Improving the quality of self-monitoring blood glucose measurement: A study in reducing calibration errors. *Diabetes Technology & Therapeutics, 9,* 347–355.

Baynes, K., McIntosh, C., & Feher, M. D. (2001). Artefactually low glycated haemoglobin is a potential pitfall in diabetes management: Consider haemolytic anaemias. *Practical Diabetes International, 18*(3), 103–106.

Centers for Disease Control and Prevention. (2007). Self-monitoring of blood glucose among adults with diabetes—United States, 1997–2006. *Morbidity and Mortality Weekly Report, 56*(43), 1133–1137.

Diabetes Control and Complications Trial Research Group. (1993). The effect of intensive treatment of diabetes on the development and progression of long-term complications in insulin-dependent diabetes mellitus. *New England Journal of Medicine, 329*(14), 977–986.

Dungan, K. M., Buse, J. B., Largay, J., Kelly, M. M., Button, E. A., Kato, S., et al. (2006). 1,5 anhydroglucitol and postprandial hyperglycemia as measured by continuous glucose monitoring system in moderately controlled patients with diabetes. *Diabetes Care, 29,* 1214–1219.

Garg, S. K., Campbell, R. K., Delahanty, L., & Halvorson, M. (2000). The role of frequent glucose monitoring in intensive diabetes management. *The Diabetes Educator, 26*(5), 3–17.

Goodall, L., Colman, P. G., Schneider, H. G., McLean, M., & Barker G. (2007). Desirable performance standards for the analysis, precision, accuracy and standardization: Consensus statement of the Australian Association of Clinical Biochemists, the Australian Diabetes Society, the Royal College of Pathologists of Australia, the Endocrine Social of Australia, and the Australian Diabetes Educators Association. *Clinical Chemistry Laboratory Medicine, 45*(8), 1083–1097.

Hinnen, D. (2002). Self-monitoring of blood glucose. In D. Guthrie & R. Guthrie (Eds.), *Nursing management of diabetes mellitus* (5th ed., pp. 182–196). New York: Springer.

Hoelzel, W., Weykamp, C., Jeppson, J. O., Miedema, K., Barr, J. R., Goodall, I., et al., on behalf of the International Federation of Clinical Chemists Working Group on HbA1c Standardization (2004). IFCC reference system for measurement of HbA1c in human blood and the National Society of Chemists in the United States, Japan, and Sweden: A method comparison study. *Clinical Chemistry, 50,* 166–174.

Kempe, K. C., Budd, D., Stern, M., Ellison, J. M., Saari, L. A., Adiletto, C. A., et al. (2005). Palm glucose readings compared with fingertip readings under steady and dynamic glycemia conditions, using the One Touch Ultra blood glucose monitoring system. *Diabetes Technology Therapy, 7*(6), 916–926.

Khaw, K. T. (2001). Glycated hemoglobin, diabetes, and mortality in men in the Norfolk Cohort European Prospective Evaluation of Cancer and Nutrition (EPECN Study). *British Medical Journal, 32*(7277), 15–18.

Lee, D., Weinert, S., & Miller, E. (2001). *Blood glucose monitoring: A study of forearm versus finger stick* (pp. 1–6). Columbus, OH: Roche Diagnostics.

Little, R. R. (2000). Recent progress in glycohemoglobin testing. *Diabetes Care, 23*(3), 265–266.

McAndrew, L., Schneider, S. H., Burns, E., & Leventhal, H. (2007). Does patients blood glucose monitoring improve diabetes control? A systematic review of the literature. *The Diabetes Educator, 33*(6), 1012–1013.

McGarraugh, G., Schwartz, S., & Weinstein, R. (2001). *Glucose measurements using blood extracted from the forearm and the finger* (ART01022 Rev.C, pp. 1–7). TheraSense, Inc.

Monnier, L., Lapinski, H., & Colette, C. (2003). Contributions of fasting and postprandial plasma glucose increments to the overall diurnal hyperglycemia of type 2 diabetic patients: Variations with increasing levels of HbA1c. *Diabetes Care, 26,* 881–885.

National Committee for Clinical Laboratory Standards. (1991). *Ancillary (bedside) blood glucose testing acute and chronic care facilities* (Document C30–T). Villanova, PA: NCCLS.

National Steering Committee for Quality Assurance in Capillary Blood Glucose Monitoring. (1993). Proposed strategies for reducing user error in capillary blood glucose monitoring, (NSCQA). *Diabetes Care, 16*(2), 493–498.

O'Connell, K. A., Hamera, E. K., Schorfheide, A., & Guthrie, D. (1990). Symptom beliefs and actual blood glucose in Type II diabetes. *Research Nursing and Health, 13*(3), 145–151.

Rodgers, J., & Wood, J. (2001). Standards for professional monitoring of capillary blood glucose. *Practical Diabetes International, 18*(3), 79–82.

Schnedl, W. J., Krause, R., Halwachs-Baumann, G., Trinker, M., Lipp, R. W., & Krejs, G. J. (2000). Evaluation of HbA$_{1c}$ determination methods in patients with hemoglobinopathies. *Diabetes Care, 23*(3), 339–344.

Schwartz, P. E., Gruhl, U., Bornstein, S. R., Landgraf, R., Hall, M., & Tuomilehto, J. (2007). The European perspective on diabetes prevention: Development and implementation of a European guidelines and training standards for diabetes patients (IMAGE). *Diabetes Vascular Disease Research, 4*(4), 353–357.

Slama, O. (2000). Clinical significance of post-prandial blood glucose excursions in type 1 and type 2 diabetes mellitus. *International Journal of Clinical Practice, 112*(Suppl.), 9–12.

U.K. Prospective Diabetes Study Group. (1998). Intensive blood-glucose control with sulfonylureas or insulin compared with conventional treatment and risk of complications in patients with type 2 diabetes. *Lancet, 352,* 837–853.

13

Psychosocial Aspects and Mental Health

Psychological problems in children and youth with diabetes are many and varied. They often result from family conflicts regarding the acceptance or denial of the child's or adult's diabetes. It does take discipline to eat nutritiously, to take multiple doses of medication, and to check for blood glucose levels frequently. Multiple tasks and the impact of the diagnosis of diabetes have led to major depression, which has been found to be more prevalent than previously considered in this population with a chronic disease (Li, Ford, Strine, & Mokdad, 2008). Depression and other psychological problems can result in dependency relationships and rebellion. Completing daily tasks requires discipline. Dependency relationships and rebellion are counter to the discipline needed to successfully manage this disease. Society requires a certain amount of discipline, that is, stopping at stop signs, going when the light turns green. It might be said that the discipline required to handle a chronic disease might contribute to a person having a better quality of life in a society that requires some discipline.

Apathy, even without depression, can also be detrimental to the person who has diabetes (Padala et al., 2008). Self-care and self-management require action and discipline. If a person "doesn't care," then the actions needed for daily care will not occur. Again, this is a problem. Whether the inactivity of depression or apathy occurs, the discipline needed for the best health outcomes will not be present. Discipline starts in childhood. Variations in approaches to discipline have led to problems that the adult with diabetes must deal with.

Practices over the past 40 years have varied from strict discipline to indulging children and adolescents and back to at least some discipline. Discipline is needed throughout the life span. The earlier practices led to pampered, immature children, rebellious adolescents, and adults with greater social and health problems. Hieronymus and Geil (2006) felt a need to give ways in which parents could raise healthy children despite having diabetes. Their book entitled *101 Tips for Raising Healthy Kids With Diabetes* gives answers to the most frequently asked questions and, therefore, becomes a very helpful resource for concerned parents.

Parents have revealed certain factors that they feel have an effect on diabetes management and outcomes (Ginsburg et al., 2005). Discipline is indirectly associated with outcome. One might say that a disciplined child who has diabetes will become a disciplined adult with better health despite having diabetes mellitus. Discipline brings length and quality of life to all who practice it.

For safety, if nothing else, children do require more discipline. When children become adolescents, the restrictions may be relaxed to a degree because adolescents are able to make increasingly responsible, mature decisions and take more responsibility for their self-care. Wysocki et al. (1997) have found that too often adolescents are given responsibility for their own care too soon. The right amount of discipline and relaxation of guidelines are often hard to balance. Self-care and self-management choices require stable emotional coping skills along with the knowledge of the choices available.

Maturity is learning self-discipline, but children do not learn self-discipline without first being disciplined. We believe that the discipline required for promoting diabetes control, rather than being psychologically damaging, may in fact have beneficial effects in promoting a mature, self-controlled, and well-disciplined adult.

A classic study by Simond (1975) of well-controlled youth observed at the University of Missouri indicates that the assumption of a dysfunctional family leads to poor control of diabetes mellitus. Simond's data indicated that, at the very least, "tighter" diabetes control does no harm psychologically. The study showed, however, that disorganized families or families with preexisting problems often cannot attain a high level of diabetes control, and that more understanding, education, and support may be needed from the health care team for these families.

Obviously, there are many individual differences, so that all management and education must be individualized, whether for a child or an adult. Psychological problems must be watched for and handled promptly by the health care team. When problems develop, they should be vigorously approached and appropriate professionals mobilized to help. For some of the minor psychological problems, group sessions, such as properly handled diabetes association meetings, camps for youths, or attendance at support groups can be helpful.

Physical Health

The growth and development of children and adolescents and their corresponding blood glucose levels have been observed in several studies. The classic study
by Jackson, Holland, Chatman, Guthrie, and Hewett (1978) found that children,
observed over a 20-year period, who were poorly controlled did not grow well,
whereas those with fair to good control grew at a normal rate. Even in identical twins, if there was a difference in the degree of hyperglycemia, there was
a difference in rate of growth. Subsequently, Clarke, Vance, and Rogol (1993)
found that growth, an important intermediate problem in childhood and adolescence, was related to control. Good control of the diabetes through careful
management and education of the individual and/or family results in children
and older youth who grow normally and follow developmental paths consistent
with their genetics.

Based on physical makeup, and age, some individuals may be more predisposed to care for themselves. If they are endomorphic, with their more often
apple shape, they are more relaxed and love to be comfortable. They enjoy the
comfort foods, from the smell of food to the actual eating. The thin person, or
ectomorph, tends to be more artistic and intellectual, so food is not such a drive.
They even have trouble gaining weight, so that when they have Type 1 diabetes (T1DM), they would rather not be bothered by exercise; in fact, their life is
more organized so that the diabetes regimen is less of a challenge except when
it interferes with their lifestyle. Then, the middle-of-the-road mesomorphs are
more energetic and muscular. If their life practice has been involved with eating
more and, as an adult, they decrease their activity level, they might experience a
little more frustration with weight control. Exercise might be welcomed if they
can fit it into their schedule. They might be more willing to participate in a self-
management program, especially if it meets their need to follow a regimen that
doesn't lead to a problem with control. If it becomes frustrating, too, then there
is another problem.

Adults with T1DM were also shown to have more difficulties when their control was not optimal. The Diabetes Control and Complications Trial (DCCT, 1993)
recognized that the more the diabetes was controlled, the fewer complications
arose. The general health of these individuals has also been noted, both from the
standpoint of fewer illnesses to the occurrence of fewer problems with mental
illness. The question as to whether brain function is disturbed when blood glucose levels are tightly controlled has been a concern. Of the original patients in
the DCCT study, 1,059 were monitored for 6.5 years beyond the end of the study
in 1993. Although people continued to experience three and a half times more
hypoglycemic events than the conventional group, there was no significant difference in mental functioning between the two groups (Musen et al., 2008).

Psychosocial Impact

This syndrome impacts not only the person involved, but also the family. Once
the diagnosis is confirmed, one can correctly assume that the individual, the
parents, and the children need considerable emotional support. They need to
have questions answered honestly. They need knowledge to put "old wives' tales"

into perspective. The first few days after the diagnosis is known, the individual and/or parents and significant others need time to adjust mentally and emotionally. The family members need to get involved with the team members; they need to learn what part the team members play in their care or the care of their loved one. When persons with the diabetes diagnosis have been experiencing diabetic ketoacidosis, friends, family, and parents see them change from being acutely ill to having a seemingly rapid recovery. These people learn that each day progress is made toward stabilization so that eventually they may easily control the diabetes at home. Individuals and family members develop confidence in themselves as they are able to participate or support the regimen under the supervision of the team's health professional.

Research on long-term adjustment and regimen adherence was reported in a one-year longitudinal study by Kovacs, Brent, Steinberg, Paulauskas, and Reid (1986). All children, regardless of severity of symptoms returned to normal levels of psychological functioning within 12 months of diagnosis. In a related study, Kovacs et al. (1985) reported that parents, mothers specifically, had come to terms with the diabetes within the first year with the greatest emotional upheaval resolved in about 6 months. Both age and gender appear to be variables relating to psychosocial functioning and diabetes adjustment. It continues to be found that older children rate their self-competence lower than younger children, and girls are observed to have better disease adjustment and peer relations than boys.

Both scientific and observational evidence further support the need for the team approach. The roles of the team members, that is, the physician, physician's assistant, nurse practitioner or nurse specialist, dietitian, exercise specialist, counselor or psychologist, play therapist, social worker, pharmacist, and so forth, are needed from the initial and ongoing adjustment to having an insulin-dependent type of diabetes, and, especially from the physician's standpoint, following a more precarious regimen on a daily basis. Adherence to a regimen needs the support of the team to aid the child or adult as they have or are developing attitudes and beliefs about their situation.

The level of adherence to the regimen is determined by one's attitudes and beliefs (Anderson, Fitzgerald, & Oh, 1993) along with involvement in health behaviors (Hanna & Guthrie, 1999). Anderson, Fitzgerald, and Oh discuss the theory of reasoned actions. This theory states that the best predictor of whether a patient will participate in an intensive regimen to get "good" blood glucose levels would be the patient's stated intentions to do so. They discuss two determinants of a patient's intention. The first is the value that others, considered to be significant in the patient's life, place on the regimen. The second determinant is how positively or negatively the patient feels about using an intensive regimen. This fits well with the views of the Health Belief Model (Bond, Aiken, & Somerville, 1992) and the measure of diabetes self-efficacy with the Perceived Diabetes Self-Management Scale (PDSMS) (Wallston, Rothman, & Cherrington, 2007).

Questions about the regimen, besides the daily self-care needs, are often focused on activities around school attendance, social activities, and athletic events for the younger children, and, for adults, on the work situation, higher education classes, and exercise. Having someone there to answer these questions and to aid in the adjustment to this chronic, potentially life-threatening syndrome assists in stabilization of both the family and the diabetes control. A social worker is also helpful as a resource person who coordinates team members for determining financial adjustment levels and for problem solving as the parents, child, adolescent, and adult return to the community. Social support does have an impact on this disease, as noted by Miller and Davis (2005). This is an expensive and complicated condition. Locating adequate resources (both material and human) helps people to be more at ease when they receive these types of assistance, especially early on after the diagnosis (Van Dam et al., 2005).

Mental Health

Depression can be found in more people with diabetes than previously thought (Rubin et al., 2006a), which prompted the need for strategies developed through the DAWN (Diabetes Attitude Wishes and Needs) study (Rubin et al., 2006b).

Some patients with diabetes exhibit subclinical eating behaviors. Regardless of whether the behavior meets the diagnostic criteria for eating disorder, the problem remains that severe caloric restriction and manipulation of insulin to promote weight loss were found to compromise glycemic control and medical management severely. Although direct or indirect self-destructive behavior often works for attaining what the people feel they need, these patients have a problem, and the causes must be found. Therapeutic intervention by a skilled therapist may help patients to cope with these destructive impulses.

These studies noted that all adults should be screened at some point for depression whether using the simple Zung Self-Rating Depression scale (1965) or the more in-depth scales: the Depression Status Inventory (Zung, 1972), the Hamilton's rating scale for depression (1960), or Beck's Depression Scale (1961). For children, there is the Children's Depression Inventory (Kovacs, 1985) and the Children's Depression Scale (Patton & Burnett, 1993; Knight, Hensley, & Water, 1988). Fisher (2006) shares a *tool chest* for assessing psychosocial variables including depression. Other tools are becoming available on user-friendly computer programs.

Diabetes does impose an emotional strain on the family, especially if the caregiver is single (Thompson, Auslander, & White, 2001), and many responses and adjustments are needed both early and throughout the different stages of the disease. If self-efficacy and regimen adherence are desired, especially for adolescents with T1DM, a positive relationship between these two must be developed (Ott, Greening, Palardy, Holderby, & DeBell, 2000). Further, from the adolescent perspective, there is a need of participation in decision making that corresponds with levels of maturity and the adolescent's increasing autonomy (Hanna & Guthrie, 2003).

There may come a time when individuals neglect or mismanage their disease. Weissberg-Benchell et al. (1995) concluded that forgetting injections and blood glucose testing are commonplace. This was also found by Polish and North American campers in a comparison study (Jarosz-Chobot, Guthrie, Otto-Buczkowska, & Koehler, 2000). They encouraged health care professionals to remember that nonadherence in adolescents with diabetes has a high prevalence. However, there are those youths who purposely mismanage their diabetes to punish or manipulate others.

A number of people have hypoglycemia without the accompanying symptoms. This can lead to fear of normalizing blood glucose levels. Signals are often present or have changed and therefore go unrecognized (Cox et al., 2001). The Blood Glucose Awareness Training (BGAT) program, which offers a solution to this problem, is discussed below. If long-term, or chronic, complications of T1DM are involved, primarily those that are caused by damage to the blood vessels and nerves, resulting in diabetic microvascular and macrovascular diseases, other counseling may be needed.

Management

Having a coach or a contact person during the early days, especially right after the diagnosis of diabetes has been made, can potentially make life a little more amiable. The use of a phone call supports many in their ongoing management (Hilton, 2006). The total involvement of family or significant others in the education and management appears to best support individuals with diabetes and their adjustment to this and other chronic illnesses (Martire, 2005).

Depression, the most common mental illness that appears to be involved with people who have diabetes, is noted with sleep disturbances, fatigue, appetite changes, and irritability, which might be confused with hypo- or hyperglycemia. People grieve for the loss of function of part of the body, some more so than others. If withdrawal and a persistent feeling of being overwhelmed are reported, consider that these might signal depression. True, they might just be symptoms of grief, but if the symptoms last two weeks to several months, then depression may be responsible.

Antidepressants are the most common medications used to treat depression and are known to have an effect on blood glucose levels (Haupt & Newcomer, 2002). If a person has a seizure history, bupropion at doses greater than 400 mg/day should not be administered. It is possible that two or more antidepressants might be needed and, if blood sugars are elevated, rather than stop this medication, the guidelines are to just raise the diabetes medication(s). Be aware that if a person has bipolar disorder and is not treated, blood glucose levels will be challenged. When the person becomes more active, there will be a need for less medication or hypoglycemia will develop.

Handling the stressors in people's lives may help to alleviate symptoms related to increased stress responses of the individuals' bodies and minds. Although the physical symptoms of stress might sound like the start of another condition or illness (headache, upset stomach, achiness, lethargy), the epinephrine (found more in acute stress) and cortisol (found more in chronic stress) both lead directly and indirectly to increased availability of glucose in the bloodstream. Relaxation training or the use of the simple self-training in the Benson Relaxation Response (BRR) will not only assist in decreasing blood pressure and pulse rate, but will also have some effect on blood glucose levels. BRR, supported with deep, abdominal breathing, has two steps: repetition of a phrase, or thought, and, two, the passive handling of intrusive thoughts (such as writing an intervening thought on a piece of paper or "self-talking" that one will deal with the item at the end of the chosen quiet time).

Determining whether the patient is getting adequate sleep is known to be associated with weight control. The right kind and right amount of sleep aid in the body functioning in the most optimal way. Sleep disturbances increase insulin resistance and decrease carbohydrate tolerance and, in people with diabetes, may be associated with arrhythmias (Yaggi, Araujo, & McKinlay, 2006). Assessment of the spirituality of the person or family may also aid in the psychological adjustment to this illness. Tanyi (2006) found that this was both a helpful and appropriate intervention for the families and that most people felt comfortable and more at ease when it was included as part of their workup.

Behavior change may be needed. A disciplined person will probably stay with the diabetes regimen more so than a laid-back type of person. The basic guidelines to change a behavior are to:

1. Identify the behavior to change,
2. Set small steps and short-term goals,
3. Determine the steps to be followed to reach the goal,
4. Implement the approach,
5. Evaluate the outcome after a predetermined period of time, and
6. Redirect with another approach if the one chosen does not work.

The key to achieving a goal is not to set the goal too high and to set the pace according to the person's ability. The BGAT program is a helpful example of a method that can be used to change behavior. The development of the BGAT program has played a role in the participation of patients in the management of their diabetes in other countries as well as the United States (Cox et al., 2004). BGAT is a psychoeducational intervention that aids in reconditioning people to recognize more subtle or different symptoms that indicate low and/or high blood glucose levels. BGAT is available on the Internet. It requires eight weeks of training, but the outcome is the ability to recognize extreme blood glucose levels, to develop an individual program to prevent such events from occurring, to treat extreme situations when needed, and to prevent situations from reoccurring. Fear of hypoglycemia has kept many patients from normalizing their blood glucose levels. Hypoglycemia Anticipation, Awareness, and Treatment Training (HAATT) appears to reduce severe hypoglycemia and lessens the fear of any hypoglycemia from using the BGAT methodology (Schachinger et al., 2005). Fifteen studies have been completed and are reviewed in *Diabetes Spectrum* (Cox et al., 2006).

Mind-body approaches have also become popular as the diabetes epidemic worsens. In 2005, Clark stated that a diagnosis of diabetes coming at a critical time in a patient's life was likely to lead to more problems with diabetes control on a long-term basis. Simple techniques such as meditation, yoga, and progressive muscle relaxation, studied more for people with Type 2 diabetes (T2DM), are useful for people with T1DM as well. Just plain mindfulness and increased awareness of one's self and the environment can be useful. Paying attention to the smaller things, such as holding a spoon or cup, and becoming more aware of its contents, for instance, the appearance and taste, seems to decrease stress responses in the body. Such a "slowing down" of life puts less emphasis on the mechanical parts of diabetes management and greater focus on the total person interacting with daily activities.

Social support is another avenue to be explored. Martire (2005) found that there are added benefits when family members are positively involved in the care of a person with a chronic illness. Positively involved does not mean doing for the person (unless the need actually arises, of course), but being a help-mate to the person involved. Nagging is out, but mutually agreed on code words are helpful. Such a statement as "Dinner will be ready in ten minutes" can be paired with "it's time for me to test my blood sugar and take my insulin." Con-trolled interventions, such as this, have been found by Van Dam et al. (2005) to contribute favorably to the total self-management program.

Another program was developed by Bayer. Bayer Health Care has a hand-out listing the top ten ways to make managing diabetes easier, from monitor-ing blood sugar to "getting with a program." The Behavioral Diabetes Institute (www.Behavioraldiabetes.org) has training workshops on "The emotional side of diabetes: 10 things you need to know." Various programs are available through other companies; go to the Internet (www.diabetes.org or http://ndep.nih.gov), or call the National Diabetes Education Program at 1-800-438-5383. They rec-ommend seven principles to enable patients to control their diabetes life (for details, go to the AADE website, www.diabeteseducator.org):

1. Learn the type of diabetes
2. Get regular care
3. Learn how to control diabetes
4. Treat high blood sugars
5. Monitor blood sugar levels
6. Prevent long-term diabetes problems
7. Get checked for long-term problems and treat them

Encourage the patient to use positive self-talk such as thinking of them-selves as successful compared to past positive occurrences. Positive self-talk especially guides the person to not dwell on failures and to consider each new day as a new beginning. Besides aiding them in identifying their support sys-tem, an important part of self-talk is telling themselves that they will keep on trying until they have the results they seek if such results are reasonable.

Perhaps they need some motivation to action that can be done only by themselves as individuals. The Patient Activation Measure (PAM) is a tool used to measure patient motivation. This is a 13-item questionnaire that indicates a person's confidence in participation in self-management. This tool, on a Strongly Disagree to Strongly Agree scale, reveals the self-reported knowledge, skill, and confidence for the management of the person's chronic condition or general health (Hibbard, Mahoney, Stockard, & Tusler, 2005). This could be any-thing from increasing exercise practice to maintaining a blood glucose test-ing system and self-management practices related to those test results. Lack of understanding or confidence could lead to or result from a state of depression. Therefore, this tool could also be used to assess a person's potential ability to participate in self-management practices.

Barriers to care must also be considered. Barriers to care, such as limited finances, poor or no health insurance program, a feeling of isolation, or a high level of stress, do have an impact on the body (mentally and physically) and, in one study, especially after food intake (Wiesli et al., 2005). When this occurs it is much more difficult to maintain or attain any type of blood glucose control.

The body changes abnormally less when it is in balance, mentally, physically, and spiritually:

> Nature's efforts are seldom purposeless. Nature, through the coordinated secretion of insulin and glucagon, makes a formidable, and in most humans a remarkably successful, effort to avoid hyperglycemia throughout life. These humans virtually always escape microangiopathy, whereas those humans in whom nature fails in its efforts to avoid hyperglycemia usually develop microangiopathy. (Unger, 1975)

The DAWN Study

The Diabetes Attitude Wishes and Needs (DAWN) study determined that the use of psychosocial strategies in diabetes care has resulted in positive outcomes in mainly the White population (other ethnic groups are being studied) (Rubin et al., 2006a). Even professionals have been affected in their use of this program (Rubin et al., 2006b). Skovkind and Peyrot (2005), as members of the International DAWN Advisory Panel, reported that the use of this program contributed to better adherence through the provision of psychological support to patients, especially the use of empowerment (the patient having educated control over the decision making and sequence of education input; Weiss, 2006).

Other Assessment and Interventions

As the DAWN study has evidenced, depression is often overlooked. Major depression is of the greatest concern, but it must occur for over two or more weeks to be diagnosed. Major depression is identified by observing or assessing one of the following: depressed mood or decreased interest or pleasure in activities and/or four of the following: suicidal ideation, problems with concentration, fatigue, problems with sleep, significant weight loss or weight gain, and restlessness or lack of movement.

De Wit, Pouwer, Gemke, Delemarre-van de Waal, and Snoek (2007) validated a simple index of emotional problems and well-being developed through the World Health Organization that gives information suitable for use with the adolescent population. It is simple to use and is available in many languages. For more focused instrument outcomes, use the pediatric Quality of Life Inventory Diabetes Module or the Diabetes Quality of Life-Youth, as noted by de Wit, Delemarre-van der Waal, Pouwer, Gemke, and Snoek (2007), or the Strength and Difficulties Questionnaire (Goodman, 1997) for more inclusive assessment. Presently, at least three evidence-based approaches are helpful for both adults and children. They are the cognitive-behavioral approach, motivational interviewing, and dialectical behavior therapy. Coping skills training is a useful example of the cognitive-behavioral approach, improving the quality of life over the period of a year, and also metabolic control (Gregg, Callaghan, Hayes, & Glenn-Lawson, 2007; Grey, Boland, Davidson, Li, & Tamborlane, 2000; Hayes, Strosahl, Follette, & Linehan, 2005).

Motivational interviewing is a counseling process to help patients change behavior by exploring and resolving concern, especially when related to treatment (Levensky, Forcehimes, O'Donohue, & Beitz, 2007). This method, as with the other approaches, indirectly involves the individual in achieving agency and a sense of empowerment over a condition they cannot change but can control. Used are the basic counseling techniques of reflective listening, asking open-ended questions, affirming positive gain, and summarizing what has been discussed. Dialectical behavior therapy, developed by Marsha Linehan in 1987, initially developed for treating borderline personality disorders, is useful for those who have problems with adjusting to having a chronic disease (emotional dysregulation) by identifying feelings, being able to communicate those feelings, being able to regulate those feelings, and taking responsibility for actions (Harley, Sprich, Safren, Jacobo, & Fava, 2008). Although developed for adults and children with borderline personalities, the exercises and approaches are very useful in daily life (Marra, 2005).

The outcomes are the potential to decrease depression, increase empowerment, and promote self-*discipline* (a word derived from the Greek word meaning to teach). Self-discipline is important for the child, the adolescent, and the adult, anyone who is involved in the techniques of self-care and self-management. As self-management is achieved through knowledge, guidance, and self-discipline, patients with diabetes are increasingly capable of taking on more responsibility of their own care. The outcome of increased self-care is the potential for a 76% decrease in risk for having retinopathy, a 60% decrease in risk for having neuropathy, a 50% decrease in risk for having nephropathy (DCCT, 1993), and a lower risk in having cardiovascular disease (Genuth, 2006).

Other Resources

More information may be obtained by going to: the American Self-Help Group Clearinghouse (http://mentalhelp.net/selfhelp), Children with Diabetes (www.childrenwithdiabetes.com), the National Board for Certified Counselors (www.nbcc.org), or the National Institute of Mental Health Public Information and Communications Branch (www.nimh.nih.gov/HealthInformation/Getting Help.cfm).

Health professionals play an important role in the way that, especially parents, handle their diabetes regimen. The way community resources are introduced, the education that is received, and the personal interaction between health professionals and patients relates to how parents perceive they can raise their child successfully despite their child having diabetes (Ginsburg et al., 2005). The positive attitude of parents and other family members and friends does influence whether the child or teenager or adult takes better care of themselves.

Summary

The cooperative effort of the entire health care team, including children, adolescents, adults, and their families, is needed to provide the level of care and education needed to accomplish the goal of normal glycemia the majority of the time, accompanied with a high degree of safety. Involvement of the total team is needed as they assess, interact, and support the person with diabetes in achieving a happier and healthier life.

With appropriate psychosocial support, the results should include less depression, less anxiety, more empowerment, improved glycemic control, and an enhanced quality of life.

Recommended Reading

Surwit, R. S. (2005). *The mind-body diabetes revolution; the proven way to control your blood sugar by managing stress, depression, anger and other emotions*. New York: Marlowe & Company.

References

Anderson, R. M., Fitzgerald, J. T., & Oh, M. S. (1993). The relationship between diabetes-related attitudes and patients' self-reported adherence. *The Diabetes Educator, 19*, 287–292.

Beck, A. T., Ward, C. H., Mendelson, M., Mock, J., & Erbaugh, J. (1961). An inventory for measuring depression. *Archives of General Psychiatry, 6*(4), 561–671.

Bond, G. G., Aiken, L. S., & Somerville, B. C. (1992). The health belief model and adolescents with insulin dependent diabetes mellitus. *Health Psychology, 11*(3), 190–198.

Clark, M. C. (2005). Managing psychosocial impacts of diabetes. *Practice Nursing, 15*(7), 334, 336, 338–339.

Clarke, W. L., Vance, M. L., & Rogol, A. D. (1993). Growth and the child with diabetes mellitus. *Diabetes Care, 6*(Suppl. 3), 101–107.

Cox, D. J., Gonder-Frederick, L., Polonsky, W., Schlundt, D., Kovatchev, B., & Clarke, W. (2001). Blood glucose awareness training (BGAT-2): Long-term benefits. *Diabetes Care, 24*(4), 637–642.

Cox, D. J., Gonder-Frederick, L., Ritterband, L., Patel, K., Schachinger, H., Fehm-Wolfsdorf, G., et al. (2006). Blood glucose awareness training: What is it, where is it, and where is it going? *Diabetes Spectrum, 19*(1), 43–49.

Cox, D. J., Kovatchev, B., Koev, D., Koeva, L., Dachev, S., Tcharatchiev, D., et al. (2004). Hypoglycemia anticipation, awareness and treatment training (HAATT) reduces occurrence of severe hypoglycemia among adults with type 1 diabetes mellitus. *International Journal of Behavioral Medicine, 11*(4), 212–218.

de Wit, M., Delemarre-van der Waal, H. A., Pouwer, F., Gemke, R. J. B. J., & Snoek, F. J. (2007). Monitoring health related quality of life in adolescents with diabetes: A review of measures. *Archives of Diseases in Children, 92*, 434–439.

de Wit, M., Pouwer, F., Gemke, R. J., Delemarre-van de Waal, H. A., & Snoek, F. J. (2007). Validation of the WHO-5 well-being index of adolescents with type 1 diabetes. *Diabetes Care, 30*(8), 2003–2006.

Diabetes Control and Complications Trial Research Group. (1993). The effect of intensive treatment of diabetes on the development and progression of long-term complications in insulin-dependent diabetes mellitus. *New England Journal of Medicine, 329*(14), 977–985.

Fisher, K. L. (2006). Tool chest: Assessing psychosocial variables: A tool for diabetes educators. *The Diabetes Educator, 32*(1), 51–52, 54, 56.

Genuth, S. (2006). Insights from the diabetes control and complications trial/epidemiology of diabetes interventions and complications study on the use of intensive glycemic treatment to reduce the risk of complications of type 1 diabetes. *Endocrinology Practice, 12*(Suppl. 1), 35–41.

Ginsburg, K. R., Howe, C. J., Jawad, A. F., Buzby, M., Ayala, J. M., Tuttle, A., et al. (2005). Parents' perceptions of factors that affect successful diabetes management for their children. *Pediatrics, 116*(5), 1095–1104.

Goodman, R. (1997). The strengths and difficulties questionnaire: A research note. *Journal of Child Psychology and Psychiatry, 38*, 581–586.

Gregg, J. A., Callaghan, G. M., Hayes, S. C., & Glenn-Lawson, J. L. (2007). Improving diabetes self-management through acceptance, mindfulness, and values: A randomized controlled trial. *Journal of Consulting Clinical Psychology, 75*(2), 336–343.

Grey, M., Boland, E. A., Davidson, M., Li, J., & Tamborlane, W. V. (2000). Coping skills training for youth with diabetes mellitus has long-lasting effects on metabolic control and quality of life. *Journal of Pediatrics, 137*(2), 107–113.

Hamilton, M. (1960). A rating scale for depression. *Journal of Neurology, Neurosurgery, and Psychiatry, 2*(23), 56–62.

Hanna, K. M., & Guthrie, D. W. (1999). Involvement in health behaviors among youth with diabetes. *Diabetes Educator, 25*(2), 211–219.

Hanna, K. M., & Guthrie, D. W. (2003). Adolescents' behavioral autonomy related to diabetes management and adolescent activities/rules. *The Diabetes Educator, 29*(2), 283–291.

Harley, R., Sprich, S., Safren, S., Jacobo, M., & Fava, M. (2008). Adaptation of dialectical behavior therapy skills training group for treatment-resistant depression. *Journal of Nervous Mental Disorders, 196*(2), 136–143.

Haupt, D. W., & Newcomer, J. W. (2002). Abnormalities in glucose regulation associated with mental illness and treatment. *Journal of Psychosomatic Research, 53*(4), 925–933.

Hayes, S., Strosahl, K., Follette, V., & Linehan, M. (Eds.) (2005). *Mindfulness and acceptance: Expanding the cognitive-behavioral tradition.* New York: Guilford.

Hibbard, J. H., Mahoney, E. R., Stockard, J., & Tusler, M. (2005). *Development and testing of a short form of the patient activation measure* (Health Services Research pp. 1–13). Eugene, OR: Department of Planning, Public Policy, and Management, University of Oregon.

Hieronymus, L. H., & Geil, P. (2006). *101 tips for raising healthy kids with diabetes.* Alexandria, VA: American Diabetes Association.

Hilton, L. (2006). Compliance may be a phone call away. *Nursing Spectrum, 18*(1), 20–21.

Jackson, R. L., Holland, E., Chatman, I. D., Guthrie, D., & Hewett, J. E. (1978). Growth and maturation of children with insulin dependent diabetes mellitus. *Diabetes Care, 1,* 96–107.

Jarosz-Chobot, P., Guthrie, D. W., Otto-Buczkowska, E., & Koehler, B. (2000). Self-care of young diabetes in practice. *Medical Science Monitor, 6*(1), 129–132.

Knight, D., Hensley, V. R., & Water, B. (1988). Validation of the Children's Depression Scale and the Children's Depression Inventory in a pre-pubertal sample. *Journal of Child Psychology and Psychiatry, 29*(6), 853–863.

Kovacs, M. (1985). The Children's Depression Inventory. *Psychopharmacology Bulletin, 21*(4), 995–998.

Kovacs, M., Brent, D., Steinberg, T. F., Paulauskas, S., & Reid, J. (1986). Children's self-reports of psychologic adjustment and coping strategies during first year of insulin-dependent diabetes mellitus. *Diabetes Care, 9,* 474–479.

Kovacs, M., Finkelstein, R., Feinberg, T. L., Crouse-Novak, M., Paulauskas, S., & Pollock, M. (1985). Initial psychologic responses of parents to the diagnosis of insulin-dependent diabetes mellitus in their children. *Diabetes Care, 8,* 568–575.

Levensky, E. R., Forcehimes, A., O'Donohue, W. T., & Beitz, K. (2007). Motivational interviewing: An evidence-based approach to counseling helps patients follow treatment recommendations. *American Journal of Nursing, 107*(10), 50–57.

Li, C., Ford, E. S., Strine, T. W., & Mokdad, A. H. (2008). Prevalence of depression among U.S. adults with diabetes: Findings from the 2006 behavioral risk factor surveillance system. *Diabetes Care, 31*(1), 105–107.

Linehan, M. M. (1987). Dialectical behavior therapy for borderline personality disorder: Theory and method. *Bulletin of the Menninger Clinic, 51*(3), 261–276.

Marra, T. (2005). *Dialectical behavior therapy in private practice: A practical and comprehensive guide.* Oakland: New Harbinger Press.

Martire, L. M. (2005). The "relative" efficacy of involving family in psychosocial interventions for chronic illness: Are there added benefits to patients and family members? *Families, Systems & Health, 23*(3), 312–328.

Miller, C. K., & Davis, M. S. (2005). The influential role of social support in diabetes management. *Topics in Clinical Nutrition, 20*(2), 157–165.

Musen, G., Jacobson, A. M., Ryan, C. M., Cleary, P. A., Waberski, B. H., Weinger, K., et al. (2008). The impact of diabetes and its treatment on cognitive function among adolescents who participated in the DCCT. *Diabetes Care,* in press.

Ott, J., Greening, L., Palardy, N., Holderby, A., & DeBell, W. (2000). Self-efficacy as a mediator variable for adolescents' adherence to treatment for insulin-dependent diabetes mellitus. *Children's Health Care, 29*(1), 47–63.

Padala, P. R., Desouza, C. V., Almeida, S., Shivaswamy, V., Ariyarathna, K., Rouse, L., et al. (2008). The impact of apathy on glycemic control in diabetes: A cross-sectional study. *Diabetes Research in Clinical Practice, 79*(1), 37–41.

Patton, W., & Burnett, P. C. (1993). The Children's Depression Scale: Assessment of factor structure with data from a normal adolescent population. *Adolescence, 28*(110), 315–324.

Rubin, R. R., Peyrot, M., Siminerio, L. M., on behalf of the International DAWN Advisory Panel (2006a). Health care and patient reported outcomes: Results of the cross-national diabetes attitude wishes and needs study. *Diabetes Care, 29,* 1249–1255.

Rubin, R. R., Peyrot, M., Siminerio, L. M., on behalf of the International DAWN Advisory Panel (2006b). Physicians and nurses use of psychosocial strategies and diabetes care: Results of the national DAWN study. *Diabetes Care, 29,* 1256–1262.

Schachinger, H., Hegar, K., Hermanns, N., Straumann, M., Keller, U., Kehm-Wolfsdorf, G., et al. (2005). Randomized controlled clinical trial of Blood Glucose Awareness Training (BGAT III) in Switzerland and Germany. *Journal of Behavioral Medicine, 28*(6), 587–594.

Simond, J. F. (1975, August). *Psychiatric status of diabetic children in good and poor control.* Paper presented at the Third International Beilinson Symposium on the Balance of Diabetes, Tel Aviv, Israel.

Skovkind, S. E., & Peyrot, M., on behalf of the International DAWN Advisory Panel. (2005). The DAWN design: A new approach to improving outcomes of diabetes care. *Diabetes Spectrum, 18*(3), 136–142.

Tanyi, R. A. (2006). Spirituality and family nursing: Spiritual assessment and interventions for families. *Journal of Advanced Nursing, 53*(3), 287–294.

Thompson, S. J., Auslander, W. F., & White, N. H. (2001). Influence of family structure among youth with diabetes. *Health and Social Work, 26*(1), 7–14.

Unger, R. H. (1975). Glucagon in the pathogenesis of diabetes. *Lancet, 3*(1), 1036–1042.

Van Dam, H. A., van der Horst, F. G., Knoops, L., Ryckman, R. M., Crebolder, H. F. J., & van den Borne, B. H. W. (2005). Social support in diabetes: A systematic review of controlled intervention studies. *Patient Education and Counseling, 59*(1), 1–12.

Wallston, K. A., Rothman, R. L., & Cherrington, A. (2007). Psychometric properties of the Perceived Diabetes Self-Management Scale (PDSMS). *Journal of Behavioral Medicine, 30*(5), 395–401.

Weiss, M. A. (2006). Empowerment: A patient's perspective. *Diabetes Spectrum, 19,* 116–118.

Weissberg-Benchell, J., Glasgow, A., Tynon, W., Wirtz, P., Turek, J., & Ward, J. (1995). Adolescent diabetes management and mismanagement. *Diabetes Care, 18,* 77–82.

Wiesli, P., Schmid, C., Kerwer, O., Nigg-Koch, C., Klaghofer, R., Seifert, B., et al. (2005). Acute psychological stress affects glucose concentrations in patients with type 2 diabetes following food intake but not in the fasting state. *Diabetes Care, 28*(8), 1910–1914.

Wysocki, T., Harris, M. A., Greco, P., Harvey, L. M., McDonell, K., Danda, C. L., et al. (1997). Social validity of support group and behavior therapy interventions for families of adolescents with insulin-dependent diabetes mellitus. *Journal of Pediatric Psychology, 22*(5), 635–649.

Yaggi, H. K., Araujo, A. B., & McKinlay, J. B. (2006). Sleep duration as a risk factor for the development of type 2 diabetes. *Diabetes Care, 29*(3), 657–661.

Zung, W. W. (1965). Self-Rating Depression Scale. *Archives of General Psychiatry, 12,* 63–70.

Zung, W. W. (1972). The Depression Status Inventory: An adjunct to the Self-Rating Depression Scale. *Journal of Clinical Psychiatry, 28*(4), 539–543.

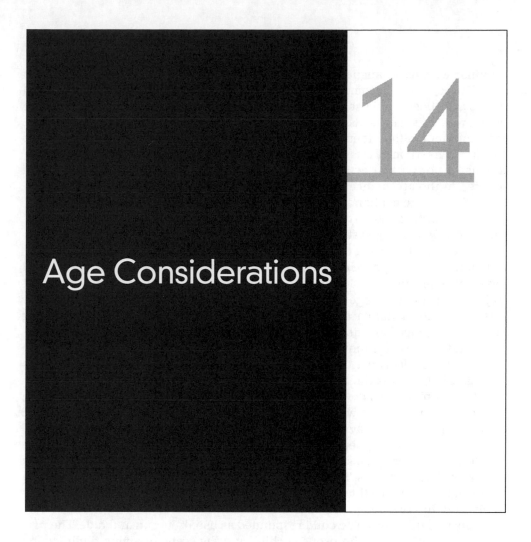

Age Considerations

All developmental stages pose unique challenges for families.

M. Harris, 2006

The continuum of life presents various obstacles and opportunities. These variations with age potentially and individually may have an impact on diabetes management. In this chapter, we address age considerations from infancy to the older population who may be unable to respond because of lack of dexterity or brain function.

Age is commonly categorized in six developmental stages: infancy through toddlers, kindergarten through preadolescence, adolescence, young adults, middle adults, and older adults. The aspects of care related to the needs of members of each age group who have diabetes mellitus are presented.

Infancy Through Toddlers

This is the time in life when the world is full of new things including walking, talking, and eating solid foods. Within the first two years of life, children become familiar with basic language skills and are able to balance, to walk, and even to run. Pureed foods become less and less a part of the stable diet and more solid foods are chosen and used as chewing (or gumming) and swallowing skills are mastered. This time is also used for controlling elimination and, because of the development of their identity, is used, especially around age two, to assert their "rights". Assertion of this level of "control", besides eating and elimination (refusing to potty train) activities, may also apply to problems with cooperation related to the acceptance of blood glucose testing and insulin injections, especially if they are not handled well by concerned parents.

A few of these concerns are as follows. Because exploration is a key part of this group's learning system, the sight of something often leads to movement, from grasping to placing the object in the mouth. A lancet, a syringe, or an insulin pump are not types of objects that should be tested in the mouth. Their usual ways of exploring are blocked, for safety reasons if nothing else, they might reject a lancet or syringe because they may feel that rejection is the only way they can control that part of their environment. This is one reason that testing and insulin injections must be given as routinely as possible. The more attention paid to these techniques, the more the child might resist. The opposite also holds true: The less attention and the more matter-of-fact way these techniques are handled, the less the child might resist.

If a problem does develop, the simplest way to handle it is to associate the activity that is invasive with the follow-up of an activity that is pleasant, such as reading a book or playing a game. The following situation is an excellent example of what can happen:

T. and L. were devastated when they learned that their already walking 1-year-old had diabetes. They did everything to please their little boy. Taking a test or giving an injection was played out as a game. The parent would laughingly find the child and proceed with the health care needed. One day, one of the parents was in a hurry. The child responded as usual—to run and hide. The parent became upset, which upset the child, and the scene of giving the injection turned into a battleground. When the father called and reported their dilemma, he was counseled to tell the child (despite the child's age) that the testing and injection were to be given at the time the doctor (a higher authority) ordered, so they, as parents, were not allowed to play any games before the test or injection. They "were told they could read a book or do something special (like a game) after the test or injection was given as there was time before or after the meal." They reported some struggling and a few tears when they first used this approach, but in a few days the child started looking forward to having a parent read the story he had chosen to hear after the procedure was completed.

Growing into toddlerhood and exploring and learning about sex differences does not seem to interfere with diabetes practices or management. Attaining physiological stability does. Going to Head Start or to preschool is a time when new organisms lead to frequent infections, which does challenge diabetes management. It also challenges beta cell function, if not all beta cells have lost their ability to make insulin. With each illness, potentially more beta cells are lost. This leads to an even greater insulin dependency. More insulin may be needed during the infectious challenge and may continue to be needed after the infection has subsided. Dosage levels of insulin often are higher at the end of the infectious process than at the beginning.

Toddlers learn simple social actions in management of elimination and eating skills. They are also learning what is acceptable and not acceptable in their own world. Cooperating with an injection or with another invasive technique, the finger (hand, arm, or ear) stick can be accepted as commonplace or may also be something over which they feel they must have control—like playing games when it is time to eat or to be tested. Parents must be aware that self-care skills regarding injections and monitoring blood glucose levels are *just a part of life*. If the children accept this approach, then self-care times can become part of the daily routine. If not, problems can arise that lead to lack of adjustment later on in life, especially during adolescence.

Kindergarten Through Preadolescence

During this time of life, learning skills for playing games, playing their male or female role, and developing the basic skills of reading, writing, and arithmetic (the three R's) aid them in forming the concepts that are needed for everyday living. They not only need to have positive self-esteem, but also a good picture of themselves when playing with siblings and friends. If this adjustment time is handled in a healthy manner, these children become able to reason and begin to develop some personal independence.

Food may or may not become an issue. Their likes and dislikes become more obvious. Tastes vary and they often mirror responses of other family members or, in their striving to be independent, act just the opposite. Likes and dislikes become part of everyday life. They may take too long to eat or keep demanding fast foods because that is what their friends are eating. Learning the skills of eating together as a family can become a real challenge to parents. This challenge increases when one child in the family (or more) refuses to eat certain healthy foods. The parents being firm in a reasonable way is helpful, but they should not push the concept of the "clean plate". Eating struggles (about eating everything on the plate) lead to a greater chance of an eating disorder later on in life. Because eating is variable at this age, it may be difficult to judge insulin doses. Using an ultrafast-acting insulin like glulisine and giving it after the meal when intake can be better judged may be a good solution.

Participation in self-care increases as dexterity and basic understanding increase. Four-year-olds may participate in a self-injection accomplished under supervision. They may become more trusting of themselves in picking a site for a finger stick or an injection. The danger is in "favorite spots". Some areas of the body may be less painful to inject or to use as a test site. The danger is that the repeated use of that same spot may lead to lipodystrophy, which includes lumps or scar tissue. Again, firm guidance is needed to get over these hurdles and trials of inappropriate independence. Parental support and education of the child with diabetes, especially by participating in a youth group or camp, aid in promoting positive self-care as an outcome.

Being accepted by their friends is also important to most of these children. Having to take a snack or stop for a shot or a test might become quite an embarrassment. These problems seem to surface when a new school semester starts. Each new semester offers new challenges, especially when a new teacher or new classroom is involved. During kindergarten and the rest of childhood education, parents must be in contact with the school health nurse and with the schoolteacher(s). Time and place must be determined for blood glucose monitoring, injection giving, snack time, and hypoglycemia treatment. Those first few days, as will be found later on in the schooling process (or in the acclimatization to a new job), are the roughest times in determining the management skills needed during that new beginning. Paperwork needs to be completed so that the regimen for that particular child is known by all personnel involved with that child. Emergency contacts need to be listed and what should be done in a real emergency related to low or really high blood sugars.

Adolescence

This is a time in and of itself. Determining one's self-worth and "who I am" plus "I am invincible" seem to rule the ages from 12 to 18. Carroll and Marrero (2006) found that, because of this internal push/pull, adolescents may have problems with developmental activities that lead to undesired consequences. Their own body is part of this adjustment, along with separating from family in their striving for independence and for transitioning into a healthy adulthood. Having a chronic disease makes this process a particularly difficult one, especially if diabetes is used as the "apron string breaker". If the earlier years have not been handled in a mature way, these years become years of resistance to self-care and diabetes management can really get out of hand. Everything from falsifying blood glucose records to gaining weight to omitting insulin in order to lose weight have been attempted.

The pressure of achieving economic independence is also an added burden. *What do I want to be when I grow up* can be a pressure, especially if the family wants the adolescent to become one type of professional or technician and the adolescent wants to become another. Preparing for an occupation is one thing. Preparing for marriage and family life is another. The general tendency is to protect (and overprotect) a child with a chronic illness. This type of stifling protection may lead to the suppression of emotional skills despite being more advanced in social skills. This means that preparation for going out into the world may be a big hardship, because they have always had someone else watching over them, caring for them, or picking up the pieces when they have had difficulty.

On the positive side, the values obtained from having a chronic disease may lay the groundwork for a more disciplined adult. Socially responsible behavior may be easily addressed as they have had to take on responsibility of self-management from choosing injection sites, to monitoring, and to treating lows and preventing high blood glucose levels. And, because diabetes is an expensive disease, it is necessary to work toward getting an education that will help adolescents to get the type of job that can best support their diabetes needs along with their social desires to advance in a field that interests them.

Adolescence is a trying time. Too much responsibility may be given too soon in the attempt of parents to relieve themselves of the perceived burden of raising a child who has a chronic problem (Wysocki, 1993). If this transition is a healthy one, the steps taken toward full self-care and self-management are safer for the adolescent. All said, having diabetes mellitus can be used to help achieve a desired goal of independence and good health or it can become the door to poor self-care and inadequate self-management practices. Raging hormone levels, self-esteem, a sense of invincibility, unwired decision-making areas of the brain, and the sense of being part of the group can lead to both good and bad consequences in adolescence. Developmental consequences must be addressed along with the technical aspects of care or progression into adulthood may be affected (Carroll & Marrero, 2006). Health care personnel must be aware of all these changes going on in the adolescent and be prepared to address them as they occur or even before they occur.

Young Adults

Ages 19–29 are considered to be in the young adult group. Young adults may or may not choose a mate and/or learn to live with another. They might be starting a family and raising children. The responsibility of managing a home and/or occupation or both must be taken seriously as they become a member of a community and social group. Without adequate education in self-management and self-care, personal health problems will potentially accelerate (Anderson, 2004).

Self-management is of the utmost importance, but consideration must also be given to priorities in life. At times, more emphasis must be placed on needs of the family versus needs of the self, but if basic self-needs are not met, then the person will not be of much help to themselves or to the rest of the family. So some measure of self-care must be met at all times, otherwise that person becomes a stumbling block to his or her own health needs and cannot be there when other members of the family are in need.

Holding down a job or being the homemaker becomes a real challenge. Too many days lost from work may mean the loss of a job. Too much time lost from higher education means that that goal might be delayed or not achieved. However, a person who practices good self-care and self-management can become one of the best workers or students. They have learned self-discipline through having a chronic illness and, therefore, are able to take on more responsibilities than the average person.

If self-care and self-management have not been good, then a likelihood exists that complications from this disease might arise. If eyes are involved, there is a greater chance that kidneys are involved. If kidneys are involved there is a greater chance that eyes will be involved along with cardiovascular problems. With or without cardiovascular problems, nerve tissue problems might occur—but are more apt to occur concurrently with cardiovascular disease. This means days lost from work or school. This also means increased expense for the family and the community as a whole. The whole living situation is more highly stressed and the potential for achieving an occupational goal is reduced.

Choice of a specialist for diabetes care and other health care professionals, especially if complications are involved, becomes a part of the lifestyle. The better part of valor is to prevent problems from occurring in the first place; seeing a specialist every three to four months is a must.

Middle Adults

This group includes the age range from 30 to 60 years old. It is the responsibility of the people in this group to assist others, especially their own children, to become responsible adults. Individually, they may be involved, to a greater extent, in social and civic responsibilities. There is a greater chance that they might have a "midlife crisis" if they have not met their own expectations. All of this is occurring at the time their body is adjusting to the physiological changes of aging.

This time in life is often called the third adolescence. The first adolescence is perceived at the ages of the 2- to 3-year-old. The second adolescence is perceived at the standard time in life. The third adolescence occurs in the mid-50s. At all three times, control becomes as important as lack of achievement, along with knowing who "I am". Self-questioning and self-doubt lead to foolish choices and, in this age range, broken marriages.

There is another problem. Weight increases when the amount of food eaten is perceived to be the same as the amount eaten when an adolescent or a young adult is growing or very active. Exercise practices are often lost in the battle of making ends meet financially. In this day and age of technology, more time is spent on gadgets than on being in the out of doors. Less exercise in the face of too much food can only result in weight gain and the potential for obesity. This is where the discipline most often lacking in the adolescent years really comes into play. If a person remains active despite decreasing exercise practices and listens to their body by decreasing the portion sizes of foods eaten, then weight gain is not an outcome.

There may be a need for more medication as the person "enlarges". The bigger the person is or the more a person eats, the more medication is needed to control blood glucose levels. If a person in this age group cuts back on food intake, then the logic is to cut back on medication as blood glucose monitoring indicates. As a professional, you can tell your patients that their own body will tell them when they need to change their medication amounts, the amount of food to be eaten, and the activity or the exercise needed if they closely observe information obtained from blood glucose level tests. This is an age, of the many others, when the professional must have blood glucose tests, not just hemoglobin A1c levels, to determine the total daily or time-of-day needs for medication for a particular patient.

Older Adults

When older than 60, even if one does not feel it, the wear and tear on the body begins to show, even if it has not shown before. Strength decreases, especially if it is not challenged by maintenance or increases in activity or exercise. Muscle mass decreases and fat mass increases. Health diminishes, especially if good health practices have not been followed. Income may be reduced with loss of work or dependence on retirement income.

If kidneys have been compromised by hyperglycemia, hypertension, or just age, all diabetes medications may become concentrated in the body, leading to the need for less medication. Insulin is especially noted to be decreased as the person's intake decreases or if the kidneys decrease in function. Such medications as sulfonylureas and biguanides are not indicated for treatment if kidney function is compromised. A 24-hour urine test is a must when kidney compromise is suspected (especially if the creatinine is over the laboratory standard for normal).

Hornick and Aron (2008) focus on the need to be very careful when working with this population. They consider that the overall goal is the best quality of life possible with healthy food intake and prevention of hypoglycemia.

Reconsidering Hypoglycemia

Perhaps the reappearance of this topic seems out of place in this chapter, but it does have special importance related to age considerations. The most damaging consideration is the potential to the youngest population whose nervous system is in the process of maturing. In the older adult, besides the glycosylation process when hyperglycemia is present, it is a ruptured blood vessel when the pulse pressure is increased by the concurrent release of epinephrine when hypoglycemia occurs. Medications are adjusted to result in less hypoglycemia (Childs, 2006). The youngest children communicate symptoms less, but older children and adults may develop hypoglycemia unawareness.

In the adult patients, problems related to hypoglycemia (and hyperglycemia) are basically found to result from errors in prescribing and monitoring (Smith, Winterstein, Johns, Rosenberg, & Sauer, 2005). Further, adults may develop problems associated with eating and drinking practices, such as the introduction of alcohol and its blocking of glycogenolysis (Richardson, Weiss, Thomas, & Kerr, 2005). The potential impact on job responsibilities was found to occur less frequently than suspected (Leckie, Graham, Grant, Ritchie, & Frier, 2005).

Similarity and differences of the signs and symptoms of hypoglycemia versus hyperglycemia are present in all age groups (refer to Table 8.1 in Chapter 8). This leads to the need for self-reporting that a person has diabetes, whether in school or at work, and what to do if an insulin reaction occurs. School personnel and work personnel must be prepared.

Summary

Whatever the age, whatever the type of diabetes, care must be taken to prevent any type of complication whether it be a physical, mental, or emotional one. Pre-preparation by carrying treatment for too high or too low a blood sugar prevents problems whether they occur at home, school, or work. Recognizing where the person is on life's continuum guides the professional to assist in the preplanning for these and other problems.

References

Anderson, B. J. (2004). A developmental perspective on the challenges of diabetes education and care during the young adult period. *Patient Education and Counseling, 53,* 347–352.

Carroll, A. E., & Marrero, D. G. (2006). The role of significant others in adolescent diabetes: A qualitative study. *The Diabetes Educator, 32*(2), 243–252.

Childs, B. P. (2006). Pramlintide use in type 1 diabetes resulting in less hypoglycemia. *Diabetes Spectrum, 19*(1), 50–52.

Harris, M. (2006). Dogs, cats, and diabetes. *Diabetes Spectrum, 19*(3), 187–188.

Hornick, T., & Aron, D. C. (2008). Managing diabetes in the elderly: Go easy, individualize. *Cleveland Clinic Journal of Medicine, 75*(1), 70–78.

Leckie, A. M., Graham, M. K., Grant, J. B., Ritchie, P. J., & Frier, B. M. (2005). Frequency, severity, and morbidity of hypoglycemia occurring in the workplace in people with insulin-treated diabetes. *Diabetes Care, 28*(6), 1333–1338.

Richardson, T., Weiss, M., Thomas, P., & Kerr, D. (2005). Day after the night before: Influence of evening alcohol on risk of hypoglycemia in patients with type 1 diabetes. *Diabetes Care, 28*(7), 1801–1802.

Smith, W. D., Winterstein, A. G., Johns, T., Rosenberg, E., & Sauer, B. C. (2005). Causes of hyperglycemia and hypoglycemia in adult inpatients. *American Journal of Health Systems Pharmacy, 62*(7), 714–719.

Wysocki, T. (1993). Associations among teen-parent relationships, metabolic control, and adjustment to diabetes in adolescents. *Journal of Pediatric Psychology, 18,* 441–452.

15

Using the Pattern Approach

> All the information in the world is wasted if not used correctly and if not used safely.
>
> D. Hinnen, 2002

There are many approaches to the management of diabetes. Before the DCCT results were announced in 1993, the argument in the diabetes world was over whether blood glucose levels needed to be well controlled. Since 1993, the argument has changed from *whether* to *how* blood glucose levels should be controlled. Argument among experts in the field suggests that no one method of control is as yet perfect. Any disease process is a deviation from what nature has created and evolved. Though nature may not be perfect either, and continued development may make us all better, it is safe to say that nature's way is the best we have now and nature's way is seldom purposeless. Consequently, the closer we can come to duplicating the way nature does what it does, the better off we will be. Restoring the individual with a disease back to physiological normality as nearly as possible should be the goal of any disease treatment. In the past we have not had good tools to restore persons with diabetes back to a physiologically normal state of metabolism. We are still not perfect, but the tools have gotten better in the past few years, so we can at least make an attempt to simulate a near-normal state.

For people with Type 2 diabetes mellitus (T2DM), the diabetes epidemic has led to a huge amount of research from the pharmaceutical industry and the development and improvement of old classes of drugs and the development of new classes of drugs. Data from the studies of the relationship of the control of diabetes to chronic complications in T2DM has also led to the concept of earlier and more aggressive use of insulin in these people. In this chapter we will discuss the use of insulin primarily in people with Type 1 diabetes mellitus (T1DM), but the same principles apply to people with T2DM, so they will not be distinguished in this discussion.

For many years after the discovery of insulin in 1921, and its introduction in 1922, only regular insulin was available. It was recognized early that a longer-acting insulin was needed. Protamine Zinc Insulin (PZI), globin, and Neutral Protamine Hagedorn (NPH) insulin were developed to meet this need. Finally, the Lente series of insulins were introduced. Many different insulin combinations and regimens were tried with these insulins with only limited success for blood glucose control. The problem with these insulins was a peak effect not correlated with the influx of food from the stomach. This resulted not in hyperglycemia when there was food but little insulin but hypoglycemia when the opposite was true. Getting the two to come out even was a real problem. Conditions began to improve with the introduction of recombinant DNA technology and with the development of human insulin and the insulin analogues. The long-acting analogues such as Glargine and Detemir provide peakless basal insulin for 24 hours in one or two injections per day. The rapid-acting analogues such as lispro, asparte, and glulisine gave us the ability to give insulin close to the meal time (for greater convenience of the patient), better coordination with food peaks, and shorter duration of action. All of these advantages of long- and rapid-acting insulins have given more physiologic control, more convenience, and less hypoglycemia for better blood glucose control with greater safety. The main problem with the analogues is price. Regular and NPH insulin and the Premixes of them can be obtained for less than $20 a vial, while the analogues may cost $65–$100 a vial. The price difference has led some physicians to advocate returning to regular and NPH insulins. We believe this is a step backward in time that is not warranted because medical insurance, Medicare, Medicaid, and State Children's Health Insurance Program (SCHIP) programs all pay for the newer insulins. When patients do not have insurance, there are programs from the companies that make insulin as well as state and local programs to provide this care. All individuals should be able to be treated to state-of-the-art medicine regardless of their financial circumstances. They are all human beings and should be treated equally. Treatment should not be compromised. The payment problem should be worked on and solved.

Even with the development of insulin analogues and the basal-bolus concept of physiologic insulin administration or even Continuous Subcutaneous Insulin Infusion (CSII), there is still not complete consensus on the best insulin regimen. There is disagreement on diet—fixed or free, high carbohydrate or low carbohydrate, carbohydrate or total calorie counting, high fat or low fat, and so on. Dietary programs are discussed in detail in Chapters 10 and 18. There other areas of lack of consensus. Do we use premeal or postmeal blood glucose measurement? Should insulin be given before or after the meal? What are the correct proportions of insulin for each meal and how does it relate to the kind of food eaten? Should long-acting insulin be given in the morning or the evening or split between both? The answers to these and many other questions await further research. Here we can give you our opinion based on more than 40 years of experience of trial and error with many thousands of patients and the best, up-to-date evidence in the literature. Our experience has validated the pattern approach to blood glucose control.

It is necessary to define what we mean by the pattern approach to diabetes management because the term is used by others with different meanings. What we try to do is administer insulin in as physiologic a manner as possible—basal-bolus administration—using insulin analogues and monitoring the results with blood glucose measurements that correspond to the peaks and valleys of the insulin and food. We then establish a pattern of glucose response over a 3-day period and then adjust the insulin, food, or activity to attain and maintain as normal blood glucose levels as possible without endangering the well-being or health of the patient. We set physiologic goals of fasting blood sugar (FBS) less than 110 mg/dl (6.1 mmol/L), 2 hr postprandial BG levels of less than 140 mg/dl (7.7 mmol/L), HbA1c at or below 6.5%, and overall daily blood glucose levels of less than 135 mg/dl (7.5 mmol/L); we know we cannot achieve these levels in all individuals. We then assess each individual and with that individual decide on the immediate and long-term goals for him or her. Patterns of blood glucose control are easy to assess if the patient is faithful in doing blood glucose monitoring. These patterns vary from individual to individual and within the same individual with changes in many of the circumstances of life (changes of activity, illness, emotional stress, travel, and so on), so looking at individual blood glucose levels and making instant adjustments will not allow for the above changes in life circumstances. Ripples of hyper- and hypoglycemia then result. Looking at the pattern over several days and making adjustments to the appropriate insulin or food intake can even out these fluctuations and result in patients who feel better as well as putting less stress on the body.

In the pattern approach, then, we use fasting and postprandial blood glucose monitoring and adjustment of the insulin preceding the abnormality found in the blood glucose level. Changing the insulin at a certain time or meal based on the blood glucose measurement at that time is retroactive management rather than proactive and is not physiologic. Blood glucose at a specific time is a measurement of the previous insulin given, not a predictor of the next insulin to be given. Thus, we look for patterns of glucose over a period of time and then correct the insulin previous to the abnormality, not the next insulin. This is not to say correction doses of insulin may not be needed at times when the blood glucose level is very high. This may certainly be necessary. If a correction dose of insulin is needed every day at a certain time, the correction doses should not be continued but rather that amount of insulin should be added to the previous dose of insulin. Here is an example: if the 2 hr postprandial glucose level after breakfast is 350 mg/dl (19.4 mmol/L), and a correction dose of insulin of X number of units is needed every day for 3 days, then that amount of insulin should be added to the morning insulin dose on a permanent basis.

Glucose monitoring is critical to pattern control. Teaching blood glucose monitoring and the use of the values to alter control to the patient will increase patient independence and flexibility of lifestyle and transfer management decisions to the well-educated, motivated patient with diabetes. This shifts the paradigm of the traditional medical model of control and decision making by the health professional to the more appropriate paradigm of empowering the person with diabetes to become the problem solver and decision maker.

Self-Care Versus Self-Management

Self-care is the minimum level of competence required for patients who have diabetes. It only includes self-injection, hypoglycemia treatment, and meal planning. The attainment of a self-management level, however, requires several additional prerequisites to be able to safely alter and manage the diabetes regimen:

1. Skills verification (return demonstration of all skills)
2. Extensive knowledge base (usually requires a minimum of 20 hr of education, guidance, and self-study)
3. Cognitive functioning (the ability to complete multiple-step processes)
4. Problem solving (the ability to evaluate and prioritize problems and solutions)
5. Support systems (personal and clinical).

Though the preceding requirements are needed and will result in improved blood glucose outcome, self-management skills can be taught to almost anyone. Pattern management takes less education and skill than knowing insulin sensitivity factors and calculating correction doses at every meal and fasting. Patterns of blood glucose over several days are usually easy to see and can be detected by people with only minimal cognitive ability or education. Simple rules can then be given to them on how to add or subtract insulin where needed based on their total daily insulin doses or body size. We usually teach them to make changes in 10%–20% increments so as to minimize the danger of too large or too small dose changes resulting in hypo- or hyperglycemia. Changes in absolute insulin amounts and contained in most insulin change algorithms may be too little for an obese person and too much for a small child. Changes in the percentage of the prescribed dose will obviate the effect of insulin sensitivity and resistance and will be safer for the patient.

Insulin adjustment is the most complex of the self-management skills. It requires extensive knowledge of the interactions among diet, activity and/or exercise, medication time action, state of physical health, and emotional state (stress level), but it can be done by most patients with quality of instruction and hands-on practice.

The use of algorithms based on carbohydrate counting or total available glucose is currently popular for determining the insulin bolus. These approaches have drawbacks. What is not factored into the decision process is the effect of total caloric intake. Some protein (about 60%) and a small amount of fat (about 17%) eventually convert to some form of glucose. So using only the carbohydrate content of the meal to calculate the insulin dose may underestimate the insulin need. Responding to the blood sugar test (i.e., giving insulin in relation to a specific blood glucose value), especially when the person is well and not hypoglycemic, without consideration for food to be eaten or activity later on in the day, may result in "roller-coaster" responses (the blood sugar is elevated, medication is increased or supplemented; the person's blood sugar drops and it is time to eat the next meal but the blood glucose is lower so less or no insulin is given even though the meal may be larger). This process—the *sliding scale* or *changing algorithm*—can often become confusing to the body and hard on the system.

Concerns Regarding the Sliding Scale

Sliding scale protocols do not consider the complex nature or multiple factors contributing to fluctuating blood glucose levels. Responding to a single problem with no consideration for preventing a recurrence of the problem is like trying to make the "insulin think backwards" (Shagan, 1990). Others have reported on these incidents and come to the same conclusion (Donihi, DiNardo, DeVita, & Korytkowski, 2006; Umpierrez, Palacio, & Smiley, 2007).

Too often, there is less emphasis on insulin timing and food needed for usual activity. The person using an insulin pump or using short- or rapid-acting insulin before each meal, with a basal insulin given once or twice a day, may be able to implement predicting insulin needs with more success if patterns are previously determined as to how much insulin covers how much food, that is, developing individualized algorithms.

Algorithms

Although algorithms may be developed for split-mixed programs, there are situation changes when mixtures of short- or rapid- and intermediate- or long-acting insulins need to be substituted. Once the mixed insulin is given, the person must be cognizant of the peak and duration of all that mixture administered. Calorie intake must be considered in relation to activity needs and the amount and timing of the insulin to be administered to prevent hypo- or hyperglycemia. Although multiple daily insulin (MDI) and insulin pump use (continuous subcutaneous insulin infusion [CSII]) may increase the flexibility of timing and composition of dietary intake, the vast majority of patients on insulin are quite different from each other, making it difficult to determine one algorithm to fit all needs.

Algorithms are tables that give patients correction or mealtime insulin doses usually based on the blood glucose level. They are far superior to sliding scales where basal insulin is often not given and gaps in coverage will appear between the insulin doses. Algorithms are usually used with basal insulin (and should be) and thus are more physiologic than a traditional sliding scale. Nonetheless, there are problems with algorithms as well. The most dangerous problem is fixed doses of insulin based entirely on the momentary blood glucose level. Differences in insulin sensitivity with differences in body weight make this practice dangerous if this is not factored in. The other problem is changes that may occur after the insulin is given. A child, for example, may eat a large or high carbohydrate breakfast and have a high blood glucose level at noon. If an algorithm is used based on the blood glucose level, a larger than normal amount of insulin may be given. If the child then decides to eat less (or sometimes with toddlers nothing) or goes out and plays harder than usual, they may get hypoglycemic. Insulin dose may be lowered at supper based on the algorithm, and the child eats a large amount, and the cycle repeats. This is a roller-coaster effect that can go on day after day and can occur in any individual in any age group. Many caregivers will then say "Well, this is a brittle diabetic and we must compromise the goals for them and go with higher blood glucose levels." This is not necessarily true. Algorithms focus on a very narrow area (a single blood glucose level) and thus miss the larger picture of changing intake, activity, and emotions. The pattern approach views the larger picture and can thus take many factors into consideration. The pattern approach also views a longer time, so fewer changes in insulin are needed. It is thus easier for the patient and can be taught in less time and to less-educated patients.

General Recommendations

Recommendations for insulin adjustments should be based on:

a. The lifestyle of the individual,
b. The food distributed throughout the day to meet the energy needs of that lifestyle,
c. The amount and type(s) of insulin needed, and
d. (for T2DM) whether or not accompanied by an oral agent or agents.

Long-term consistency in glucose levels is most likely attained with routine schedules and consistent calorie intake but that often does not represent reality. Assessment of glucose patterns will allow for insulin or calorie corrections. For example, reviewing all fasting blood sugars during the past 3–5 days will give an indication of the appropriateness of the bedtime snack and nighttime insulin, whether that insulin is an intermediate- or long-acting variety.

Hypoglycemia Unawareness

One of the physical problems that confuse the issue of using patterns obtained from blood glucose monitoring is hypoglycemia unawareness. Duration of the disease and tightness of blood glucose control may lead to hypoglycemia unawareness. Cryer, Davis, and Shamoor (2003) were some of the first to document this occurrence. Frequent blood glucose monitoring not only relieves the fears that might be associated with this phenomenon, but also assists in directing the person to the health care professional for the guidance needed to alter this physiological response. The program most evidence-based is the blood glucose awareness training for the purpose of reestablishing hypoglycemia awareness (Clarke et al., 1995; Cryer, 1993). This training is especially useful in preventing severe hypoglycemia (Cox, Gonder-Frederick, Ritterband, Clarke, & Kovatchev, 2007). Continuous glucose monitors (CGMs) are also useful in alerting the individual to impending hypoglycemia. If hypoglycemia unawareness is present, and CGMs are not available, more frequent blood glucose monitoring by meter may be needed. We usually recommend blood glucose monitoring fasting and 2 hours postprandial, but with unawareness blood glucose may need to be monitored fasting, 2 hour postprandial, premeal, and bedtime. In some individuals, nighttime monitoring may be needed on occasion as well.

To Review

- Short- (regular) or rapid-acting (analogue) insulin given before breakfast covers the breakfast and midmorning snack (the snack is needed only if short-acting insulin [regular] is used) and is reflected in the blood glucose value after breakfast (before the snack—rapid-acting insulin) or before lunch (short-acting insulin). If this value is too high or too low, the morning short- or rapid-acting insulin, the food at breakfast, or the midmorning snack should be modified.

- Intermediate-acting insulin (NPH) given before breakfast or short- or rapid-acting insulin given before lunch covers the lunch and afternoon snack (if short-acting insulin is used), and is reflected in the after-lunch glucose value (before the afternoon snack—rapid-acting insulin) or the before-supper blood glucose value (the short-acting insulin or the intermediate-acting insulin given before breakfast). If the values are too high or too low, the morning intermediate-acting insulin (or noon short- or rapid-acting insulin, if in a multiple-dose system), or the lunch or midafternoon snack should be modified to correct this blood glucose outcome.

Note: The presupper blood glucose value should never be used alone to judge the supper insulin dose, because that blood glucose level is a reflection of the previous dose in relation to food and activity, not a full predictor of the next dose. Expected intake and proposed activity with consideration as to why the blood glucose level is elevated or depressed can only aid as a predictor of an insulin dose.

- Short- or rapid-acting insulin given before supper covers the supper food intake (and snack, if short-acting insulin is used) and is reflected in the postprandial (taken before the snack, reflecting the rapid-acting insulin) or bedtime blood glucose level measurement (reflecting the short-acting insulin). Any change in blood glucose levels that are too high or too low reflect a needed change in the insulin or food for supper or postsupper snack.

- Intermediate-acting insulin, if given before supper or at bedtime, provides basal insulin through the night and is reflected in the fasting blood glucose value in the morning. Alterations in the bedtime snack or insulin may be needed to correct the Somogyi (rebound) effect or the Dawn phenomenon (early morning elevated blood sugars due to growth hormone release after midnight), or lack of insulin coverage during the late evening or night, or too large or too small a bedtime snack.

- Long-acting insulin (analogue), usually given at bedtime or before breakfast or both, represents the basal insulin, recognizing that the insulin production of a person without diabetes is never at a level of zero insulin secretion. The long-acting analogue insulins form more stable basal insulin and therefore logically fill the need of a basal insulin. They also have no peak in most people and thus usually will not cause nighttime hypoglycemia, a profound fear of most people including caregivers. If this insulin is given at bedtime, the fasting blood glucose level determines whether the right dose has been given. If this insulin is given the first thing in the morning, the bedtime blood glucose level is the one to observe. Premeal blood glucose levels may also be found to relate to basal insulin if rapid-acting insulin is used.

Note: If the fasting blood glucose value is elevated, the morning insulin is not altered. Instead, the evening intermediate-acting insulin or long-acting insulin is changed. If the basic long-acting analogue insulin (Glargine or Detemir) demonstrates hypoglycemia or hyperglycemia during the night or early morning hours, then an alteration is needed in this medicine (whether given at bedtime or at the time of a meal, always in a separate syringe). To change the morning insulin, when using an intermediate- or long-acting insulin at bedtime, is to make a change after the fact that could potentially result in trouble over time. It is critical in diabetes management to remember which insulin covers which period, and which blood glucose level values are indicative of that coverage. If those principles are known and understood, and the appropriate blood glucose measurements are available, then the adjustments are a matter of simple mathematics. See Chapter 9 for insulin time actions.

Remember that sliding scales, however, are not rational therapy because they give insulin after the fact and do not use the appropriate blood glucose values to adjust the insulin dosage(s). They will not provide physiologic control and may cause serious hypoglycemia—this caution is being repeated to emphasize that sliding scale management is archaic and should be discarded. The regimen as outlined is physiologic. It duplicates the insulin secretion pattern of individuals without diabetes that produce a small amount of insulin continuously (basal insulin), and a bolus of insulin with each meal. When intermediate-acting insulins are used, one-third to twice as much intermediate-acting insulin as short- or rapid-acting insulin is given because the intermediate-acting insulins must cover a longer period of time and more than one meal. (An exception to this rule may occur in persons who eat very little food during the day and a very large meal in the evening. Here a 50/50 mixture of short- and intermediate-acting insulin may be needed.)

A four or more insulin daily dose schedule (MDI) or CSII increases the ability of the person with diabetes to have a more flexible lifestyle and is more physiologic than regular and NPH regimen. MDI or CSII are more effective, especially when the fasting blood glucose levels become elevated or there is a problem of high or low blood sugar occurrences during the day. Whatever the regimen, three principles must remain the same:

1. Basal insulin must last for the entire 24 hr with little if any peak during that time especially at night.
2. A bolus of insulin needs to be given with each meal and any large snack.

3. The regimen of insulin and/or food related to activity adjustment is based on the blood glucose pattern or the way that a particular person responds to a specific regimen.

In our experience, parents, supervised teenagers, and adults have effectively learned to use blood glucose data and to effectively and safely make adjustments in food and insulin after self-management education.

If a behavioral eating problem exists with a preschooler or toddler or an adult is not sure of the total amount and types of foods to be eaten, rapid-acting insulin may be administered just after eating, and the amount of insulin given is based on the predetermined food to insulin ratio, that is, the amount of insulin per unit calculated to cover each calorie point or CHO to be ingested. Smaller children, with their increased sensitivity to the insulin, may require the smaller ratio versus the adult or teenager requiring more insulin to cover the same amount of food. Consideration as to how much and what type of carbohydrate foods are included in the meal aids in recognizing the rapidity in which the blood glucose level will be raised after the meal. If the insulin does not get there at the time of the elevated blood sugar, the outcome will, of course, be a higher reading. This is why rapid-acting insulins are more effective, flexible, and convenient than a short-acting insulin. Food peaks in 1–2 hours after ingestion, so a short-acting insulin, like regular insulin, must be given at least 1 hour before the meal, while a rapid-acting insulin analogue can be given just before, with, or, in some individuals, after the meal.

To obtain patterns, the blood sugar is measured four or more times a day, usually at set times. Especially if rapid-acting insulin is in use, fasting and 2-hr postprandial testing is best, because this insulin peaks in 1 hr or so and is gone in 3 hr or so. In most cases, then, the rapid-acting insulin will be gone long before the next meal. The premeal blood sugar will better reflect the basal insulin given, rather than the rapid-acting insulin, and therefore should not be used to adjust the latter.

Because present data indicate that a high degree of metabolic control is necessary to prevent the acute-, intermediate-, and long-term complications of the disease, many alternate regimens are needed to meet individual needs. An increasing number of diabetologists in this country and especially in Europe are adopting multiple-dose programs. A high level of control is desirable and is safely achievable with three, four, or more insulin doses per day or CSII regimens.

Self-Management

As noted earlier, the procedure for self-management involves more than self-care. Self-management requires participation and teamwork and frequent glucose monitoring especially for intensive diabetes management (Garg, Campbell, Delahanty, & Halvorson, 2000). The full response to rapid- and short-acting insulin from one day's use may not be observed the following day. Responses to intermediate-acting insulin are better noted on the second or third day. Long-acting insulin may be altered daily with the majority of its effect noted by the fasting blood glucose level. In the home, the patient should preferably wait three or more days to see whether the change in dosage(s) meets the altered physiologic needs.

Considering this information, the following sequence of steps may be used to develop a protocol for teaching self-management regarding dosage changes:

1. Adjust the insulin that controls the fasting blood glucose value (intermediate-acting insulin administered at supper or bedtime or preferably a long-acting insulin analogue also administered the day before) until the fasting blood glucose value is in the normal range. An adjustment of 10%–20% each day is made until the desired fasting blood glucose level is achieved.
2. Next, adjust the short- or, preferably, the rapid-acting insulin administered at breakfast until the blood glucose values between breakfast and lunch are in the normal range.
3. Now, adjust the short- or rapid-acting insulin taken at lunch or intermediate-acting insulin taken at breakfast until the blood glucose values after lunch and before supper are in the normal range.
4. Then, adjust the short- or rapid-acting insulin taken before supper until the blood glucose values after supper and at bedtime are in the normal range.

Initial or starting doses are given in Chapter 6 as transition doses from oral hypoglycemic agents or IV insulin to subcutaneous insulin. Adjustment of an insulin dosage is in 1–2 Units or 10%–20% increments every 1–3 days until blood glucose levels are normal. Exceptions are as follows:

- Daily adjustments are made for pregnant women in whom it is urgent to establish and maintain control quickly.
- Daily adjustments of 2 or more unit increments are used when significant hypoglycemia warrants rapid reduction in insulin prior to the time the reaction occurred on the next day.
- Changes in dosage may exceed 2 Units per change when the blood glucose values are grossly out of the normal range, especially if ketones are present in the urine. This would be an indication if there is a markedly inadequate insulin dosage for illness and for more rapid control.
- Changes in dosage may be less than 2 Units per change in small children, in whom 2 Units may represent a change in percentage too great to be tolerated. In children, a change of 5%–10% in insulin dosage may be a better guide than the use of absolute units.
- Any of these insulin doses can be changed for long-term therapy by the caregiver or the patient every 3–5 days based on the patterns of the blood glucose as follows:
  1. Change the evening long-acting insulin based on the fasting blood glucose level.
  2. Change the breakfast rapid-acting insulin based on the pattern of the 2 hour postprandial blood glucose level.
  3. Change the noon rapid-acting insulin based on the afternoon blood glucose level.
  4. Change the supper rapid-acting insulin based on the 2 hour postprandial level after supper.

This approach is simple and easy for the caregiver and patient and is flexible and safe.

Useful Approaches

The following three approaches have been very useful for dietary therapy with insulin:

1. The first is the more common CHO counting method, with the added caveat that a protein is counted as a ½ CHO rather than just counting the CHO alone. This is close to the number used in the ADA's advanced carb counting, though few patients go beyond basic carb counting, and therefore protein intake is usually not counted. The usual insulin carbohydrate ratio is 15 g of CHO equal to one carb point or to 1 Unit of insulin. Though protein is not counted in basic or intermediate carb counting, it is frequently unconsciously adjusted for. The 15:1 carb-to-insulin ratio that is used to start is often adjusted to 12 or 10 or 8 to 1 ratio. This adjustment is often said to be due to insulin sensitivity, and in some cases it may be, but it is usually needed to adjust for the protein content of the diet. We have observed that people need to adjust the ratio downward as the protein content of the diet increases (for example, people on the Atkins' high protein low carbohydrate diet or children who need high protein diets for growth). We therefore use the protein content of the diet in initial calculations and therefore do not need to change the ratio if the diet changes. This also prevents the underdosing of insulin that we frequently see when only carbohydrates are counted.

   As blood glucose levels demand, changes from 5 to 25 g of CHO may be needed in relation to a person's insulin sensitivity. The 1,700 rule can be used to change insulin glucose ratios or to calculate correction doses. This is the rule used in most insulin pumps for correction insulin doses. The rule is as follows: 1,700 divided by the total daily dose of insulin equals the milligrams per deciliter of blood glucose that will be changed by 1 Unit of insulin. This is called the insulin sensitivity factor (ISF). Based on this formula, a correction factor is the ideal blood sugar (usually 140) subtracted from the blood glucose obtained divided by the ISF. Many of the CSII programs include the ability to calculate this number within the pump program.

2. The second approach is the food/insulin ratio. This is based on the concept that people eating at home eat about the same way daily. This is defined in three steps: (1) Determine the average calorie points eaten at each meal over a 3- to 5-day period. (2) Stay on that average food intake, altering the premeal insulin until the 2-hr postprandial blood glucose reading is in an acceptable range. (3) Once that occurs, divide the number of calorie points into the insulin given to determine the food/insulin ratio for each meal. Then, if the person is not sure how much is going to be eaten and only eats half the meal, then only half the number of previously calculated units are given after the meal. If ¾ is eaten, then ¾ of the units are given after the meal, and so on. During illness when blood sugars are more than 250 mg/dl (13.8 mmol/L) or higher, 10% of the total daily dose (or 20% if ketones are present) is given with the premeal insulin. For hourly insulin use, 0.05 Unit/kg of body weight

(or 0.1 Unit if ketones are present) is given until the blood glucose levels are below 250 mg/dl (13.8 mmol/L). This method can be used as a correction factor (although increasing fluid intake is better) using 0.025 Unit/kg of body weight (or 0.05 Unit if ketones are present) for blood glucose levels the same as above, but without illness.

3. The third approach is to determine how much insulin (an algorithm determined between the patient's information and the professional guidance) to add to the premeal insulin when the blood glucose values are above the desired level. The basal insulin remains (unless it is the insulin that needs to be changed) and no insulin is held except in unusual circumstances. When this added insulin is needed over a 2- to 3-day period, then the insulin is added to the previous dose to be given on a routine basis.

Summary

Intensive diabetes management cannot be achieved unless blood glucose levels are monitored. Intensive management may be achieved with multiple doses of insulin and with CSII. Persons on CSII must monitor blood glucose values four to eight times a day to be safe so that too much or too little insulin is not released into the person at an inappropriate time. Self monitoring of blood glucose (SMBG) is needed four times a day in everyone taking insulin so that insulin doses can be properly adjusted to whatever regimen is used and to ensure patient safety.

Keep the following in mind: If you don't aim for the center of the target (normal blood glucose levels as safely tolerated—without any *significant* hypoglycemia), you won't be able to hit it. The center of the target will not be hit in everyone all the time. Frequent blood glucose monitoring, the use of MDI with insulin analogues, CSII, and a pattern approach will come closer to the target with greater safety than can be achieved with other therapies.

The important issues are:

1. Safety first
2. Control second
3. Quality of life integrated.

Recommended Patient Resource

Deitz, P. W. (2000). Be proactive with patterns. *Diabetes Forecast, 54*(7), 55–60.

References

Clarke, W. L., Cox, D. J., Gonder-Frederick, L. A., Julian, D., Schlundt, D., & Polonsky, W. (1995). Reduced awareness of hypoglycemia in adults with IDDM: A prospective study of hypoglycemic frequency and associated symptoms. *Diabetes Care, 18*(14), 517–522.

Cox, D. J., Gonder-Frederick, L. A., Ritterband, L., Clarke, W., & Kovatchev, B. P. (2007). Prediction of severe hypoglycemia. *Diabetes Care, 30*(6), 1370–1373.

Cryer, P. E. (1993). Hypoglycemia unawareness in IDDM. *Diabetes Care, 16*(Suppl. 3), 40–47.

Cryer, P. E., Davis, S. N., & Shamoon, H. (2003). Hypoglycemia in diabetes. *Diabetes Care, 26*(6), 1902–1912.

Donihi, A. C., DiNardo, M. M., DeVita, M. A., & Korytkowski, M. T. (2006). Use of a standardized protocol to decrease medication errors and adverse events related to sliding scale insulin. *Quality of Safe Health Care, 15*(2), 89–91.

Garg, S. K., Campbell, R. K., Delahanty, L., & Halvorson, M. (2000). The role of frequent glucose monitoring in intensive diabetes management. *The Diabetes Educator, 26*(5), 3–17.

Hinnen, D. (2002). Self-monitoring of blood glucose. In D. Guthrie & R. Guthrie (Eds.), *Nursing management of diabetes mellitus* (5th ed., p. 182). New York: Springer Publishing Company.

Shagan, B. P. (1990). Does anyone here know how to make insulin work backwards? Why sliding-scale insulin coverage doesn't work. *Practical Diabetology, 9*(3), 1–4.

Umpierrez, G. E., Palacio, A., & Smiley, D. (2007). Sliding scale insulin use: Myth or insanity? *American Journal of Medicine, 120*(7), 563–567.

16

Problems and Solutions: Type 1 Diabetes

Different patients have different degrees of insulin sensitivity. In general children are more insulin sensitive than adults. But there are adults who are or become extremely sensitive to insulin and children who are insulin resistant because of obesity. In general, obese individuals are insulin resistant regardless of age. The following case studies are intended to demonstrate the differing patterns and problems that can occur for an individual taking insulin.

Cases

Case #1

CB is a 27-year-old, slightly overweight for height, female that had not felt well and had seen her obstetrician because she was pregnant. She had an abnormal random blood sugar. The glucose tolerance test identified a fasting blood glucose level of 88 mg/dl (4.8 mmol/L), and after a glucose load of 100 g, a half-hour blood glucose value of 154 mg/dl (8.5 mmol/L); a 1-hr value of 189 mg/dl (10.5 mmol/L); and a 2-hr value of 192 mg/dl (10.6 mmol/L).

The diagnosis? Gestational diabetes. The goal for blood glucose levels with pregnancy is 90 mg/dl (5.0 mmol/L) or less premeal and less than 120 mg/dl (6.6 mmol/L) 2 hr postprandial. She was into her second trimester and, therefore, she was started on low-dose insulin therapy. Hopefully, her blood glucose levels had not been elevated during her first trimester.

Ideally, she would have had this glucose assessment during the first trimester, but she had little if any nausea that even indicated that she was pregnant. With the recognition that there was a great possibility of increased glucose intolerance as the pregnancy progressed, the need for insulin or other treatment was likely.

The options could have been a few weeks' trial on diet alone and/or the use of metformin or glyburide. Because insulin was chosen, the decision would be to start just a basal insulin such as 10 Units at bedtime with a limitation of sweets in her food intake. Another approach would be just to go ahead and start a more flexible sequence of insulin. This most often is the use of four doses of rapid-acting insulin analog before each meal, for example, 2 Units before breakfast, 1 Unit before lunch, 2 Units before supper, and 50% or 5 Units basal or long-acting insulin at bedtime. The fasting blood glucose level would determine whether the bedtime basal needed to be raised or lowered. The postprandial blood sugars would determine whether the previous rapid-acting insulin would need to be changed the next day. It is possible that initially a 70/30, a 75/25, or a 50/50 insulin premix could be given before breakfast and supper. Then, when the blood sugars became higher, the woman could be switched to multiple doses. Oral hypoglycemic agents are usually not recommended in pregnancy. See Chapter 23 for a discussion of pregnancy and gestational diabetes.

A high degree of blood glucose control (overall average blood glucose levels were between 90 and 110 mg/dl [5.0–6.1 mmol/L]) was achieved and the woman delivered a 7 pound 6 ounce daughter at 39 weeks' gestational age.

Case #2

AL is a 15-year-old moderately obese girl complaining of fatigue. She received a diagnosis of Type 1 diabetes mellitus (T1DM) 9 years ago. Ongoing treatment has been with insulin. The family said her diabetes had been fine and they only "needed to see the doctor" when there was a problem. She has had episodes of diabetic ketoacidosis approximately 5 times during those 9 years. Her usual insulin dose has been 22 Units of neutral protamine Hagedorn (NPH) and 15 Units of regular insulin in the morning, 5–10 Units of regular before supper, and 4 Units of NPH at bedtime. She was following no set meal plan. She was told to just restrict her sweets. The patient has had insulin reactions several times a month. Her mother reported that AL had a moderately severe insulin reaction about 3 a.m. which was undocumented by a blood sugar measurement.

The patient felt sick this morning when she awoke. She ate breakfast and took her usual insulin doses of NPH and regular. The patient continued to feel ill throughout the morning. She ate some macaroni and cheese at approximately 1 p.m. During the afternoon, she began to become more nauseated and began to vomit at 4 p.m. Her mother gave her 20 Units of regular insulin but her condition became worse so that her mother brought her to the emergency room.

There, her blood sugar was documented at 620 mg/dl (34.4 mmol/L). She had a sodium level of 131, potassium of 4.0, chloride of 101, CO_2 of 7, blood urea nitrogen (BUN) of 18, pH of 7.25, Pco_2 of 24, and Po_2 of 112. Normal saline was started intravenously at 300 cc/hr (she weighed 181 lbs or 53.6 kg). The specialist was consulted and insulin was started at 0.1 $Unit \cdot kg^{-1} \cdot hr^{-1}$ by infusion pump (on a 1:1 dilution of regular insulin to saline). By standing orders in the intensive care unit, the nurse regulated the drip to keep the blood glucose levels from falling faster than 100 mg/dl (5.5 mmol/L) per hour. When AL's blood sugar reached 250 mg/dl (16.6 mmol/L), the IV was changed to D5 and ½ normal saline. Hourly blood sugars were maintained until blood glucose levels had fallen below 200 mg/dl (11.1 mmol/L) and the CO_2 value was more than 18.

She has no known drug allergies. There is a history of the patient being caught smoking a few years ago. Her parents are divorced and she is currently living with her mother and two siblings. Her mother does not know her family history because she was adopted as a child.

On the review of systems, she was found to be negative for everything except a sore throat and a tender abdomen (at first, the emergency room resident thought she had appendicitis, but another resident, who had just rotated off the diabetes rotation, recognized this as a sign of diabetic ketoacidosis and recommended that the lab work be done before surgery). A throat culture was obtained.

Within 6 hr, the blood glucose levels were in an acceptable range and the nausea and abdominal tenderness had subsided. The throat culture came back positive for strep and an antibiotic was started. The basal insulin (glargine or detemir) was started 2 hr before the IV (1 Unit/kg) was stopped. Rapid- (lispro, aspart, or glulisine) acting insulin was prescribed for premeal dosing in relation to the dietary intake. She was discharged from the hospital within 48 hr once the education on the new insulin was given.

Follow-up phone calls scheduled her and family members for class and for their first specialist appointment. Once she was released from the hospital and throughout her diabetes management, 24-hr hotline information was made available to them for immediate questions.

Case #3

BL was a 55-year-old, 5 ft 11 in., 215-lb (97.7-kg) male. He had been married for 11 years. He and his wife had 2 children, ages 4 and 9. His employment was full-time as a cellular telephone sales representative. He jogged three times a week (approximately 3 miles each time). He was still following a 2,000 calorie ADA diet prescribed to him two years ago when he saw a dietitian to assist him with weight loss.

He had received a diagnosis of T1DM 10 years before. He presented with an HbA1c of 10%. He was self-administering a 70/30 mixture before breakfast, a rapid-acting insulin before supper, and an intermediate-acting insulin at bedtime. Hypoglycemia was reported as being infrequent. He stated any episodes of hypoglycemia were usually related to increased activity. He was able to self-treat each reaction, but noted he had a history of overtreating himself or treating himself when he just *felt* he was low. He also reported a history of background retinopathy and mild peripheral neuropathy. Hyperlipidemia was present with the total cholesterol at 245, the high-density lipoprotein (HDL) at 39, the low-density lipoprotein (LDL) at 157, and the triglycerides at 240.

BL said that he had not been concerned about his blood glucose control because he was "feeling fine." However, since he found that he had complications developing, he felt a need to change. He recently increased his SMBG to four times a day, premeal and bedtime. He self-adjusts his insulin based on self-monitoring of blood glucose SMBG by using his own system. BL admitted not following any meal plan, including the one given to him two years ago. His job is currently becoming more stressful because of pressure to increase sales.

At the start of his new program, he was given a meal plan of 2,100 calories with 30% fat, 15% protein, and 55% carbohydrate. Because he was on 24 Units of a basal insulin (50% of 0.05 Unit/kg), he was comfortable not to have snacks in the morning or afternoon, but did want to have a snack at bedtime. The points were distributed as 9 points for breakfast; 8 points for lunch; 10 points for supper; and 1 point for a bedtime snack. If he ate a snack of 2 points or more, he was instructed to cover it with 1–2 Units of a rapid-acting insulin.

His basic insulin dosages were based on half a unit per kilogram, 50% of which would be the basal and the other insulin divided between the three meals as rapid-acting insulin. The dosages were 20% before breakfast (10 Units), 13% before lunch (6 Units), and 17% before supper (8 Units).

On return, in two weeks, his self-care history (completed at each visit) included a dietary intake history for breakfast of a large banana (1½ points), toast with margarine (1½ points), a bowl of oatmeal (1½ cups or 3 points), 1 cup of skim milk (1 point), 1 small orange (1 point), and 1+ teaspoon of peanut butter (about 1 point). For lunch he had a sandwich with four pieces of meat and mustard (5–6 points), 2 pieces of fruit (2 points), and some carrot sticks (not counted) and water. For supper he reported having a lean piece of steak (5–6 ounces or 5–6 points), a small potato (1 point), 1 cup of green beans (1 point), ¼ of a melon (1 point), and a small roll (1 point) with a small amount of butter (½ point) and ice tea. His bedtime snack was two peanut butter crackers (1 point) (refer to Table 16.1).

He had eaten a bowl of ice cream the night before. His fasting blood glucose obtained in the office at his 2-week check was 303. He said he had learned that lesson. It should have been a few bites not the whole thing or he needed to take some rapid-acting insulin to cover it.

His home blood glucose measurements were a little high, so his bedtime basal was increased 2 Units and his premeal insulin was increased by 1 Unit each (he had maintained his weight).

After a month had passed, he returned to the clinic. He had some contact with the nurse On-Call to problem solve and adjust treatment. Blood glucose levels had improved. He tried adjusting his insulin as instructed when blood glucose levels were too high. He reported that he had made some healthier food choices but said he continued to have some problems at lunch and supper, with extra snacking on the weekends. He also wondered why he had not lost weight. He did try to exercise more, but had noticed some low blood glucose levels during the night after his increased exercise days (see Table 16.1 for his blood sugar history).

Blood sugars had improved, but there was no weight loss. His desired weight was 200 lbs. 2,100 calories appeared to be a maintenance meal plan, but he needed fewer calories for weight loss. It was determined that he would eat two less points at lunch and supper, which would put his calorie level at a little more than 1,900 calories (1,900 divided by 75 = 25 points) with the expectation that when he was more active on weekends he could eat about 2,100 calories or 28 points. He was to take one more unit of basal insulin at bedtime and keep the other insulin the same.

When he returned on the next visit, he had lost 6 pounds over a two-month period (see Table 16.2 for the blood sugars for the last two months). He had learned that if he increased his exercise time or frequency, to decrease the previous dose of insulin 1–2 Units. His printout recorded one blood sugar less than 60 (59) the first day that he exercised, forgetting to decrease the previous dose of insulin. He reported he has trouble following his meal plan all the time, but he was doing better. He was still working toward the goal weight of 200 lbs (90.9 kg). He reported feeling better.

At the next visit (three months later—or the routine rotation of clinic visits—see Table 16.3), he had his lipid profile repeated (he had been put on a statin). All values were normal except for the LDL which was at 104 (with the desired level being less than 100, or preferably 70) and he was closer to his desired weight.

16.1 Blood Sugar History: 2 Week Visit

Breakfast	2 hr PP	Lunch	2 hr PP	Supper	2 hr PP	Bedtime
172	183	178	176	202	198	272
141	157	146	166	173	199	202
303	204	166	166	185	170	199

16.2 Blood Sugar History: 2 Month Visit

Breakfast	2 hr PP	Lunch	2 hrs PP	Supper	2 hr PP	Bedtime
172	111	–	166	–	174	–
104	121	–	156	–	183	–
113	108	–	168	–	166	183

16.3 Blood Sugar History: 3 Month Visit						
Breakfast	2 hr PP	Lunch	2 hr PP	Supper	2 hr PP	Bedtime
95	–	101	–	127	–	118
102	–	111	–	119	–	121
98	–	121	–	117	–	120

Case #4

SD is a 50-year-old male who has had T1DM since age 20. He has had retinopathy that required laser treatment, hyperlipidemia, and no known microalbuminuria. He reported problems with sexual dysfunction and depression. He was referred for assessment and follow-up.

He was on four shots of insulin with the use of a basal and three doses of rapid-acting insulin. His physical history and foot exam revealed peripheral neuropathy. He did not have a regular physical activity program. Most of his noon meals were eaten in a restaurant. He does not smoke but drinks "a few" alcoholic beverages in the evening.

SD has no history of diabetes on either side of the family. His mother had hypothyroidism and his father was being treated for hypertension.

The medications he takes are as follows: an aspirin a day (low dose); an antidepressant; erectile dysfunction treatment as needed; and alpha lipoic acid three times daily. He is receiving 16 Units of a basal insulin in the morning and 20 Units in the evening. His rapid-acting insulin includes 2 Units per calorie point for breakfast and 1 Unit per calorie point for lunch, supper, and snacks. He tried the 2 Units per carb at breakfast and 1 Unit per carb for the other times, but his postprandial blood glucose levels were not as well controlled when he used his units per carb only, and he gained weight. A trace protein was found intermittently in his urine so he was placed on an angiotensin-converting enzyme inhibitor (ACEI) for renal protection. He took a daily statin.

Dietary history revealed an intake of 2,400 calories with a 35% of total fat, 13% of protein, and 52% of CHO. He was 5 ft 2 in tall and weighed about 171 lbs. His body mass index (BMI) was 23 and his lipid levels were essentially normal on his present treatment level. His creatinine was gradually increasing (1.1 mg/dl). His hemoglobin A1c was 7.5%. Electrocardiogram (ECG) results were within normal limits, but his blood pressure was elevated, as noted previously. His depression appeared to be only moderately controlled by the antidepressant. His blood pressure was not controlled, and his HbA1c was not below the desired level of 7.0% (ADA) or 6.5% (International Diabetes Federation [IDF]/American Association of Clinical Endocrinologists [AACE]). His blood glucose levels averaged about 145 mg/dl (8.0 mmol/L) before breakfast, 155 mg/dl (8.6 mmol/L) 2 hr after breakfast, 168 mg/dl (9.3 mmol/L) 2 hr after lunch, and 177 mg/dl (9.8 mmol/L) after supper. It was very important to get both his blood sugars and blood pressure controlled in the light of his upper limit of normal creatinine level.

Further assessment of the depression indicated a need for referral to a mental health specialist. His ACEI medication was increased to see if this would control the blood pressure. His evening basal insulin was increased by 3 Units at bedtime, and if his postprandial blood glucose levels did not then fall into acceptable ranges, he was to increase from 1 to 3 Units before each meal. His attendance at a review class for diabetes self-management was encouraged.

The outcome was positive. His creatinine lowered to 1.0 and his blood pressure decreased to 128/75. All other measures appeared to be controlled without any problems other than two blood sugars in the upper 60s.

Case #5

EB is a 36-year-old female who had had diabetes for 5 years. She had been insulin dependent but was well until a week prior to admission when she began to note arthralgias and anorexia. A few days before admission she began vomiting and stopped her insulin because her physician stated she might get hypoglycemic since she could not keep food down. The day before her hospitalization she awoke confused, was seen in an emergency room and given an antibiotic, Tylenol with codeine was given for her discomfort, and Compazine was given for the nausea. The following day the confusion persisted and she was admitted to the hospital.

On arrival, she was noted to be mildly icteric, with dry mucous membranes and right upper quadrant tenderness. Her blood glucose level was 529 mg/dl (29.4 mmol/L). Ketones were positive; arterial pH was 7.1, sodium was 137, potassium 5.2, chloride 95, CO_2 11, white blood count 8.800, hemoglobin 13.7, hematocrit 35.42. The urinalysis showed a pH of 5, a trace of protein (15 mg/dl), 2% glucose, and large ketones. She was treated with IV fluids and insulin. She soon felt better, and improvement was noted in her mental status.

Two days later, her fasting glucose level was 124 mg/dl (6.8 mmol/L), ketones negative, the bilirubin 14.0 total, 5.9 direct; the alkaline phosphatase was 45 (4.5 to 11, within normal limits), serum glutamic-oxaloacetic transaminase (SGOT) 10,275 (normal, 8 to 30), serum glutamic-pyruvic transaminase 8,325, albumin 2.8, and cholesterol 172. The next day the SGOT was 860. The patient was given 20 mg of vitamin K, apparently for a prolonged prothrombin time.

The next day she became agitated, closely followed by obtundation, responding only to severe pain. A lumbar puncture revealed normal pressure and clear fluid. The arterial pH was 7.07, blood ketones positive, lactic acid was greater than 40. Treatment with $NaHCO_3$ was begun, and after approximately 350 mEq of bicarbonate was slowly injected, the pH was 7.5.

The next day, the patient was transferred to a specialty center hospital. Prior to the initial hospitalization, the patient had been receiving intermediate-acting insulin twice a day. She did smoke and drank the equivalent of a case of beer per week. She was married and worked as a chemical engineer.

Findings at the center revealed a blood pressure of 147/74, a pulse of 108, with shallow, rapid respirations (42 per minute). Her temperature was in the normal range. She had generalized icterus, multiple ecchymoses, no adenopathy, a supple neck, but had right upper quadrant abdominal tenderness. The liver was 12 cm below the rib edge. No rectal masses were palpated. She was responsive only to name, and otherwise disoriented. Motor and sensory responses were normal. Deep tendon reflexes were symmetrical.

The lab results at this admission were the following: bilateral lower lobe infiltrates were present; the ECG was normal. The white count was 22,800 (66% granulocytes, 24% bands, 6% lymphocytes, 3% monocytes, 1 myelocyte, 1+ toxic granulocytes). The hemoglobin was 14.2; the hematocrit 41.8, the platelets 147,000, and the urinalysis with a pH of 5.5, specific gravity 1.027, ½% glucose, 30 mg protein, 5,010 white blood cell count, 20–25 red blood cells, and 4+ bilirubin. The arterial blood gases on 4 L of O_2 were pH 7.56, Po_2 72, Pco_2 31, Na 137, K 4.5, Cl 90, CO_2 27, glucose 250, BUN 31, creatinine of 2.5, Ca^{2+} of 7.4, Po_4 of 1.3, prothrombin time 19.1 (control 11), partial thromboplastin time 42, bilirubin 17.5 total, 13.5 direct, and amylase 152.

The patient was placed in the intensive care unit. Upper gastrointestinal bleeding was manifest by "coffee-ground" nasogastric suction. Two units of fresh-frozen plasma were given. Oliguria and hypotension were noted and fluids were increased. A Swan-Ganz catheter was placed and the wedge pressure was 10. Fluid challenge and dopamine were given. Progressive hypotension and hypoxia ensued. Solu-Medrol was given. The patient went into a cardiorespiratory arrest that was reversed. She was intubated and ventilation controlled. The patient did not regain consciousness. At that time she was noted to have a calcium of 4.2 mg/dl. Liver size was measured at 10 cm, SGOT fell from 725 to 370. Creatinine rose from 2.5 to 6.0. Pupils became fixed and dilated and the patient was pronounced dead after subsequent cardiac arrest, less than 37 hr after arrival at the center.

What is to be learned from this experience? The initial pH was too high for bicarbonate use; she had lactic acidosis and should never have been given bicarbonate. The bicarbonate controversy is discussed further in Chapter 6.

Case #6

NS was an emergency room (ER) case. NS is a 4-year-old boy who was having trouble breathing. The team did a complete physical examination and blood pressure and heart rate. He was found to have an obvious state of dehydration. A plasma expander was started. Blood was drawn and sent stat to the lab. A neurologic assessment began. The blood pressure was 90/62. The pulse was 102 bpm and the temperature was 103°F (39.4°C). He was unresponsive to verbal stimuli. His eyeballs were sunken and soft. He was found to have a mild pharyngitis, bilateral otitis media, and bilateral enlarged cervical lymph nodes. There was a fruity odor to the breath. The respirations were deep and labored. No rebound tenderness was noted on the abdomen. The skin was dry. The skin turgor was poor. The deep tendon reflexes were depressed, but the superficial reflexes were within normal.

This child weighed 30 lbs (13.6 kg) and was 40 inches tall (101.6 cm) (one should expect a 4-year-old who was 40 inches tall to weigh about 40 lbs [18.2 kg]). The mother reported that the patient had unusual thirst and frequent urination with accompanying bedwetting and some slight daytime incontinence. The parents thought the thirst was the result of the temperature and the frequent urination due to the increased fluid intake.

A throat culture had been done in the physician's office the day before. No report was given at that time of the otitis media. The child had been noticeably quite tired acting over the past few weeks. His clothes were noticeably looser. The parents noticed his fever getting higher and when they could not awaken him, after what they believed was an appropriate length of time for a nap, they brought him to the ER.

In the ER, a complete blood count (CBC), electrolytes, urinalysis, BUN, creatinine, and arterial blood gases were ordered. They obtained a bedside glucose determination and found that it was greater than 400 mg/dl (18 mmol/L) with large ketones. Insulin was started by perfusion based on 0.1 Unit/kg of body weight per hour in a dilution of 1 Unit/cc of normal saline placed in a 20-cc syringe and given by pump. Fluids were normal saline. A cardiac monitor was connected.

The laboratory's significant data were: hematocrit 33%, white blood cells 15,200, sodium 145 mEq/L, chloride 100 mEq/L, potassium 2.5 mEq/L (a U wave was noted on the cardiac monitor readout), HCO_3 2 mEq/L, BUN 88 mg/dl, creatinine 3.2 mg/dl, arterial blood gases were Po_2 85 mm/Hg, Pco_2 12 mm/Hg, blood glucose 782 mg/dl (43.4 mmol/L), and throat culture positive for beta hemolytic Streptococcus, ketones on a 1:11 test on a dark, straw-colored urine specimen.

Fluids were calculated as 3,000 to 3,500 cc per square meter per day; electrolytes were added (40 mEq/L of potassium per bottle of fluid). Once the blood glucose was down to 250 mg/dl (13.1 mmol/L), the IV was changed to D5 and ½ sodium chloride, also with potassium, because electrolytes indicated a continued need. An antibiotic was started. Once the child was able to eat, insulin was given prior to each meal and a basal insulin given at bedtime. The starting injections were based on 1 Unit/kg of body weight or 36 Units (doses were 7 Units before breakfast; 5 Units before lunch; 6 Units before supper; and 18 Units of basal insulin at bedtime). Basal insulin was started 2 hours before the IV was discontinued.

Diagnoses that were considered, besides diabetic ketoacidosis, were hyperosmolar coma (except he required 0.1 $Unit \cdot kg^{-1} \cdot hr^{-1}$ to initially lower his blood glucose levels while hyperosmolar coma usually requires much lower insulin doses), salicylate intoxication, some form of meningitis, possibly encephalitis, or head injury (he had fallen a week ago and hit his head).

Things to consider would be adequate insulin doses, adequate insulin distribution, response of infection to antibiotic, adequate food and fluid intake for growth and development, psychologic support for family and child, and education for care. Diabetic Ketoacidosis (DKA) is discussed in Chapter 6.

Case #7

LL was a 56-year-old woman referred for diabetes control (HbA1c 9.8%). Income was low and the ability to pay for any medications was a problem. She qualified for drug company support, so the papers were submitted.

She voiced that she did not want to change the types of insulin she was getting: 70/30 before breakfast, short-acting before supper, and intermediate-acting at bedtime. Her doses were 12 before breakfast, 5 before supper, and 10 at bedtime: completely inadequate based on body weight (90 kg; 5 ft 5 in.), length of time having diabetes (diagnosed 11 years ago), and elevated blood glucose levels.

She was in the hospital for some tests so she was administered four doses of short-acting insulin. This was based on ½ Unit per kilogram of body weight or a total of 44 Units/day or 11 Units every 6 hours while NPO for tests. Because she was on short-acting insulin, her blood glucose testing was to be every 6 hr while nothing by mouth (NPO) then premeal and bedtime when diet was resumed (refer to Table 16.4 for follow-up: Day 1).

Based on 1 Unit of insulin covering 30 to 50 or so mg/dl (1.6–2.7 mmol/L), each insulin dose was raised 2 Units (refer to Table 16.4: Day 2).

The following day, her doses were converted to the previous types of insulin that she had used, recognizing that effective control and flexibility of control was not as easy as with four doses of short-acting insulin or the use of the new analogue insulin. She received 28 Units of 70/30 before breakfast; 13 Units of short-acting insulin before supper; and 7 Units at bedtime (see Table 16.4: Day 3).

Recognizing that it takes 24–48 hr to determine a truer response from the intermediate-acting insulin, but also taking into consideration that the person would be more active on discharge, she was told to decrease her breakfast insulin to 24, and to increase her supper insulin to 15 and her bedtime insulin to 8.

Over the next three days, she reported (by phone) and the blood sugars were averaged for those three days (see Table 16.4: Day 7).

She was told to hold her insulin at those last prescribed levels and to attend class on a scholarship. Subsequently, she needed a unit less at each dosing time as she was able to decrease her caloric intake about 200 calories or roughly three points as part of her plan to lower her weight to at least 150 lbs (68.1 kg).

Hemoglobin A1c at the three-month clinic visit was 7.2%, or well on the way to less than 6.5% if she could safely tolerate it. She said the testing of her blood glucose levels when she felt hungry or symptomatically low really helped—for she found that her blood sugars were in a normal range and that if she sat down, did some deep breathing, and rechecked her blood sugars in 15 min or so, the symptoms stopped or, at a few other times, a couple of crackers handled the lowered outcome results of the blood sugar test.

Therefore, this last case illustrates that even with the older insulins, a high degree of control is possible without needing to treat each blood sugar at the time of testing—not knowing at the time (unless continuous monitoring is used) whether the blood sugar is increasing or decreasing.

16.4 Blood Sugar History: As Reported by Day

Breakfast		2 hr PP	Lunch	2 hr PP	Supper	2 hr PP	Bedtime
Day 1	140	–	155	–	162	–	172
Day 2	94	–	101	–	89	–	105
Day 3	112	–	76	–	64	–	145
Day 7	88	–	91	–	86	–	106

One Final Case

MT called at 12:04 a.m. She had taken 30 Units of rapid-acting insulin instead of her long-acting insulin. What should she do? The nurse on call asked her what her food-to-insulin ratio was. She did not know as she was another physician's patient and she had not taken the self-management class yet. The nurse then asked her how much insulin she usually took for supper. She usually took 10 Units. This was followed by a question about what she ate or usually ate at supper. It turned out to be about 7 points. Therefore, the calculated assumption was to take three times the food usually eaten at supper time (30 divided by 10 = 3; 3 times 7 points = 21 points). The discussion that followed included what foods were available and how she would distribute these points over a 2- to 3-hr period to cover the rapid-acting insulin time action. The basal insulin could have been given then or half the dose of the basal given in the morning and the full dose the following night.

The outcome? No hypoglycemia. The blood sugar in the morning was reported to be 128 mg/dl (7.1 mmol/L).

Summary

Diabetes, in most instances, is a logical disease that is controllable. We, too, have misinterpreted the needs of the individual by not asking the right questions. Determining the right amount of the insulin needed for a person's food intake and activity is the challenge. With CSII/continuous glucose monitoring, the phone, the computer (Marrero, 2000), and the Internet (Kwon et al., 2004; McMahon et al., 2005), the possibility for closely controlled blood glucose levels becomes even greater. Following the basic principles of safety first, control second, and quality of life integrated, a person can lead an active and healthy lifestyle, free or slowing the development of complications throughout his or her life.

References

Kwon, H. S., Cho, J. J. H., Kim, H. S., Song, B. R., Ko, S. H., Lee, J. M., et al. (2004). Establishment of blood glucose monitoring system using the Internet. *Diabetes Care, 27*(3), 478–483.

Marrero, D. G. (2000). Computer assisted dietary self-management counseling: A technique for addressing public health needs. *Medical Care, 38*(11), 1059–1061.

McMahon, G. T., Gomes, H. E., Hohne, S. H., Hu, T. M., Levine, B. A., & Conlin, P. R. (2005). Web-based care management in patients with poorly controlled diabetes. *Diabetes Care, 28*(7), 1624–1629.

IV

Type 2 Diabetes in Children and Adults

17

Medications for Type 2 Diabetes Mellitus

The vast majority of the people that we serve are people with Type 2 diabetes mellitus (T2DM), metabolic syndrome, prediabetes, and now children with T2DM (Geiss et al., 2006). T2DM, metabolic syndrome, and prediabetes are metabolic defects and medications are available that tackle the problem. Helping people understand what is causing their blood glucose to elevate is an important task; we will integrate teaching tips for patients throughout this chapter.

T2DM in Review

The blood glucose is elevated from the intake of food and the subsequent breakdown and absorption of nutrients in the stomach and jejunum of the intestinal tract. The brain, as an obligate glucose user, utilizes some of this available glucose in the 3–4 hr after the meal. The remaining glucose is stored in hepatic, muscle, and adipose sites. High insulin levels after meals suppress glucagon and facilitate triglyceride storage in adipose tissue. Insulin prevents the breakdown of glucose from glycogen and triglycerides. Glucose storage occurs. Amylin, a hormone cosecreted by the beta cells of the pancreas, is also stimulated by calorie intake. Amylin facilitates glucose utilization by decreasing postmeal glucagon secretion, slowing gastric emptying, and suppressing appetite.

Several hours after eating, the insulin levels decrease and glucagon levels increase. This ends glucose storage and begins the period of glucose breakdown. This shift in decreasing insulin and increasing levels of glucagon triggers a release of glucose (energy) from glycogen stores and increases gluconeogenesis in the liver. Additional energy production occurs with fat breakdown of adipocyte triglyceride and free fatty acids (FFAs) that provide primary energy to the liver and skeletal muscle. As the time without food intake increases, early starvation occurs. Glucose continues to come from hepatic sources of gluconeogenesis and glycogenolysis. Counterregulatory hormonal responses include increased levels of glucagon, cortisol, growth hormone, and epinephrine. Insulin is suppressed. And finally as this starvation continues, renal gluconeogenesis contributes to maintaining plasma glucose levels (DeFronzo & Ferrannini, 1995; Ratner, 1998).

This complex process of glucose regulation includes interaction between insulin, counterregulatory hormones such as glucagon, the brain, the liver, and the gut. The role of the gut hormones is a relatively new area in the understanding of the physiology of T2DM. The impact of the gut peptide hormones was identified when it was discovered that insulin secretion was increased when a person ate a meal compared with having that same amount of glucose delivered intravenously. This increased secretion of insulin from intestinal response to glucose was identified as the *incretin* effect (Drucker, 2006; Elrick, Stimmeler, Hlad, & Arai, 1964).

Although there are many incretin hormones, glucagon-like peptide 1 (GLP1) and glucose-dependent insulinotropic polypeptide (GIP) have had the most research. Not only do these hormones stimulate insulin release in response to a meal, they also promote beta cell neogenesis and therefore proliferation, decrease apoptosis (beta cell death), and inhibit glucagon secretion from the alpha cells, which has an impact on decreasing glucose production and release from the liver. GLP1 additionally has an effect on normalizing gastric emptying and increasing satiety, therefore enhancing the potential for weight loss (Drucker, 2007).

Other hormones are known to affect fuel metabolism. Ghrelin, secreted from the stomach, has been demonstrated to promote food consumption (Druce et al., 2005).

Cholecystokinin (CCK) and gastrin, secreted in the small and large bowel, have actions in addition to control of gallbladder contraction that increase insulin concentration and reduce glucose excursion following meal ingestion in healthy people and people with T2DM (Ahren, Holst, & Efendic, 2000).

The endocannabinoid system, which has receptors in the brain, adipose tissue, gastrointestinal tract, and other organs, contributes to food intake and lipid and glucose metabolism. When activated, this system increases food intake and thus increases weight gain. Stimuli, such as excessive food intake, may overactivate this system leading to more overeating. Research in blocking these receptors has produced weight loss, improved lipids, and improvement in metabolic defects (Scheen et al., 2006). See Appendix K to read how nurse educator Debbie Hinnen explains this complex information to patients.

Changes When a Person Gets T2DM

People with a strong familial predisposition for T2DM develop abnormal beta cell secretion and eventually beta cell failure as well as concomitant severe insulin resistance. Multiple hormones impact glucose homeostasis. Insulin resistance exists for years before the onset of hyperglycemia. Insulin sensitivity in both the liver and peripheral muscle tissue is diminished. Despite high fasting insulin levels, hepatic glucose release occurs nocturnally. This glucose release is primarily from gluconeogenesis.

The other component of insulin resistance is peripheral glucose utilization. If peripheral glucose utilization is diminished, circulating glucose levels remain elevated. Because insulin binding to the receptor, insulin receptor number, and insulin receptor activity appear to be essentially normal in T2DM (Reaven, 1988), other mechanisms such as the internal signaling mechanisms are implicated in insulin resistance. Many other abnormalities in the glucose uptake by muscle and fat cells may exist and continue to be evaluated.

The beta cell increases secretion of insulin in response to hepatic glucose release and insulin resistance. Beta cell mass is depleted in T2DM, the beta cells die (apoptosis) at a faster rate, and insulin secretion is impaired. A loss of beta cell function of about 50%–70% is identified at the time of diagnosis of T2DM (U.K. Prospective Diabetes Study, 1998). Some research suggests that the ability to reproduce beta cells and islet formation may be unaffected in people with T2DM, but the rate of beta cell death outpaces restoration at a rate of 3- to 10-fold (Butler et al., 2003).

Autoimmune issues and positive antibodies attributed to Type 1 diabetes mellitus (T1DM) are not typically present in T2DM, though GAD 65 antibodies may be present in some people with T2DM.

Dysfunctional fat cells break down at a rapid pace in T2DM, increasing FFA levels. These FFAs are toxic to the beta cells and increase liver and muscle insulin resistance. Additionally, prolonged hyperglycemia and exposure to FFAs lead to glucose toxicity. Glucose toxicity suggests that the beta cell is progressively less efficient at responding to glucose elevations (again, see Appendix K for patient wording).

T2DM in Children

Children with a familial predisposition for diabetes are developing insulin resistance and, in epidemic proportions, T2DM. Obesity and inactivity are considered toxic trends in today's society that lead to diabetes. A strong clinical marker for insulin resistance is acanthosis nigricans. This darkening of the skin folds and velvety texture to the skin is particularly evident on the back of the neck. Mothers embarrassed to "not be able to get their kids' necks clean" are unaware that this is often a precursor to overt diabetes. Acanthosis nigricans can occur in the axilla and groin and is related to insulin resistance.

Part of the toxic environment is attributed to increased consumption of fast food. More was spent on fast food in the year 2000 in the United States than was spent on higher education. Larger portion sizes and excessive calories in high-density foods contribute to the weight gain that leads to insulin resistance and diabetes. Schools are reducing the amount of physical education required and increased computer, video games, and television time contribute to sedentary lifestyles for our youth. Add to this the normal insulin resistance of puberty, and many children are not able to increase the endogenous insulin secretion enough to maintain normoglycemia.

Clinicians are struggling to develop education and exercise programs to combat this alarming trend. Camps for children with T2DM are starting to appear around the country. The Centers for Disease Control and Prevention and other organizations such as the American Diabetes Association, the Juvenile Diabetes Research Foundation, State Diabetes Control Programs, and school systems are adapting the Diabetes Prevention data into materials for implementation for interventions for children as well as adults.

The only oral hypoglycemic medication approved for use in children is metformin. If this doesn't maintain glycemic control, insulin use is started (again, see Appendix K for suggested wording).

What if Diet and Exercise Do Not Get the Blood Sugars in Target Range?

Then diabetes medications are needed (see Table 17.1). Understanding the metabolic defects of T2DM helps connect the dots of medication management. The target actions of each family of medications is directly connected to the defects of the disease. First steps *always* are healthy eating and increasing activity.

If the beta cells of the pancreas are not making enough insulin, and glucose levels are all elevated, treat with insulin secretagogues (to increase endogenous insulin secretion) like glimepiride, glipizide, glyburide, and/or incretins, such as exenatide-4 or sitagliptin.

If the insulin resistance is affecting peripheral glucose utilization, demonstrated by elevated postmeal glucose levels, treat with insulin sensitizers like the thiazolidinediones (TZDs), such as pioglitazone or rosiglitazone. (Note: There is some controversy with rosiglitazone as of this printing. This drug has been implicated by meta-analysis of previous studies in increasing the risk of heart disease. This risk remains to be proven by prospective studies.)

If hepatic glucose release is dominant, as demonstrated by "leaky liver" and high fasting glucose levels, treat with a biguanide, that is, metformin. If peripheral insulin resistance is the primary defect, then a TZD should be used. Exactly when to introduce exenatide-4 and sitagliptin into the mix is to be determined. Because these drugs may have an effect on the preservation of beta cell mass, their use early in diabetes therapy may be indicated, but human data are not yet available to support this use.

The pathophysiology of T2DM has demonstrated that several metabolic defects are usually present simultaneously. In clinical practice, pharmacotherapy increasingly begins with metformin or a combination of metformin and a TZD. Successfully treating multiple defects requires treatment by multiple agents. Several protocols and guidelines are available to guide treatment decisions. One of the best protocols is the updated American Association of Clinical Endocrinologists (AACE) Roadmap. (Find this roadmap by going to http://www.aace.com/pub/roadmap/index.php.) In this protocol, HbA1c is

Trade name	Generic name	When to Take[a]	Doses
Alpha-glucosidase Inhibitors			
Precose	Acarbose	Take with first bite	20, 50, 100 mg
Glyset	Miglitol	Take with first bite	20, 50, 100 mg 300 mg max
Biguanides			
Glucophage	Metformin	Take with meals	500, 850, 1,000 mg
Glucophage XR	Fortamet	Take with meals	500, 1,000 mg 2,500 mg max
Glucovance	Glyburide/ Metformin	Take with meals	1.25/250, 2.5/500, 5/500 mg
Metaglip	Glipizide/ Metformin	Take with meals	2.5/250, 2.5/500, 5/500
Avandamet	Rosiglitazone/ Metformin	Take with meals	1/500, 2/500, 4/500, 2/1,000, 4/1,000 mg
Actoplusmet	Pioglitazone/Metformin	Take with meals	15/500, 15/850
Avandaryl	Avandia/Amaryl	Take same time/day	4/1, 4/2, 4/4 mg
Sulfonylureas			
Diabeta or Micronase	Glyburide	30 min before meals	1/25, 2.5, 5 mg, 20 mg max
Glynase	Glyburide press tab	30 min before meals	1.5, 3, 6 mg, 12 mg max
Glucotrol	Glipizide	30 min before meals	5, 10 mg, 40 mg max
Glucotrol XL	Glipizide	Before or with meals	5, 10 mg, 20 mg max
Amaryl	Glimepiride	Before or with meals	2, 3, 4 mg, to 16 mg max
Meglitinides			
Prandin	Repaglinide	Take right before meals	0.5, 1, 2 mg, to 16 mg max
Starlix	Nateglinide	Take right before meals	60, 120 mg
Thiazolidinediones			
Actos	Pioglitazone	With or without meals	15, 30 mg, to 45 mg max
Avandia	Rosiglitazone	With or without meals Once (or twice) daily	2, 4, 6, 8 mg, to 8 mg max
DPP-4 Inhibitors			
Januvia	Sitagliptin	With or without meals Once daily	100 mg, 50 mg (moderate renal insufficiency), 25 mg (severe renal insufficiency, ESRD[b])

[a] Initially do a liver function study and then yearly.
[b] ESRD, end-stage renal disease.

used as the guide as to whether to use diet, diet and insulin alone, oral agent monotherapy, or multiple drug therapy. This protocol also includes points for the introduction of insulin therapy either with oral agent therapy or alone.

Clinical considerations exist for each category of medications.

Secretagogues

1. Sulfonylureas. Second generation of sulfonylureas have fewer side effects associated with them than are associated with first-generation drugs. Although older medications like diabinase and tolbutamide are available, most insurance companies provide coverage for second-generation agents because they are now available in generic formulations. The duration of action of the agents is the distinguishing characteristic of these pills. The 24-hr pills are glimepiride (Amaryl) and glipizide ES (Glucotrol XL). Pills that last 10–12 hr and thus must often be prescribed twice a day, before breakfast and before supper, are glipizide and glyburide. All the medications in this family lower the blood glucose by increasing the endogenous insulin secretion. Hypoglycemia and weight gain are the primary side effects to consider. Renal and hepatic excretion of these drugs requires that liver and kidney studies verify that the patient is able to tolerate these drugs.
2. Meglitinides (nateglinide [Starlix] and repaglinide [Prandin]) are rapid-acting agents that cause a burst of insulin to be released from the pancreas, thus having time actions similar to rapid-acting insulins. They must be given before each meal. As with the other agents in this category, hypoglycemia may occur if the patient takes the medication and misses a meal.

Patients should understand that these are the medications that help squeeze more insulin out of the pancreas and in today's therapy are usually the last oral drugs added to the regimen before insulin.

Biguanides

Metformin (Glucophage) is a medication that was tested and used in Europe for several decades before reaching the United States. The metformin family has now become the most widely prescribed medication for T2DM. Metformin is an insulin sensitizer and improves blood glucose by reducing gluconeogenesis and glycogenolysis by the liver. Biguanides also have a mild effect on the peripheral uptake of glucose. The primary benefit is seen in its reduction of fasting glucose levels. Even with Glucophage XR (Fortamet, Glumetza) this medication often needs to be prescribed twice daily with food. Because the initial side effects may be gas, diarrhea, or cramping, this medication is best prescribed to be given with supper for a day or two and then increased to being given with breakfast and supper. The clinical therapeutic dose is 1,000 mg twice daily. An alternate dosing schedule might be 850 mg three times daily with meals. Patients having gastrointestinal problems may benefit from Glucophage XR, which has an enteric coating. Other side effects are rare, but creatinine levels should be checked to assure kidney function. This drug is excreted exclusively by the kidney. If kidney function is compromised the drug can accumulate in the bloodstream and have a deleterious effect on the liver, causing lactic acidosis. Creatinine should be less that 1.4 in men and less than 1.3 in women to assure renal clearance. In older patients, creatinine clearance (CrCl) would be a better indicator of sufficient kidney function than just the serum creatinine level. CrCl should be above 50 ml/min for the safest use of metformin, the only biguanide available in the United States.

Good oxygenation is another consideration in safe metformin use. Someone who has recently had a myocardial infarction, is preparing for surgery, or is otherwise experiencing compromised oxygenation should not take metformin. Patients having testing with iodinated contrast media should be off metformin 24–48 hr before and after the dye. The dye may exacerbate any renal dysfunction. Metformin can be restarted 24–48 hr after the dye testing, preferably after testing for serum creatinine.

Metformin is weight neutral, improves glucose levels, especially fasting blood glucose levels, and is available in the generic form. Metformin alone will not cause hypoglycemia. It is used in almost all the combination drugs for treating diabetes.

Patients should understand that metformin is the medication that helps "plug the leaky liver" and therefore helps to fix the fasting blood sugar.

Insulin Sensitizers

Pioglitazone (Actos) and rosiglitazone (Avandia) are thiazolidinediones (TZDs) or glitazones. These drugs stimulate peroxisome-proliferator-activated receptor gamma (PPAR-gamma), an enzyme in the cell nucleus that activates a transcription gene for the synthesis of glucose-transporting hormone (GLUT 4) to cause the transport of glucose into the cell. This allows more efficient glucose transport and therefore improved peripheral glucose utilization. The patient would see the best improvement in postprandial glucose levels after about 6–8 weeks of therapy. These medications can be taken with or without food.

Troglitazone (Rezulin) was the first drug in this category. Liver problems caused this drug to be removed from the market and worries about this problem carried over for this family of medications even after Rezulin was removed. In 2005, the boxed warning for checking liver function studies (LFTs) for pioglitazone and rosiglitazone was lifted as these two drugs proved to be nontoxic to the liver. The difference was that troglitazone was lipid soluble and thus penetrated the mitochondrial membrane and damaged cell function. Pioglitazone and rosiglitazone are water soluble and thus will not penetrate the lipid membranes of the mitochondria.

Side effects that have become most evident for these agents are edema and weight gain. Patients and providers should monitor for peripheral edema and unwanted weight increases. More than 3–4 lbs of weight gain should be reported to the provider. The edema and weight gain is due to fluid retention and thus could lead to congestive heart failure (CHF). A box warning is now included in the package insert for these drugs, indicating that the drugs should not be used in patients with CHF or who have any risk factors for CHF. Both TZDs and metformin increase ovulation and, consequently, may benefit patients with polycystic ovary syndrome (PCOS), but they may also increase fertility. These drugs should be used with caution if the patient does not desire pregnancy and is not using contraceptives.

The Diabetes Reduction Assessment With Ramipril and Rosiglitazone Medication (DREAM) Trial (Gerstein et al., 2006; Lubsen & Poole-Wilson, 2006) and the Diabetes Prevention Program (Knowler et al., 2005) both have suggested that TZDs may improve beta cell function and protect beta cell mass.

Alpha Glucosidase Inhibitors

Precose and Glyset inhibit the enzyme that breaks down the carbohydrate in the gut. These medications should be started with low doses at meals and titrated slowly. Hypoglycemia should be treated with dextrose, because this monosaccharide is not affected by the action of the drug. The mechanism of action causes the delay in carbohydrate breakdown until it reaches the lower gut where it is acted on by yeast and bacteria causing a fermentation of the carbohydrate throughout the intestine, resulting in unacceptable levels of flatulence for most patients.

Incretins—Gut Hormones

Glucagon-like peptide 1 (GLP1) and glucose-dependent insulinotropic polypeptide (GIP) are intestinal hormones that have an impact on glucose metabolism and therefore diabetes. Both are decreased in patients with prediabetes and T2DM (Abdul-Ghani, Tripathy, & DeFronzo, 2006). Secreted in the L and K cells of the intestine, the primary function of these hormones is to stimulate insulin secretion. Secondarily, they decrease alpha cell release of glucagon and consequently reduce postmeal hyperglycemia from hepatic sources. Hypoglycemia should be prevented by decreasing the sulfonylurea dose given to patients receiving these agents at the beginning of their treatment.

The first agent in this category to be marketed was exenatide (Byetta). Exenatide is an incretin mimetic, with greater that 50% homologous amino acid structure between exendin-4 and GLP1. Slight changes to the amino acid structure of exenatide allow a longer half-life than GLP1 and thus provide a greater therapeutic benefit. In addition to glucose-stimulated insulin release and hepatic glucose decrease after meals, the mechanism of action includes normalizing gastric emptying after meals and increasing satiety. Increasing satiety leads to lower caloric intake and weight loss is often the side effect. Data at 2 years show continued weight loss, averaging about 12 lbs (American Diabetes Association [ADA], 2008). A1C reduction is maintained, with more than 60% of trial patients reaching the ADA goal of less than 7%.

Byetta is initiated with 5-µg subcutaneous injections within an hour of the two largest meals of the day. The pen holds doses for a month. The 10-µg twice daily dose is the maintenance dose. Byetta is approved for use with metformin, sulfonylurea, both, or TZDs. Refrigeration is not necessary after starting the pen as long as maximum temperatures do not exceed 77°F (25.3°C). Mild to moderate nausea is a side effect seen sometimes, but it usually decreases over time. This drug cannot be used with insulin because it is a glucose-activated chemical. Insulin suppresses glucose levels, thus preventing the activation of the drug.

Sitagliptin (Januvia) is a dipeptidyl peptidase 4 (DPP-4) inhibitor. This agent inhibits the enzyme that breaks down native GLP1 and GIP in the gut. The action of this drug consequently makes more GLP1 available, and available for a longer period, and therefore reduces postprandial glucose levels by stimulating insulin release and decreasing glucagon levels to reduce hepatic glucose release after meals. No effect on gastric emptying or satiety has been documented. So, although this medication is in pill form and is thus easier to take than injectable exenatide, there is no associated weight loss with its use, so it may not be as useful as exenatide. Side effects to this drug are minimal. The dosage is 100 mg once a day. The dosage should be reduced to 50 mg a day if renal impairment is present.

Both of the incretins have demonstrated a decrease in beta cell apoptosis and an increase in ductal beta cell regeneration in animals. Although research mechanisms do not allow verifying this in humans, there is some consensus that beta cell regeneration along with decreased beta cell workload, weight loss, and other factors may contribute to long-term glucose control.

Summary

Oral hypoglycemic agents have proved to be safe and effective if used appropriately in the therapy of T2DM (Bolen et al., 2007). Therapy of T2DM always includes diet, weight control, and exercise. Choices of other treatment agents are varied. Initiating therapy for T2DM is often begun with metformin or metformin and a TZD. If postprandial glucose levels remain elevated, an incretin or insulin secretagogue to increase or replace first-phase insulin may be indicated. More frequently, combination therapy is used at the beginning of treatment. TZDs or insulin might then be a choice. A combination of oral hypoglycemic agents and insulin might be next (Janka, Hessel, Walzer, & Ma Ller, 2007; Robbins et al., 2007) demonstrating few hypoglycemic events and improved control.

The debate about whether to start insulin with the second or third oral hypoglycemic agent is ongoing among thought leaders. ADA/European Association for the Study of Diabetes (EASD) Type 2 treatment protocols suggest basal insulin as a second-line therapy after metformin (ADA, 2008). This protocol was developed before incretin therapies were available. If the HbA1c is very high (over 8.5% in the AACE Roadmap) or the FPG is > 300 mg/dl (16.67 mmol/L), beginning therapy with insulin, usually in combination with metformin, is indicated. People with T2DM are nearly always trying to lose weight, and because TZDs and secretagogues may increase weight, they are not always a welcome addition to the treatment protocol. Now there is the choice to include an incretin (Peters & Miller, 2007; Raz et al., 2008) or even U500 insulin by injection or insulin pump therapy in severely insulin-resistant individuals (Bulchandani, Konrady, & Hambrug, 2007). Insulin therapy in individuals with T2DM is always indicated when oral hypoglycemic agents are no longer effective because of beta cell exhaustion. A few patients with T2DM may have sufficient beta cell reserve for a time to get by with using insulin mixtures of regular and NPH (70/30 or 50/50 mixtures) or rapid-acting NPL (Novolog 70/30 or Humalog 75/25 mixtures). Most people with T2DM will require basal-bolus insulin therapy no different from that of people with T1DM.

In the prediabetes population, a biguanide might be chosen to treat people at risk. This intervention reportedly improved "weight, lipid profiles, insulin resistance, and reduced new-onset diabetes by 40%" (Salpeter, Buckley, Kahn, & Salpeter, 2008).

There is no longer a question concerning whether or not to control blood glucose levels. The American College of Physicians concluded that guidance statements needed to be made to assist in increasing education and improving the prescribing habits of physicians. These statements are highlighted as follows:

1. The goal for glycemic control should be blood glucose levels as low as feasible in order to prevent complications of diabetes . . .
2. The goal for hemoglobin A1c level should be based on individualized assessment . . .
3. There still is a need for further research to assess the optimal level of glycemia control (Qaseem et al., 2007)—but normal values for blood glucose and HbA1c are physiologic and can't hurt if safely achieved.

A consensus is forming that the older method of *step therapy*, starting with a secretagogue and adding other drugs one by one in a step manner, is probably not the therapy of choice. The early insulin resistance is best treated with an insulin sensitizer (metformin, a TZD, or both). Because metformin works at the level of the liver with some peripheral effect and TZDs work at the peripheral cell level with some effect on the liver, a combination of these two drugs makes good physiologic sense. Another consensus developing in diabetes thought leaders is that oral agent therapy should be pushed harder toward maximum doses and that insulin should be introduced earlier in T2DM treatment to attain and maintain the best blood glucose control possible.

References

Abdul-Ghani, M. A., Tripathy, D., & DeFronzo, R. A. (2006). Contributions of β-cell dysfunction and insulin resistance to the pathogenesis of impaired glucose tolerance and impaired fasting glucose. *Diabetes Care, 29*(5), 1130–1139.

Ahren, B., Holst, J. J., & Efendic, S. (2000). Antidiabetogenic action of cholecystokinin-8 in type 2 diabetes. *Journal of Clinical Endocrinology & Metabolism, 85*(3), 1043–1048.

American Diabetes Association. (2008). Standards of medical care in diabetes-2008. *Diabetes Care, 31*(Suppl. 1), S23–S54.

Bolen, S., Feldman, L., Vassy, J., Wilson, L., Yeh, H. C., Marinopoulos, S., et al. (2007). Systematic review: Comparative effectiveness and safety of oral medication for type 2 diabetes mellitus. *Annals of Internal Medicine, 147*(6), 383–399.

Bulchandani, D. G., Konrady, T., & Hamburg, M. S. (2007). Clinical efficacy and patients satisfaction with U-500 insulin pump therapy in patients with type 2 diabetes. *Endocrine Practice, 13*(7), 721–725.

Butler, A. E., Janson, J., Bonner-Weir, S., Ritzel, R., Rizza, R. A., & Butler, P. C. (2003). Beta-cell deficit and increased beta cell apoptosis in humans with type 2 diabetes. *Diabetes, 52*(1), 102–110.

DeFronzo, R. A., & Ferrannini, E. (1995). Regulation of intermediary metabolism during fasting and fed state. In L. J. DeGroot (Ed.), *Endocrinology* (3rd ed., pp. 1395–1397). Philadelphia: WB Saunders.

Druce, M. R., Wren, A. M., Park, A. J., Milton, J. E., Patterson, M., Frost, G., et al. (2005). Ghrelin increases food intake in obese as well as lean subjects. *International Journal of Obesity, 29*(9), 1130–1136.

Drucker, D. J. (2006). The biology of incretin hormones. *Cell Metabolism, 3*(3), 153–165.

Drucker, D. (2007). The role of gut hormones in glucose homeostasis. *Journal of Clinical Investigation, 117*(1), 24–32.

Elrick, H., Stimmeler, L., Hlad, C. J., Jr., & Arai, Y. (1964). Plasma insulin response to oral and intravenous glucose administration. *Journal of Clinical Endocrinology & Metabolism, 24,* 1076–1082.

Geiss, L. S., Pan, L., Cadwell, B., Gregg, E. W., Benjamin, S. M., & Engelgau, M. M. (2006). Changes in incidence of diabetes in U.S. adults, 1997–2003. *American Journal of Preventive Medicine, 30*(5), 371–377.

Gerstein H. C., Yusuf, S., Bosch, J., Poque, J., Sheridan, P., Dinccaq, N., et al. (2006). Effect of rosiglitazone on the frequency of diabetes in patients with impaired glucose tolerance or impaired fasting glucose: A randomized controlled trial: DREAM (Diabetes Reduction Assessment With Ramipril and Rosiglitazone Medication). *Lancet, 368*(9541), 1096–1105.

Janka, H. U., Hessel, F., Walzer, S., & Ma Ller, E. (2007). Insulin glargine added to therapy with oral antidiabetic agents improves glycemic control and reduces long-term complications in patients with type 2 diabetes—a simulation with the Diabetes Mellitus Model (DMM). *International Journal of Clinical Pharmacology Therapy, 45*(12), 623–630.

Knowler, W. C., Hamm, R. F., Edelstein, S. L., Barrett-Connor, E., Ehrmann, D. A., Walker, E. A., et al., Diabetes Prevention Program Research Group. (2005). Prevention of type 2 diabetes with troglitazone in Diabetes Prevention Program. *Diabetes, 54*(4), 1150–1156.

Lubsen, J., & Poole-Wilson, P. A. (2006). The DREAM trial. *Lancet, 368*(9552), 2050–2051.

Peters, A. L., & Miller, D. (2007). New insights: Clinical pearls for using incretin mimetics in type 2 diabetes. *The Diabetes Educator, 33*(Suppl. 1), 14S–19S.

Qaseem, A., Vijan, S., Snow, V., Cross, J. T., Weiss, K. B., Owens, D. K., Clinical Efficacy Assessment Subcommittee of the American College of Physicians. (2007). Glycemic control and type 2 diabetes mellitus: The optimal hemoglobin A1c targets. A guidance statement from the American College of Physicians. *Annals of Internal Medicine, 18*(6), 417–422.

Ratner, B. (1998). The pathophysiology of the diabetes disease state. In M. Funnel (Ed.), *A core curriculum for diabetes education* (3rd ed., pp. 169–184). Chicago: American Association of Diabetes Educators.

Raz, I., Chen, Y., Wu, M., Hussain, S., Kaufman, K. D., Amatruda, J. M., et al. (2008). Efficacy and safety of sitagliptin added to ongoing metformin therapy in patients with type 2 diabetes. *Current Medical Research Opinion, 24*(2), 537–550.

Reaven, G. M. (1988). Banting lecture: Role of insulin resistance in human disease. *Diabetes, 37*(12), 1595–1607.

Robbins, D. C., Beisswenger, P. J., Ceriello, A., Goldberg, R. B., Moses, R. G., Pagkalos, E. M., et al. (2007). Mealtime 50/50 basal + prandial insulin analogue mixture with a basal analogue, both plus metformin, in the achievement of target HbA1c and pre- and postprandial blood glucose levels in patients with type 2 diabetes: A multinational, 24 week, randomized, open-label, parallel-group comparison. *Clinical Therapy, 29*(11), 2349–2364.

Salpeter, S. R., Buckley, N. S., Kahn, J. A., & Salpeter, E. E. (2008). Meta-analysis: Metformin treatment in persons at risk for diabetes mellitus. *American Journal of Medicine, 121*(2), 149–157.

Scheen, A. J., Finer, N., Hollander, P., Jensen, M. D., Van Gaal, V. F., & RIO-Diabetes Study Group (2006). Efficacy and tolerability of rimonabant in overweight or obese patients with type 2 diabetes: A randomized controlled study. *Lancet, 368*(9548), 1660–1672.

U.K. Prospective Diabetes Study Group. (1998). Intensive blood glucose control with sulfonylurea or insulin compared with conventional treatment and risk of complications in patients with type 2 diabetes mellitus. *Journal of the American Medical Association, 284,* 363–365.

18

Nutrition and Weight Loss: Type 2 Diabetes Mellitus

Medical nutrition therapy (MNT) is an integral component of the treatment of Type 2 diabetes (T2DM). Because approximately 80%–90% of patients with T2DM are obese, weight loss is a primary treatment goal. The combination of a sedentary lifestyle and excess calories leading to weight gain is the primary factor in the development of insulin resistance and, ultimately, T2DM. With an oversupply of calories relative to energy expenditure, insulin resistance progresses to the point in which insulin secretion cannot compensate and impaired glucose tolerance results, then diabetes. In many patients with T2DM MNT and physical activity may be the only therapeutic intervention needed to control the metabolic abnormalities of diabetes.

Obesity is becoming a challenge worldwide. More than 1.1 billion adults are overweight. Of them, 312 million are obese. Added to this number are the 155 million children who are overweight or are obese, as found by the International Obesity Task Force of the World Health Organization (Deitel, 2002). Hossain, Kawar, & Nahas (2007) stated that in the past 20 years the obesity rate has tripled in many of the developing countries that have adopted western lifestyles—which involved a decrease in physical activity and overconsumption of high-fat foods. The challenge worldwide, then, is to address this situation before it becomes even greater.

Health professionals have the opportunity to address the challenges of leading people to develop a healthier lifestyle and to maintain and manage diabetes control. A coordinated team effort, with the patient as the center of the team, is optimal in helping the patient learn to implement nutrition recommendations and lifestyle changes. Consultation with a registered dietitian is recommended to individualize meal planning according to food preferences, cultural influences, physical activity, schedules, and family eating patterns. When a physician addresses and encourages weight loss, patients are more likely to make positive changes than patients who do not receive a physician's advice (Galuska, Will, Serdula, & Ford, 1999).

The goals of MNT for prevention and treatment of diabetes presented in Chapter 10 also apply to T2DM. These include maintaining normal blood glucose levels as safely as possible, normalizing blood pressure and lipid levels, and by doing so preventing or slowing the rate of development of chronic complications of diabetes. This is assisted through the individualizing of nutrition therapy, especially for those with metabolic syndrome (Lorenzo, Williams, Hunt, & Haffner, 2007).

Nutrition interventions for T2DM (American Diabetes Association [ADA], 2007) include:

- Individuals with T2DM are encouraged to implement lifestyle modifications that reduce intakes of energy, saturated and trans fatty acids, cholesterol, and sodium, and to increase physical activity in an effort to improve glycemia, dyslipidemia, and blood pressure.
- Plasma glucose monitoring can be used to determine whether adjustments in foods and meals will be sufficient to achieve blood glucose goals or if medication(s) needs to be combined with MNT.

The fundamental principle that underlies nutritional therapy is a plan based on the normal nutritional needs of the person for good health. Energy intake in the diet is constantly balanced with energy output in work and exercise and metabolic body processes. The appropriate calorie and nutrient needs are the basis for the diet for diabetes. The ADA (2007) nutrition recommendations for energy balance, overweight, and obesity include:

- In individuals who are overweight, obese, and insulin resistant, modest weight loss has been shown to improve insulin resistance. Thus, weight loss is recommended for all such individuals who have or are at risk for diabetes.
- Structured programs that emphasize lifestyle changes, including education, reduced energy and fat (about 30% of total energy) intake, regular physical activity, and regular participant contact, can produce long-term weight loss on the order of 5%–7% of starting weight. Thus, lifestyle change should be the primary approach to weight loss.
- Low-carbohydrate diets (restricting total carbohydrate to less than 130 g/day) are recommended with care in the treatment of overweight or obesity. The long-term effects of these diets are becoming known (Clifton, Keogh, & Noakes, 2008; Nuttall & Gannon, 2006) and, although such diets produce short-term weight loss, maintenance of weight loss

is similar to that from low-fat diets and the impact on cardiovascular risk profile and nephropathy is still somewhat uncertain.

■ Physical activity and behavior modification are important components of weight loss programs and are most helpful in maintenance of weight loss.

■ Weight loss medications may be considered in the treatment of overweight and obese individuals with T2DM and can help achieve a 5%–10% weight loss when combined with lifestyle modification.

■ Bariatric surgery may be considered for some individuals with T2DM and body mass index (BMI) ≥ 35 kg/m² and can result in marked improvements in glycemia. The long-term benefits and risks of bariatric surgery in individuals with diabetes continue to be studied.

Body Weight

Most patients with T2DM present with weight and BMI above goal so weight loss is a primary therapeutic goal to improve blood glucose, hypertension, and cardiovascular risk. BMI is a practical measure defining body weight relative to health risk. BMI is weight in kilograms divided by the square of height in meters (kg/m²). A healthy BMI is 19–24.9 according to the U.S. Department of Health and Human Services Dietary Guidelines for Americans (2005), a BMI greater than 25 is generally defined as overweight, and a BMI greater than 30 is obesity. (There are exceptions to the BMI standards. Weight lifters, body builders, football players, etc., will have a high BMI because of muscle mass rather than fat.) Body weight profoundly influences insulin resistance, insulin requirements, and blood glucose control, so appropriate calories and nutrition recommendations are integral to treating T2DM. Excess body weight, particularly abdominal fat, is associated with increasing risk of T2DM (Rana, Li, Manson, & Hu, 2007). Intraabdominal or central obesity refers to fat deposited around abdominal organs and this visceral fat contains more capillaries, making it more metabolically active than subcutaneous fat or fat in the hips and thighs. As a result, there is a greater turnover of free fatty acids (FFAs), which in the liver contributes to insulin resistance (lipotoxicity). These FFAs also may be used as fuel instead of glucose which causes hyperglycemia (American Association of Diabetes Educators [AADE], 2006). Central obesity is measured as a waist circumference greater than 102 cm (40 inches) in men or greater than 88 cm (35 inches) in women (National Heart, Lung and Blood Institute, 1998) or as an increased waist-to-hip ratio. Intraabdominal fat is also more active in producing hormones that stimulate appetite than is subcutaneous fat.

Nutrition Management

Individual assessment, lab data, and monitoring provide the basis for medical nutrition therapy including a meal plan that guides the patient in what to eat. Assessment of what the patient typically eats for breakfast, lunch, dinner, and snacks, where the patient eats, and how much is eaten provides the basis for setting goals. Depending on the assessment, the emphasis may be on reducing fat, reducing portions, controlling carbohydrates, increasing fiber, or rearranging the timing or frequency of meals. Options for meal planning include basic eating guidelines, sample menus, or counting calories, points, carbohydrate, or fat. Most commonly, portion sizes are a central issue in weight loss and food records with accurate measurements of food portions may be a key component in identifying where change can be most effective. *Portion distortion* was a key element noted in the young adults Schwartz and Bydr-Bredbenner (2006) studied.

Calorie restriction alone may improve glucose tolerance and as little as 5%–10% loss of body weight improves insulin sensitivity, increases glucose uptake, reduces insulin secretory requirements, and decreases hepatic glucose production. Eating low glycemic indexed foods, such as high-fiber foods, have shown positive effect on blood glucose levels in both long-term and short-term studies (Riccardi, Riveliese, & Giacco, 2008).

Weight loss may be most beneficial in the early stages of T2DM when beta cells are secreting large amounts of insulin (Anderson, Kendall, & Jenkins, 2003; Hamman et al., 2006). A 3,500 calorie deficit will result in a loss of 1 pound of body fat. Standard weight loss strategies provide 500–1,000 fewer calories than the estimated daily requirement for weight maintenance and result in a 1–2 pound weight loss per week. A meal pattern that includes carbohydrate from fruits, vegetables, whole grains, legumes, and low-fat milk is encouraged for good health. Saturated fat is limited to less than 7% of total calories, trans fat should be minimized, cholesterol should be limited to less than 200 mg/day, and two or more servings of fish per week are recommended. The protein intake of 15% of energy in the average adult is appropriate for patients with normal renal function. There is no evidence of benefit from vitamin or mineral supplementation in patients with diabetes who do not have underlying deficiencies. More extensive information is included in Chapter 10 and in the ADA (2007) evidence-based nutrition recommendations.

The optimal distribution of carbohydrate, protein, and fat for diabetes meal plans has not been established. The ratios of carbohydrate, fat, and protein are individualized and based on recommendations by the American Diabetes Association, the American Heart Association, the American Dietetic Association, and Guidelines for Healthy Americans. Recent reports have guided the associations to support education on the restriction of carbohydrate intake for weight loss for some in this T2DM population. This is the outcome of a meta-analysis (Kirk et al., 2008) and the Canadian Trial of Carbohydrates in Diabetes (CDD) (Wolever et al., 2008).

A registered dietitian (RD) is an essential member of the diabetes health care team and uses skills to assess, plan, and recommend a plan for healthy eating that promotes blood glucose control and health. Outcome studies have demonstrated that MNT provided by a registered dietitian can achieve a 1%–2% decrease in A1C in patients with diabetes (Pastors, Franz, Warshaw, Daly, & Arnold, 2003) and can improve dyslipidemia (Yu-Poth al., 1999) and hypertension (Whitworth & Chalmers, 2004). The registered dietitian will generally require two to three appointments to design and monitor an individualized plan with continued follow-up to reassess and revise the plan to meet the goals of diabetes management. After initiation of MNT, improvements were apparent in three to six months (Whitworth & Chalmers, 2004). All members of the diabetes team should be knowledgeable about nutrition and supportive of the patient in making lifestyle plans to accomplish diabetes goals.

Studies demonstrate that structured, intensive lifestyle programs involving patient education, individualized counseling, reduced dietary energy and fat intake, regular physical activity, and frequent patient contact are necessary to produce a sustained weight loss of 5%–7% (Franz et al., 2002). Options for weight loss diets are endless, so professional resources that provide tools to provide collaboration between the patient and health care team to address the issue are valuable (Adolfsson & Arnold, 2006). Helping patients to begin implementing healthy lifestyle choices is the core concept. Weight control is a long-term commitment so the patient must make the decision to change and take responsibility for behavior change and mobilize their own internal resources. If the health professional is working harder in the process than the patient, a paradigm shift is required. The patient must be central in defining the problem, establishing goals, and creating success with the professional as the consultant for planning, encouraging success, providing feedback, empowering the patient in improving health, and making referrals as needed. Chart reviews in one clinic revealed that 17% of obese patients had dietitian referrals and 36% had an indication of physician weight loss recommendation. However, at the same clinic in the patient survey, 64% of obese patients wanted a dietitian referral and 62% felt that their physician could help with weight loss. If weight was discussed, the patient was more likely to have a dietitian consultation (Davis, Emerenini, & Wylie-Rosett, 2006). Physician counseling and advice can be an effective intervention to promote behavioral change. Huang et al. (2004) found that patients who recalled receiving weight loss counseling from their physician were more motivated to attempt weight loss and had a better understanding of their health risk. It is important to place as much, or more, emphasis on meal planning and physical activity than on pharmacologic interventions.

Barriers to following dietary recommendations must be explored and readiness to change must be addressed to improve success in weight loss therapy. Communication between patient and provider depends on mutual respect and positive attitude, which is often a problem in lifestyle change. Dietary change is seen as a greater burden than taking pills, but less a burden than insulin therapy, and self-reported adherence was much higher for both pills and insulin than for a diet (Vijan et al., 2005). Barriers such as cost, portion sizes, family issues, schedules, support, and quality of life require time to provide adequate nutrition counseling and follow-up for lifestyle change and successful outcomes.

The physician, dietitian, and health care team can translate the patient's follow-up data, such as BMI, HbA1C, and other lab results, to encourage the patient to eat healthy, exercise, and control glucose levels. See Table 18.1 for some of these quick messages that can impact behavior change.

Type 2 Diabetes in Children

Because of the increase in numbers of overweight children, the diagnosis of T2DM in children is increasing dramatically (Kim et al., 2006; Nader et al., 2006). In the presence of excess fat cells, the initial metabolic abnormality in glucose intolerance is insulin resistance, which leads to deterioration of pancreatic beta cell function and progression to clinical diabetes. Insulin receptors in the liver, muscle, and adipose tissue are normally exquisitely sensitive to insulin, but as

18.1 Quick Messages to Encourage Nutrition Health

- You are in control. The choices of what you eat will influence your blood sugar and your health.
- How much you eat affects your blood sugar increase after eating.
- With diabetes knowledge comes power. Learn how food affects your blood sugar – the more you know, the better you can manage your diabetes.
- Include several vegetables, salads, fruit, and whole grains each day to reduce your risk for heart disease.
- Modest weight loss improves insulin resistance and improves your blood sugar, blood pressure, and cholesterol levels.
- When you have diabetes, what you eat is very important, so I will have a dietitian help you choose what to eat.

adiposity increases, cells become resistant to insulin and the body is unable to maintain blood glucose in the normal range. Visceral adiposity promotes insulin resistance to a higher degree than subcutaneous adiposity. The first few years of life are a key period in the development of overweight children and long-term health consequences. An analysis of published evidence concludes that breastfeeding in infancy is associated with a reduced risk of T2DM, including marginally lower insulin concentrations in later life and lower blood glucose and serum insulin concentrations in infancy (Owen, Martin, Whitcup, Smith, & Cook, 2006). Maintaining a healthy weight is the best way to prevent T2DM in children (Hannon, Goutham, & Arslanian, 2005) because, unfortunately, overweight children are likely to become overweight adults with long-term health implications. Television watching rather than active play is just one of the culprits (Gable, Change, & Krull, 2007).

The American Academy of Pediatrics Committee on Nutrition (Krebs & Jacobson, 2003) published recommendations for preventing pediatric overweight and obesity:

Major Recommendations

Health Supervision

- Identify and track children at risk because of family history, birth weight, socioeconomic status, or ethnic, cultural, or other environmental factors.
- Calculate and plot BMI once a year in all children and adolescents.
- Use change in BMI to identify rate of excessive weight gain relative to linear growth.
- Encourage, support, and protect breastfeeding.

- Encourage parents and caregivers to promote healthy eating patterns by offering nutritious snacks, such as vegetables and fruits, low-fat dairy foods, and whole grains, encouraging children's autonomy in self-regulation of food intake, setting appropriate limits on choices, and modeling healthy food choices.
- Routinely promote physical activity, including unstructured play at home, in school, in child care settings, and throughout the community.
- Recommend limitation of television and video time to a maximum of 2 hr/day.
- Recognize and monitor changes in obesity-associated risk factors for adult chronic disease, such as hypertension, dyslipidemia, hyperinsulinemia, impaired glucose tolerance, and symptoms of obstructive sleep apnea syndrome.

Advocacy

- Help parents, teachers, coaches, and others who influence youth to discuss health habits, not body habits, as part of their efforts to control overweight and obesity.
- Enlist policy makers from local, state, and national organizations and schools to support a healthful lifestyle for all children, including proper diet and adequate opportunity for regular physical activity.
- Encourage organizations that are responsible for health care and health care financing to provide coverage for effective obesity prevention and treatment strategies.
- Encourage public and private sources to direct funding toward research into effective strategies to prevent overweight and obesity and to maximize limited family and community resources to achieve healthful outcomes for youth.
- Support and advocate for social marketing intended to promote healthful food choices and increased physical activity.

The management of T2DM in children must be appropriate for the age of the child. All children and/or caregivers with T2DM should receive comprehensive self-management education including nutrition. Referral to a dietitian knowledgeable in the nutritional management of children with diabetes is necessary (ADA, 2000). Calories must be adequate for the child to reach full potential in height, so monitoring and follow-up are essential. The expert committee convened by the Maternal and Child Health Bureau (Barlow & Dietz, 1998) recommends that for children from 2 to 7 years of age with a BMI in the 85th–94th percentile, the goal is weight maintenance. For 2- to 7-year-olds with a BMI over the 94th percentile without complications, the treatment should also be weight maintenance. However, if the BMI is over the 94th percentile with complications, the treatment should include gradual weight loss. For children over 7 years of age with a BMI in the 85th–94th percentile without complications, treatment is weight maintenance, but with complications or a BMI over the 94th percentile, treatment should include weight loss and medications. The only oral medication approved for children is metformin.

Nutrition education and counseling should be age appropriate, culturally appropriate, and sensitive to socioeconomic resources and include the family and caregivers. Obesity and diabetes disproportionately affect certain minority groups including Black and Mexican American children. The most promising approaches to weight and lifestyle modifications are through schools and families. One approach to weight control counseling in pediatric obesity is motivational interviewing. This approach is used extensively in addiction counseling and assumes that behavior change is affected more by motivation than information (Resnicow, Davis, & Rollnick, 2006).

The entire household is important in implementing healthy eating habits. Strategies for decreasing high-calorie, high-fat food choices and increasing physical activity are important components of therapy. Physical activity can improve insulin sensitivity and improve weight management. In a study of Mexican children, the risk of becoming overweight increased by 12% for each hour of daytime television viewing. The risk of becoming overweight decreased by 10% for each hour of moderate or intense exercise (Hernandez et al., 1999). Because physical activity and nutrition affect weight, goals must be planned according to the patient and family preferences.

Research evaluating the relationship of soft drink consumption and body weight found clear association of soft drink intake with increased calorie intake and body weight. Soft drink intake was also associated with lower intake of nutrients and an increased risk of several medical problems including diabetes (Vartarian, Schwartz, & Brownell, 2007). Specific recommendations by health professionals to reduce soft drink intake are prudent to improve health outcomes.

Summary

Strategies for weight control are best implemented in small steps. One easily implemented goal at a time should be recommended, such as eating a healthy breakfast for a week, taking a 30-min walk daily, or drinking water in place of sweet drinks for a week. Just implementing one exercise goal or one nutrition goal successfully may improve self-confidence to start lifestyle change and improve health.

Readiness to change will affect the outcome of any recommendations (see the options listed in Table 18.2). The art and science of obesity management (Franz & Dokken, 2007) and how to maintain weight loss (Craig, 2007) are reviewed in *Diabetes Spectrum*, from research to practice.

Controlled blood glucose levels are less of a challenge for weight gain with the availability of new medications, but Krentz (2008) found that how these medicines will be used most effectively is still to be established.

Because diabetes is primarily a self-managed disease, education is fundamental so that the patient understands the diabetes treatment plan and is empowered to collaborate with health care providers to make informed decisions about daily diabetes self-management. Information, resources, and support are the foundation of diabetes self-management in nutrition therapy. Patients must learn the skills to effect change in their personal behavior, in social situations, and in decisions that impact diabetes care. Certified diabetes educators,

18.2 Specific Options

Skip the fries

Eat a fruit with breakfast, lunch, and dinner

Eat fast food no more than once a week

Eat a vegetable and/or salad with lunch and dinner

Eat breakfast

Eat 500 calories or less after 5 P.M.

Keep video and TV time to 2 hr or less daily

Take a 30-min walk 5 days a week

Use low-fat milk and dairy items

Skip fried food

Avoid the super size

Avoid soda and drinks that have sugar

physicians, dietitians, and every person on the health care team are educators and coaches to help the patient succeed as a diabetes self-manager.

References

Adolfsson, B., & Arnold, A. S. (2006). *Behavioral approaches to treating obesity: Helping your patients make changes that last.* Alexandria, VA: American Diabetes Association.

American Association of Diabetes Educators. (2006). *The art and science of diabetes self-management education.* Chicago: Author.

American Diabetes Association. (2000). Type 2 diabetes in children and adolescents. *Diabetes Care, 23,* 381–389.

American Diabetes Association. (2007). Nutrition recommendations and interventions for diabetes. *Diabetes Care, 30,* S48–S65.

Anderson, J. W., Kendall, C. W., & Jenkins, D. J. (2003). Importance of weight management in type 2 diabetes: Review with meta-analysis of clinical studies. *Journal of the American College of Nutrition, 22,* 331–339.

Barlow, S. E., & Dietz, W. H. (1998). Obesity evaluation and treatment: Expert committee recommendations. *Pediatrics, 102*(3), 1–11.

Clifton, P. M., Keogh, J. B., & Noakes, M. (2008). Long-term effects of a high protein weight loss diet. *American Journal of Clinical Nutrition, 87*(1), 23–29.

Craig, J. (2007). Nutrition FYI: How to maintain lost weight. *Diabetes Spectrum, 20*(3), 186–188.

Davis, N. J., Emerenini A., & Wylie-Rosett, J. (2006). Obesity management: Physician practice patterns and patient preference. *The Diabetes Educator, 32,* 557–561.

Deitel, M. (2002). The International Obesity Task Force and "globesity." *Obesity Surgery, 12*(5), 623–624.

Franz, M. J., Bantle, J. P., Beebe, C. A., Brunzell, J. D., Chiasson, J. L., Garg, A., et al. (2002). Evidence-based nutrition principles and recommendations for the treatment and prevention of diabetes and related complications. *Diabetes Care, 25,* 148–198.

Franz, M. J., & Dokken, B. B. (Guest Eds.). (2007). From research to practice: The art and science of obesity management. *Diabetes Spectrum, 20*(3), 133–176.

Gable, S., Chang, Y., & Krull, J. L. (2007). Television watching and frequency of family meals are predictive of overweight onset and persistence in a national sample of school-aged children. *Journal of the American Dietetic Association, 107,* 53–61.

Galuska, D. A., Will, J. C., Serdula, M. K., & Ford, E. S. (1999). Are health care professionals advising obese patients to lose weight? *Journal of the American Medical Association, 282,* 1576–1578.

Hamman, R. F., Wing, R. R., Edelstein, S. L., Lachin, J. M., Bray, G. A., Delahanty, L., et al. (2006). Effect of weight loss with lifestyle intervention on risk of diabetes. *Diabetes Care, 29,* 2102–2107.

Hannon, T. S., Goutham, R., & Arslanian, S. A. (2005). Childhood obesity and Type 2 diabetes mellitus. *Pediatrics, 116,* 473–480.

Hernandez, B., Gortmaker, S. L., Colditz, G. A., Peterson, K. E., Laird, N. M., & Parra-Cabrera, S. (1999). Association of obesity with physical activity, television programs and other forms of video viewing among children in Mexico City. *International Journal of Obesity Related Metabolic Disorders, 23,* 845–854.

Hossain, P., Kawar, B., & El Nahas, M. E. (2007). Obesity and diabetes in the developing world: A growing challenge. *New England Journal of Medicine, 356*(3), 213–215.

Huang, J., Yu, H., Marin, E., Brock, S., Carden, D., & Davis, T. (2004). Physicians' weight loss counseling in two public hospital primary care clinics. *Academic Medicine, 79,* 156–161.

Kim, J., Peterson, K. E., Scanlon, K. S., Fitzmaurice, G. M., Must, A., Oken, E., et al. (2006). Trends in overweight from 1980 through 2001 among preschool-aged children enrolled in a health maintenance organization. *Obesity, 14,* 1107–1112.

Kirk, J. K., Graves, D. E., Craven, T. E., Lipkin, E. W., Austin, M., & Margolis, K. L. (2008). Restricted-carbohydrate diets in patients with type 2 diabetes: A meta-analysis. *Journal of the American Dietetic Association, 108*(10), 91–100.

Krebs, N. F., & Jacobson, M. S. (2003). American Academy of Pediatrics Committee on Nutrition. Prevention of pediatric overweight and obesity. *Pediatrics, 112,* 424–430.

Krentz, A. J. (2008). Management of type 2 diabetes in the obese patisent: Current concerns and emerging therapies. *Current Medical Research Opinion, 24*(2), 401–417.

Lorenzo, C., Williams, K., Hunt, K. J., & Haffner, S. M. (2007). The National Cholesterol Education-Adult Treatment Panel III, International Diabetes Federation, and World Health Organization definitions of the metabolic syndrome as predictors of isncident cardiovascular disease and diabetes. *Diabetes Care, 30,* 8–13.

Nader, P. R., O'Brien, M., Houts, R., Bradley, R., Belsky, J., Crosnoe, R., et al., National Institute of Child Health and Human Development Early Child Care Research Network. (2006). Identifying risk for obesity in early childhood. *Pediatrics, 118,* 594–601.

National Heart, Lung, and Blood Institute. (1998). *Clinical guidelines on the identification, evaluation and treatment of overweight and obesity in adults.* Bethesda, MD: Author.

Nuttall, F. Q., & Gannon, M. C. (2006). The metabolic response to a high-protein, low-carbohydrate diet in men with type 2 diabetes mellitus. *Metabolism, 55*(2), 243–251.

Owen, G. O., Martin, R. H., Whitcup, P. H., Smith, G. D., & Cook, D. G. (2006). Does breastfeeding influence risk of type 2 diabetes in later life? A quantitative analysis of published evidence. *American Journal of Clinical Nutrition, 84,* 1043–1054.

Pastors, J. G., Franz, M. J., Warshaw, H., Daly, A., & Arnold, M. (2003). How effective is medical nutrition therapy in diabetes care? *Journal of the American Dietetic Association, 103,* 827–831.

Rana, J. S., Li, T. Y., Manson, J. E., & Hu, F. B. (2007). Adiposity compared with physical activity and risk of type 2 diabetes in women. *Diabetes Care, 30,* 53–58.

Resnicow, K., Davis, R., & Rollnick, S. (2006). Motivational interviewing for pediatric obesity: Conceptual issues and evidence review. *Journal of the American Dietetic Association, 106,* 2024–2033.

Riccardi, G., Riveliese, A. A., & Giacco, R. (2008). Role of glycemic index and glycemic load in the healthy state, in prediabetes, and in diabetes. *American Journal of Clinical Nutrition, 87*(1), 269S–274S.

Schwartz, J., & Bydr-Bredbenner, C. (2006). Portion distortion: Typical portion sizes selected by young adults. *Journal of the American Dietetic Association, 106,* 1412–1418.

U.S. Department of Health and Human Services & U.S. Department of Agriculture. (2005). *Dietary guidelines for Americans.* Washington, DC: Author.

Vartarian, L. R., Schwartz, M. B., & Brownell, K. D. (2007). Effects of soft drink consumption on nutrition and health: A systematic review and meta-analysis. *American Journal of Public Health, 97,* 667–675.

Vijan, S., Stuart, N. S., Fitzgerald, J. T., Rones, D. L., Hayward, R. A., Slater, S., et al. (2005). Barriers to follsowing dietary recommendations in type 2 diabetes. *Diabetic Medicine, 22,* 32–38.

Whitworth, J. A., & Chalmers, J. (2004). World Health Organization-International Society of Hypertension (WHO/ISH) hypertension guidelines. *Clinical Experience of Hypertension, 26,* 747–752.

Wolever, T. M., Gibbs, A. L., Mehling, C., Chiasson, J. L., Connelly, P. W., Josse, R. G., et al. (2008). The Canadian Trial of Carbohydrates in Diabetes (CCD), a 1-y controlled trial of low-glycemic-index dietary carbohydrate in type 2 diabetes: No effect on glycated hemoglobin but reduction in C-reactive protein. *American Journal of Clinical Nutrition, 87*(1), 1–4.

Yu-Poth, S., Zhao, G., Etherton, T., Naglakon, M., Jonnalagadda, S., & Kris-Etherton, P. M. (1999). Effects of the National Cholesterol Education Program's Step I and Step II dietary intervention programs on cardiovascular disease risk factors: A meta-analysis. *American Journal of Clinical Nutrition, 69,* 632–646.

19

The Power of Exercise

Exercise or increased activity is a need for everyone, especially a person with Type 2 diabetes (T2DM). The Diabetes Prevention Program Trial (DPPT I) (2002) demonstrated that changes in lifestyle that include increasing activity or adding exercise have a role in preventing the diagnosis of T2DM. Daly (2005) stated that lowered blood pressure, lowered triglycerides, decreased weight, and the increase in high-density lipoprotein (HDL), fibrinolysis, and insulin sensitivity contributed to a decrease in cardiovascular risk. "Epidemiological and laboratory evidence shows that regular exercise not only decreases blood glucose levels and increases insulin sensitivity, but may be instrumental in reducing the development of Type 2 diabetes" (Fodor & Adamo, 2001). Insulin sensitivity only continues as long as exercise continues, but will rapidly decrease if exercise is stopped (Albright et al., 2000). Whether they have T2DM or Type 1 diabetes (T1DM), it is important to aid people with diabetes to select the form of exercise(s) they will continue to do for the remainder of their life.

Depending on age, any type of exercise or increased activity will do. The key is to start out slowly, and the older the person, the slower that person should start (see Mullooly, 2006, p. 299, on current terminology as addressed by the President's Council on Physical Fitness).

Individuals who have T2DM have less risk of exercise-induced hyper- and hypoglycemia. They will usually have insulin on board, which allows for fewer large swings or changes in blood glucose levels. The major concern for people with T2DM is insulin resistance at the cellular level along with impaired insulin production from the pancreas. Excessive weight, a high body-fat composition, and lack of physical activity are promoters of insulin resistance. When weight increases, fat cells increase in size and can lose their ability to either receive or bind insulin to the cell receptors. This leads to insulin resistance. As weight and body fat are decreased, the number and affinity of the cell receptor sites appear to improve, which can then be translated to better utilization of blood glucose in the body.

Exercise of moderate intensity can be of importance for the person with T2DM especially when reduction of hypertension can be an outcome. To aid in the prevention and treatment of T2DM in children, exercise is considered one of the best interventions (Berry, Urban, & Grey, 2006; Wolfsdorf, 2005).

Initial Assessment

Any adult with T2DM should have a full evaluation before starting an exercise program because blood vessel damage may have occurred long before T2DM was diagnosed. Exercise is a stressor, so heart, eye, and kidney evaluations are needed. If cardiovascular vessels have been damaged, there is a greater chance that a myocardial infarction might occur. Neurologic damage might be expressed by changes in proprioception or by problems related to polyneuropathy or autonomic neuropathy. On the other hand, documented complications such as these might be changed as circulation improves throughout the body along with normalization of blood glucose levels.

If a person has advanced nephropathy, even without documented heart deficits, the results of a treadmill stress test along with blood pressure and heart rate monitoring must be acceptable before the level of exercise can be determined. The mode of exercise could be walking, the use of the stationary bike, cycling, water exercises, and chair exercises. If the person's endurance level is very low, an interval walking program of alternating 5 min of walking with 5 min of rest might be tolerated. As for precautions, no involvement in long-distance events should occur until a level of flexibility and strength is achieved.

When in doubt, assess, even though asymptomatic, when the person is a man older than 45 years of age or a woman older than 55 years of age with no more than one risk factor. Screen everyone who has two or more risk factors regardless of age. At high risk are individuals who have a sign or symptom suggesting cardiovascular disease or who have had pulmonary disease, metabolic disease, or cardiovascular disease (Harris & White, 2007). The risk factors are high blood pressure, dyslipidemia, diabetes, cigarette smoking, obesity, a family history of diabetes, older age, masculine sex (except in women with diabetes, who are post-menopausal), sedentary lifestyle, poor exercise ability, personal history of vascular disease, or history of sudden death in a first-degree relative.

The Exercise Program

Once the evaluation is completed and the green light has been given to start, then there is a need for guidance and education for anyone embarking on an exercise program. Popular programs are usually within easy reach for most people (Christian et al., 2008). Other programs may be found on television. Encourage people to start slowly. The older the person is the slower they should start, meaning fewer numbers of repetitions or a shorter length of time exercising. An out-of-condition 80-year-old should start with 5 min or shorter time. If this rule is not followed, it is possible that the person will feel sore and be less willing and able to exercise for a number of weeks. It is possible that the person will be reluctant to exercise at all. A 70-year-old might begin with 5–8 repetitions or 5–8 min of exercise, whereas a 60-year-old might start out with 8–10 repetitions or 8–10 min of exercise during the first week. Adding only one or more repetitions or minutes per week is a wise plan.

Fluid volumes should be maintained to prevent dehydration. Blood glucose monitoring is necessary to prevent hypoglycemia, especially when on oral hypoglycemic agents and/or insulin is involved. It is also necessary to monitor for any joint or bone soreness to eliminate the potential of stress fractures that could occur. No high-intensity exercises should be part of this program. If standing or walking is a problem, chair exercises can be quite useful. There are rubber-type bands that can be stretched when working on more advanced muscle action. It might be useful to recommend that a person use a personal trainer so that progress will be monitored appropriately. DVDs and CDs are easily obtainable along with various books on exercise.

> Scientists now regard this nation as an aging society, with the fastest growing minority in the United States being those who reach or pass the age of 65. (Nieman, 1995)

Without question, the health habits of today's generation will be reflected on life expectancy and the quality of that life as old age approaches. Exercise and regular physical activity are the gateway to healthy aging.

The red flags for people with T2DM are the same red flags needed for people with T1DM, especially if the blood glucose levels are 300 mg/dl (16.6 mmol/L) or above, or 60 mg/dl (3.3 mmol/L) or lower. There should be no exercise until proper adjustments in food and/or medication are made.

A Useful Program

The American Academy of Family Physicians suggests doing the following both before and at various intervals throughout the program that is chosen: assessment of age, weight, clothing size, waist and hips in inches, waist-to-hip ratio, body mass index (BMI), calculation of percent body fat, resting pulse rate, resting blood pressure, blood glucose measurements before and after exercise, triglyceride level, total cholesterol, low-density lipoprotein (LDL), high-density lipoprotein (HDL), cigarettes (number per day smoked), alcohol (number of drinks per day), and a medication list.

They also recommend measuring the person's rate, on the scale of 1 to 10, with 1 being low and 10 being high, for the following: stress level, coping skills ability, self-nurturing activities, and support system(s).

They include a booklet that can instruct the person to write down his or her food intake, goals, and progress. The other useful sheet is the paper that is called *Fitness Prescription*. Here, persons are instructed to list their physical activity, their healthy eating, and their emotional well-being in relation to what they want to do, their target or goal, how much and/or how often the person would exercise, medication dosage, any changes in medication, and the benefit(s) for doing what they have chosen. They recommend that each person involved should share this information with their physician at the time of their clinic visits.

A home-based exercise program should be monitored by the clinic visits, and BMI measured at each visit has been found the most useful interaction to follow changes in the person's response to the program (Krousel-Wood et al., 2008). This is especially true for those with T2DM who are at potential risk for cardiovascular disease if the program is not appropriately followed (Mathieu, Brochu, & Beliveau, 2008).

There is a fun side to this personalized fitness prescription. It gives AIM as the brand name for this fitness program and the generic names as physical activity, healthy eating, and emotional well-being, including the indications, benefits, side effects, precautions, and dosage as a professional would direct for any prescription. The directions "Start small, increase slowly and repeat often. Adjust to fit your needs" and the warning—"Likely to become habit-forming when used regularly!"—that they used with permission are from *Am I Hungry? What to Do When Diets Don't Work*, by May, Galper, and Carr (2005). This might be a resource to share with your patients to supplement the AIM program.

Other Ideas

If exercise is reported as too boring, suggest cross-training or choosing two or more exercises from which to alter from day to day or week to week. Suggest that for exercise to be more enjoyable, the exercise time may be accompanied by music that has a brisk beat. Remember the FITT principle—frequency, intensity, time, and type of exercise to be chosen.

And, for those that are not into exercise no matter what, help them plan increases in activity from parking away from an entrance to using the steps instead of the elevator or escalator. Also, as an important reminder, the older the person is, the slower they should start—or take small steps in order to attain the final goal of 20–30 min three to five times a week. If they are sensitive to their oral agent or insulin, be sure they decrease the dose prior to the time they plan to participate in increased activity. One or two units of insulin or one-half of a tablet less of an oral hypoglycemic medication may keep the person from responding to exercising with low blood glucose levels.

Always teach people to warm up and cool down in their exercise program. They can stretch the back of the legs by alternately placing one leg forward as they lean against the wall, stretching the opposite leg. Alternately hold up and stretch each leg toward the back. Then, if physically able, they can bend over and stretch the back. Next, they should sit on the floor and pull both legs toward themselves. While they are sitting, teach them to cross one leg over the other and have them hold the bent knee close to the chest. This could be followed by stretching, alternately, their hand toward the opposite foot. Have them shrug their shoulders both together and separately. Reach each arm up and bend it, reaching toward the back of the opposite shoulder. Follow this by having them move both arms backward, away from the chest. All of these positions should be held for 10–20 seconds or more and not stretched more than the tightness allows.

Walking is best, but weight lifting, tai chi, yoga, qigong, swimming, or any aerobic activity would be useful. Just dancing to music around the house is great, still accompanied with the warm-up and cool-down stretches. Other exercises can be used for specific parts of the body: circling the upper part of the body to the right and to the left (if they are free of back problems). Side bends and lunges are also useful. Circle the arms in both directions and push and pull an imaginary bar in all directions. Finish with the person swinging their arms up as high as possible and back and low as possible, touching their fingertips together at each point. Recommend that they do any or all of these at a special workout time or when cleaning house or cooking. Some of these can be even done while driving (keeping their eyes on the road) or while watching TV. Using barbells or exercise bands increases energy output, but they should be instructed to gradually increase the weights used in the position shifts and arm swings and other movements.

Kubota et al. (2006) found that therapeutic or mechanical horseback riding was useful for older patients and induced glucose uptake for individuals with T2DM. It may also be useful in T1DM. Tai chi, even after only 12 weeks, improved balance, strength, and flexibility in individuals who also had cardiovascular disease, whether the person had T1DM or T2DM (Taylor-Piliae, Haskell, Stotts, & Froelicher, 2006). For individuals 60 years of age or older, walking 45 min, 3 days a week, improved blood pressure and lipid metabolism and lowered BMI in those that had T2DM (Fritz, Wandell, Aberg, & Engfeldt, 2006).

Children and Exercise

A special note must be made about children who have T2DM or are obese and may have prediabetes. Exercise is a mandate for these kids. Wolfsdorf (2005) emphasized the fact that all children with diabetes reap many benefits from exercise. Among these benefits are weight loss, improved circulation, and an increased sense of well-being. Games that require physical activity allow any type of exercise to be fun. Just plain movement from Hip-Hop to Capture the Flag involves a range of movement appropriate to burning calories and having fun at the same time.

The goal is to have children spend 30 min or more per day in active play. Whether it is right after school, which is the best time to increase creativity for the homework to be done later, or after supper, active participation in play is needed and should be part of the treatment regimen.

Schools should be supported in keeping recess times—so long as they are not just stand-around times, but involve some type of activity. Even more important, schools should seek and obtain funding to reinstitute mandatory physical education.

Physical activity is one of the best preventions for youth-onset T2DM (McGavock, Sellers, & Dean, 2007). Such activity should also be a part of daily care for youth who are already diagnosed as having T2DM.

Exercise and Pregnancy

Mottola (2007) reports that, to date, there are no specific guidelines for those with gestational diabetes or those who have T1DM and are pregnant. Mild to moderate exercise has not been reported as detrimental to the woman who is pregnant. Guidance and caution must be exercised in any high-risk population. Guidance and observation from a health professional are especially needed.

Summary

The Look AHEAD clinical trials demonstrated not only the characteristics of overweight patients with T2DM (Ribisl et al., 2007), but also the risk factors in relation to fitness versus fatness and the response of the cardiovascular system (Wing et al., 2007). Sinclair, Conroy, and Bayer (2008) also found how older people responded in general health and fitness.

There are numerous books that are easily available in most bookstores that can help guide an individual or school program toward more active exercise or play. Sometimes, the intensity of the exercise needs to be questioned. For more information on prescribing exercise intensity, read the article by Sykes (2004) on promoting health through physical activity. Gleeson-Kreig (2006) reported on exercise and its relation to self-efficacy and behavior in any person with T2DM. It is recommended that a person plan a daily activity program as part of enhancing self-efficacy levels (see Tables 19.1, 19.2, and 19.3 for further resources).

19.1	Suggestions for Getting Your Patients Moving

As they are physically able:

1. Gently—touch the toes—from a standing or sitting position.
2. Sit, bend the knees, and hold the knees to the chest.
3. Sit, rotate the upper body to the left and then to the right.
4. Stand away from a table and bend over, touching the table with both hands.
5. Lie down, put a book on the abdomen and breathe so that the book goes up when breathing in and down when breathing out.
6. Tell them about or obtain, "Growing Stronger: Strength Training for Older Adults" (free) through www.cdc.gov

Finally, be sure there is a good match of medication with exercise or play. Omari, Yue, and Twigg (2005) reported a case of hypoglycemia induced by exercise in a patient taking metformin, one medication often prescribed for children with prediabetes, dysmetabolic syndrome, or T2DM, even though this medication is not considered a hypoglycemic agent.

Exercise is powerful. It helps young and old to feel better if they do not overdo the exercise chosen or exercise too much or too often. Again, exercise increases circulation. It decreases depression (those endorphins really work). It helps in being creative and more organized. And, when used appropriately, it acts to lower and control blood glucose levels and has played a role in both the prevention and management of T2DM (Zoeller, 2007).

19.2 Online Resources

Americans in Motion (AIM)—Includes a fitness prescription and a personal assessment form for the patient (www.americansinmotion.org)

American Family Physician (2003)—Counseling for physical activity in patients who are overweight and obese (www.aafp.org/afp/20030315/1249.html)

American Family Physician Monograph (2003)—Advice to help patients who are overweight (www.aafp.org/x24060.xml)

Information on Combating Childhood Obesity (www.ahrq.gov/child/dvdobesity.htm)

Growth and BMI Charts—Centers for Disease Control and Prevention (CDC) (www.cdc.gov/bmi and www.cdc.gov/growthcharts)

Children and family-friendly interactive website that promotes healthy eating and active living (www.kidnetic.com)

Motivational interviewing—Information to assist the health professional in getting patients to motivate themselves (www.motivationalinterviewing.org)

19.3 Levels of Exercise Intensity

Light: Walking, sitting, and activities of daily living

Moderate: Brisk walking, bicycling, swimming, dancing, sports (30 min, 5 times a week)

Vigorous: Very brisk walking, jogging, hiking, shoveling, tennis (20 min, 3 times a week)

Strength and endurance: Leg lifts, knee and arm extensions, overhead presses

References

Albright, A., Franz, M., Hornsby, G., Kriska, A., Marrero, D., Ullrich, I., et al. (2000). American College of Sports Medicine position stand: Exercise and type 2 diabetes. *Medical Science and Sports, 32*(7), 1345–1360.

Americans In Motion. (2005). Retrieved June 29, 2008, from www.americansinmotion.org

Berry, D., Urban, A., & Grey, M. (2006). Understanding the development and prevention of type 2 diabetes in youth. *Journal of Pediatric Health Care, 20*(1), 3–10.

Christian, J. G., Bessesen, D. H., Byers, T. E., Christian, K. K., Boldstein, M. G., & Bock, B. C. (2008). Clinic-based support to help overweight patients with type 2 diabetes increase physical activity and lose weight. *Archives of Internal Medicine, 168*(2), 129–130.

Daly, A. (2005). Healthy lifestyle changes: Food and physical activity. In B. P. Childs, M. Cypress, & G. Spollett (Eds.), *Complete nurse's guide to diabetes care* (pp. 20–32). Alexandria, VA: American Diabetes Association.

Diabetes Prevention Program Research Group. (2002). Reduction in the incidence of type 2 diabetes with lifestyle intervention or metformin. *New England Journal of Medicine, 346,* 393–401.

Fodor, J. G., & Adamo, K. B. (2001). Prevention of type 2 diabetes mellitus by changes in lifestyle. *New England Journal of Medicine, 345*(9), 696–697.

Fritz, T., Wandell, P., Aberg, H., & Engfeldt, P. (2006). Walking for exercise—Does three times per week influence risk factors in type 2 diabetes. *Diabetes Research and Clinical Practice, 71*(1), 21–27.

Gleeson-Kreig, J. M. (2006). Self-monitoring of physical activity: Effects on self-efficacy and behavior in people with type 2 diabetes. *Diabetes Educator, 32*(1), 69–77.

Harris, G. D., & White, R. D. (2007). Exercise stress testing in patients with type 2 diabetes: When are asymptomatic patients screened? *Clinical Diabetes, 25*(4), 126–134.

Krousel-Wood, M. A., Berger, L., Jiang, X., Blonde, L., Myers, L., & Webber, L. (2008). Does home-based exercise improve body mass index in patients with type 2 diabetes? Results of a feasibility trial. *Diabetes Research in Clinical Practice, 79*(2), 230–236.

Kubota, M., Nagasaki, M., Tokudome, M., Shinomiya, Y., Ozawa, T., & Sato, Y. (2006). Mechanical horseback riding improves insulin sensitivity in elder diabetic patients. *Diabetes Research and Clinical Practice, 71*(2), 124–130.

Mathieu, M. E., Brochu, M., & Beliveau, L. (2008). DiabetAction: Changes in physical activity practice, fitness, and metabolic syndrome in type 2 diabetic and at-risk individuals. *Clinical Journal of Sports Medicine, 18*(1), 70–75.

May, M., Galper, L., & Carr, J. (2005). *Am I hungry? What to do when diets don't work.* New York: Nourish Publishing.

McGavock, J., Sellers, E., & Dean, H. (2007). Physical activity for the prevention and management of youth-onset type 2 diabetes. *Diabetes Vascular Disease Research, 5*(4), 283–284.

Mottola, M. F. (2007). The role of exercise in the prevention and treatment of gestational diabetes mellitus. *Current Sports Medicine Report, 6*(6), 381–386.

Mullooly, C. A. (2006). Physical activity. In C. Mensing (Ed.), *The art and science of diabetes self-management education: A desk reference for healthcare professionals* (pp. 297–330). Chicago: American Association of Diabetes Educators.

Nieman, D. (1995). Physical activity and aging. In *Fitness and sports medicine: A health related approach* (pp. 425–449). Palo Alto, CA: Bull.

Omari, A., Yue, D. K., & Twigg, S. M. (2005). Exercise, metformin and hypoglycemia: A neglected entity. *British Journal of Diabetes & Vascular Disease, 5*(2), 106–108.

Ribisl, P. M., Lang, W., Jaramillo, S. A., Jakicic, J. M., Steward, K. J., Bahnson, J., et al., Look AHEAD Research Group. (2007). Exercise capacity and cardiovascular/metabolic characteristics of overweight and obese individuals with type 2 diabetes: The Look AHEAD clinical trial. *Diabetes Care, 20*(10), 2679–2684.

Sinclair, A. J., Conroy, S. P., & Bayer, A. J. (2008). Impact of diabetes on physical function in older people. *Diabetes Care, 31*(2), 233–235.

Sykes, K. (2004). Promoting health through physical activity—update 2003: Prescribing exercise intensity. *Journal of the Association of Chartered Physiotherapists, Spring*(94), 35–38.

Taylor-Piliae, R. E., Haskell, W. L., Stotts, N. A., & Froelicher, E. S. (2006). Improvement in balance, strength, and flexibility after 12 weeks of tai chi exercise in ethnic Chinese adults with cardiovascular disease risk factors. *Alternative Therapies in Health and Medicine, 12*(2), 50–58.

Wing, R. R., Jakicic, J., Neiberg, R., Lang, W., Blair, S. N., Cooper, L., et al., Look AHEAD Research Group. (2007). Fitness, fatness and cardiovascular risk factors in type 2 diabetes: Look AHEAD study. *Medical Science in Sports Exercise, 39*(12), 2107–2116.

Wolfsdorf, J. I. (2005). Children with diabetes benefit from exercise. *Archives of Disease in Childhood, 90*(12), 1215–1217.

Zoeller, R. F., Jr. (2007). The role of physical activity and fitness in the prevention and management of type 2 diabetes mellitus. *American Journal of Lifestyle Medicine, 1*(5), 344–350.

20

Monitoring for Type 2 Diabetes

Monitoring for Type 2 diabetes mellitus (T2DM) is a little more difficult than for Type 1 diabetes mellitus (T1DM), not because of the procedure, but because of the availability of strips through third-party payers. Although it is known that control of blood glucose levels, whether with T1DM or T2DM, is important to prevent or delay complications associated with having diabetes (Albisser, Alejandro, Meneghini, & Ricordi, 2005), there is still controversy as to the frequency, timing, and number of tests to be completed. The result is that the number of blood glucose strips approved for those with T2DM is often less than what should be used to maintain blood glucose control, especially during illness, extended emotional stress, or with changes in medication. In T1DM, daily self-monitoring of blood glucose (SMBG) is needed to alter insulin doses on a daily basis to meet the daily changing needs of self-management. In T2DM, patients usually do not change their oral hypoglycemic agent or dose except on a physician's order, so many people assume that daily monitoring is not needed.

Some support was given by Medicare with the occurrence of the Balanced Budget Act of 1997. Patients with Medicare who were taking oral agents were and are still able to receive coverage for 100 test strips and supplies for a 3-month period. This can be translated to testing 4 times per day; fasting and postprandial, less than 1 day per week. Some clinicians recommend testing 2 times per day at alternate times. Our program recommends 4 times a day, one day a week, for those who are diet controlled; 4 times a day, three days a week, for those on oral agents; 4 times a day daily for those on insulin; or 4–6 times a day daily for those on a pump. These needs must be specified on the prescription and the pharmacist can ask for verification. Medicare and Medicaid may require submission of glucose monitoring logs.

Why Four Times a Day?

Foods and oral hypoglycemic agents have various time actions. Knowing a person's response to food or medicine leads, ideally, to closer and safer blood glucose control. When patients arrive in the clinic without their blood sugar log book, it presents a problem for the health care team. When they arrive with blood glucose levels monitored only once a day (usually fasting), that presents another problem. We can see problems, if any, in the overnight control, but still know nothing about any postprandial problems. Overnight control may be acceptable with the medication used but after eating blood sugars may be elevated. We need data from the whole day to adjust medications. HbA1c levels are helpful but tell us only whether there is a problem, not where the problem is. The Kumamoto Study (Wake et al., 2000) and the U.K. Prospective Diabetes Study Group (Gray et al., 2000) have both found that there is cost effectiveness in intensive control for those people that have T2DM.

In general, when patients learn that the one-time-a-day testing only lets them know their physiologic response at that time, they often try to do more tests, especially the week or so before a clinic visit. It is recognized that if finances are a problem, less frequent testing might have to be accepted, except when the person is ill or experiencing high stress levels. If blood sugars are stable, even once a week, four times a day gives more information than taking a test once a day. It is assumed that if that one time a day is at different times of the day, that would probably, compressed (i.e., average blood sugars at different times of the day), give the information needed to safely increase or add medication for that person's particular diabetes regimen.

When patients come to the clinic without a log book, there are two choices: (1) to reschedule when they can bring the log book to the clinic, or (2) to test their memory. Our clinic often takes the second choice. What we ask is: When is the first time of the day that you test? What is the lowest and the highest blood glucose level you remember? When is the next time of day you test? What is the lowest and highest blood sugar you remember at that time? And so forth. Whatever the process, it contributes to overall management of diabetes care (Rizvi & Sanders, 2006).

Truthfulness?

Truthfulness by the patient to the health care professional is often a problem, especially with medicine taking and blood glucose monitoring. Patients wish to look good in the eyes of their health care professionals. Each person should be given some latitude with questions that do not point to incrimination or accusation, such as "What percentage of the time do you take your medicine (or test your blood sugar)?" instead of "Why didn't you take all your medications?" or "You didn't take all your medications, did you?" This type of questioning allows for a variety of answers and does not push anyone into the corner to lie. It is their body, and their body (the blood sugars) will let us know when one or more diabetes medications are needed. Making the patients' responses the basis for the medical decisions helps them to recognize that they are being included in the decision-making process. In this and other ways, it is worth monitoring diabetes blood glucose levels (Hicks, 2005). Patients will then be more truthful.

General Procedures

Testing for blood glucose levels in an individual with T2DM is not as stringent as for T1DM, but it is still very important. The following are considerations for monitoring T2DM:

1. Testing should be accomplished on a schedule that includes at least three or more tests at each time of the day during a week. Ideally, this should be fasting and 2-hr postprandial (Goal: less than 110 premeal and less than 140 mg/dl or 6.1–7.7 mmol/L 2 hr after a meal).
2. If a person is being controlled by diet alone, a four times a day, once a week, would be adequate unless the individual is ill.
3. Illness should usually require a need for blood sugar testing four times a day.
4. If the person is on oral hypoglycemic agents, request testing four times a day, three days a week. Fasting and postprandial is preferable but premeal and bedtime can be used (second choice).
5. Since T2DM is more often found in older individuals, ask the person if it is easier to remember to test before breakfast and two hours after a meal or testing before meals and at bedtime. Unless there is something to remind the person (like an alarm wristwatch) when it is time to test, the testing process is too often overlooked.
6. If the person chooses the premeal/bedtime test routine, request two or three days before the next clinic visit to focus on remembering to test some postprandial blood glucose levels.
7. If or when insulin is added or the oral agents are replaced by insulin, ask for added cooperation (more frequent testing) until stability of blood glucose levels is attained and blood sugars are normal most of the time. Then it may be possible, except during illness, to test just three times a week—but, again, documenting four times even on different days of the week.
8. If the Somogyi effect or rebound effect is suspected, which is still possible when taking a secretagogue, monitoring could be done at 1, 2, and 3 or more hours after a meal to determine whether the blood sugars go up rather than down when responding to the diabetes medication.
9. Elevated fasting blood sugars may indicate the need for the addition of another diabetes medication or the need to rule out the Dawn phenomenon

(if suspected, the 4 a.m. blood glucose level will usually be found to be lower than the fasting blood glucose level).

10. It is as important for people of all ages who have T2DM to have normal blood glucose levels the majority of the time.

What to Look for in a Meter

Because many of those who receive a diagnosis of T2DM will be older individuals, it is important that eyesight and the sense of feeling are considered when choosing a machine. Therefore, the machine itself should have a large-print readout. For others, a talking meter might be needed. A backlight is also desirable for easier readability, especially at night. Capillary action, found with the strips for most meters, increases ease of use in obtaining a sample of blood. The buttons on the monitor should be easily felt, and having a timing device to remind the person when the next test should be done would be ideal. The 800 number (or other toll-free number) to the manufacturer (located on the back of the meter) should be easy to read so that questions and concerns plus technical support are readily available.

Have the patients find the expiration date on the container of strips and help them to understand that when the strips are out of date they may not be as accurate. Have the patient find the expiration date on the control solution(s), if they come with that particular machine. Again, if the control solution has expired, emphasize the need to buy updated solution(s).

There is concern regarding use of the testing procedure even after many years of testing. At least once a year, the patient should perform the blood test in front of the health professional or at least be questioned about the procedure expected. For best results, the manufacturers recommend following the procedure for that meter to the letter.

Have patients bring their machine into the office at the time of the office visit. Test it with the "same drop of blood" to see whether the office machine and their machine are no farther apart than 10%. If they have a backup machine at home, recommend that they compare the two machines to determine whether both of the machines are working correctly. Some machines, albeit fewer and fewer, tend to read higher or lower when the machine is wearing out.

One thing that seems to be overlooked, in particular, is what to do once a battery is changed. Some machines have a backup electrical supply so there is no need to recalibrate or reset the date and time. Other machines at least need the date and time reset. It is possible to still get timely blood glucose tests without resetting the machine, but if the machine is to be off-loaded to a computer at the office, there is a chance it will not print out or it will print out with all the numbers averaged together rather than being averaged at specific times of the day.

The use of a meter memory versus use of a log book is an important issue. Or the use of both? Does the meter have a memory? Most meters today do have a memory, but how much memory? Depending on the type of memory, does it average for each period of time (a day) or does it include this information, but also give the averages per time of day; the response to food eaten, the exercise or activity completed (Gleeson-Kreig, 2006)? Does it give error messages if there is an error with not enough blood on the sample or the battery is running low? Some meters tell if the trend of blood glucose levels is going up or down. Some meters may even be set to alarm if the blood glucose reading level is above or below a set number.

Some or all of the above may be on a meter. What advantage does a meter with lots of bells and whistles have over writing down a specific blood sugar at a specific time? It depends on the individual. Some people do not like to write down their values, so they need a meter with lots of memory. Other people like to write down their blood glucose values so they can see them and pick out patterns and make corrections. Evaluation of each individual's needs is vital to selecting the right meter for them.

Because the numbers represent information about the possible need to change medication, then referring to the numbers needs to be part of the regimen at least one or more times a week, especially if insulin is involved. The clinic visit gives an opportunity to view the printout or the person may contact the company and get the connectors and program to print out their own copy at home. If this is done once or twice a week and the results are used in self-management, it will be to the patient's advantage. If not, this extra equipment could be considered a waste.

When patients write down the results of a test in a log book, they can immediately recognize that the blood glucose levels are not as normal as they were or they are higher or lower at a particular time of day. Then they can call or make changes as instructed at home or bring the results to the health professional to discuss and direct those changes at the time of their clinic visit (Hall, 2005).

If people know how important their testing process is to themselves and to the professional, it is possible that they more likely will complete the testing process and document the results. Size of blood sample (down to 0.3 µl); size of the meter (down to about the size of a container of strips or a large pen); the ability to use the fingertip, outer palm of the hand, or arm (or ear); the length of time of the test (down to 3 seconds), combined with a blood pressure monitor; self-coding; low cost (often the meter is available through an office visit, leaving just the cost of obtaining the strips); large storage (over 400 tests); determination of average test per time of day or time of meal and overall for weekly to monthly intervals; talking capabilities (for those who are sight impaired); warning when blood sugar is too high or too low; plus ease of use of the meter contribute to more people using blood glucose testing and more health professionals being able to attain and maintain greater control of their patients' blood sugars.

New products that are Food and Drug Administration (FDA) approved are able to telemonitor the diabetes results from a meter. The meter can download in seconds through a device that sends the information directly to a health professional's office (Kovatchev, Otto, Cox, Gonder-Frederick, & Clarke, 2006). This test may also be useful for those patients who are unable to afford more than once a day or less testing and can be an adjunct to the measurement of 2–3 months of hemoglobin A1c's overall averaging results in the health professional's office (Dugan et al., 2006).

Being able to interpret these results, whether in a person's log book or by a meter's memory or telemonitoring, becomes a doorway to the prevention of problems. Actions may be taken to alter the diabetes management sooner than later. Participation in self-management leads to a person feeling like a part of the process rather someone who is being "done to."

This reminds me of a particular patient who told us the following story: After completing the education course to which her family physician had referred her, she continued to meticulously test and record her daily tests. She took the paper with her test results to the next clinic visit. When she had her clinic visit, the doctor took the paper of her blood sugar values, glanced at it briefly, and then told her to continue on with what she was doing, even though her fasting blood sugars had become higher since the last clinic visit. As the patient left the office, he was noticed throwing the paper into the wastebasket. She immediately turned around, grabbed her paper from the wastebasket, and said, by her report, "I gave blood for those tests. They mean more than just being thrown into the round file. I guess I need to see another doctor." And so she found a physician who "respected the testing she had done."

Key Principles in Testing

The following should be done when testing at any time:

1. Assemble what is needed for testing: machine, strips, log book, and pencil (if they are used).
2. Wash hands with warm, soapy water—Many people do not do this and have not had any infection occur, but this is a part of general hygiene that should be adhered to, especially in this day and age. Some people have chosen to use alcohol wipes, but it has been found that these individuals often have fingertips that have become dry and scaly. Alcohol is cold and constricts blood vessels, making the obtaining of blood more difficult. Warm water dilates blood vessels, creating an easier and more voluminous blood flow.
3. Insert a strip into the machine—This turns on most machines; the machines indicate when the instrument is ready for the blood to be tested. (Note: For some machines, a code must be changed to match the particular new container of strips before a test is considered accurate.)
4. Pierce the finger—The sides of the finger or the sides of the palm of the hand may be used at all times; if the person is not perceived to be symptomatic of having a low blood sugar, it is permissible to use the arm (or alternate site). When using an alternate site, it is necessary for the person doing the test to view whether an adequate blood sample has been obtained. When using an alternate site, the person is instructed to hold the lancing device in place (even after the lancet has punctured the skin) and to milk it up and down until a sizable drop of blood is observed on the skin.
5. Hold the section of the strip to receive the blood at the edge of the drop (if a hanging drop of blood is to be used, the patient must be sure that enough blood is available—and, therefore, the fingers or ear is usually the only site capable of doing this).
6. Allow the machine to count down and then record the results (or allow the machine to process this—but still encourage the patient to assess these results at a predetermined number of days).
7. Place the sharps in a hard plastic or metal container and instruct the patient to take this container, when full, to the nearest pharmacy for disposal.

Ketone Testing

Although T2DM has also been termed nonketone-prone diabetes, this test should be kept in mind. During illness or during prolonged emotional stress, there is the possibility of decompensating to an insulin-dependent or insulin-requiring state. If this occurs, it is possible that the person may need to test for ketones in the blood or urine when blood glucose levels are elevated above 240 or 250 mg/dl (13.3 or 13.8 mmol) or higher.

One meter is available that tests for blood glucose levels and also converts to testing for ketones in the blood. Otherwise, urine testing for ketones is available with the use of strips. Note that once a bottle is opened, it is possible that the strips will become less accurate beyond a four-month period. These strips are available, usually on special order, individually wrapped in aluminum foil. This certainly extends the stability of the strips over a longer period of time.

Even though those with T2DM are not ketosis prone, they still need to be educated about this possibility. These strips might also come in handy when they are losing weight. Ketones may occur in blood and urine if a person is fasting, is experiencing a gastrointestinal illness, is starving, or does not have enough insulin to process glucose into the cells of the body.

Patients having these strips on hand, if so directed, should be able to identify the expiration date on the package or bottle of strips. They should be aware of the timing required after the strip is dipped and removed from the urine and the excess urine tapped off. Color comparisons may be done with a card or the label on the side of the bottle. As with T1DM, the presence of ketones in the urine (or blood) accompanying high blood sugars is an indication for insulin and, if already on insulin, there might be a need to double the dose of insulin to get the best results.

Summary

Self-monitoring of blood glucose (SMBG) is part of the daily care for the person who has diabetes. It is a guide to determine whether changes need to be made or if decisions were not as appropriate as desired. A person is not good or bad if blood glucose levels are normal or high. Diabetes management is difficult at best. Associating poor control with bad blood sugars often signals to the patients that they are bad. Assuring the patient that these numbers are only information from which to work, and that an assessment of these numbers is a necessary part of the clinic visit, will help them to obtain accurate numbers.

Medicare support has made a difference in the frequency of testing (Li, Zhang, & Narayan, 2008) even though many people with T2DM do not have the number of blood glucose test strips to actually be able to complete the multiple tests that we ask them to. Most of those testing are testing more frequently before meals than after meals. Choe and Edelman (2007) found, as did we, that postprandial testing can give more guidance to the health care professional, especially if a rapid-acting pill (a meglitinide) or a rapid-acting insulin is being used by the patient.

Then there is the importance of taking those blood glucose level test results to the clinic visit. Every so often, a person will attend the clinic and either not have their meter with them or not have their listing of blood glucose readings. One person in our office, who has had diabetes for a number of years, offered this reminder, "Blood glucose level tests taken to the clinic visit are as valuable as taking their dog to the vet. For instance, you wouldn't go to a vet without your animal; so you shouldn't go to a diabetes specialist without your blood glucose meter or log book."

Patients should be assured that if their blood sugars are elevated, that it is the time they should not miss the appointment, rather than what too often happens—the person misses or cancels an appointment because the blood sugars did not show that he or she was a "good person."

The direction and approach to SMBG are important to support the patient in recognizing how this information is used. Care in obtaining and interpreting this information will lead to the safe attainment of the normalization of blood glucose levels.

References

Albisser, A. M., Alejandro, R., Meneghini, L. F., & Ricordi, C. (2005). How good is your glucose control? *Diabetes Technology & Therapeutics, 7*(6), 863–875.

Choe, C., & Edelman, S. V. (2007). The role of self-monitoring of blood glucose during the treatment of type 2 diabetes with medications targeting postprandial hyperglycemia. *Southern Medical Journal, 100*(11), 1123–1131.

Dugan, K. M., Buse, J. B., Largay, J., Kelly, M. M., Button, E. A., Kato, S., et al. (2006). 1,5-Anhydroglucitol and postprandial hyperglycemia as measured by continuous glucose monitoring system in moderately controlled patients with diabetes. *Diabetes Care, 29*(6), 1214–1219.

Gleeson-Kreig, J. M. (2006). Self-monitoring of physical activity: Effects on self-efficacy and behavior in people with type 2 diabetes. *The Diabetes Educator, 32*(1), 69–77.

Gray, A., Raikou, M., McGuire, A., Fenn, P., Stevens, R., Cull, C., et al.; U.K. Prospective Diabetes Study Group. (2000). Cost effectiveness of an intensive blood glucose control policy in patients with type 2 diabetes: Economic analysis alongside randomized controlled trial (UKPDS 41). *British Medical Journal, 320*(7246), 1373–1378.

Hall, G. (2005). Choosing and teaching the use of blood glucose monitors. *Practice Nurse, 30*(7), 46, 49–51.

Hicks, D. (2005). Is it worth monitoring blood glucose levels in type 2 diabetes? *Journal of Diabetes Nursing, 9*(10), 369–372.

Kovatchev, B. P., Otto, E., Cox, E., Gonder-Frederick, L., & Clarke, W. (2006). Evaluation of a new measure of blood glucose variability in diabetes. *Diabetes Care, 29*(11), 2433–2438.

Li, R., Zhang, P., & Narayan, K. M. (2008). Self-monitoring of blood glucose before and after Medicare expansion among Medicare beneficiaries with diabetes who do not use insulin. *American Journal of Public Health, 98*(2), 358–364.

Rizvi, A. A., & Sanders, M. B. (2006). Assessment and monitoring of glycemic control in primary diabetes care: Monitoring techniques, record keeping, meter downloads, tests of average glycemia, and point-of-care evaluation. *Journal of the American Academy of Nurse Practitioners, 18*(1), 11–21.

Wake, N., Hisashige, A., Katayama, T., Kishikawa, H., Ohkubo, Y., Sakae, M., et al.; The Kumamoto Study. (2000). Cost-effectiveness of intensive insulin therapy for type 2 diabetes: A 10 year follow-up of the Kumamoto study. *Diabetes Research in Clinical Practice, 48*(3), 201–210.

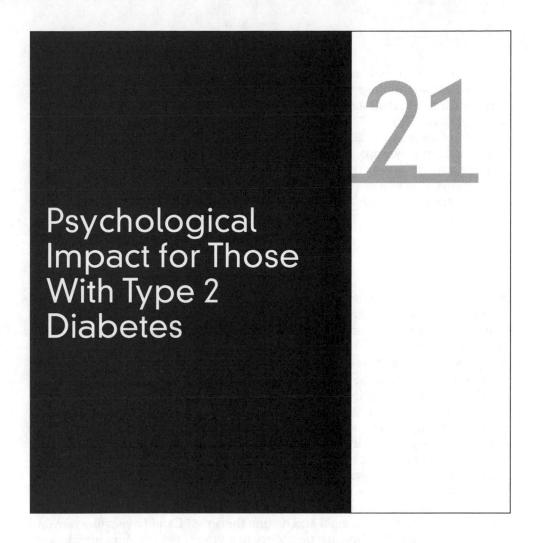

21

Psychological Impact for Those With Type 2 Diabetes

The very nature of diabetes whether Type 1 or Type 2, the regimen, and the potential complications increase the psychosocial demands on the individual and the family. These demands include permanent changes in lifestyle, threats to self-esteem, threats to social and vocational roles, disruption to normal life transitions, uncertain and unpredictable futures, increased expenses, and potentially decreasing resources. Whether the individual can cope with these demands or not often depends on the ability of the health care team to assess individual difficulties and to intervene before crisis and needless morbidity develop.

This chapter looks at one's adjustment to having and living with diabetes, psychopathology and diabetes, the social implication of the disease, and possible interventions.

Adjustment to Living With Type 2 Diabetes

The adjustment to living with Type 2 diabetes mellitus (T2DM), once called adult-type diabetes, calls for adjustment in multiple areas: diagnosis, following the regimen, emphasis on tight control, dependency on others, and the possible adjustment to the complications of diabetes. A correlation has also been found with a "negative mood" and postmeal, rapid rise in blood glucose levels with insulin-requiring T2DM (Cox et al., 2007). This finding is similar to the findings of Yaffe et al. (2004) of cognitive impairment in older women associated with hyperglycemia. For this and other reasons, the family will also need to make adjustments as they too live with diabetes and their quality of life and perceptions of health are affected, just as the quality of life and perceptions of health of the person with a diagnosis of diabetes are affected (Magwood, Zapka, & Jenkins, 2008).

Diagnosis

Persons with newly diagnosed diabetes may not immediately feel the impact or the implications of the disease. They may be in shock and are trying to make sense of the diagnosis, especially those who were fairly asymptomatic. "I felt tired all the time." "I went to the doctor because I thought I had a urinary tract infection." "I just had these terrible leg pains." These are the types of statements often heard, revealing the disbelief in the diagnosis.

Feelings commonly induced by a diagnosis of diabetes include fear, anger, anxiety, and depression. Initially, persons with newly diagnosed diabetes may not know what having diabetes will mean in their lives. Anxiety levels may be high as they try to take in all that is happening. As they receive education on the regimen, anxiety may increase as they realize the demands and imposed restrictions of the regimen. Anxiety may also be heightened when one begins contemplating the future with diabetes. Patients have many questions, some of which may even be too scary to ask: How long will I live? Will I go blind? What if I pass out from hypoglycemia and no one finds me? Can I have children? Can I really do all this? Health care providers need to provide reasonable answers to these questions and not assume that if the question is not asked that it does not exist.

There are two concepts about diabetes that are very difficult to grasp at diagnosis. One is permanence. It is difficult to think about living one's entire life with additional demands that may determine the very quality of life. The second is unpredictability. It is frustrating to know that even on days that all demands are met or exceeded, euglycemia is not guaranteed. A person with newly diagnosed diabetes seeks reassurance by understanding diabetes in a very concrete cause-and-effect relationship. "Now if I just do all these things, my blood sugars will be okay." This expectation fails to take into account the many variables that affect blood glucose.

Regimen and Metabolic Control

Impact on Quality of Life

Diabetes is a disease in which a major part of the treatment is performed by the patient. The results of the Diabetes Control and Complications Trial (1993), which only included people with Type 1 diabetes mellitus (T1DM) and which was brought to a close in 1993, gives resounding evidence to the value of tight control of blood sugars. But what are the challenges? The diabetes regimen is demanding, challenging, and often contrary to one's previously chosen lifestyle.

Persons with T2DM (as well as those with T1DM) must, in a way, learn to be their own diagnosticians, laboratory technicians, and nurses. They must also know when and where to call for help. All of these requirements have the potential to alter lifestyle.

The changes in one's lifestyle may create resistance and initiate other feelings. When one is told not only what can be eaten, how much can be eaten, and when it is to be eaten, then resistance makes sense. Everyone wants to feel that they have some control over their life. One must now sometimes forego food when one has the munchies and is told at other times to eat, even though the person is not hungry. This is done under the goal of weight maintenance, maybe weight loss, and glucose control. With a demanding regimen, life loses some of its spontaneity. The need for planning, scheduling, and consistency challenges the freedom of flexibility that one used to take for granted. The unforeseen change in schedules, the request to stay late at work, or the delayed meal has new and sometimes severe consequences.

Overwhelmed by anxiety or depression, the individual may deny the illness and neglect or refuse to take responsibility for self-care. The person with diabetes might also deny the seriousness of the disease and be haphazard about the timing of medication, meals, snacks, or the quantity of food. Those persons may do glucose monitoring rarely or just prior to doctor visits or may not keep doctor's appointments.

For the person with diabetes, the task of change and adaptation may produce resentment, hostility, and anger. Just the idea of cutting back on meat or pizza or other favorite, high-caloric foods, may evoke a wide gamut of feelings, not to mention the possibility of backsliding. Because decreasing caloric content is often a key element in good control, enough flexibility must be provided in the management program for individual tastes, preferences, and ethnicity. Teaching patients how to allow for some of their favorite foods will add to a sense of freedom and increase adherence.

The attitudes and beliefs that influence people to choose preventive health behaviors and comply with medical regimens fit with the following factors and contribute to the person's success in following the prescribed regimen:

1. The health and willingness of the patient to accept medical recommendations.
2. The patient's subjective estimate of susceptibility, vulnerability, and extent of negative consequences.
3. The degree to which the regimen interferes with the patient's lifestyle.

If a patient's perspective is the inability to complete a task (self-efficacy), more than likely the task will not be done and poor control is the possible outcome. As an example: Apply the concepts of health beliefs and self-efficacy (which is expected to occur at some point) to the person with T2DM who needs to start insulin. Resistance to starting insulin is common (Peyrot et al., 2005). Patients often see it as a crisis. Many believe that insulin will make their diabetes worse or complications will develop or become worse. Patients often experience a sense of failure when told that they need to be on insulin. In this multinational study, patients from the United States thought insulin was less efficacious than patients from other countries did. Patients from the United States also reported more self-blame for requiring insulin. They also showed poorer exercise adherence and greater amounts of diabetes distress. The interesting correlate was that the greater the distress, the greater the patient's sense that insulin might be helpful in their management. The sense of feeling more desperate about the management might open one up to more desperate means.

Similarly, a large group (>700) of persons with diabetes, not taking insulin, were surveyed regarding their willingness to begin insulin therapy if it were prescribed (Polonsky, Fisher, Guzman, Villa-Caballero, & Edelman, 2005). The survey indicated that persons who were unwilling (28.2%) had several reasons for not wanting to start insulin therapy, but the most common was a sense of personal failure at their previous regimen.

Issues of Dependency and Support

Although persons with diabetes are encouraged to be self-reliant in managing their illness, diabetes creates a need for increased support. Because the demands of the regimen are extensive, things seem to go better if support is available and accepted. It is obvious that when there is a supportive family member or friend, there is a better psychosocial adjustment to the illness. Support also takes other forms such as informational, financial, and medical. Support may be to act as a sounding board, be a cheerleader, actually help with the mechanics of diabetes, or contribute to structuring the environment to be more conducive to diabetes management.

Sometimes, the person with T2DM may decompensate to severe hyperglycemia or even diabetic ketoacidosis. In these situations, the person with diabetes depends on others for help. Family members and coworkers need to know how to respond to such an emergency.

Family members may accentuate and encourage dependency by being overly solicitous, excessively concerned, and overly protective. This type of behavior has many disadvantages. It may have the tragic effect of increasing the person's sense of being handicapped, abnormal, and particularly vulnerable to premature death. The individual often interprets such behavior as "I must really be sick." On the other hand, if family members or friends develop the habit of monitoring the diabetes-related behaviors of the person with diabetes, they can become what William Polonsky (1999) calls in his book *Diabetes Burnout: What to Do When You Can't Take It Anymore*, the *diabetes police*.

As the individual with diabetes works even harder to maintain independence, diabetes self-care may suffer. The person with diabetes and their loved one may become polarized in their relationship around diabetes care with neither being happy about the outcome and potentially damaging the relationship.

Adjustment to Complications

For those persons who develop complications, feelings may again become intense. Feelings of anger, depression, and hostility are common among those with peripheral retinopathy during the first 2 years after diagnosis. These persons also show an increase in negative life experiences and psychiatric distress. This is true regardless of the severity of the complication. In fact, the poorer adjustment may occur with the individual who has a partial loss of vision but fluctuating impairment compared with those who have a more severe disability. The recognition of the challenges faced beyond the diagnosis of the disease is of utmost importance, as noted by Ruggiero, Wagner, and Groot (2006).

Obviously, recent vision loss for persons with diabetes is associated with increased difficulties in daily activities, a diminished sense of well-being, and symptoms of depression. Although persons with diabetes who are visually impaired have more stressors with which to cope, they seem to do so with no more psychologic distress than the control subjects without diabetes who have visual impairment. Persons facing laser treatment for the first time often experience high anxiety associated with worry as to what the treatment will be like (Scanlon et al., 2005). This study out of the United Kingdom reports that those who have had multiple laser treatments over time expressed the mixed feelings of dissatisfaction of progressing disease and a decline in their vision, but the satisfaction that there was technology available to prolong their vision.

The following should be of assistance to the health care professional working with persons who have complications:

1. If patients with complications are frustrated, angry, and fearful, guide them to seeking support and information on how to do the best with what they have.
2. If patients experience a lack of control and an awareness of the severity and perpetuity of the complications, aid them in finding new levels of normality, making practical adjustments, reevaluating what is worthwhile in life, and organizing daily schedules to avoid unpredictable demands.
3. If patients have difficulty making sense of the consequences of having diabetes and complications, direct them to create positive meaning, for example, pride in oneself, reappraising life, or being grateful for what one has left; and explain diabetes complications by external factors, that is, by long diabetes duration, or the unknown, rather than by personal factors.

Family Adjustment

Regardless of one's role in the family, diabetes affects each one in a different way. The spouse and other family members may experience similar feelings to those of the patient. Fears, feelings of loss, and anxiety may exist. The loved one as known to them is undergoing some very dramatic changes in health and lifestyle. The greater the changes, the greater the impact may be on the relationship. The partner now feels the effect of the changes and faces the possibility of increased dependency by the loved one with diabetes.

Couples who bring to this situation a solid foundation in their relationship based on trust and communication will have better tools for a healthy adjustment. But for those whose relationship was already experiencing difficult times, possibly in the form of unmet expectations, poor communication, or decreased trust, diabetes may well exacerbate or exaggerate the difficulties. Diabetes may be one more way either partner can try to control the other.

Does the person with diabetes really comprehend the nature and cause of the illness? Often, all the patient really understands is the pain or physical symptoms of the disease. Unfortunately there are times when a person may interpret these as signs of mistreatment, punishment, or simply being bad. It is often difficult to deal with these feelings in a rational and objective manner. Compounding the difficulties is the fact that certain behavior evident in some adults is difficult to distinguish from some symptoms of diabetes. For example, awkwardness or irritability may be confused with low blood glucose levels, or the reverse might be true. The result of such confusion might be the start of educational problems. A spouse may not recognize whether the patient is ill or some other difficulty exists.

To help families cope with these problems and promote healthy personality development in the one who has diabetes, the health care worker must be able to identify some of the signs of dysfunction. The following behaviors are some clues that may indicate difficulties in personal coping or dysfunctional family interaction:

1. Perfectionistic and aggressive attitudes on the part of the spouse. Such attitudes may lead to good control of diabetes, but the outcome may be inappropriate behavior problems.
2. Change in the spouse's attitudes toward the patient. The spouse may become more loving, and indulgent, or may become rejecting, hostile, or blaming.
3. Fearfulness, inactivity, and lack of outside interests on the part of the patient.
4. Dependency of the patient or a constantly worried and overprotective spouse.
5. Overly daring and blatantly antisocial behavior manifest by the patient.

Any or all of the preceding behaviors may result from a family system that is tense, resentful, hostile, guilt ridden, or even overly solicitous. Such a family situation may, in the long run, stifle mastery of the skills and the competence necessary for healthy maturation.

Optimally, the person with diabetes mellitus should not be reduced to a state of helpless dependence. The adults or child with T2DM should be encouraged to take the primary responsibility for their care with age-appropriate expectations and only necessary and realistic restrictions should be enforced. Regular work or school attendance and reasonable physical activity should be promoted. To achieve these goals for adults or children who have T2DM requires a strong therapeutic alliance between the patient, the family, and the health care team. Health care professionals should pay particular attention to those with lower social economic status, prior psychopathology, and longer duration of diabetes. These people are the most vulnerable to negative health outcomes.

Dysfunctional and Maladaptive Adjustment

Although many persons with diabetes cope well, some exhibit more intense problems, some of which may be due to psychopathology. This section examines two areas of dysfunctional or maladaptive behavior in diabetes: depression, eating disorders, and self-destructive behaviors.

Depression

The number of research articles that include information about depression in diabetes has increased. In a review of the literature in 2001, Anderson, Freedland, Clouse, and Lustman reported that diabetes doubles the odds of depression in comparison with the population without diabetes. Depression is also associated with an increased risk of complications from hyperglycemia.

The relationship between diabetes and depression is complex. Persons with a family history of depression are apt to be more prone to depression than those persons with diabetes and no family history of depression. The challenge of coping with the regimen, dietary restrictions, increased financial burden, and risk of complications increases the vulnerability to depression for many. Regardless of the cause, depression has the potential to negatively affect diabetes. Depression is often connected to poor glycemic control and to factors that contribute to poor glucose control such as obesity and physical incapacity. Depression also limits the success of lifestyle interventions, such as smoking cessation, weight loss programs, and diabetes treatment regimens.

Many of the current assessments and screens for depression may obtain skewed scores for the person with diabetes whose blood glucose is in poor control. Noticeable signs and symptoms are fatigue, appetite, sleep disturbances, weight loss, irritability, and loss of sexual interest that may be associated with either depression or hyperglycemia. However, the presence of any depressive signs and/or symptoms, even if the criteria for major depressive disorder or dysthymia are not met, increases the risk for morbidity for a person with diabetes (Black, Markides, & Ray, 2003). In the population that they studied, Black et al. found that the effects of untreated depression in a person with diabetes are greater than the impact of poor glycemic control.

The relationship of depression and self-care is interwoven. The patient with depression may present with the typical symptoms of low energy, worthlessness, hopelessness, and helplessness that manifest in a "why bother" attitude and poor follow-through. The patient may get labeled as noncompliant with the diabetes self-care regimen. The underlying problem of depression may go undiagnosed. When diabetes and depression coexist, the effects are synergistic. This is especially true in populations already at risk such as older people and some ethnic groups such as Hispanics, Native Americans, and African Americans.

Self-Destructive Behavior

Those individuals who present as noncompliant and experience numerous hospital admissions frequently require psychotherapeutic intervention. This is true whether the source of the problem is individual, the psychopathology of a dysfunctional family, or both. These patients may get caught up in game playing and manipulation. They are very good at explaining away their behavior so that it sounds logical to them.

The dependency dilemma (discussed earlier) may contribute to self-destructive behavior. One way of expressing the desire to be cared for is willful abandonment of the medical regimen. If persons can become really sick and go to the hospital, there they find the desired attention and security. Unfortunately, the reality of this behavior is that it is sure to enhance the vulnerability to disability and premature death. Working with persons exhibiting this type of behavior is often difficult. It is not uncommon for professional health care workers to feel that these people are deliberately jeopardizing their health and well-being and thus sabotaging the efforts to keep them out of the hospital and functioning normally. It is extremely important that the health care workers explore these persons' behavior and motives. Often these people can be interrupted in their flight toward excessive dependency by early identification of the behavior and the development of a therapeutic milieu under the guidance of a skilled professional. Such guidance will provide these persons with an opportunity to explore the universality of their feelings and subsequent behavior.

Another destructive type of behavior is motivated by depression rather than excessive dependency. The individual may abandon the medical regimen in an attempt to escape a troubled home or work situation or an intolerable life. At the same time, the person may be ambivalent about taking his or her own life.

Some patients with diabetes exhibit subclinical eating behaviors. Regardless of whether the behavior meets the diagnostic criteria for an eating disorder, the problem remains that severe caloric restriction or purposefully overeating or eating and binging plus the manipulation of medication will compromise glycemic control and medical management.

Although direct or indirect self-destructive behavior often works for obtaining what the person feels a need for, it is not more constructive than alcoholism or drug addiction. These patients have problems and the roots must be found. Therapeutic intervention by a skilled therapist may help the patient cope with these destructive impulses.

Social Implications

The impact of diabetes on one's social life may be tremendous. It can affect both the interpersonal and social life. Diabetes may limit one's career and one's financial opportunities. Those individuals with fewer community and personal resources usually experience the social implications of diabetes more profoundly. They may already face limited possibilities economically, vocationally, and educationally. They are further constrained by diabetes.

In addition, the general public is poorly educated regarding diabetes, and this lack of information often perpetuates misunderstanding about diabetes. Myths, distortions, and fallacies also accentuate the difficulties individuals encounter in training and education, employment, insurance, health care, and social relationships. Despite the less-than-desired formal education, there are a number of strategies to facilitate lifestyle changes, for example, becoming a participant in a diabetes support group. Such interaction gives people ideas to try that have worked for others and might work for them.

Vocational Challenges

Having a means of financial support may be complicated by the presence of diabetes. Those with T2DM that have become insulin-requiring may find certain occupations closed to them. On the positive side, legislation is in effect to allow truck drivers taking insulin to drive under the U.S. Department of Transportation regulations as long as they can document that they are closely monitoring their blood glucose levels and that they are in good control. Legislation is pending to decide on an individual basis if a pilot on insulin will be allowed to fly if accompanied by an individual who is not taking insulin. The military restricts the activities of someone who starts on insulin after entering the service. The military will not recruit or sign anyone already on insulin as the military cannot guarantee the availability of insulin around the world, making that person ineligible for worldwide duty. Many local law enforcement agencies have their own restrictions limiting the hiring of persons on insulin, but depending on the responsibilities of the job, these persons may find themselves qualified and hired.

Unskilled workers with diabetes have a particularly rough time gaining and holding onto employment. Success in finding and keeping a job may depend on company regulations and stipulations rather than on the person's ability and motivation. Many employers have cut the number of full-time positions to cut costs in benefits, which then increases the number of persons who do not have access to group health insurance coverage. And the part-time hours available are often just 4–6 hr, often over a meal time, and often inconsistently scheduled from one day to the next. This makes scheduling meals and snacks more challenging for an employee who has diabetes. It is important for persons with diabetes to know their rights under the American Disabilities Act of 1990.

Some employers are very open to hiring a well-disciplined person who has diabetes. They listen and work with the employee and are sensitive and accommodating to employees with chronic illnesses. At the same time, employers find that no employee needs special consideration. In some companies, the responsibilities or type of work may make it difficult for the persons with diabetes to maintain their treatment regimen. Things for employees to consider are the company's ability to give sufficient time at breaks, to allow breaks as needed, to arrange temporary coverage by a coworker, to encourage workers to set their own break and meal schedules, and to get appropriate coverage during the time of health care appointments.

Persons with diabetes often worry about how others will view their competency. Many persons with diabetes have indicated that they have lost jobs or job opportunities because they have diabetes. In this classic review using a job performance survey, supervisors rated employees with diabetes better than the norm in all categories (Greene & Geroy, 1993). The categories included composite job performance, task behaviors, interpersonal behaviors, down-time behaviors, and hazardous behaviors. This may be an indicator that persons with diabetes do feel a need to overcompensate for what they fear may be seen as a deficit in their performance. This may also indicate a well-disciplined person who takes care of his or her health needs appropriately should make a well-disciplined employee.

Financial Burdens

The individual who has diabetes often faces financial strain, as if occupational and physical complications were not enough, The person with diabetes may have many prescriptions to fill at the local pharmacy, plus the added cost of an adequate and nourishing diet, increased doctor's visits, including ophthalmologists and possibly podiatrists. How will these expenses be met? If the person is fortunate enough to qualify for group medical insurance coverage, it may still not be enough to cover the costs. For those persons without group coverage the options narrow to no medical insurance coverage, prohibitively high insurance premiums, inadequate health care plans, or government-assisted programs.

Assessment

There are a variety of tools available for assessment of depression or lack of quality of life. A number of these tools were discussed in Chapter 13. One tool that is useful in the older populations is the Geriatric Depression Scale: short form (Greenberg, 2007). This 15-item questionnaire can be found at http://www.stanford.edu/~yesavage/GDS.html and should be useful for all adults. If the score is greater than 5, depression is most likely possible, and a score greater than 10 usually indicates a depressive state.

Just hearing negative answers to questions about quality of sleep, patterns of eating, changes in behavior, and difficulty in concentration should make one suspicious of depression. Problems with blood glucose level control usually, but not always, precede depressive symptoms. Depression has a possibility of affecting their ability to make appropriate decisions in self-management care. Anderson et al. (2007) used Patient Health Questionnaire-9 as a screening tool for depression as the first step in developing an individualized management program. This short form was found to identify populations at risk. The results enabled them to tailor their interventions to meet both situational and cultural needs.

One of the self-care behaviors that appears to trigger depression is the fear of having to self-inject. The Diabetes Attitudes, Wishes, and Needs (DAWN) study found that two variables lowered belief in self-efficacy: (1) lack of belief that insulin would help them and (2) self-blame that they were not "doing it right" (Peyrot et al., 2005). Haas (2007) summarizes this resistance by stating four beliefs—the belief, among others, that insulin will lead to weight gain, that the diabetes is worse, that life will be more restricted, and that diabetes will be less easy to manage. Overcoming psychologic insulin resistance is an important part of overcoming depression.

Interventions

Education

One of the most powerful ways to help patients is to share information about diabetes. Health care professionals can make sure that persons with diabetes are well aware of the results of the Diabetes Control and Complications Trial (1993) and the U.K. Prospective Diabetes Study (1998). These patients should also be knowledgeable about self-care. They need to understand the relationship between blood sugars, diet, exercise/activity, medication, and coping. People are helped when they understand the relationship between their attitudes and behaviors and their success with diabetes. The myths about diabetes can be dispelled and the scary questions about the future addressed. Patients are best served by being prepared to make informed decisions.

Empowerment

The term empowerment encapsulates the idea that the persons with diabetes should be the primary decision maker in their diabetes care (Anderson, Funnell, Barr, Dedrick, & Davis, 1991). This approach makes some basic assumptions. The first is that to be healthy, individuals must be able to bring about changes in personal behavior, social situations, and the institutions that influence their lives. The empowerment view requires that the costs and benefits of diabetes self-care be viewed in the broader context of patients' personal and social lives. The approach also assumes that most patients with diabetes are responsible for making important and often complex decisions while carrying out the daily treatment of their diabetes. The final assumption is that because patients are the ones who experience the consequences of both having and treating diabetes, they have the right to be the primary decision makers regarding their own diabetes care.

The patient empowerment approach to diabetes education seeks to maximize the self-care knowledge, skills, self-awareness, and sense of personal autonomy of patients to enable them to take charge of their own diabetes care.

Work With Older Persons Who Have Diabetes

Older persons with diabetes may need to be assessed for physical impairment related to diabetes complications in addition to level of cognitive functioning and the presence of depression (Sinclair, 2006). The complexity of diabetes management needs to be assessed for relevance of each older patient and weighed against quality of life and helping the patient to remain independent.

Stress Management

Stressors have a deleterious effect on blood sugar control and other health factors. This effect can be minimized through more effective coping. Good coping skills can help to minimize the impact of diabetes. These skills can assist in maintaining blood glucose control as other stressors come along. Part of the coping process needs to involve the education of others and the acceptance of their support.

Referral for Mental Health Treatment

Referral to a mental health professional is appropriate for those persons or families that are thrown into a crisis by the diagnosis or anytime that the health care provider is concerned that daily functioning and diabetes management are compromised. This would also be true if indicators of psychopathology are seen.

The DAWN study reported that nurses were more comfortable addressing psychosocial issues than physicians. They were also more likely to make referrals (Peyrot, Rubin, & Siminerio, 2006). Diabetes specialists among both nurses and physicians were more likely to use psychosocial strategies than nonspecialists (Peyrot et al., 2006).

Cognitive behavioral therapy is effective in the treatment of mild depression (Lustman, Griffith, Kissel, & Clouse, 1998). Williams et al. (2004) found that treating depression in older persons with diabetes (more than 60 years of age) resulted in an increase in the number of exercise days. The population they studied started with diabetes control near target with baseline Hgb A1c of 7.28 ± 1.43 ($n = 293$). At 6 and 12 months Hgb A1c values had improved but not significantly despite the improvement in the number of exercise days.

But do antidepressants pose another threat to those that are trying to prevent T2DM? Another finding, which needs further research, is the potential hyperglycemic effect of antidepressants. Rubin et al. (2008) reported that, for those individuals in the intensive control group and the placebo group in the Diabetes Prevention Program study, there was no other confounding variable, other than the taking of an antidepressant, resulting in higher blood glucose levels. The question then arises, should antidepressants be excluded from the management of someone in need who has prediabetes? Obviously, no.

Summary

People with diabetes are challenged by struggles to cope with the disease and its regimentation. Snoek and Skinner (2000), in their *Psychology in Diabetes Care*, reviewed a variety of problems and concerns, especially the fear of the unknown. Patients face the fear of an unknown future because diabetes may affect their physical abilities, their social relationships, and their careers. Many people with diabetes adjust well and lead productive lives. Complications to adjustment to having diabetes or developing a complication will be worse if the individual or the family is dysfunctional.

Diabetes in older adults has been noted to lead to early death. Bogner, Morales, Post, and Bruce (2007) found that instituting a depression-care-management plan were less likely to die over a 5-year interval. This is the outcome from a randomized controlled prospective study (Prevention of Suicide in Primary Care of the Elderly [PROSPECT]) in which they compared the management plan group with the standard depression-treated group. As the DAWN study (see Chapter 13) indicated for youth, this study suggests that assessment and intervention are also needed for the older adult.

Possible interventions that the health professional can provide include emotional support, education, movement toward empowering the patient, and stress management. A useful resource is Anderson and Rubin's book (1996) *Practical Psychology for Diabetes Clinicians*. It takes a team approach and the early assessment and intervention by first-line health care professionals and specialists to result in the best benefits for patients.

References

Anderson, B. J., & Rubin, R. R. (1996*). Practical psychology for diabetes clinicians: How to deal with the key behavioral issues faced by patients & health care teams*. Alexandria, VA: American Diabetes Association.

Anderson, D., Horton, C., O'Toole, M. L., Brownson, C. A., Fazzone, P., & Fisher, E. B. (2007). Integrating depression care with diabetes care in real-world settings: Lessons from the Robert Wood Johnson Foundation Diabetes Initiative. *Diabetes Spectrum, 20*(1), 10–16.

Anderson, R., Freedland, K., Clouse, R., & Lustman, P. (2001). The prevalence of comorbid depression in adults with diabetes: A meta-analysis. *Diabetes Care, 24,* 1069–1078.

Anderson, R. M., Funnell, M. M., Barr, P. A., Dedrick, R. F., & Davis, W. K. (1991). Learning to empower patients: Results of professional education program for diabetes educators. *Diabetes Care, 15,* 584–590.

Black, S. A., Markides, K. S., & Ray, L. A. (2003). Depression predicts increased incidence of adverse health outcomes in older Mexican Americans with type 2 diabetes. *Diabetes Care, 26,* 2822–2828.

Bogner, H. R., Morales, K. H., Post, E. P., & Bruce, M. L. (2007). Diabetes, depression, and death: A randomized controlled trial of a depression treatment program for older adults based in primary care (PROSPECT). *Diabetes Care, 30*(12), 3005–3010.

Cox, D. J., McCall, A., Kovatchev, B., Sarwat, S., Ilag, L. L., & Tan, M. H. (2007). Effects of blood glucose rate of changes on perceived mood and cognitive symptoms in insulin-treated type 2 diabetes. *Diabetes Care, 30*(8), 2001–2002.

Diabetes Control and Complications Trial (DCCT) Research Group. (1993). The effect of intensive treatment of diabetes on the development and profession of long-term complications in insulin dependent diabetes mellitus. *New England Journal of Medicine, 329*(14), 957–985.

Greenberg, S. A. (2007). The Geriatric Depression Scale: Short form. *American Journal of Nursing, 107*(10), 60–70.

Greene, D. S., & Geroy, G. D. (1993). Diabetes and job performance: An empirical investigation. *The Diabetes Educator, 19,* 293–298.

Haas, L. (2007). Psychological insulin resistance: Scope of the problem. *The Diabetes Educator, 33*(Suppl. 4), 228S–231S.

Lustman, P., Griffith, L., Kissel, S., & Clouse, R. (1998). Cognitive behavior therapy for depression in type 2 diabetes mellitus. A randomized, controlled trial. *Annals of Internal Medicine, 129,* 613–621.

Magwood, G. S., Zapka, J., & Jenkins, C. (2008). A systematic review evaluating diabetes interventions: Focus on quality of life and disparities. *The Diabetes Educator, 34*(2), 242–265.

Peyrot, M. F., Rubin, R. R., Lauritzen, T., Skovlund, S. E., Snoek, F. J., Matthews, D., et al. The International DAWN Advisory Panel. (2005). Resistance to insulin therapy among patients and providers: Results of the cross-national diabetes attitudes, wishes, and needs (DAWN) study. *Diabetes Care, 28,* 2673–2679.

Peyrot, M. F., Rubin, R. R., Lauritzen, T., Skovlund, S. E., Snoek, F. J., Matthews, D. R., et al. (2006). Patient and provider perceptions of care for diabetes: Results of the cross-national DAWN study. *Diabetologia, 49*(2), 279–288.

Peyrot, M. F., Rubin, R. R., & Siminerio, L. M. (2006). Physician and nurse use of psychosocial strategies in diabetes care: Results of the cross-national Diabetes Attitudes, Wishes and Needs study. *Diabetes Care, 29*(2), 1256–1262.

Polonsky, W. H. (1999). *Diabetes burnout: What to do when you can't take it anymore*. Alexandria, VA: American Diabetes Association.

Polonsky, W. H., Fisher, L., Guzman, S., Villa-Caballero, L., & Edelman, S. V. (2005). Psychological insulin resistance in patients with type 2 diabetes. *Diabetes Care, 28,* 2543–2545.

Rubin, R. R., Ma, Y., Marrerro, D. G., Peyrot, M., Barrett-Connor, E. L., Kahn, S. E., et al. (Diabetes Prevention Program Research Group). (2008). Elevated depression symptoms, antidepressant medication use, and risk of developing diabetes during the diabetes prevention program. *Diabetes Care, 31*(3), 420–426.

Ruggiero, L., Wagner, J., & Groot, M. (2006). Understanding the individual: Emotional and psychological challenges. In C. Mensing (Ed.), *The art and science of diabetes self-management education: A desk reference for healthcare professionals* (pp. 59–96). Chicago: American Association of Diabetes Educators.

Scanlon, P. H., Martin, M. L., Bailey, C., Johnson, E., Hykin, P., & Keightley, S. (2005). Reported symptoms and quality-of-life impacts in patients having laser treatment for sight-threatening diabetic retinopathy. *Diabetic Medicine, 23,* 60–66.

Sinclair, A. (2006). Special considerations in older adults with diabetes: Meeting the challenge. *Diabetes Spectrum, 19*(4), 229–233.

Snoek, F. J., & Skinner, T. C. (2000). *Psychology in diabetes care*. New York: Wiley.

U.K. Prospective Diabetes Study Group. (1998). UKPDS28: A randomized trial of efficacy of early addition of metformin in sulfonylurea treated type 2 diabetes. *Diabetes Care, 21*(1), 87–92.

Williams, J., Jr., Katon, W., Lin, E., Noel, P., Worchel, J., Cornell, J., for the IMPACT Investigators. (2004). The effectiveness of depression care management on diabetes-related outcomes in older patients. *Annals of Internal Medicine, 140,* 1015–1025.

Yaffe, K., Blackwell, T., Kanaya, A. M., Davidowitz, B. A., Barrett-Connor, E., & Krueger, K. (2004). Diabetes impaired fasting glucose, and development of cognitive impairment in older women. *Neurology, 63,* 658–663.

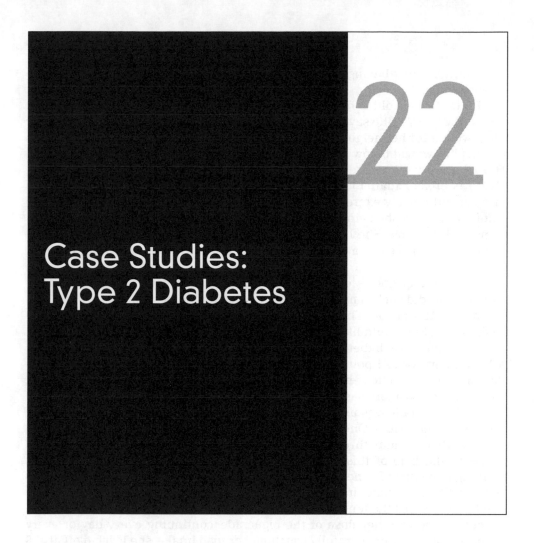

Case Studies: Type 2 Diabetes

22

Type 2 diabetes mellitus (T2DM) can appear and/or manifest in people in various ways, either because of the genetics of the individual, the absorption of medication, the sensitivity to the medication, the absorption of food, the glucagon response, and/or the person's emotional or illness state. One or more causes can result in one or more physiologic outcomes. In most cases, it is a combination of causes that lead to the varied physiologic responses.

The following case studies are examples of various responses to medication in relation to the individual's mental, emotional, or physical status. As with the cases presented for Type 1 diabetes, these cases are combinations of real situations with random initials used as part of the narrative:

Case #1

When LL first received a diagnosis she could not believe that she was ill. She did have some frequent urination and some weight gain but really didn't feel different. It was determined that she had T2DM. Her diabetes was "so mild" that her doctor misnamed it borderline diabetes—a diagnosis still used today despite the education that having diabetes is like being pregnant. It is an all-or-none phenomenon.

LL is 47 years old, 5 ft 4 in., weighs 160 lbs (72.7 kg), and has a body mass index (BMI) of 29. She says she has tried everything but cannot lose weight. Her ideal weight for her height and build is 130 lbs (59.1 kg), but realistically, if she can get her weight below 140 lbs (63.6 kg) she should have a BMI of 25 or less. Her laboratory values are insignificant except that her low-density lipoprotein (LDL) is greater than 130 and her HbA1c is 7.2%. She has a high-stress job and gets little if any exercise. Her food intake history ranges from 900 to 2,500 calories. She says she gains weight on any food intake above 1,200, but she feels hungry all the time. She has tried four different programs and they all helped at first. Then, if she has a crisis at work or at home the cycle of eating starts all over again.

A specific diagnosis of depression was ruled out because her periods of "feeling low" did not last more than 3 or 4 days. Her blood sugar in the office was 220 mg/dl (12.2 mmol). The urine specimen was negative except for 1% glucose in the urine. She would like to lose weight and is willing to try again.

She attended a diabetes education class and the nutritionist recommended a 1,200 calorie or 16½ point meal plan with a range of 1,000 to 1,400 calories per day. She agreed to check her blood glucose levels four times a day, three days a week. Her medication was 500 mg of a biguanide twice a day. Perhaps the best part of her therapy was meeting and making friends when she attended a diabetes education class. One classmate and she planned to walk together in the mall for about 45 min, three to four times a week.

With the help of this new friend as a support person and her focus on wanting to be there for her grandchildren, she was gradually able to lose 15 lbs (6.8 kg). She hit a plateau at 145 lbs (65.9 kg) for about two weeks even though she had increased the length of time she was walking. Then, little by little, with a need to decrease her dose of the biguanide, continuing every day or every other day walking, and carefully watching her food intake, she leveled off at 138 lbs (62.7 kg) and has maintained that lifestyle and weight for more than four years.

Case #2

DD was a 72-year-old male who had had a history of impaired glucose tolerance since his 30s. His blood glucose levels appeared to gradually rise until he was having premeal blood sugars in the high 90s (5 mmol) and low 100s (5.5 mmol/L) and his postmeal blood sugars in the 150s to 190s (8.3–10.5 mmol/L). He received a diagnosis of prediabetes. When the blood glucose levels increased to a fasting of 132 mg/dl (7.3 mmol), he received a diagnosis of T2DM.

His treatment regimen included biguanide dose increases to maximum (1,000 mg twice daily of metformin), plus eventually the addition of a sulfonylurea until he reached the maximum doses of each. His HbA1c gradually increased. Weight gain became a problem. He found that when he ate over 1,800 calories, he gained weight. He exercised almost daily for he found that if he missed more than three days of exercise he would feel depressed and hungrier than he usually did. Although the addition of a thiazolidinedione (TZD) was considered, DD discussed and agreed to try extenatide twice a day.

He reported a lessening of hunger, but the occurrence of mild dyspepsia, with exenatide. This dyspepsia went away over a period of two weeks. Blood glucose levels decreased to the point that he reported some high 50s (2.7 mmol/L) along with more normal blood glucose levels. The exenatide eventually resulted in a lowering and stopping of his biguanide and sulfonylurea. The following months led to the decision to decrease his exenatide to once a day with his blood sugars continuing to normalize the majority of time. After about a year, with more of normal weight versus height, he even needed to stop the one dose a day.

He continued to maintain his weight with his blood glucose levels no higher than the lower 90s (5 mmol) premeal and no higher blood sugars than the lower 120s (6.6 mmol) 2 hr after a meal. Hemoglobin A1c remains in the normal range.

Time will tell whether or when the blood glucose levels will elevate and when or if the restarting of the exenatide at that time will result in his body responding as it has before.

Case #3

MT is a 37-year-old man who was working as a salesman. He first presented in the office with complaints of tiredness and severe headaches. Neurologic and other laboratory tests, except for mildly elevated blood glucose levels, were not supportive of any specific pathologic findings except prediabetes. The physician recommended lifestyle changes and stress management therapy.

At the time of the first appointment, MT was found to be very tense. He described his health situation, his home environment, and his workplace—all high stressor sites. A pending divorce from his second wife had an effect on him and his two children from a previous marriage, making life "miserable" for him. His parents were living at a distance (low socioeconomic and educational level). Her parents were living close by (high socioeconomic and educational level). He was also in a job he disliked.

He recognized, in his primary appraisal, that his stressors were causing him to have potentially harmful health problems. He was not eating right. He had stopped going to the gym. He was not sleeping well. He also had a family history of T2DM on his dad's side (a history of cardiovascular disease on his mother's side). Increasing his exercise at that time, he thought, would help him as it had in the past, but he found that his tiredness and headaches became worse rather than better. In discussion, he recognized that his stressors at home and at work were related to his physical responses: heightened blood pressure and blood sugars, high lipid levels, and weight gain. His mental state exacerbated the outcomes.

Primary Appraisal: Initially, his work environment proved challenging. It eventually became physiologically threatening and then proceeded to be potentially harmful (his blood pressure was getting out of control). His home situation, because of background circumstances, aided in the deterioration of his cardiovascular state (his heart rate increased).

Secondary Appraisal: He had retried a method that had worked before (exercise) but his environmental stressors were too overwhelming to be controlled by this reintervention. Resilience was noted in him, restarting his exercise in a more appropriate manner, but he still was not facing or addressing the social issues at home and at work.

Attending diabetes education classes both gave him a time to regroup and also directed him to coping strategies that were more effective than the ones he had tried before. Exercise was included, but not in the stressful and driven way he had reinstituted it. Dietary practices were addressed and reformed. Self-monitoring of blood glucose (SMBG) gave him direction and a reminder that he could change his lifestyle, decrease his stress levels, and possibly prevent or delay the frank diagnosis of diabetes. Elevated blood pressure and lipid levels were controlled with medication.

All in all, the various interventions resulted in him learning more about himself (he took the Myers Briggs Personality Inventory), learning negotiation skills and conflict resolution skills, learning newer ways to problem solve, and learning how to purposefully relax. He was also referred to a marriage and family counselor.

Outcome: The marriage relationship improved once he was able to persuade his wife to attend counseling sessions with him. His work situation improved. His blood glucose levels improved. His headaches subsequently diminished.

Case #4

AR, a 27-year-old female with obesity, presented with complaints of increased weight, fatigue, and constipation. She lives alone and has a sedentary job as an accountant for a grocery chain.

She reported that she did not participate in physical activity, ate two meals a day, and snacked in the evening and on weekends. She frequently eats at a fast food restaurant at lunchtime. She smokes less than a pack a day since her workplace became a no-smoking building. Alcohol intake is mainly beer ". . . while watching game shows on weekends." She has noticed a darkened area on the back of her neck that she reports she is unable to wash off.

The family history included people with diabetes, obesity, and hypertension. She was not taking any medication and did not take vitamins, minerals, or supplements. At home, her dietary history revealed a frequent intake of high-carbohydrate foods with a total caloric intake per day of about 2,500 calories. History demonstrated that this intake was composed of carbohydrate (60%+), fat (28%+), and protein (12%+).

Her height was 5 ft 7 in.; her weight, 290 lbs (13.2 kg); and her BMI 45. A random blood sugar was 169 mg/dl (9.3 mmol); blood pressure, 140/92; lipids: total cholesterol, 221; high-density lipoprotein (HDL), 39; LDL, 126; triglycerides, 276; and the results of her thyroid panel were normal.

This woman was identified as having the metabolic syndrome. This was evidenced by the acanthosis nigricans (the darkened, velvet-like appearance on the back of her neck, which was also found under her arms) and "apple" obesity along with hypertension and hyperlipidemia. The random blood glucose level indicated a need for further testing that resulted in the diagnosis of T2DM. She had a trace of protein in her urine. Her lifestyle, current health history, and family history put her at high risk for cardiovascular disease.

Once her history of past attempts at weight loss and of the barriers to physical activity were detailed, she was educated as to appropriate dietary needs, given guidance for future food choices, and assessed for the potential for joining a group-based physical activity program. She was advised to get a pedometer and to make a goal for walking, or dancing (she loved to dance), or exercising to at least 5,000 steps a day during the week and to try for more than 8,000 steps on weekends.

Because of her accompanying, elevated glycosylated hemoglobin test (7.9%), she was started on a combination of a TZD and a biguanide. The purpose for this combination was to focus her body on using its insulin in a more effective manner, to block her liver from making excessive glucose, and to support weight loss so that her triglyceride levels, total lipid levels, and blood glucose levels would be normalized. Dosage levels for the diabetes treatment were altered once higher than acceptable blood glucose levels were attained. Hypertension medications were introduced once a history of blood pressure levels was taken over the next few weeks. An angiotensin-converting enzyme inhibitor (ACEI) was started since there was no indication of excessive exercise or menses or infection present that might have contributed to the slightly elevated protein content found in her urine.

At the third month visit, after a trial of dietary and lifestyle changes alone, the lipid levels were reassessed and, with the still elevated LDL, a statin was indicated and started. Weight was slightly less and blood glucose levels were more stable. She reported she was smoking only one or two cigarettes a day and was trying to quit. Her alcohol intake was diminished to one "lite" beer a day, if she drank one at all.

Case #5

This 55-year-old Hispanic man, RR, has had T2DM for about six years. His BMI was greater than 40, his weight was 265 lbs (120.5 kg), and his height 5 ft 8½ in. His blood pressure was measured at 142/88. His abnormal lipid levels were triglycerides over 300 and LDL over 150. His fasting blood glucose measure was 202 mg/dl (11.2 mmol/L). His hemoglobin A1c was 9% and he had 100 mg of protein in the urine.

His accompanying diagnoses were arthritic knees (which also prevent him from walking) and hypertension. He was working and volunteered for a variety of community projects. He was no longer drinking any alcohol (he had been dry for 3 years) and had stopped smoking when he was told it might lead to heart disease.

Medications included one to treat his hypertension (an ACEI), one to treat his hyperlipidemia (a statin at bedtime), and one to treat his "sugar" diabetes (glyburide, 10 mg twice daily). His caloric intake appeared to be more than 3,000 calories with 15% of that protein and 15% of that saturated fat. He reported periods of tiredness and blurred vision, but nothing else that would indicate neuropathic or cardiovascular problems other than some chest tightness. There was a history of heart problems in the family.

He stated that he finally wanted to do something about his physical condition. He has not been taking the statin or the sulfonylurea on a regular basis.

Because he did most of his eating in a restaurant, he said that he is really help-less in controlling his food intake.

Education helped him to handle his restaurant eating and also his activity. He was taught chair exercises and encouraged to attend a YMCA that included water aerobics. He had a microwave in his apartment, so he learned to choose some lower caloric, more nutritional frozen dinners for his meals and to limit his outside eating when he could.

Medication for the diabetes treatment was discussed and, because he understood that when his blood glucose levels needed to be "more normal," it was decided to start him on basal insulin that did not challenge his desire to eat. After a month on basal insulin, a meglitinide was administered premeal, because, although premeal blood sugars were within the desired range, the post-prandial blood sugars were still higher than desired.

(An aside: Using rapid-acting oral agents with basal insulin has come of age. If a person wants a more rapid way of getting blood sugars under control and does not need insulin to control postprandial blood glucose levels, this approach is quite useful. The basal insulin was based on 50% of the total insulin calculated. For instance, if a person is taking a total of two or three oral agents and their diabetes is moderately controlled, a choice, rather than going completely to insulin, which would solve the immediate problem, is to use a long-acting insulin, based on 50% of ⅓ to ½ Unit/kg of body weight and starting with 0.5 or 1 mg of Pramlin or 60 mg Starlix (meglitinides) before each meal. These oral agents would be raised to 4 mg premeal (or the Starlix to 120 mg) before each meal depending on the 2 hr postmeal blood glucose response. Again, the basal insulin would be raised or lowered based on the fasting blood sugar. Careful dietary monitoring and regulation prevented weight gain.

Reassessment three months later revealed he still needed the statin but the triglycerides were now within normal range. He also was found to have had a significant weight loss and his blood pressure was controlled.

Case #6

TR was first seen in the clinic with the initial diagnosis of uncontrolled T2DM. His secondary diagnoses were diabetic neuropathy and retinopathy.

TR was a 65-year-old White female with a history of over 16 years' duration of T2DM. During this time, she had been treated with a variety of oral agents. Her overall blood glucose control had been poor as indicated by a hemoglobin A1c of 9.8%. It was determined that she needed to start on insulin.

Initial laboratory data revealed a serum creatinine of 1.1 with normal cho-lesterol and triglyceride levels. Creatinine clearance was 132 ml/min indicating that her kidneys were working overtime to normalize her output. A random urine protein level was 30 mg, but it was found that she had a mild bladder in-fection. A complete blood count and thyroid profile were indicated with the his-tory of tiredness and periods of feeling hot and cold. The serum iron was found to be 17 (markedly low) and the hemoglobin 10.2, with a mean cell volume of 71, consistent with the diagnosis of iron deficiency anemia. A thyroid profile was completed, but the results were normal.

The chronic anemia secondary to nutritional deficits was treated with di-etary guidance and ferrous sulfate 200 mg (65 mg of elemental iron) three times a day. The insulin dosing was based on kilograms of body weight with consideration that the anemia might have altered the results of her hemoglobin A1c, even though the standardized testing process made this less of a possibility (abnormal iron content in the blood has been documented to lead to higher hemoglobin A1c, whereas hemolytic and other anemias have led to falsely low hemoglobin A1c).

The total insulin was based on ½ Unit of insulin per kilogram (she weighed 152 lbs; approximately 69 kg). The dose was divided in half for the basal: 35 Units of basal insulin and the premeal doses were based on the percentages of 20% before breakfast (to aid in covering the Dawn phenomenon), 13% before lunch (her smallest meal of the day), and 17% before supper (her largest meal of the day).

Subsequent blood sugars were elevated before breakfast, but appropriate 2 hr after meals. This prompted an increase of 2 Units of her basal insulin at bedtime.

The outcome? A normal fasting blood sugar, but the premeal insulin needed to be decreased by a unit each so that the postprandial blood sugars would not be lower than 80 mg/dl (4.4 mmol).

Case #7

TT was taking the maximum dose of both a TZD daily and a biguanide three times a day. She was still having postprandial blood sugars that were a little higher than desired. She was given a choice of including a meglitinide before each meal and bedtime or going on insulin. She still wanted to try the oral agent program. In her decision making, she was educated that once the three agents were not able to control her blood glucose levels, "Thank goodness there was insulin" and "Your body will tell you when it is time to start insulin."

Watchful guidance was used to aid her in not gaining weight during the period her body became accustomed to more normal blood glucose levels. Along with routine four-times-a-day, three-days-a-week self-monitoring, blood sugars were to be taken when she felt hungry or had other possible hypoglycemic symptoms. This gave her guidance as to whether to deep breathe and relax (adrenergic symptoms were experienced from a drop in blood sugars), or to treat the possible hypoglycemia if the blood glucose levels were below normal.

Gradually, blood glucose levels were less controlled on maximum doses of the three agents. At the time of her next visit she stated, before being told, she knew that it was time to begin treatment with insulin. Careful monitoring of blood sugars and her weight and concurrent dietary adjustment (she found she did not need to eat as much food with her more acceptable blood glucose levels) prevented her from gaining weight after going on insulin.

Case #8

BB is a 14-year-old, obese, African American male, taking a biguanide twice a day. He goes to school and is a good student, by his mother's description. His major complaint is that his fingers are sore and "he needs his fingers to work on the computer." He also hesitates to complete much of the requested blood glucose testing.

He was educated as to alternative site testing and became more faithful in completing the requested testing program. When he found out that his alternative test site machine also had available a computer program, he became quite excited about the possibilities of completing his test results and putting them on a computer.

BB understands that if he has symptoms of low blood sugar, he was to document his blood glucose level by fingertip rather than by the alternative site. He did state that sometimes there was difficulty in obtaining enough blood at the alternative site and sometimes there was bruising, but most of the time this method of testing became acceptable to him.

He appears to enjoy bringing in his records printed out in pie graphs, histograms, and basic tests with their average numbers per time of day and for the past 14 days.

Summary

Not all cases have such happy endings. These individuals were willing to obtain the supportive and necessary education to participate in self-management. Others were not or it was unsafe for them to participate in self-management alone, that is, a child or adult with mental challenges. Other cases had problems with willingness to consistently take good care of themselves or had too many outside distracters or stressors that could become barriers in their self-care. Whatever the situation, all these cases demonstrated continued support by the professionals; maintaining timely clinic visits and ongoing education are a must.

Our mentor, the late Dr. Robert Jackson, was Catholic—he said, "Attending a clinic visit is just like going to confession. The person confesses their 'sins' and then resolves to do better—and this lasts for a while and dwindles down until the next clinic visit when things get stimulated again and the self-care improves."

These two statements have been most helpful to us:

1. Your body will tell us (you) when insulin is needed.
2. Thank goodness there is insulin.

With these two statements included in the initial and ongoing education process of people having diagnoses of T2DM, there has been little if any resistance when it is time to take injections.

V

Intermediate
Complications
and Their
Management

23

Pregnancy

Having diabetes and being pregnant is viewed by some as opposing factors. It is true that pregnancy is like climbing a mountain. It is very difficult; it takes lots of planning and hard work. There may be moments of depression and moments of sheer joy. Every step must be carefully thought out and precisely taken. The journey has hazards and dangers, most of which can be avoided with careful planning. The exhilaration, the feelings of wonder and accomplishment when reaching the mountaintop or giving birth compare to precious few experiences on this earth.

D. Hinnen, 2002

Reece (2008) describes the scope of the problem and, therefore, the importance of normalization of blood glucose levels (as safely as possible) before and during pregnancy. The tools, knowledge, and skills of the team approach have continued to improve with the addition of research and technologic growth. A successful pregnancy begins with careful planning and strict glycemic control *before* conception.

A number of the following referenced statements relate to the history of diabetes and pregnancy and contribute to the recognition of the great strides that have been made in this field that result in a healthy pregnancy and a healthy baby.

Pregnancy counseling and family planning should begin before the person becomes sexually active. Preconception counseling is readily available in health care (family practice, primary care, community health clinics, and diabetes specialty care programs). Strategic blood glucose control in the preconception period and during the first trimester of pregnancy has demonstrated dramatic reductions in rates of fetal malformations compared with the infants of women with diabetes who did not participate in preconception care.

Unger (2007) noted that healthy lifestyle choices in the prepregnant and pregnant woman influence the prevention or delay of onset of Type 2 diabetes mellitus (T2DM) in children and adolescents. It has also been documented that prepregnancy weight, as found in women with obesity, more than doubles the occurrence of stillbirths and neonatal deaths (Kristense, Vestergaard, Wisborg, Kesmodel, & Secher, 2005) and increases the chance of the baby being born with congenital malformations (Garcia-Patterson et al., 2004).

The key to the prevention of problems is adequate education, preconception counseling, and excellent supportive medical management by a knowledgeable team. Care should still be taken for women with advanced vascular disease who should be aware of the increased risk related to the potential accelerating effects of pregnancy (Volpe et al., 2007). In fact, Bo et al. (2007) suggests that the reader consider gestational diabetes as a vascular risk factor for the woman who is identified as being pregnant.

Retinopathy and nephropathy are the most common complications that occur in women with Type 1 diabetes mellitus (T1DM) during the childbearing years. Although there may be a greater risk of accelerating the microvascular changes of retinopathy and nephropathy during pregnancy, that same risk also exists while using high-dose contraceptive medications to prevent pregnancy. Women with normal urinary albumin excretion (less than 30 mg/24 hr) are not at the same clinical risk as those who show evidence of microalbuminuria or overt proteinuria (more than 300 mg/24 hr). Decreased creatinine clearance and hypertension further jeopardize maternal health. Although women with microalbuminuria may have an increase in urinary albumin excretion rates during pregnancy or even transient nephrotic syndrome and increased preeclampsia, there is no evidence of long-term effects on kidney function (Reece, 2008).

The use of angiotensin-converting enzyme inhibitors, known as ACE inhibitors (ACEIs), in patients with diabetes who are not pregnant has demonstrated a decrease in proteinuria as improving metabolic control does. ACEIs are used to reduce proteinuria and prevent hypertension. ACEIs are contraindicated in pregnancy because they can cause fetal abnormalities. As soon as the urinary protein or albumin excretion is achieved, and metabolic control has been optimized, the patient may more safely become pregnant. Because the use of ACEIs is contraindicated in pregnancy, this treatment must be discontinued immediately if menses stops or a positive pregnancy test occurs.

Diabetic nephropathy may complicate 5% of pregnancies in T1DM (Landon, 2007). Retinopathy, if proliferative at the time of pregnancy, may worsen. Laser treatment prior to pregnancy prevents worsening of the retinopathy. T1DM with a duration longer than 15 years, poor glycemic control, and hypertension put the woman at high risk for the occurrence or progression of retinopathy during pregnancy (Rahman, Rahman, Yassin, Subeirman, & Rahman, 2007).

If maternal health is adequate to maintain pregnancy, genetic considerations remain. Some authorities once discouraged pregnancy on genetic grounds. That recommendation, however, is not frequently given today because the risk of T1DM is less than might be expected in genetically susceptible individuals. The occurrence of T1DM in the offspring of parents who have diabetes is too low to warrant counseling against pregnancy. In fact, the Position Statement from the American Diabetes Association (ADA) on Preconception Care of Women With Diabetes (2008) does not even mention genetics as a consideration. The healthy woman with well-controlled diabetes who does not have advanced vascular disease not only can plan a family today, but with the help of recent developments in attaining glycemic control, she can often deliver vaginally a healthy, normal-weight infant.

Perinatal Morbidity and Mortality

The survival rate of infants of diabetic mothers has improved from less than 70% a number of years ago to nearly 98%, the same rate as seen in the general population. This figure is attainable only with the best of care in tertiary centers with interdisciplinary care specializing in diabetes and pregnancy, especially in women with T1DM.

When the diabetes is well controlled, age of the patient at onset, duration, and degree of vascular disease are no longer thought to be correlated with outcome. Persons with poor control may have severe complications in the early stages of the disease, whereas persons with good control may be free of serious complications for many years. Women with documented complications before or during pregnancy have fetal survival rates similar to women with T1DM without complications if fetal congenital malformations are excluded. Because there may be a linkage between glycosuria and ketonemia during organogenesis and the development of congenital malformations, it is imperative that glycemic control is attained well before conception. If diabetes is poorly controlled and conception occurs, the chance of congenital malformation such as neural tube defects, caudal regression syndrome, and major heart abnormalities greatly increases.

If the fetus escapes damaging levels of ketonemia but is exposed to intermittent or continuous hyperglycemia, it is likely hyperinsulinemia of the fetus will occur. Fetal hyperinsulinemia inhibits pulmonary maturation, thus contributing to respiratory distress syndrome of the neonate. Fetal hyperinsulinemia and maternal hyperglycemia also cause macrosomia (a large infant) and may result in hypoglycemia after birth. Macrosomia has also been associated with maternal serum insulin-like growth factor (Lauszus, Klebe, & Flyvbjere, 2001).

Hypocalcemia may be another complication for the infant of the diabetic mother. Polycythemia leading to hyperbilirubinemia may be an additional concern. The congenital malformations in the infant of the diabetic mother are related to poor glycemic control during the initial weeks of gestation when organogenesis occurs. Poor glycemic control throughout the pregnancy will cause problems of macrosomia and respiratory immaturity.

Physiology

The same physiologic changes occur in pregnant women with diabetes as in those who do not have diabetes. Diabetes imposes additional metabolic changes so that the patient and health care professionals must be aware of these changes to plan for a successful pregnancy. These changes are more dramatic in the late pregnancy than in the early pregnancy in this population (Lain & Catalano, 2007).

Most women who are pregnant are concerned about their metabolic changes. The most notable of these changes is the increase in body weight. A woman of average size should gain about 11 kg. The woman usually gains 1 kg in the first trimester and 5 kg in each of the second and third trimesters. The weight increase comes from (a) the fetus, placenta, amniotic fluid, uterus hypertrophy, and breast tissue expansion; (b) water retention, secondary to hormone effect; and (c) fat and protein deposits.

In the pregnancy of a woman with diabetes these changes are enhanced. There is an expansion of blood volume by human placental lactogen, which is a substance similar to a growth hormone and a product of the placenta. Placental lactogen can increase blood glucose levels in the mother and increase insulin needs. Amounts of this hormone increase as the pregnancy progresses. It has been used as an indicator of placental well-being, and its increase in late pregnancy explains the higher incidence of gestational diabetes in the mid-second and third trimesters. Increases in estrogen, progesterone, and cortisol also have an effect on increased insulin needs. Protein metabolism is important because no fetal protein can be synthesized if the proper amino acids are not present at the time of synthesis. Protein also is the secondary energy source because less energy is required to metabolize protein to glycogenic substances than to metabolize fat. The pregnant woman must take in quality protein, which will be discussed more fully under the subject of nutrition.

The cardiovascular system changes significantly in the woman who is pregnant. This not only represents a change in the amount of work it must perform, but also reveals an anatomic change. Because of the elevation of the diaphragm, the longitudinal axis of the heart shifts to the left on the electrocardiogram (ECG). The apex of the heart moves to the left and lateral to its position in the nonpregnant state. The heart increases its activity following the arterial-venous shunt of the placenta. The pulse rate increases 10–15 beats per min. Cardiac output increases steadily in the first and second trimesters and then levels off near term. Total blood volume increases 45% to compensate for (a) increased vascularity and expansion of the uterus, (b) increased subcutaneous circulation to dissipate heat, (c) impaired venous return, and (d) blood loss at parturition. Blood volume change is made up of increases in plasma protein and erythrocytes. Some increase in clotting factors occurs, producing a hypercoagulation state. Mechanical changes in the heart also occur. A systolic murmur occurs in 96% of mothers, as well as a more prominent split-second sound in 5%.

The renal system is probably the most important organ system in the pregnant woman—especially in the woman with diabetes who is pregnant. Diseases of the kidneys and collecting system create the highest number of premature infants and small-for-gestational-age babies. Anatomically, the kidney undergoes general enlargement. The collecting system shows dilatation of the ureters below the pelvic brim; the right ureter shows greater dilatation than the left.

Kidney function increases in the first trimester. This is noted by a 50% increase in the glomerular filtration rate (GFR) and a lesser increase in renal plasma flow (RPF). This may be a result of placental lactogen production. With an increase in GFR and RPF, there is an increase in amino acids and water-soluble vitamins in the urine. Creatinine clearance increases to above-normal levels in women who are pregnant and can give the physician a prognostic tool should the level drop during the second trimester. Associated with the increase in clearance is a lowering of serum creatinine and blood urea nitrogen levels of 75% and 50%, respectively.

Glycosuria can result from an increase in GFR and poor glucose tubular reabsorption. This can reduce the renal glucose threshold in some patients. Lactose can also cause a positive urine reduction reaction and is found in moderate amounts in the urine of the woman who is close to term. An increase in the glomerular filtration rate results in a lowering in the renal threshold—the results being glucose in the urine at lowered blood glucose levels. Because of threshold changes, blood glucose monitoring becomes paramount for maintenance of euglycemia in the woman with diabetes who is pregnant (Henry, Major, & Reinsch, 2001).

Changes in the gastrointestinal system are not major but are uncomfortable for the patient. The patient with diabetes requires good control of dietary intake and may find it difficult to keep the intake adequate. These changes include hyperemic gingiva, which causes bleeding of the gums, and compression of the stomach and intestines, which produces significant heartburn and a full feeling. Also contributing to this condition is the decreased motility of the intestine and stomach because of high progesterone levels.

The endocrine system changes by producing more hormones from glands. The thyroid gland is the best example. Histology shows a hypertrophy of gland tissue and an increased iodine uptake. The basal metabolic rate is elevated, but most of the increased levels of thyroxine circulate in the plasma in bound form, because estrogen elevates the hormone-binding protein. Growth hormone from the pituitary gland decreases, secondary to increasing levels of placental lactogen, which is similar in activity to growth hormone. Prolactin increases to 10 times its normal amount to prepare the mammary glands for lactation. Cortisol and aldosterone are produced in the adrenal gland. Total serum cortisol, like thyroxine, increases in serum owing to increased protein binding, so despite increased production, the free hormone level is normal. The aldosterone increase is secondary to changes in the angiotensin-renin system and becomes a significant problem in pregnancy-induced hypertension.

An understanding of these normal changes in physiology helps us to understand the problems of the woman who has diabetes. Increases in human placental lactogen and cortisol, for example, will increase blood glucose levels. Insulin must then be increased to maintain glycemic control. Insulin requirements frequently decrease in the first trimester of pregnancy. When placental maturation and human placental lactogen production occur in the mother in the second trimester, insulin requirements begin to increase and may more than double by the end of pregnancy. Careful attention to these physiologic principles will greatly facilitate diabetes control. At about 37 weeks, insulin needs decrease as placenta function decreases.

Classification

Because pregnancy can cause a diabetogenic state even in women that have not been diagnosed with diabetes, but are potentially diabetic, the American College of Obstetrics and Gynecology (ACOG, 2008) has presented a classification for the identification and evaluation of diabetes mellitus and pregnancy (Table 23.1). White's Class A diabetes is now called gestational diabetes—women who develop abnormal glucose tolerance during pregnancy. (Note: Many professionals now prefer to use this updated form of classification for diabetes in pregnancy and no longer use the White classification).

Screening

Because of the high incidence of gestational diabetes (variously estimated between 2% and 12% of all pregnancies depending on the diagnostic criteria used) and potential fetal and neonatal abnormalities, the ADA and ACOG suggest that

23.1 Classification of Diabetes in Pregnancy

Class	Age of Onset (Year)	Duration (Year)	Vascular Disease	Therapy
A	Any	Any	0	A1, diet only* A2, insulin*
B	>20	<10	0	Insulin
C	10–19	10–19	0	Insulin
D	10 or 20	Any	Benign retinopathy	Insulin
F	Any	Any	Nephropathy	Insulin
R	Any	Any	Proliferative retinopathy	Insulin
H	Any	Any	Heart disease	Insulin

Class	Fasting glucose	Postprandial glucose level
*A1	FBS <95 mg/dl; 5.3 mmol/L	2 hr PC <120 mg/dl; 6.7 mmol/L
*A2	FBS <105 mg/dl; 5.8 mmol >95 mg/dl; 5.3 mmol/L	2 hr PC >120 mg/dl; 6.7 mmol/L

all pregnant women be screened for elevated levels of glucose at 24–28 weeks. The ADA Preconception Care of the Women with Diabetes (2004) state:

> Risk assessment for gestational diabetes mellitus (GDM) should be undertaken at the first prenatal visit. Women with clinical characteristics consistent with high risk of GDM (marked obesity, glycosuria, or strong family history of diabetes) should undergo glucose testing as soon as feasible. If negative, they should be re-screened at 24–28 weeks. Women at average risk should have testing at 24–28 weeks.

If there are suggestive signs or symptoms of diabetes at the initial history and physical examination, blood glucose screening should be carried out immediately and repeated later if the initial screen is negative. Initial screening criteria are (a) a strong family history of diabetes (such as a maternal and paternal family history), (b) a history of fetal wastage or stillbirth, (c) a history of large babies weighing more than 9 lbs, (d) a history of previous gestational diabetes or carbohydrate abnormalities, or (e) obesity.

The initial metabolic screen is performed at the first visit if there is a positive history or physical examination or later if there is a negative history or physical examination. When there is some question whether to test or not for gestational diabetes mellitus, consider testing (Reece & Homko, 2005). The most positive outcomes correlate with early screening and intervention (Pennison & Egerman, 2001). The screen consists of a 1-hr blood glucose value of more than 140 mg/dl (7.8 mmol) on venous plasma after a 50-g oral glucose load. This screen should be done routinely on all women who are pregnant between the 24th and 28th week of gestation (ACOG Education Pamphlet APH2, 2008). If the results of the screen are positive, a 3-hr oral glucose tolerance test using 100 g of glucose is performed and interpreted according to the criteria of O'Sullivan and Mahan (1964) (see Table 23.2).

Women with proven gestational diabetes should be vigorously treated to avoid fetal and neonatal abnormalities. Once having a diagnosis of gestational diabetes, they should be monitored by a team familiar with diabetes and

23.2 Detection of Diabetes in Pregnancy

Test	Time	Plasma Glucose Concentration	
Screening test:			
50 g glucose (no prep) load	1 hr	140 mg/dl	7.8 mmol
Oral glucose tolerance test (for diagnosis)			
100 g glucose load (after overnight fast)		95 mg/dl	5.3 mmol
FBS (2 abnormal values)	2 hr	155 mg/dl	8.6 mmol
	3 hr	140 mg/dl	7.8 mmol

managed similarly to the woman with T1DM who is pregnant. Initially, an ADA diet of 1,800–2,200 calories is prescribed, self-monitoring of blood glucose is started, and an HbA1c obtained, which should be in the low-normal range (3.4%–6.2%). As the HbA1c rises or self-monitoring of blood glucose indicates blood glucose values above the range described for pregnancy and diabetes, usually a fasting blood glucose of more than 90 mg/dl (5.0 mmol/l) or a 2 hr postprandial value of more than 120 mg/dl (6.6 mmol), medication is initiated and continued until the end of the pregnancy.

According to Russell, Carpenter, and Coustan (2007), there is little scientific evidence to determine the best way to screen women who are pregnant, but the preceding practice is the most acceptable at this writing.

Management and Control

Oral Agents

Some health professionals are using metformin but others use glyburide (Langer, 2007a), both off label, until the blood glucose levels reach the criteria noted above with no reported untoward responses occurring in the mother or the infant. Most authorities believe that there are insufficient data to support the use and safety of these drugs and recommend insulin as a safe and proven method of management of the woman with diabetes who is pregnant but who cannot be managed by diet alone (Jovanovic, 2007). Langer (2007a) takes the opposite view that no harm is done and Langer (2007b) reports that this practice is accepted by many. These two papers indicate that the use of oral agents, in pregnancy, remains controversial. The studies reported are basically retrospective because it would be difficult to obtain permission from human subjects to do prospective studies with this population. Until hard scientific evidence is forthcoming, we do not recommend using oral agents during pregnancy.

Insulin Management

Goals for glycemic control in the woman with diabetes should be tighter than those of her nondiabetic counterpart. Optimal goals for glycemic control are as follows (Table 23.3).

23.3 Glycemic Goals		
	Whole Blood Samples	Plasma Samples
Fasting	60–95 mg/dl, 3.3–5.3 mmol	70–110 mg/dl, 3.8–6.1 mmol
Preprandial	<105 mg/dl, 5.8 mmol	120 mg/dl, 6.6 mmol
1 hr postprandial	<140 mg/dl, 7.8 mmol	160 mg/dl, 8.8 mmol
2 hr postprandial	<120 mg/dl, 6.7 mmol	140 mg/dl, 7.8 mmol

Data suggest that fasting blood glucose should be kept below 90 mg/dl (5.0 mmol/l) and 2-hr postprandial below 120 mg/ml (6.6 mmol/l) in all women who are pregnant whether they have diabetes or not.

Gestational diabetes is most often controlled with multiple insulin injections. Frequently, in early pregnancy, two injections a day of short- and intermediate-acting insulins are used. The first injection given before breakfast is the largest (two-thirds of total) dose, consisting of two parts intermediate-acting insulin with one part short- or rapid-acting insulin. The smaller, evening injection, one-third of total, may be a 2:1 ratio or a 1:1 ratio of intermediate-acting insulin to short- or rapid-acting insulin. A premixed insulin may be used. As the fasting blood glucose level rises, then the presupper dose may be split into a rapid- or short-acting insulin before the evening meal and the intermediate-acting insulin at bedtime. When adequate control can no longer be maintained, as is usually the case by the end of the first trimester, four injections per day will be needed, often with rapid-acting insulin before each meal and long-acting insulin at bedtime and possibly before breakfast. Women with T1DM will usually need a basal-bolus regimen or a pump, from preconception.

Numerous insulin regimens to achieve multiple insulin peak actions while maintaining basal insulin levels (simulating normal physiology) have been devised. Multiple-injection therapy or pump therapy allows tighter control and greater flexibility in the timing and amounts given than other methods of administering insulin. Insulin analogs, albeit off label, have effectively been used, with no untoward side effects reported for use in this population (Gamson, Chia, & Jovanovic, 2004). The use of glargine insulin in pregnancy has been questioned because of the high affinity of this insulin for insulin-like growth factor-1 (IGF1) receptors. The high affinity of glargine for this receptor could produce abnormal growth or malignant lesions of the placenta. We have used glargine in women who are pregnant since it became available in 2002. We have seen no placental changes or abnormalities in the babies because this insulin was used. A detailed analysis of data from these deliveries is currently underway. Preliminary analysis reveals no problem in over 100 deliveries of women with T1DM and over 300 women with gestational diabetes (Guthrie, Childs, & Prey-Dede, 2008). For those who are concerned about the use of glargine, insulin detemir can be used for the basal insulin because this insulin has a very low affinity for the IGF1 receptor.

For individuals with T1DM or T2DM, the four-injections-of-insulin-per-day program is the most frequently prescribed protocol in our clinic. This regimen, which has been used with great success, is the same one that has been used for many years for acute diabetes control in patients who are not pregnant. The regimen consists of the establishment of a presumed total daily insulin requirement in units per day based on body weight or on previous insulin requirements. Insulin aspart was studied in comparison with human insulin with successful outcomes (Hod et al., 2008). This insulin or other rapid-acting insulin is used premeal (Guthrie, 1988; Jovanovic, 2007b) (see Table 23.4).

In this four-dose schedule, the total daily dose or the individual doses can then be altered as needed to establish control during the time interval controlled by that dose. If the premeal blood glucose levels are too high or too low (especially the fasting blood sugar), the long-acting insulin is altered; if the 1- or 2-hr postprandial blood glucose level after meals is too high or too low, then the rapid-acting insulin taken before the meal is altered to bring these glucose values into

23.4 Comparison of Management Approaches: Jovanovic/Guthrie

Average Percentage Insulin Needs: Premeal/Bedtime	
Jovanovic	Guthrie
18% before breakfast (rapid-acting)	20% before breakfast (rapid-acting)
15% before lunch	13% before lunch or smaller meal
17% before supper	17% before supper or larger meal
50% at bedtime (long-acting)	50% at bedtime (long-acting)

the normal range. For example: the afternoon blood glucose level is used to determine the noon insulin dose; the evening value used to determine the presupper insulin; and the fasting blood sugar is used to determine the bedtime insulin.

All these changes are determined by careful blood glucose monitoring. Self-monitoring of blood glucose (or bedside blood glucose monitoring in the hospital) is then performed beginning with the fasting value each morning. The bedtime long-acting insulin dose is then increased or decreased in 1-unit increments daily (more if initial blood glucose values are markedly out of the expected range) until the fasting blood glucose value is in the desired range (70–90 mg/dl [3.3–5.0 mmol/L]).

Once the fasting value for blood glucose is normal, monitoring of the postprandial value after meals can be used to alter the premeal doses in 1–2-unit increments daily until the blood glucose values are in the desired range. We use, as a goal, a fasting blood glucose level less than 90 mg/dl (5 mmol) and a 2-hr postprandial goal less than 120 mg/dl (6.6 mmol) without any significant hypoglycemia occurrences. Once the morning blood glucose values are in the normal range, the process is repeated with afternoon measurements and adjustments of the rapid-acting insulin taken before lunch. The process is then repeated with the blood glucose values that occur after supper. All these insulins can, of course, be changed simultaneously.

If only short-acting insulin is available, the same level of control may be achieved using four doses (every six hours) of 25% each of short-acting (regular) insulin or 30%, 22%, 28% for the premeal dosing of short-acting insulin with 15% of the short-acting insulin at midnight. If a culture is used to having "high tea," some of the noon dose (1–2%) and part of the supper dose (1%) can be given with the afternoon "tea."

If the woman is using a pump, 50% of the total of the daily insulin needs are used as basal, and the remainder apportioned with meal bolus per meal size.

The preceding process must be done slowly, for patients at home, to avoid an overshoot that would result in hypoglycemia. Alteration in insulin as outlined earlier, however, may be too slow for the person who is both pregnant and diabetic when performed in the home. It is urgent to establish control in the pregnant woman with diabetes to prevent fetal damage. More rapid insulin adjustment may be achieved in a hospital and may be desirable for some women.

Other regimens for diabetes control during pregnancy can be used. The preceding regimens are most useful in attaining and maintaining glycemia control in most pregnant women who have diabetes in any form. When there is careful medical supervision, a motivated patient and close glucose control should be expected.

An analysis of 100 deliveries in our center has demonstrated the value of the system we use. Only two babies had congenital anomalies (a 1% rate). Deliveries occurred at an average of 38 weeks' gestation, with average birth weight of 3,037 g. There was only one premature infant, one death, and one baby more than 4,000 g (this woman arrived and was first seen during her third trimester). This good pregnancy outcome exceeds the national average for diabetic pregnancies (Guthrie, 1988). We continue to recommend the use of a four-injection-a-day regimen from early in pregnancy.

Testing for Ketones in the Urine

Urine testing for ketones continues to be important and should not be omitted. The ketone levels are routinely checked with the fasting blood sugar. If ketones are found in the urine on the first void, other checks for ketones may be requested during the day. This information would be used to indicate whether the changes made with increased calorie intake have been adequate. Ketones in the system are a signal that not enough calories are being ingested or that the person is going into diabetic ketoacidosis and, therefore, should not go unattended. Ketones detected in the early morning indicate starvation ketosis. An increased bedtime snack or a snack during the night will need to be implemented.

Dietary Management

The nutrient and energy needs of the woman increase dramatically during pregnancy. The time when it is necessary to increase the amount of a specific nutrient varies considerably. Increases in energy needs relate to increased maternal metabolism, added maternal tissues, and growth of the fetus and placenta. Caloric needs during pregnancy may be from 400 to 600 kcal more per day than for the same period in the nonpregnant state.

Weight gain, which is a crude indicator of energy expenditure, should be minimal in the first trimester, with an average of 0.4 kg/week in the last two trimesters. Total pregnancy weight gain of 11 to 12.5 kg should not be altered because of glucose intolerance. The end of the first trimester marks the beginning of the increased energy requirements, which remain relatively constant until term. Second-trimester energy expenditures are primarily related to expansion of blood volume, uterus and breast growth, and fat accumulation. Third-trimester energy is primarily devoted to fetal and placental growth.

Weight reduction programs implemented during pregnancy potentiate ketonemia, which creates great physical and mental risks to fetal development. Pregnancy is not the time to lose body fat by going on a diet. Calorie restriction is not usually implemented during pregnancy, and there is even controversy about whether women who are obese should gain some weight for optimal fetal development. Restriction of carbohydrates to 35%–40% of calories has been shown to decrease maternal glucose levels and improve maternal and fetal outcomes, but CHO restriction in a person with diet-controlled gestational diabetes has been of some concern. A gradual, steady weight gain is optimal and is as important as the total weight gained (Reader et al., 2006).

Specific nutrient increases include protein, iron, folic acid, minerals, and fat-soluble and water-soluble vitamins. Protein needs to be increased to assist with growth, particularly of the maternal breasts, uterus, extracellular fluid, and fetus. Experimental and theoretical methods for calculating protein requirements are available; however, protein metabolism is generally thought to be adequate if calorie consumption is maintained at 36 kcal·kg^{-1}·day^{-1}. Additional protein requirements for the mature gravid woman would be 1.3 g·kg^{-1}·day^{-1}, whereas the pregnant adolescent may require 1.5–1.7 g·kg^{-1}·day^{-1}.

The goals of dietary management in pregnancy include meeting nutritional requirements while eliminating hyperglycemia. Distribution of meals and snacks must coincide with peaks of insulin given by injection. Because of nausea and hyperemesis in early pregnancy, the size of snacks may begin to equal the size of meals. Three meals and three to four snacks per day with equal timing between periods of food intake are optimal. Eating every 3–4 hr may become necessary to prevent ketonemia. Daily calories of 36–50 kcal/kg of ideal body weight should meet a majority of the previously mentioned nutrient needs. This increase may average about 300 kcal/day above the prepregnancy meal plan.

Alcohol consumption during pregnancy is strongly discouraged because of fetal alcohol syndrome. In the woman with diabetes who is pregnant, alcohol consumption may increase the risk of immediate hyperglycemia and potential hypoglycemia, and it may lead to a lack of nutrient intake and an inhibition of gluconeogenesis.

On a side note, one study found that milk consumption during pregnancy was associated with a higher birth weight for gestational age which correlated with the protein rather than the fat in the milk (Olsen et al., 2007). What probably is more important, at this point, is that women with diabetes who are obese and are pregnant not only beget obesity in their children, but also a tendency for a multitude of complications (Reece, 2008).

The Team Approach

The woman with diabetes who is pregnant or thinking about becoming pregnant should be monitored carefully before and during pregnancy by a competent team of people trained not only in the management of pregnancy but of diabetes as well. This team should consist of an obstetrician with experience in high-risk pregnancy, a diabetes specialist with experience in managing women with diabetes who are pregnant, and an appropriate support team of nurse practitioners, nurse educators, dietitians, counselors or psychologists, and social workers. This is best done in a tertiary care center that is equipped with appropriate laboratory support and a tertiary care newborn center with trained neonatologists. Developing and sustaining a quality diabetes-in-pregnancy program requires continuous evaluation and updating (Pagano, Luerssen, & Esposito, 2006). The emphasis on "prepregnancy counseling" and multidisciplinary team management is the key to achieving good pregnancy outcomes (Kapoor, Sankaran, Hyer, & Shehata, 2007).

Contraception

Fastidious and scrupulous control of the diabetes during pregnancy will decrease perinatal morbidity and mortality. The risk of congenital abnormalities during the first few weeks of gestation can be reduced by correct glycemic control. Blood glucose control and metabolic equilibrium must be attained well before the time of conception and maintained throughout the pregnancy. Considerations and planning for pregnancy consequently begin with contraception as an initial step in family planning.

Low-dose oral contraceptives have a minimal effect on glycemic control and a reduced effect on vascular complications compared with their earlier predecessors. Norplant is used with some success when the compliance of taking a daily pill is in question. The nausea from the daily pill, which occurs in some cases, may be a limiting factor. Natural family planning is also an alternative to consider but is less effective than oral contraceptives or mechanical devices (condoms, diaphragms, intrauterine devices, etc.).

Stages of Care

Preconception Management

Management begins before conception with a comprehensive education in diabetes and pregnancy. This high-risk pregnancy necessitates careful planning and early intervention by health professionals. Any education should also include the woman's significant other. Education and emotional factors will be easier to deal with if the patient develops support systems early.

Education must include more than the survival skills of injection technique, blood testing, ketone testing, and meal planning for this woman who is pregnant. A comprehensive self-management course is imperative. Working from predetermined protocols, the patient must make precise insulin and calorie adjustments. The desire for a successful pregnancy is often enough of a motivating factor to ensure a high degree of patient compliance with the recommended regimen. If the woman has T2DM, there should be a change from oral hypoglycemic agents to insulin before pregnancy. In this instance, in particular, the patient joins the physician, nurse, and dietitian as a member of the health care team. Pregnancy in the woman with diabetes is a difficult and risky task, requiring increased patient compliance. More frequent blood glucose and urine ketone testing and more frequent visits to the physician or other health professional are needed. All of this requires time, patience, and more, before the decision to undertake the risk of pregnancy.

Antepartum Care

Antepartum care for any woman who is pregnant should begin soon after the first missed menstrual period. Although detection of a pregnancy is much earlier, most women will enter care at about 5–6 weeks of gestation. This should not be the case for the woman who has diabetes. Normalization of blood glucose values should ideally be attained before the actual conception.

The first prenatal visit for the pregnant woman with diabetes should include a complete history and physical examination including an ophthalmologic and neurologic examination. A consultation with a dietitian about adjustment of calorie intake and food distribution for the pregnant state is also important.

Evaluation of the fetus can begin with measurement of uterine size and noninvasive ultrasonography. A schedule for ultrasonography can be found in Table 23.5. Measurements should include fetal biparietal diameter, head circumference, abdominal circumference, and femur and humerus lengths. Because of the increase in spontaneous abortion in diabetic pregnancies, first-trimester assessment of embryonal fetal development is a most important evaluation.

Gestational dating can be performed simultaneously and repeat testing assesses progress of the glucose intolerance and the pregnancy. Ultrasonography at 16–18 weeks can give an excellent assessment of the presence or absence of gross congenital malformations. Another test of congenital malformations, especially neural tube defects, is the maternal serum alpha-fetoprotein (MSAFP) determination, which should be performed at least once in every diabetic pregnancy.

Assessment of fetal growth is often followed with serial sonography every 10–14 days beginning at the 28th week of gestation. Umbilical blood flow studies are now being used to evaluate the function of the uteroplacental unit. This test is used especially when there is ultrasound evidence of intrauterine growth retardation.

Monitoring fetal well-being in the third trimester can begin at 32 weeks' gestation by using the fetal monitor and the nonstress test (NST). The NST looks for acceleration in the fetal heart rate (FHR) with fetal movement. An increase in FHR for more than 15 seconds with fetal movement indicates a reactive or positive test and is reassurance of good fetal health. If this test is negative, uterine contraction can be stimulated to see if there is deceleration in the FHR. If deceleration occurs there may be fetal distress, and the baby may need to be delivered. Biophysical parameters are assessed and the delivery date effected. The biophysical profile is detailed in Tables 23.6 and 23.7. Each positive finding in the profile is equal to 2 points, each negative finding to zero points. A drop in amniotic fluid may be the earliest sign of fetal illness.

Women with diabetes who are pregnant should have an obstetric management plan before delivery. Before delivery, fetal lung maturity should be assessed. Amniocentesis can be safely performed to determine fetal lung maturity. Measurement of surfactant and its precursors are available at most Level 3 centers. The lecithin sphingomyelin ratio should be 3:1 with phosphatidylglycerol present.

The mother should be seen frequently—usually monthly during the first trimester, every two weeks during the second trimester, and weekly during the third trimester. Home blood glucose monitoring and HbA1c are the tests to be used. HbA1c should be in the low-normal range. The fructosamine test can be alternated monthly with the HbA1c test. It assesses shorter term control (8–10 days or 1–2 weeks) than the HbA1c.

All patients with T1DM need a renal evaluation. This can be done early in pregnancy and then at 28–30 weeks by a 24-hr urine for total protein and creatinine clearance or, now, a random urine to calculate an estimated glomerular filtration rate (eGFR). If the test results are normal in the nonpregnant state, it is still possible for the woman who is pregnant to show increasing renal compromise in the third trimester, requiring increased bed rest to obtain a successful pregnancy.

23.5   Schedule for Ultrasonography

Determination	Number of Weeks
Embryonal-fetal viability and dating	8 to 12
Fetal anomalies and size	16 to18
Fetal echocardiogram	28 to 30
Fetal growth and weight with an interval of 10–14 days between studies	28 to 38
Doppler studies for uteroplacental flow	28 to 38

23.6   Biophysical Profile Scoring: Technique and Interpretation

Biophysical Variable	Normal Score	Abnormal Score
Fetal breathing movements (FBM)	At least 1 episode FBM in a duration in 30-min. observation.	Absent FBM or no episode of >30 sec in 30 min.
Gross body movements	At least 3 discrete body-limb movements in 30 min. (episodes of active continuous movement considered as a single movement).	2 or fewer episodes of body-limb movements in 30 min.
Fetal tone	At least 1 episode of active extension with return to flexion of fetal limb(s) or trunk, opening and closing of hand considered normal tone.	Either slow extension with return to partial flexion or movement of limb in flexion or movement of limb in full extension or absent fetal movement.
Reactive fetal heart rate (FHR)	At least 2 episodes of FHR acceleration of >15 sec duration associated with fetal movement in 30 min.	Less than 2 episodes of acceleration of FHR or acceleration of <15 beats/min in 30 min.
Qualitative amniotic fluid volume (AFV)	At least 1 pocket of AFV that measures at least 1 cm in 2 episodes of FHR.	Either no AFV pockets or a pocket <1 cm in 2 episodes of FHR.

23.7 Biophysical Profile Scoring: Management Protocol

Score	Interpretation	Recommended Management
10	Normal infant, low risk for chronic asphyxia	Repeat testing at weekly intervals; repeat twice weekly in patients with diabetes and patients with pregnancies of > 42 weeks' gestation.
8	Normal infant, low risk for chronic asphyxia	Repeat testing at weekly intervals; repeat twice weekly in patients with diabetes and patients with pregnancies of > 42 weeks' gestation; oligohydramnios is indication for delivery.
6	Suspected chronic asphyxia	Repeat testing in 4–6 hours; deliver if oligohydramnios is found.
4	Suspected chronic asphyxia	If pregnancy is > 36 weeks and favorable, then deliver; if < 36 weeks and L/S[a] < 2, repeat test in 24 hours; if repeat score is < 4, deliver.
0–2	Strong suspicion of asphyxia	Extend testing time to 120 min; if persistent score < 4, deliver regardless of gestational age.

[a]L/S = lecithin-sphingomyelin amniotic fluid ratio.

Labor and Delivery

Labor and delivery of the woman with diabetes require planning and continuous monitoring. In the person with poorly or loosely controlled diabetes in the gestational or pregestational state, there is a higher incidence of such women giving birth to macrosomic infants, who require long inductions for vaginal delivery and present a risk to both mother and infant. This has led to a high incidence of caesarean sections in patients with diabetes, because the occurrence of fetal and maternal morbidity from macrosomia and cephalopelvic disproportion in vaginal delivery is higher. The person with more tightly controlled diabetes can carry to term and potentially deliver vaginally, providing the following requirements are present:

1. Small- to average-sized infant.
2. Inducible cervix.
3. Emergency caesarean section capabilities with anesthesia in hospital.
4. Neonatal intensive care in hospital.
5. Ability to maintain normal glycemia in mother through infusion pump or multiple-dose insulin therapy.
6. No perinatal complications.
7. No previous fetal wastage.

The women who should be considered for caesarean section are those who meet the following criteria: (a) previous fetal wastage, (b) poor prenatal glucose control, (c) renal complications, (d) premature fetus, (e) unfavorable cervix (Bishop score 1–4), and (f) fetal distress in utero.

Maintenance of normal glycemia during delivery or caesarean section leads to only mild blood glucose problems in the neonate. Normal glucose control during labor can be achieved in many ways. Intravenous insulin throughout labor and delivery is the simplest method of control. Blood glucose levels are to be maintained between 80 and 120 mg/dl (4.4–6.6 mmol/L). Regular insulin every 6 hr or a rapid-acting insulin every 4 hr can also be used. In women with gestational diabetes taking insulin, the long-acting insulin (glargine or detemir) should be given at bedtime the night before delivery. With the long-acting insulin on board for 24 hr, usually no insulin is needed during labor. Blood glucose should be monitored at least every 2 hr and maintained at less than 120 mg/dl (6.6 mmol/L).

Along with close control of blood glucose levels during labor and delivery, evaluation of urine ketones should be performed. If ketonuria occurs, the patient should be given more glucose intravenously to eliminate the problem.

Postpartum Care

Insulin requirements decrease during the postpartum period. This is a result of the removal of the insulin antagonist, human placental lactogen, as well as changes in estrogen and progesterone levels.

Lactation

Breast-feeding should be encouraged for mothers with diabetes. Knowledge of the benefits of lactation has been increasing, influencing the acceptance of more breast-feeding. Many mothers recognize the advantages of breast-feeding as both nurturing and nourishing. The presence of diabetes is no contraindication to breast-feeding.

Lactation does impact the glycemic control of diabetes. This is one additional area clinicians must be aware of when helping the woman with diabetes who is pregnant attain euglycemia. There may be more difficulties in breast-feeding if the delivery has been by caesarean section or if the infant is in the intensive care unit. The mother with diabetes can and should be assisted in maintaining lactation and breast-feeding by maintaining a healthy fluid intake and pumping the breasts, if needed.

Adjusting insulin dosages during lactation is a challenge for the individual and the health professional. Glucose transferred from serum to breast for conversion to lactose and the energy expenditure of milk production explains the lowering of blood glucose levels in the mother usually seen during lactation. Hypoglycemia is to be prevented. The secretion of epinephrine, during hypoglycemia, can lead to the reduction in lactose in the milk, inhibit milk production, and adversely affect the mother's ejection reflex. Generally, insulin is reduced about 25%–30% during lactation.

Calorie increases during lactation may be even more dramatic than during pregnancy. The caloric needs may increase 500–800 cal/day above basal levels. Higher calorie needs may occur quickly as insulin needs drop after delivery. There is an adjustment period of several days.

The potential for mastitis and breast abscess should be no greater for the woman with well-controlled diabetes than for the general population. If sore nipples, plugged ducts, and breast infections do occur, the mother should continue breast-feeding her baby (i.e., a pump could be used) and seek appropriate treatment (infections may affect glycemia control very quickly).

The weaning process presents a time of fluctuation in glycemic control for the woman with diabetes. As the baby takes less milk, the maternal blood glucose level again rises. If the weaning process is slowly accomplished during weeks or months, this adjustment is gradual and more easily controlled. Frequent contact with health professionals and close daily monitoring should help minimize problems of diabetes control. Assistance offered by health professionals should include insulin and calorie adjustment in the form of education regarding self-management and emotional support during the breast-feeding period. In general, the mother who is breast-feeding increases her calories and decreases her insulin, and does the opposite while weaning.

Infant of the Diabetic Mother

The infant of the diabetic mother has in the past (and still too frequently today) had many problems, including an increased incidence of congenital malformation, a high incidence of perinatal mortality, hypoglycemia, hypocalcemia, hyperbilirubinemia, and other problems. Most if not all of these problems are due to poor maternal diabetes control, and can be reduced or eliminated by meticulous maternal glucose control.

Summary

The future is not determined and it lies in our own hands.

—Margaret Mead

This quotation is so very true in our work with diabetes and pregnancy. Our ability to educate and motivate the women with diabetes who are planning a pregnancy will let us help determine and shape the future. Perinatal outcomes continue to be positive with normalization of blood glucose levels whether the woman has T1DM or T2DM (Gonzalez-Gonzalez et al., 2008). Only in the rarest of cases (women with severe vascular complications) should pregnancy be discouraged. Before they undertake conception, women and their partners should be carefully counseled concerning risks to the mother and fetus, the requirements of management and need for compliance, increased surveillance during pregnancy, and increased costs of pregnancy (Pagano et al., 2006). Properly supported and supervised by a competent and well-trained medical team, a healthy baby should be expected as the happy outcome in the pregnancy of a motivated patient with diabetes mellitus. Climbing the highest of mountains is an incredible experience if proper equipment is used and ideal care is given.

Because women with gestational diabetes are at high risk for developing T2DM, it is important to consider using all prevention measures (encouraging exercise, weight control, and stress management) and periodically screening these individuals (Case, Willoughby, Haley-Zitlin, & Maybee, 2006).

References

American College of Obstetrics and Gynecology. Education pamphlet APH2 (2008). *Diabetes and women: Clinical guidelines on the identification, evaluation, and treatment.* Retrieved March 24, 2008, from www.ACOG.org

American Diabetes Association. (2004). Preconception care of the women with diabetes. *Diabetes Care, 27*(Suppl. 1), S6–S18.

American Diabetes Association. (2008). Preconception care. In Executive summary: Standards of medical care in diabetes. *Diabetes Care, 31*(Suppl. 1), S10.

Bo, S., Valpreda, S., Menato, G., Bardelli, C., Botto, C., Cambino, R., et al. (2007). Should we consider gestational diabetes a vascular risk factor? *Atherosclerosis, 194*(2), 72–79.

Case, J., Willoughby, D., Haley-Zitlin, V., & Maybee, P. (2006). Preventing type 2 diabetes after gestational diabetes. *The Diabetes Educator, 32*(6), 877–886.

Coetzee, K. E. J. (2007). Counterpoint: Oral hypoglycemic agents should be used to treat diabetic pregnant women. *Diabetes Care, 30*(11), 2976–2979.

Gamson, K., Chia, S., & Jovanovic, S. (2004). Review of the safety and efficacy of insulin analogs in pregnancy. *Journal of Maternal-Fetal Neonatal Medicine, 15*, 26–34.

Garcia-Patterson, A., Erdozain, L., Ginovart, G., Adelantado, J. M., Cubero, J. M., Gallo, G., et al. (2004). In human gestational diabetes mellitus congenital malformations are related to pre-pregnancy body mass index and the severity of diabetes. *Diabetologia, 47*(3), 509–514.

Gonzalez-Gonzalez, N. L., Ramirez, O., Mozas, J., Melchor, J., Armas, H., Garcia-Hernandez, J. A., et al. (2008). Factors influencing pregnancy outcome in women with type 2 versus type 1 diabetes. *Acta Obstetria et Gynecologica Scandinavia, 87*(1), 43–49.

Guthrie, R. (1988). *Diabetes and pregnancy at the University of Kansas School of Medicine at Wichita.* Presented at the 13th International Diabetes Federation Conference on Diabetes in Pregnancy, University of Auckland, Auckland, New Zealand.

Guthrie, R., Childs, B., & Prey-Dede, E. (2008). [Research in progress] Unpublished data.

Henry, M. J., Major, C. A., & Reinsch, S. (2001). Accuracy of self-monitoring of blood glucose: Impact on diabetes management decisions during pregnancy. *Diabetes Educator, 27*(4), 521–529.

Hinnen, D. (2002). Pregnancy. In D. Guthrie & R. Guthrie (Eds.), *Nursing management of diabetes mellitus* (5th ed., p. 308). New York: Springer Publishing Company.

Hod, M., Damm, P., Kaaja, R., Visser, G. H., Dunne, F., Demidova, I., et al.; Insulin Aspart Pregnancy Study Group. (2008). Fetal and perinatal outcomes in type 1 diabetes pregnancy: A randomized study comparing insulin aspart with human insulin in 322 subjects. *American Journal of Obstetrics and Gynecology, 198*(2), 186–187.

Jovanovic, L. (Guest Ed.). (2007b). Diabetes and pregnancy. *Diabetes Spectrum, 20*(2), 82–107.

Kapoor, N., Sankaran, S., Hyer, S., & Shehata, H. (2007). Diabetes in pregnancy: A review of current evidence. *Current Opinion in Obstetrics and Gynecology, 19*(6), 586–590.

Kristense, J., Vestergaard, M., Wisborg, K., Kesmodel, U., & Secher, N. J. (2005). Pre-pregnancy weight and the risk of stillbirth and neonatal death. *The International Journal of Obstetrics and Gynecology, 112*(4), 403–408.

Lain, K. Y., & Catalano, P. M. (2007). Metabolic changes in pregnancy. *Clinical Obstetrics and Gynecology, 50*(4), 938–948.

Landon, M. (2007). Diabetic nephropathy and pregnancy. *Clinical Obstetrics and Gynecology, 50*(4), 998–1006.

Langer, O. (2007a). Oral anti-diabetic drugs in pregnancy: The other alternative. *Diabetes Spectrum, 20*(2), 101–107.

Langer, O. (2007b). From educated guess to accepted practice, the use of oral anti-diabetic agents in pregnancy. *Clinical Obstetrics and Gynecology, 50*(4), 959–971.

Lauszus, F. F., Klebe, J. G., & Flyvbjerg, A. (2001). Macrosomia associated with maternal serum insulin-like growth factor I and II in diabetic pregnancy. *Obstetrics and Gynecology, 97*(5), 734–741.

Olsen, S. F., Halldorsson, T. I., Willett, W. C., Knudsen, V. K., Gillman, M. W., Mikkelsen, T. B., et al. (2007). Milk consumption during pregnancy is associated with increased infant size at birth: Prospective cohort study. *American Journal of Clinical Nutrition, 86*(4), 1104–1110.

O'Sullivan, J. B., & Mahan, C. M. (1964). Criteria for the oral glucose tolerance test in pregnancy. *Diabetes, 13,* 278–285.

Pagano, M., Luerssen, M., & Esposito, E. (2006). Sustaining a diabetes in pregnancy program: A continuous quality improvement process. *The Diabetes Educator, 32*(2), 229–234.

Pennison, E. H., & Egerman, R. S. (2001). Perinatal outcomes in gestational diabetes: A comparison of criteria for diagnosis. *American Journal of Obstetrics and Gynecology, 184*(6), 1118–1121.

Rahman, W., Rahman, F. Z., Yassin, S. A., Subeirman, S. A., & Rahman, J. (2007). Progression of retinopathy during pregnancy in type 1 diabetes mellitus. *Clinical Experiment in Ophthalmology, 35*(3), 231–236.

Reader, D., Splott, P., Gunderson, E. P.; Diabetes Care and Education Dietetic Practice Group. (2006). Impact of gestational diabetes mellitus nutrition practice guidelines implemented by registered dietitians on pregnancy outcomes. *Journal of American Dietetic Association, 106*(9), 1426–1423.

Reece, E. A. (2008). Perspectives on obesity, pregnancy and birth outcomes in the United States: The scope of the problem. *American Journal of Obstetrics and Gynecology, 198*(1), 23–27.

Reece, E. A., & Homko, C. J. (2005). How, when, and why to test for gestational diabetes mellitus. *Contemporary OB/GYN, 50*(8), 42, 45–46, 48.

Russell, M. A., Carpenter, M. W., & Coustan, D. R. (2007). Screening and diagnosis of gestational diabetes mellitus. *Clinical Obstetrics and Gynecology, 50*(4), 949–958.

Unger, J. (2007). Management of diabetes in pregnancy, childhood, and adolescence. *Primary Care, 34*(4), 809–843.

Volpe, L., DiGianni, G., Lencioni, C., Cuccuru, I., Benzi, L., & Del Prato, S. (2007). Gestation diabetes, inflammation, and late vascular disease. *Journal of Endocrinology Investigation, 30*(10), 873–879.

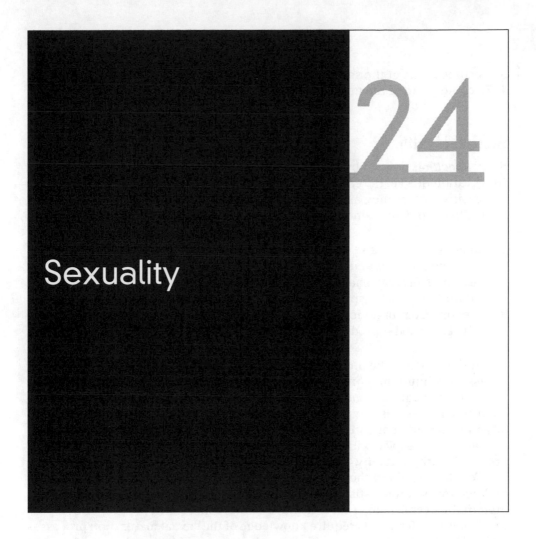

Sexuality

If you do not ask, they will not tell. This seems to be especially true if one has diabetes. Even with "sexual dysfunction" listed with a yes or no answer on the intake physical assessment form, people may not reveal this information and even if they do, they may not consider this something to question during the clinic visit. Sexuality is a dynamic physical and emotional reality of life that is interwoven with every aspect of being human. It is an expression of the self, an awareness of who a person is—biologically, psychologically, and socially—throughout the lifespan. Sexuality is impacted by gender, age, ethnicity, culture, and religious beliefs. The foundations for a healthy sexuality begin in infancy and continue through puberty. As a person matures, self-concept, body image, and gender identity forge links with a sexual value system to support each individual's unique manner of being male or female.

A healthy sexuality underlies the complete range of human experience and offers opportunities to:

1. Develop a sexual identity as a male or female.
2. Develop physical and emotional intimacy with another person.

3. Become aware of the sensuality of sexual pleasure.
4. Become a part of the genetic future, through reproduction and parenting.

Sexual Health

Sexual health is defined by the World Health Organization (WHO, 1975) as the "integration of somatic, emotional, intellectual, and social aspects in ways that are positively enriching and that will enhance personality, communication, and love." This definition identifies three essential elements:

1. Capacity to enjoy and control sexual and reproductive behavior in accordance with a social and personal ethic.
2. Freedom from fear, shame, guilt, false beliefs, and other psychologic factors that inhibit sexual response and impair sexual relationships.
3. Freedom from organic disorders, diseases, and deficiencies that interfere with sexual and reproductive functions.

Maintaining sexual health throughout the life cycle is an important goal, yet illness and injury may interfere. In addition, such factors as anxiety, stress, and fear may have a negative impact on sexual integrity. Diabetes mellitus, as a chronic illness, has the potential of interfering with sexual health. Additionally, the discomfort of patients, partners, and health professionals in discussing sexual issues, coupled with a lack of awareness and information, become barriers to a healthy sexuality.

For the client and the client's partner to maintain or regain sexual health and achieve sex role satisfaction during illness, sexual needs must be considered in the overall plan of care. To place sexual concerns in the proper perspective, health professionals require knowledge of the sexual maturation processes and behaviors and normal sexual response patterns. Keeping abreast of current sexuality research will also assist the health professional in meeting patient needs.

Sexual Response Cycle

To understand sexual dysfunction, it is necessary to have some understanding of the normal sexual response. At least four systems of the body, the circulatory, endocrine, neurologic, and psychologic, must be coordinated in this phenomenon. Currently, three models exist that demonstrate and explain the human sexual response cycle. Masters, Johnson, and Kolodny (1992) divide the sexual response into four phases: excitement, plateau, orgasm, and resolution. The sexual response is divided into three stages: desire, excitement, and orgasm; sexual dysfunction occurs when one of these stages is impaired. The *Diagnostic and Statistical Manual of Mental Disorders (DSM-IV)* (American Psychiatric Association, 2000) describes the stages of the sexual response cycle as follows:

1. Desire: This phase consists of fantasies about sexual activity and the desire to have sexual activity.

2. Excitement: This phase consists of a subjective sense of sexual pleasure and accompanying physiologic changes. The major changes in the male consist of penile tumescence and erection. The major changes in the female consist of vasocongestion in the pelvis, vaginal lubrication and expansion, and swelling of the external genitalia.

3. Orgasm: This phase consists of a peaking of sexual pleasure, with release of sexual tension and rhythmic contraction of the perineal muscles and reproductive organs. In the male, there is the sensation of ejaculatory inevitability, which is followed by ejaculation of semen. In the female, there is contraction (not always subjectively experienced as such) of the wall of the outer third of the vagina. In both genders, the anal sphincter rhythmically contracts.

4. Resolution: This phase consists of a sense of muscular relaxation and general well-being. During this phase, males are physiologically refractory to further erection and orgasm for a variable period of time. In contrast, females may be able to respond to additional stimulation almost immediately.

The sexual response cycle is a highly rational and orderly sequence of physiologic events, in contrast to the more sensitive psychologic component. Sexual stimulation elicits neurologic, vascular, muscular, and hormonal reactions that affect the entire body. As has been emphasized before, biologic, psychologic, environmental, social, and cultural factors affect the capacity of all individuals to function sexually.

Parameters of Sexual Function With Diabetes Mellitus

Sexual Dysfunction in Men With Diabetes

In a classic early investigative study of men with diabetes, Rubin and Babbot (1958) found that almost all the men reported the libido or desire had continued beyond the time they first noticed any loss of erectile function. Most of the younger men reported little or no change from their prediabetic libidinal state. These men were unable to obtain or maintain an erection sufficient to complete coitus or masturbation. Later, Rubin (1967) also found that men with diabetes older than 55 years with erectile dysfunction reported diminished or complete absence of libido. The continuation of libido after erectile dysfunction may be highly indicative of an organic cause as opposed to a psychogenic cause, in which diminished libido generally precedes the loss of erectile function.

To determine whether the lack of erection is a psychologic or physiologic response, a simple question may be asked: "Do you have night time erections?" In most instances, if the person says yes, then focus should not be on performance, but on hyper- or hypoglycemia, and psychologic problems as the probable reasons why sexual functioning during other hours of the day is presently not possible. If the person says no, then other tests might need to be done to determine whether physiologic activity is not possible because of diabetes complications.

Clinical depression is not unexpected when a person with diabetes, who would be more vulnerable, has to deal with the diagnosis of this chronic syndrome. This depression not only results in reduced desire for food and sleep but also in the reduced desire for sex. The loss of libido in this type of situation leads to erectile dysfunction. These individuals may voluntarily report an inability to achieve an adequate erection for coitus, yet when questioned, will admit to nocturnal and/or morning erections. Whether the erections are adequate for vaginal penetration remains to be determined, but without this type of questioning, the health professional may erroneously interpret the erectile dysfunction as an organic manifestation of diabetes. If the cause is depression, erectile function may be restored after treatment with psychotherapy and/or antidepressants. It is recommended that each clinician routinely evaluate people with diabetes for signs of clinical depression.

In the past, the term *impotence* had been used to signify the inability of the male to attain and maintain erection of the penis sufficient to permit satisfactory sexual intercourse. However, this term has often led to confusing and uninterpretable results in both clinical and basic science investigations because desire and orgasmic and ejaculatory capabilities were not included in the definition. At the 1992 National Institutes of Health (NIH) Consensus Development Conference on Impotence, the panel concluded that the more precise term *erectile dysfunction* should replace the term impotence. Accordingly, this chapter will follow their recommendation.

Etiologic factors for erectile disorders may be categorized as neurogenic, vasculogenic, or psychogenic, but they most commonly appear to act in concert in all three areas. Although the majority of patients with erectile dysfunction are thought to demonstrate an organic component, psychologic aspects of self-confidence, anxiety, partner communication, and conflict are often important contributing factors. These psychologic processes can impair erectile functioning by reducing erotic focus or otherwise reducing awareness of a sensory experience. These factors may lead to the inability to initiate or maintain an erection.

Other sexual dysfunctions may appear in men who have diabetes, including premature, retarded, or retrograde ejaculation, and loss of orgasmic sensations. The timing of premature and retarded ejaculation may have subjective connotations because of individual expectations and desires. However, a more precise definition is possible with retrograde ejaculation. Reproductive capacity may diminish secondary to retrograde ejaculation. On occasion, male patients may also complain of loss of orgasmic sensations and still expel semen. Anecdotal reports confirm that the loss of orgasm awareness creates significant distress for the male patient.

Causes

The causes of sexual dysfunction follow the classic headings listed by Ellenberg (1971):

 I. Psychogenic
II. Organic

    a. Congenital abnormality
    b. Trauma

    c. Systemic disease
    d. Vascular disease
    e. Endocrine deficiency
    f. Neurologic disease

       i. Central
      ii. Spinal
     iii. Peripheral

III. Drug induced

Psychologic Aspects

Although past research supported the notion of psychogenic factors causing erectile dysfunction, marital disharmony, medical treatment, and peripheral vascular disease were the main etiologic and pathogenic factors that appeared to be psychologic contributors or correlates of sexual dysfunction in men with diabetes. Although patients with diabetes had significantly lower levels of erotic drive, sexual arousal, enjoyment, and satisfaction, there was no evidence that psychologic distress or psychiatric disorders were associated with diabetes or with its effects on sexual function, but there was some concern with an individual's view on masculinity and having a chronic, possibly life-threatening disease (Jack, 2005).

From the material presented, one can see that the cause of sexual dysfunction in the man with diabetes requires more study; still it is concluded that organic factors are mainly responsible. Congenital abnormality, trauma, and systemic disease are obvious reasons why sexual functioning is limited or absent. The other aspects will be dealt with in turn.

Vascular Aspects

Because adequate arterial supply is critical for erection, any disorder that impairs blood flow may be implicated in the etiology of erectile disorder. The corporal venous occlusive mechanism may be interrupted and blood may fail to be trapped within the penis, or leakage may occur so that an erection cannot be maintained or is easily lost. The most common lesion in diabetic erectile dysfunction is probably vascular. Atherosclerosis of the peripheral penile arteries is the earliest and most common factor. Hypertension adds to the risk of erectile dysfunction, partly because the underlying atherosclerotic process affects the penile blood supply and partly because of the direct effect of most antihypertensive medications on erectile function. There is greater sexual dysfunction in patients suffering from both diabetes and hypertension, especially if they are taking antihypertensive drugs, particularly diuretics and beta blockers.

Endocrine Aspects

The endocrine system itself, particularly the production of androgens, appears to play a role in regulating sexual interest, and may also play a role in erectile function. Few conceptions and a greater number of miscarriages are associated with diminished erectile functioning.

Endocrine studies showed two-thirds of the men complaining of erectile dysfunction had decreased urinary excretion of pituitary gonadotropin. Conversely, urinary excretion of 17-ketosteroids was increased. One-third of the men with erectile dysfunction had low sperm counts or absence of sperm, and one half had low concentrations of fructose in the semen; both findings are indicative of androgen deficiency. Instances of complete absence of sperm are frequently explained by retrograde ejaculation.

According to a study by Kapoor, Clarke, Channer, and Jones (2007), men with diabetes with erectile problems had higher values of glycosylated hemoglobin than sexually functional men with diabetes. Both groups had lower bioavailable testosterone than control subjects and, in this study, had visceral adiposity. Other associated factors included age and hypertension in Type 1 diabetes mellitus (T1DM) in men. According to Spark (2007), one-third of men with Type 2 diabetes mellitus (T2DM) "are now recognized as testosterone deficient." This author found that use of testosterone therapy opened the possibility to reverse some responses found in the metabolic syndrome.

Most patients younger than 40 years responded to the combined therapy of testosterone and chorionic gonadotropin. A positive outcome of the results of this treatment was conception in the participating female. Improvement of sexual functioning is noted when testosterone alone is used in the treatment of patients older than 40. Sexual dysfunction (erectile dysfunction and diminished fertility) in men with diabetes may lead to a need to rule out hypogonadotropic hypogonadism.

Neurologic Aspects

Damage to the autonomic pathways innervating the penis may eliminate psychogenic erections initiated by the central nervous system. Visceral symptoms like intermittent diarrhea, postural hypotension, diminished sweating in the legs, and urinary bladder dysfunction suggest the presence of autonomic neuropathy. Lesions of the somatic nervous pathways may impair reflexogenic erections and may interrupt tactile sensation needed to maintain psychogenic erections. Peripheral neuropathy occurs from impaired neuronal innervation of the penis. Autonomic neuropathy is less frequently noted. Both peripheral neuropathy and autonomic neuropathy that accompany erectile dysfunction may be accompanied by neurogenic vesicle paralysis, neuropathic ulcer, Charcot's neuroarthropathy, enteropathy, and orthostatic hypotension. The fact is neuropathy plays a significant role in sexual dysfunction in men with diabetes mellitus.

Drug Effects

Drugs, prescription and numerous over-the-counter products, alcohol, and tobacco inhibit sexual response. Examples of these medications include tranquilizers and psychoactive drugs; antihypertensive and cardiovascular agents, such as thiazides, beta blockers, clonidine, digoxin, methyldopa, hydralazine, prazosin, and reserpine; antidepressants; antihistamines; analgesics including narcotics and nonsteroidal anti-inflammatory drugs; and others. Caffeine and other stimulants may inhibit erectile function. It is imperative that a review of medications be done to rule out iatrogenic causes of sexual dysfunction.

Sexual Dysfunction in Women With Diabetes

Does diabetes also have an effect on sexuality of women? Most research on sexuality and diabetes has been done on male patients. West, Vinikoor, and Zolnoun (2004) presented a review of the history of sexual dysfunction as reported for females as a whole; Rutherford and Collier (2005) focused on diabetes and female sexuality and sexual function. According to their study, there is still little research into the physical effects of hyperglycemia on sexual functioning in women. Problems with vaginal lubrication leading to dyspareunia have been reported but rarely documented as a sexual problem.

In a retrospective study, 127 Turkish women who were married, about one-fourth with T1DM, one-half with T2DM, and the rest without the diagnosis of diabetes, were evaluated via a questionnaire. The investigators found no particular factor that predicted sexual dysfunction in the population with diabetes, but age, poor education, absence of occupation, and menopause did (Doruk et al., 2005).

To view the sexual function of women with diabetes in specific studies, three parameters have been selected: libido, orgasm, and fertility. Intrinsic to these parameters are the psychologic factors that may contribute to sexual drives and urges, coital response, and the ability to procreate.

Libido and Orgasm

Researchers found various sexual disturbances noted in the literature concerning the libido of women with diabetes. They reported that the subjects experienced a change in sexual life. For example, the women experienced a reluctance to have sexual intercourse, an increase in menstrual disorders, and a loss of orgasm and clitoral erectility. Problems reported were usually fatigue, changes in perimenstrual blood glucose control, vaginitis, decreased sexual desire, decreased vaginal lubrication, and an increase in time to reach orgasm. There appears to be no correlation of libido and orgasmic response whether neuropathy is present or not. Vaginal lubrication, leading to painful intercourse, lower sexual interest, and lethargy are reported the most.

Although much less research is reported on women's sexuality and diabetes than on men, the following two studies do contribute important knowledge that still is found to be current in clinical practice.

Sexual arousal in females with diabetes was researched by Wincze, Albert, and Bansai (1993). They determined that the women demonstrated significantly less physiologic arousal to erotic stimuli than the controls, whereas their subjective responses were comparable. These objective, physiologic findings support and extend previous subjectively based research that found potential diabetes-related sexual dysfunction in female patients with diabetes. The study groups did not differ in the recorded occurrence of sexual difficulties.

Another study indicated a significant difference between the subjects with diabetes and without diabetes in relation to orgasmic function (Dunning, 1993). In the group of 125 women with diabetes, 44 (35%) reported an absence of orgasmic response in the year preceding the study. Only 6 of the 100 women without diabetes made the same report. Of the 44 women with diabetes without orgasm, 40 had previously been orgasmic prior to their diagnosis of diabetes mellitus.

Sexual dysfunction in women with diabetes, as in men with diabetes, can originate, despite one study previously cited, on the basis of neurologic changes. Masters et al. (1992) support the concept that orgasm in women derives from clitoral stimulation. Alteration of the nerve fibers of the clitoris has been found in women with diabetes. When the fibers of nervus pudendus clitoridis were examined microscopically in the 1970s, degenerative changes of this nerve were revealed in females having diabetes in all age groups. Particularly severe changes were found in women with a long duration of diabetes, that is, more than 10 years. The changes that occurred in this nerve could alter the orgasmic status of women who had diabetes. Diabetes may not be the culprit that prevents women from being orgasmic. It is important to remember that only 30% of females in the general population report reaching orgasm during intercourse without direct stimulation of the clitoris; female patients with diabetes should be no different. However, arousal phase disturbances, from whatever cause, such as a decrease in lubrication during sexual activity or the tiredness response due to hyperglycemia, may decrease the orgasmic response. Other factors associated with diabetes, such as urinary bladder dysfunction or vaginitis, may also have an impact on the sexual function of women with this metabolic disease.

Although the potential for alteration in sex drive exists in women with diabetes, it must be remembered that the sex drive differs from person to person and may also vary in the same person periodically. Age, culture, physical wellness, and psychologic status may influence desire. Although discussion of the effects of culture and age on sex drive is beyond the scope of this chapter, it is important to consider their contribution to sex drive when examining the sexual function of women with diabetes. Consideration must also be given to how the individual adapts to the disease and the potential physiologic changes that result from this metabolic disorder. Both factors may contribute to sexual dysfunction.

Fertility

Although evidence abounds that euglycemia during pregnancy will support a positive outcome, a preponderance of literature about women with diabetes concerns the problems women encounter during pregnancy. Among these problems are difficulty in controlling diabetes, increased danger to toxemia and fetal loss, termination of the pregnancy before due date, possibility of the offspring becoming diabetic, and congenital malformations. All of these factors could affect the sex drive of this population. Thus, women of childbearing age, faced with the potential of a multitude of problems resulting from diabetes and pregnancy, may wish to limit the number of their pregnancies. These components could lead to a decrease in sex drive and consequently an alteration in sexual response. Because of lack of data, it is impossible, at this time, to be certain that the aforementioned factors associated with pregnancy are major determinants of sexual dysfunction in this population.

Diagnosis

The appropriate evaluation of patients with sexual dysfunction should include a medical and detailed sexual history, a physical examination, a psychosocial evaluation, and basic laboratory tests. The general medical history is important in identifying specific risk factors that may account for or contribute to patients' problems. These include additional vascular risk factors, such as hypertension, smoking, coronary artery disease, peripheral vascular disorders, pelvic trauma or surgery, and blood lipid abnormalities. Decreased sexual desire or history suggesting a hypogonadal state could indicate a primary endocrine disorder. Neurologic causes may include a history of alcoholism, with associated peripheral neuropathy in addition to the known diabetes. It is also essential to obtain a detailed medication and illicit drug history, because an estimated 25% of cases of erectile dysfunction may be attributable to medications for other conditions.

For erectile dysfunction complaints, an endocrine evaluation consisting of a morning serum testosterone is generally indicated. It is also recommended that serum prolactin should be measured. It is important to note that decreased testosterone levels are not commonly identified in patients with diabetes. A low testosterone level merits repeat measurement, together with assessment of luteinizing hormone (LH) and follicle-stimulating hormone (FSH). Other tests may be helpful in excluding unrecognized systemic disease. A complete blood count, urinalysis, creatinine, fasting lipid profile, hemoglobin A1c, and thyroid profile with thyroid-stimulating hormone (TSH) tests are all relevant.

Quantification of erectile function may be evaluated by (a) the use of a snap gauge fastener for measurement of maximum penile rigidity, or (b) continuous nocturnal penile tumescence and rigidity monitoring by recording of circumferential penile expansion and concurrent rigidity during sleep. These definitive measures are particularly useful in differentiating psychogenic and organic erectile dysfunctions.

The outcome of measurements of nocturnal penile tumescent episodes should be compared with lack of metabolic control and the presence of other diabetes-related complications to determine the possible source of erectile dysfunction. Comparison with psychogenic measures related to self-image should then be taken into account.

Treatment

Medications

Several therapeutic options, which depend on the nature of the erectile dysfunction, are available for male patients. With uncontrolled diabetes, the focus of treatment must begin with euglycemia.

In cases of endocrine dysfunction, replacement measures are directed at restoring maximum physical health. Although testosterone therapy has been a somewhat controversial subject, it is commonly recommended for patients with clear-cut hypogonadism if there are no other contraindications. If androgen therapy is indicated, it can be given by a daily testosterone transdermal patch, in the form of intramuscular injections every 2–3 weeks, or by the implant of testosterone pellets every 3 months (Testosterone Facts and Comparisons, 2000). This therapy has been associated with side effects such as gynecomastia, liver dysfunction, prostatic hypertrophy, polycythemia, and water retention; therefore, its use should be monitored closely. Treatment of men with hyperprolactinemia, bromocriptine therapy, often is effective in normalizing the prolactin level and improving sexual function.

Oral pharmacologic treatment of erectile dysfunction has been successful with the advent of sildenafil citrate (Viagra). In the largest study of men with T2DM taking Viagra, 56% reported improved erections after 12 weeks. Viagra was equally effective for these men regardless of age or duration of diabetes or erectile dysfunction (Sandovsky, Miller, Moskowitz, & Hackett, 2001). Viagra creates an erection with sexual stimulation by blocking phosphodiesterase 5, an enzyme that breaks down the erection-producing chemical, cycle guanosine monophosphate. Viagra is taken an hour before sexual relations. Only one treatment of 25, 50, or 100 mg in 24 hr is recommended because of the potential for hypertension. Viagra is contraindicated in men with cardiovascular disease who take medications containing nitrates, such as nitroglycerin, because interaction of those drugs with Viagra can cause life-threatening hypotension.

Research results have been released on vardenafil, Bayer Pharmaceuticals' phosphodiesterase-5 inhibitor (Levitra). The study of 580 men, ages 21–70 years, found that the oral treatment not only improved erections in up to 80% of men, but also increased their ability to complete sexual intercourse with ejaculation regardless of age or the cause or severity of their problem. Adverse events were generally mild, for example, headache, flushing, rhinitis, and dyspepsia, and related to dosage (Bayer Pharmaceuticals, 2001). It is available in 2.5, 5, 10, and 20 mg tablets. It also must be taken 1 hr before activity. Again, it must not be taken with nitrates or sodium nitroprusside. It is not for the person with cardiovascular disease or liver disease.

Cialis (Tadalafil) is an erectile dysfunction treatment that lasts up to about 36 hr. It is only to be taken once daily, but at no specific time before sexual activity. It is available in 5, 10, and 20 mg tablets. It has similar warnings: It should not be used in individuals with known cardiac disease (especially when the person has to use nitroglycerine for self-treatment) or hepatic disease. Headache, nasal congestion, dyspepsia, muscle pain, flushing, and visual disturbances are some of the adverse reactions noted.

Another pharmacologic treatment of erectile dysfunction and/or decreased desire involves the oral use of the alpha-adrenergic antagonist, yohimbine. This herb, available by prescription, has been reported to have limited success in patients without diabetes as well as in patients with diabetes, but it is an option for men who cannot take Viagra, Levitra, or Cialis. Although the treatment with yohimbine is painless, it must be continuous and side effects have been reported. The recommendation is not to take this herb unless under the direct supervision of a health professional.

Two forms (injectable [Caverject] and transurethral pellet [MUSE]) of alprostadil (prostaglandin E1) have been approved by the U.S. Food and Drug Administration (FDA) for the treatment of erectile dysfunction. Alprostadil, like other prostaglandins, causes relaxation of smooth muscle and vasodilation. The drug increases arterial inflow through vasodilation and decreases venous outflow by causing relaxation of corporal smooth muscle that occludes draining venules.

After unilateral intracavernous injection (Caverject), alprostadil acts bilaterally through cross-circulation; dosage is arrived at by titration in the physician's office. The endpoint is an erection suitable for intercourse that does not last more than 1 hr. The site of injection recommended by the manufacturer is along the dorsolateral aspects of the proximal third of the penis, alternating sides and sites for each injection. The manufacturer warns against using the drug more than 3 times per week or more than once in 24 hr. The main adverse effects of alprostadil injections into the corpus cavernosum, all dose related, have been pain after injection, prolonged erection or priapism and, with continued use, penile fibrosis, including Peyronie's disease. Orthostatic hypotension rarely has occurred and, if so, usually with higher doses.

MUSE is a single-use, medicated transurethral system for the delivery of alprostadil to the male urethra. Alprostadil is formed into a medicated pellet (microsuppository) and is administered by inserting the applicator stem into the urethra after urination. MUSE system is packaged in an individual foil pouch and is available in four dosage strengths to be determined by the physician. The lower dosages are recommended for initial dosing and titrated in a stepwise manner until the patient achieves an erection that is sufficient for sexual intercourse. The onset of effect is within 5–10 min after administration and the duration is 30–60 min. Each patient should be instructed by a medical professional on the proper technique prior to self-administration. The maximum frequency of use is recommended to be no more than two systems per 24-hr period. Reported adverse reactions include penile pain, urethral burning, minor urethral bleeding and spotting, testicular pain, and dizziness. Orthostatic hypotension may be caused by overdosage. Vaginal burning or itching was the most common drug-related adverse event (5.8%) reported by female partners during placebo-controlled clinical studies (MUSE package insert, VIVUS, Inc., 1997).

In cases of neurogenic and some vasculopathic causes of erectile dysfunction, vacuum constriction devices may be effective. These devices are rigid plastic tubes placed over a well-lubricated penis, creating a vacuum and inducing negative pressure, which results in blood flow into the penis and subsequent erection. A rubber ring is then placed at the base of the penis to restrict venous outflow. These devices have been used with some success to maintain erection sufficient for vaginal penetration. Although a low incidence of side effects is documented, penile ecchymosis and petechiae have occurred. Generally, no treatment is required. Additionally, patients have reported some difficulty with ejaculation. Partner involvement in training with these devices would help ensure a successful outcome and a more mutually satisfying level of sexual activity.

Surgical Implantation

Surgical implantation of silicone prostheses in some men with diabetes who have complete erectile dysfunction has been undertaken successfully. All types of penile prostheses have two cylinders that are placed within the two chambers of the penis that would normally fill with blood during an erection. It is important to inform the patient that every surgical procedure involves some risks such as infection. With the patient with diabetes, normalization of blood glucose levels prior to surgery and during the healing must be emphasized. Medical risks can vary from patient to patient and should be discussed with the implanting urologist prior to surgery. Sexual activity may usually be resumed

4–6 weeks postprocedure. Men with penile implants are usually able to achieve an orgasm, ejaculate, and impregnate a female if they were able to do so before the need of an implant.

Penile prostheses are available in four forms for patients who fail with or refuse other forms of therapy: the semirigid rod, the inflatable penile prosthesis, the self-contained inflatable penile prosthesis, and the positional penile prosthesis. Desirable components of a penile prosthesis include extended size range; simple implantation procedure, requiring only local anesthesia; positional stability (no spring back); excellent rigidity and less pain during the healing process. It is easy for patients to use and gives a good cosmetic result (Stanley, Bivalacqua, & Helistrom, 2000).

Revascularization

Revascularization of the penis has been attempted, using the inferior epigastric artery to the corpus cavernosum or the dorsal penile artery. In addition to increasing arterial inflow, venous outflow has also seemed to be reduced.

Hormone Replacement Therapy

For the female patient with diabetes, an endocrine workup may also be helpful. Hormone replacement therapy (HRT) for the surgically or chronologically menopausal woman may relieve desire and/or lubrication issues. Conflicting research reports continue to confound health care professionals and the general public with regard to possible benefits or problems of HRT related to osteoporosis, heart disease, Alzheimer's disease, and colon cancer. Each patient must be carefully evaluated by her physician to determine whether she is a candidate for HRT. Estrogen alone or a combination of estrogen, in low dosage, and testosterone may be prescribed for the menopausal patient with a surgically removed uterus. To protect against endometrial cancer, progesterone will be added to these regimens if the patient has an intact uterus.

Blood Glucose Level Control

Yeast- or bacterial-caused vaginitis and/or urinary tract infections in the female can be significant deterrents to sexual interaction. Judicious control of blood glucose and prompt identification and treatment of infections are a must. It is also important to evaluate and treat the sexual partner to prevent cross- or reinfection in those sexually transmitted diseases.

In the individual with poorly controlled diabetes, sexual dysfunction may be a manifestation of malnutrition and associated weakness. Correction of the metabolic aspect of diabetes control will restore a more normal nutritional state and strength, and may alleviate the sexual arousal for both men and women. It is appropriate to advise testing blood glucose levels before and after sexual activity, noting the time of day in relation to the peak action of insulin, meal time, and the duration of sexual activity.

Counseling

If it is determined that the sexual dysfunction is psychogenic in origin, appropriate sexual counseling or therapy is indicated. Sexual counseling is a process of education and advisement grounded in knowledge of biologic, psychologic, and social sciences. Sexual therapy includes this process but is a form of psychotherapy. The purpose of both sexual counseling and therapy is to resolve personal and interpersonal conflicts that may result in some degree of sexual dysfunction.

According to the American Association of Sex Educators, Counselors, and Therapists (AASECT) (2008), the promotion of sexual health goals in therapy can be wide. The goal of the therapist and the patients may vary from the reassurance and relief gained from accurate information imparted in a half-hour discussion to a fundamental reorientation of the personality after long years of intense therapy. Most individuals who enter therapy are merely confused or anxious about their sexual identity or their sexual roles. The goal of sexual therapy then becomes one of providing increased understanding and awareness of the wide range of possibilities for expressing sexual desire.

Sexual therapy seeks to enable individuals to grow in their capacity to:

a. Manage sex creatively and without exploitation of others in their own life situations;
b. Improve their sexual function, thus enriching their own lives and those of others;
c. Communicate effectively with their sex partners; and
d. Increase their joy and fulfillment.

Sexual Interviewing and Responsibilities of Health Professionals

Obtaining accurate information to assess the sexual status of an individual is the prelude to counseling and treating sexual difficulties. Topics of a sexual nature tend to evoke discomfort in the person who is receiving the content and in the person who is disclosing. Professionals may be desensitized through education. Interviewing is not an art, but rather a professional skill that can be learned. Although this chapter does not contain an in-depth exploration of the process of the sexual interview, several major considerations are included.

Foremost, the interviewer has the responsibility to be objective and nonjudgmental and to establish a relationship with the client that demonstrates response. Aside from objectivity and rapport, one must consider other components as part of the interviewing process. Among these is the setting, which should be private, free from distractions, and conducive to an atmosphere of comfort. The elements of therapeutic communication must also be incorporated. Attention must be given to the approach being used. When specific information is needed, the interviewer leads the individual in that direction. If the interviewer is uncomfortable, the patient will be uncomfortable.

The language employed by the professional and the patient presents another consideration. The fact that different terms are used to mean the same thing presents the problem of which expression to use when interviewing so that personal affronts, patronization, and misunderstandings are prevented. There is no common agreement as to words or phrases to be used in discussing sexuality. The interviewees need to be provided the opportunity to express themselves in their own words; however, meanings must be clarified.

Interview Outline

The PLISSIT model developed by J. S. Anion (1976) was one of the first interview guides developed for this field. This interview guide provides for four intervention levels with the client, allows the health professional to direct the approach on a personal level of confidence, and establishes guidelines for referral to a more specialized professional:

> P—Permission giving: Establish trust, offer reassurance of normalcy
> LI—Limited Information: Educate about diabetes and sexuality
> SS—Specific Suggestions: Give accurate, pertinent information about specific concerns.
> IT—Intensive Therapy: Refer to a sex therapist certified by the American Association of Sex Educators, Counselors, and Therapists.

Certain areas should be addressed whether or not the interviewer uses a form when compiling a sexual history. In general, the interview can be divided into three basic questions that can be modified to specifically deal with illness, hospitalization, life events, and any other element that may influence or interfere with sexual health:

1. How has diabetes affected the way you see yourself as a man or woman?
2. How has diabetes affected your role as a single man or woman, husband, wife, mother, father?
3. How has diabetes affected you or your ability to function sexually?

These questions are nonthreatening and place sexuality in its proper context of self-concept, self-esteem, and role performance. If sexual problems are found to exist, it is important that the patients describe them in their own words, including onset, nature, and duration. It is often helpful to categorize questions around the sexual response cycle, determining if the problem is in the desire, excitement, orgasm, or resolution phase. At this point, it is vital to determine the understanding of the person in relation to the problem and the history of any previous evaluations or treatments. Finally, explore the individual's desires and expectations related to treatment so that a common ground is established before any interventions are discussed.

Health Professional Responsibilities

With recognition that sexual health is a right of all individuals, it is no longer debatable that health professionals have a role in the sexual counseling of patients. For professionals to help facilitate sexual adaptation, they will need to increase their knowledge and assessment skills and evaluate their own attitudes and beliefs concerning human sexuality.

In the past 30 years, many health care providers have made a concentrated effort to develop new knowledge about the methods of assistance in the areas of human sexuality and sexual dysfunction. Yet our society is still plagued with much misinformation and trouble about sexual function. As awareness increases in our society, more health care consumers will be requesting help with sexual problems.

Professional health care involves addressing the totality of patient needs, including sexuality. Clinical practice will change with the advancement of knowledge and change of attitudes. Health care providers can prepare themselves to deal with sexuality as a vitally important aspect of health care by being willing to be educated to assist in this long-neglected area. Consideration must be given to the following:

1. One's own values, attitudes, and beliefs toward sexual function must be examined closely. The person must be willing to separate sexual myth from fact to provide accurate information.
2. If they are to maintain a sensitive and nonjudgmental position toward individuals who are experiencing sexual problems, health professionals must become familiar with the wide range of values, attitudes, and beliefs of other persons.
3. Health professionals must take advantage of educational opportunities to increase their knowledge of sexual growth and changes that occur during the life cycle.
4. If the health professional wishes to become directly involved in counseling or therapy with persons who are experiencing a sexual problem, he or she must receive further education and proper certification in the techniques and methods of assistance for treating specific problems.
5. Sexual health programs should be affiliated with reputable health care agencies that are supervised by qualified individuals. All health professionals need to acquaint themselves with reputable sexual health programs in their communities to make appropriate referrals for the person with sexually associated problems.

Certification in both sexual counseling and therapy is currently available through the AASECT. Although certification requirements of the association are specific and stringent, most states have no regulations pertaining to these fields. Thus, in most states anyone can claim to be a sexual therapist. There must be an awareness of the qualification of the individual therapist before referring any patient for sexual concerns.

Summary

Hyperglycemia may lead to sexual dysfunction. Problems and concerns about sexual functioning may contribute to hyperglycemia. Whether male or female, education (e.g., *Diabetes for Guys: A Guy Flick*, 2000) and appropriate support will assist the person with diabetes to become more knowledgeable about this normal side of life and, in turn, assist the individual to live a more balanced and joyful existence.

References

American Association of Sex Education, Counselors, and Therapists (AASECT). (2008). *Promotion of sexual health.* Retrieved September 10, 2008, from www.AASECT.org

American Association of Sex Educators, Counselors, and Therapists (AASECT). (2008). *Certification; Professional standards.* Retrieved August 29, 2008, from www.aasect.org

American Psychiatric Association. (2000). *Diagnostic and statistical manual of mental disorders* (4th ed.). Washington, DC: Author.

Anion, J. S. (1976). *Behavioral treatment of sexual problems: Vol. 1, Brief therapy.* New York: Harper & Row.

Bayer Pharmaceuticals. (2001). *Study shows vardenafil improved erectile function regardless of age or severity of erectile difficulty.* Princeton, NJ: Author.

Bradley, W., Timm, G., Johnson, B., & Gallager, J. (1985). Continuous penile tumescence and rigidity monitoring in the evaluation of impotence. *Urology, 26,* 4.

Diabetes for guys: A guy flick. (2000). Alexandria, VA: American Diabetes Association.

Doruk, H., Akbay, E., Cayan, S., Akbay, E., Bozlu, M., & Acar, D. (2005). Effect of diabetes mellitus on female sexual function and risk factors. *Archives of Andrology, 51*(1), 1–6.

Dunning, P. (1993). Sexuality and women with diabetes. *Patient Education Counseling, 21*(1–2), 5–14.

Ellenberg, M. (1971). Impotence in diabetes: The neurologic factor. *Annals of Internal Medicine, 75,* 213.

Intracavernous injection of alprostadil for erectile dysfunction. (1995). *The Medical Letter, 37*(9), 58.

Jack, L., Jr. (2005). Professional development: A candid conversation about men, sexual health, and diabetes. *Diabetes Educator, 31*(6), 810–817.

Kapoor, D., Clarke, S., Channer, K. S., & Jones, T. H. (2007). Erectile dysfunction is associated with low bioactive testosterone levels and visceral adiposity in men with type 2 diabetes. *International Journal of Andrology, 30*(6), 500–507.

Masters, W., Johnson, V., & Kolodny, R. (1992). *Human sexuality* (4th ed.). New York: Harper Collins.

MUSE. (1997). Package insert. VIVUS, Inc.

National Institutes of Health. (1992). *Consensus development conference on impotence.* Bethesda, MD.

Rubin, A. (1967). Sexual behavior in diabetes mellitus. *Medical Aspects of Human Sexuality, I,* 23.

Rubin, A., & Babbot, D. (1958). Impotence and diabetes mellitus. *Journal of the American Medical Association, 168,* 498.

Rutherford, D., & Collier, A. (2005). Sexual dysfunction in women with diabetes mellitus. *Gynecological Endocrinology, 21*(4), 189–192.

Sandovsky, R., Miller, T., Moskowitz, M., & Hackett, G. (2001). Three-year update of sildenafil citrate (Viagra) efficacy and safety. *International Journal of Clinical Practice, 55*(2), 115–128.

Spark, R. F. (2007). Testosterone, diabetes mellitus, and the metabolic syndrome. *Current Urological Repertoire, 8*(6), 467–471.

Stanley, G. E., Bivalacqua, T. J., & Helistrom, W. J. G. (2000). Penile prosthetic trends in the era of effective oral erectogenic agents. *Southern Medical Journal, 93*(12), 1153–1156.

Testosterone pellets and testosterone transdermal system. (2000). *Facts and comparisons.* St. Louis: Wolters Kluwer.

West, S. L., Vinikoor, L. C., & Zolnoun, D. (2004). A systematic review of the literature on female sexual dysfunction, prevalence and predictors. *Annual Review of Sex Research, 15,* 40–172.

Wincze, J., Albert, A., & Bansai, S. (1993). Sexual arousal in diabetic females: Physiological and self report measures. *Archives of Sexual Behavior, 22*(6), 587–601.

World Health Organization. (1975). *Education and treatment in human sexuality: The training of health professionals* (Report of a WHO meeting, Technical Report Series, No. 572).

25

Surgery

Several complications of diabetes can be alleviated by surgical procedures. Surgery is risky at any time. Physicians, at times, disagree in their evaluation of the surgical risk of the person with diabetes. More and more surgeons believe that patients with diabetes encounter a surgical risk no greater than that of the general population so long as blood glucose levels are controlled. It is expected that if blood glucose levels are maintained in the normal range, the person with diabetes should heal like a person without diabetes, whether the surgery is for repair, after an accident, for an infection, or for a need related to one of the diabetes complications. Data from many sources support the need for normalizing the blood glucose levels before, during, and after surgery (Funary, Zerr, Grunkeineier, & Starr, 1999; Krinsley, 2003; Pomposelli et al., 1998; Umpierrez et al., 2002; Zerr et al., 1997). Normalizing blood glucose levels is important in surgery of any kind whether the patient is known to have diabetes or has previously not had a diagnosis of diabetes.

"Standards of Medical Care in Diabetes" (ADA, 2008) includes recommendations for blood glucose level control during surgical procedures.

Cardiovascular Status and Surgery

Diabetes mellitus is a condition that more frequently occurs in the middle-aged and the elderly. Vascular changes not only associated with advancing age, but also with diabetes mellitus, should not be overlooked when the patient is considered for surgery. To estimate the vascular age (or functional age) of the individual, one adds together the number of years the individual has had diabetes plus the chronological age (especially if the individual has had poorly controlled diabetes).

The outcome of any surgery in the individual with diabetes mellitus may be influenced by the probable existence of premature arteriosclerosis with resulting cardiac, renal, and cerebral complications. Even if control can be maintained and the risk of microvascular disease decreased, preventing macrovascular changes in the older population continues to be more of a problem. Attaining and maintaining normalization of blood glucose levels as much as safely tolerated remains the best hope for the person who has diabetes undergoing a surgical procedure.

Surgical Procedures in Person With Diabetes

There are several surgical procedures performed more frequently in people with diabetes than the population without diabetes. The surgery most often performed is the amputation of a part or all of a limb as a result of foot ulcers, osteomyelitis, or gangrene. Gangrene or ulcers of the lower extremities are caused by peripheral vascular disease and diabetic neuropathy. Sophisticated surgical procedures such as vascular grafts can benefit the person who has diabetes who has developed peripheral vascular disease (PVD). Coronary bypass grafts, femoral popliteal bypass grafts, balloon angioplasty, endarterectomy, and laser angioplasty are examples of procedures that are being used in people with diabetes in whom macrovasculopathy is present. Added to this are the procedures deemed important for individuals that are obese. These have been the lap-band procedures for individuals of gross obesity, plus the past surgical procedures such as stomach stapling or intestinal bypass.

Abscesses, such as furuncles and carbuncles, are not observed as often as they were in past years. Better diabetes control, better hygiene, and the use of antibiotics have brought about the decline in the occurrence of this once serious problem. When abscesses do occur, however, some of them require normalized glucose levels and extensive surgical incisions to promote debridement, drainage, and healing.

Acute and chronic cholelithiasis and cholecystitis must be mentioned. The progression of cholelithiasis or cholecystitis to necrosis and sepsis increases the indications for early surgery in the person with diabetes. Controversy exists only about when the surgical procedure should be done, not if it needs to be done, and with today's microsurgical procedures (laparoscopic surgery) and good diabetes control, most patients are out of the hospital the same day as the surgery.

Physiologic Considerations

Diabetes control is affected by stressors, which may be caused by both emotional and/or physiologic upheavals. Surgery and the anesthetic agents themselves are physiologic stressors. The body reacts to these stressors to maintain homeostasis. The homeostatic reaction involves the release of at least two hormones, epinephrine and the glucocorticoids, which cause a rise in the blood glucose level, an increase in free fatty acids, and a fall in the serum insulin levels in persons with endogenous insulin-secreting ability.

A decrease in glucose tolerance has been observed in most people undergoing a surgical procedure. The greatest degree of glucose intolerance was noted on the third postoperative day. In 1973, Wright and Johnson observed the glucose tolerance returning to normal by the eighth postoperative day. Later, Keith and Pieper (1989) studied the effect of perioperative blood glucose levels and their effect on surgery and reached a similar conclusion.

It is commonly recognized now that getting through the third day is the hardest whether the person has diabetes or not. Since more discomfort is experienced during these days, it is logical that pain itself will influence glucose levels and result in a need for supplemental doses of diabetes medication. The healing time of those without diabetes is usually seven to ten days. If blood glucose levels are controlled, this same healing time should apply for the person with diabetes.

Preoperative Preparation

The outcome of any surgery is a result of the combined effort in planning, execution, and follow-up of four key medical professionals: the internist (or pediatrician, in the case of children), the nurse, the surgeon, and the anesthesiologist.

Preoperative preparation must proceed with detail. Preferably, most surgery should be performed on an elective rather than an emergency basis. Preparing the patient for elective surgery should allow adequate time to ensure that the diabetes is under reasonable control and the patient is educated as to the expectations prior to, during, and after the surgical procedures. Reasonable control means the absence of symptoms of hyperglycemia (polydipsia and polyuria) and a presurgical blood glucose level of less than 150 mg/dl (8.3 mmol/L).

The medical workup should include, but is not limited to, all of the following:

1. Detailed diabetes history.
   a. Date of diagnosis.
   b. Medical management program.
   c. Diet and dietary habits.
   d. Recent history of diabetic ketoacidosis and/or severe hypoglycemia.
   e. Weight vs. height—BMI.
2. Evaluation of vascular status and complications of diabetes mellitus.
   a. Renal status.
   b. Cardiovascular status.
   c. Peripheral vascular status.
   d. Cerebral vascular status.
3. Previous illnesses, accidents, infections, and surgeries.
4. General history and physical examination.

5. Diagnostic tests, particularly those whose results reflect the diabetes control and the absence or presence of complications.
   a. Fasting and postprandial blood glucose levels for three to five days.
   b. Hemoglobin A1c.
   c. Electrolytes, i.e., sodium, potassium; and the acid-base deficit (HCO3).
   d. Complete metabolic profile.
   e. Fasting lipid profile.
   f. Complete blood count.
   g. Urinalysis.
   h. Electrocardiogram.
6. Other medications including over-the-counter drugs, vitamins, minerals, and herbs.
   a. Drug allergies, response to past anesthetics (if appropriate), and any use of social drugs including alcohol and tobacco.

Preoperative preparation (see also Appendix L) of the person also includes careful consideration of the choice of the anesthetic agent to be used (Aviles-Santo & Raskin, 1998). The ability of a drug to raise or lower the blood glucose level is not the sole criterion in choosing or rejecting the anesthetic gas or injectable. The type of surgery to be performed is a definite determinant in the choice of anesthesia. The age of the patient is another. The physiologic state of the individual is yet another; for example, if the lower extremity is involved, spinal anesthesia may be what is chosen.

Management During Surgery

Understanding the management and care of the patient undergoing surgery is facilitated if one knows the patient's needs and the criteria of maintaining blood glucose levels between 110 mg/dl (6.1 mmol) and 140 mg/dl (7.8 mmol) are maintained (ADA, 2008).

Type 2 Diet Controlled

The patient with diet-controlled Type 2 diabetes mellitus (T2DM) requires little more preoperative preparation than does the individual without diabetes. The extensive workup is usually done in the physician's office. An attempt is made for the individual to be in optimal blood glucose control.

On the day of surgery, the past diabetes history and admission blood glucose level are obtained. These serve as starting points from which subsequent blood glucose values are obtained and assessed during surgery and postoperatively.

The complications one watches for, during the postoperative period, are hyperglycemia, diabetic ketoacidosis (DKA), and hyperglycemic hyperosmolar nonketotic syndrome (HHNS). The latter is a particular danger in the very elderly. Surgery, physiologic stress, and fluid and electrolyte losses may hasten the onset of the complications mentioned. These problems are rare in the patient with diet-controlled diabetes, but should be observed through careful blood glucose monitoring in the postoperative period.

Type 2 Oral Agent Controlled

The patient taking any oral agent should at least check blood glucose levels 3–5 days before surgery. If the person's control of diabetes is poor, it may be advisable to institute insulin therapy before, during, and for a while after the surgical period. On the day of surgery, all oral agents (i.e., insulin secretagogues [sulfonylureas and meglitinides more apt to result in hypoglycemia than other oral agents], hepatic glucose production blockers [metformin], thiazolidinediones and insulin sensitizers [pioglitazone; rosiglitazone], and alpha-glucosidase inhibitors [acarbose; miglitol], or any mixture of these) should be withheld. Close observation for signs and symptoms of hypoglycemia during and after surgery is most important so blood glucose monitoring must be maintained at specified intervals.

The previous day's blood glucose level tests may be used as a baseline. Intravenous feedings with a solution of D5 and one-half normal saline or D5LR as dictated by the individual's condition should be started in the morning on the day of surgery. Hypoglycemia during surgery in this group is rare. Conversely, hyperglycemia could occur secondary to the administration of dextrose solutions in combination with loss of fluids and electrolytes, anesthesia, and the stress of surgery.

In the postoperative period, it may be necessary to administer small amounts of insulin at regular intervals to maintain control. As soon as the patient is able to eat and normal glycemic levels have been established, oral hypoglycemic agents may be reinstituted. If major surgery is performed, IV insulin should be used in surgery and the postoperative period until feeding is resumed.

Type 1 or Type 2 Insulin Controlled

The patient who depends on insulin for control requires closer observation and careful monitoring of the diabetes status. Ideally, such patients should enter the hospital at least one or more days before surgery, but this does not fit the admission criteria unless the person's blood glucose levels are 250 mg/dl (13.8 mmol) or higher. If control is less than reasonable—that is, if blood glucose levels are higher than 200 mg/dl (11.1 mmol), intensive work should be done to assist the patient to have normalized blood glucose levels more of the time before entering the hospital for surgery or before having the surgical procedure. Patients dependent on insulin and patients requiring insulin should be free of the symptoms of hyperglycemia (polydipsia and polyuria) before surgery.

Ketoacidosis or ketosis must be brought under control before any consideration for surgery, except in the most extreme, life-threatening circumstances. Dehydration and electrolyte imbalance secondary to glycosuria and ketoacidosis can be expected to develop within a 24-hr or sooner period if a person dependent on insulin is without the availability of exogenous insulin. Surgery is extremely hazardous in the presence of these complications and should almost always be deferred until the ketoacidosis and accompanying electrolyte imbalance are under control.

During surgery, both hypoglycemia and hyperglycemia should be prevented. Hypoglycemia could go unnoticed if close attention is not paid to vital signs and blood glucose values. Hyperglycemia might result from dehydration, electrolyte imbalance, and ketoacidosis, which can also be devastating and life threatening. The balance lies in determining the most appropriate amount of insulin to prevent both hypoglycemia and hyperglycemia.

It is important that the diet and dosage of insulin that the patient takes at home on a regular basis be ascertained. On entering the hospital, the patient receives a concise calorie and/or carb counted diet, so insulin requirements may drop drastically.

On the morning of the surgery, a fasting blood glucose value should be obtained. Intravenous feedings are started: preferably D5 and one-half normal saline (anesthesiologists often use Ringer's lactate, but will accept D5 and Ringer's lactate when they don't agree to use D5 and one-half normal saline).

There is some disagreement among surgeons and diabetologists regarding how much insulin, what kind of insulin, and at what time insulin should be administered during and after surgery. This disagreement suggests that the ideal system of management has not yet been devised. Machines for continuous blood glucose monitoring are becoming increasingly available. Flexibility and sensitivity to the patient's changing needs are required.

The following are various regimens:

1. Short-acting (regular) insulin is given every 6 hr, based on the total amount of daily insulin divided by four (i.e., 25% of total daily insulin is given as regular insulin every 6 hr). No long-acting insulin is given the day of surgery. Additional insulin is given as indicated by blood glucose determinations monitored before each insulin dose.

2. One-half of the usual dosage of intermediate-acting insulin is administered before surgery. The remaining half is given in the recovery room after surgery or one third of this type of insulin is given before surgery and one third is given after surgery.

3. The following are procedures for children and adults dependent on or requiring insulin:

   a. Insulin is given by IV infusion (0.05 Unit$\cdot$kg$^{-1}\cdot$hr^{-1} of rapid- or short-acting insulin) during the surgical procedure with the insulin started once the IV is in place. Insulin may be titrated up or down depending on the blood glucose readings on an hourly basis using an approved protocol (there are a number of protocols available: Markowitz protocol, Portland protocol, Yale protocol, and others; Van den Berghe et al. [2001]; and there are many locally designed or modified protocols in use; Wilson, Weinreb, & Hoo, 2007). We use a slight modification of the Yale protocol in which the starting insulin dose is based on body weight, not on blood glucose level, to reduce the risk of under- or overdosing because of differences in insulin sensitivity from thinness or obesity,

   b. Basal insulin (glargine; detemer) is usually given on a daily basis or the basal on a pump setting may be used along with IV fluids (English & Young, 2005). Electrolytes may be added as parameters determine. Rapid-acting analogs (or short-acting insulin) are added once the person is in recovery and a blood sugar level is obtained and reported. If a 5% dextrose solution does not maintain the blood glucose levels at normal infusion rates, 10% solutions may be used (see Appendix L for presurgery orders).

When injected insulin is to be started (i.e., when being given either as a basal insulin going to a basal-bolus program or other type of injected insulin programs), the rapid-acting insulin is to be injected 10–15 min before the IV is stopped; the short-acting insulin is to be injected 30 min before the IV is stopped; the intermediate-acting insulin is to be injected 45–60 min before the IV is stopped; and the long-acting insulin is to be injected 2 hr before the IV is stopped. A transitional insulin protocol can be found in Appendix E.

Postoperatively, immediately and every 1–6 hr finger-stick blood glucose specimens should be tested, especially before each insulin dose, and the insulin dosage should be adjusted as needed. If dietary intake is started, it is recommended that blood glucose levels are checked prebreakfast and 2 hr (or 1 hr for some programs) after eating.

The infusion of dextrose solution must be continuous to cover the long-acting, rapid- and/or short-acting insulins and to cover the patient's caloric need when the patient is taking nothing by mouth (NPO). It is possible for patients who have diabetes and are undergoing surgery to have documented severe hypoglycemia on regimens using any insulin, such as intermediate-acting insulin, that has a peak action. The regimens using intermediate-acting insulin are now considered inappropriate therapy for most patients, particularly in the pre- and postoperative period.

Insulins that are peakless and are long-acting lead to a reduced possibility of severe hypoglycemia occurring, but consideration must be given as to variability of needs during extensive surgery and of a surgery of long duration if these insulins are used. These insulins are usually given in full dose the night before the surgery. If the surgery is to be of long duration, the IV insulin drip approach is usually the one chosen.

Most surgeons and anesthesiologists believe that the greatest danger for the person with insulin-dependent diabetes is hypoglycemia (Maser, Eller, & DeCherney, 1996). The paradox is that almost everything done raises rather than lowers the blood glucose levels during and after surgery. Unrecognized and untreated hypoglycemia will endanger the patient's life, but is rare during and after surgery. Because hypertension or hypotension are signs of hypoglycemia, any such change during surgery must be recognized as a potential sign of hypoglycemia. If an error in the diabetes control is inevitable, the error should occur on the side of hyperglycemia rather than hypoglycemia.

Van den Berghe et al. (2006) reported that medical intensive insulin therapy definitely had an effect on morbidity but not mortality when targeting blood glucose levels to below 110 mg/dl (6.1 mmol). In contrast, if patients stayed in the intensive care unit for 3 days (as might be needed postsurgery), there was a reduction in both the morbidity and the mortality. More studies are needed to confirm these preliminary data.

Postoperative Period

Dextrose solution should be administered intravenously during and after surgery as long as there is no oral food intake. In the adult, 150–200 g of dextrose or 50 g of dextrose for every missed meal or 2–4 g/kg^{-1}/day^{-1} for children, evenly distributed throughout the 24-hr period, should be administered. Insulin is best administered during this period in four equal doses of regular crystalline insulin given at approximately 6-hr intervals. The dosage can be altered as needed. These changes should be based on blood glucose determinations at the bedside and urine ketone determinations as necessary.

If the surgery will require a period of more than a few hours, NPO, then IV insulin per protocol should be used. Many institutions now have nurse-initiated IV insulin protocols that the nurse may initiate in the intensive care unit (ICU) on a monitored patient without a direct doctor's order. These IV protocols are initiated if the postoperative blood glucose is high or if, on the judgment, the patient will be NPO for a long period. These IV insulin protocols would be initiated in the ICU if they had not already been started in the pre- or operative period.

The following paragraph is repeated to emphasize the fact that, too often, IV insulin is stopped without consideration of the onset of the time of action of the injectable insulin to be started:

When injected insulin is to be started (i.e., when being given either as a basal insulin going to a basal-bolus program or other type of injected insulin programs), the rapid-acting insulin is to be injected 10–15 min before the IV is stopped; the short-acting insulin is to be injected 30 min before the IV is stopped; the intermediate-acting insulin is to be injected 45–60 min before the IV is stopped; and the long-acting insulin is to be injected 2 hr before the IV is stopped. The half-life of IV insulin is about 4 min so subcutaneous insulin *must* be on board before the IV insulin is stopped. If this is not done, a very high blood glucose level will occur requiring catch-up therapy (see Appendix E for insulin transition orders).

It should be pointed out that, although calorie intake is decreased postoperatively, thus decreasing insulin needs, stress may counteract this effect and elevate insulin requirements. The net effect of these counteracting forces may be an immediate postoperative insulin requirement that is similar to the preoperative requirement or higher. Complications directly related to diabetes mellitus are, on the one hand, the undertreatment of hyperglycemia with resulting ketoacidosis and, on the other, the overtreatment of hyperglycemia with resulting hypoglycemia.

The stability of a person's metabolic state may be altered if nausea, vomiting, anorexia, or the possible use of nasogastric suctioning occurs during and after the surgery. Diabetes control can very well fluctuate, requiring varying amounts of insulin. That is why testing in the intensive care unit (Peaston, 1998) and recovery room is important. The dosage of insulin must be determined on an individual basis. IV insulin or frequently administered, small doses of rapid-acting insulins (using a long-acting basal insulin) are always safer than short-acting and intermediate-acting insulins when used in the postoperative period, especially in the pediatric patient.

Inpatient Care

The patient undergoing surgery presents a challenge. To provide care for this patient, the health professional must be familiar with the needs of the surgical patient in addition to being knowledgeable of the specific needs of having diabetes. Basic to care are all of the following:

1. Assessment of the physical, emotional, and psychologic needs preoperatively.
2. Care and observation during surgery and the immediate postoperative period.
3. Maintenance of optimal glucose levels throughout hospitalization.
4. Care during the postoperative period, with emphasis on control of infection and promotion of wound healing.
5. Health promotion, which includes diabetes education.

Assessment of the physical, emotional, and psychologic needs the day before surgery is used to prepare the patient for surgery. Reasonable control of the diabetes must be maintained for the least complications and the best healing to occur (Lober, 1995; Tao, Mackenzie, & Charlson, 2008). A review of the patient's medical history will provide a sketch of the medical background. Assessment of needs should include a complete diabetes history. This information is used to develop a plan during hospitalization and to establish a baseline for teaching and making plans for posthospitalization.

With some patients, the diagnosis of diabetes mellitus is made at the time of admission for surgery. These patients will not only have to be prepared for the forthcoming surgery but will also require basic knowledge regarding self-care before discharge. "Bridging" to an outpatient clinic and an in-depth education program should be part of the planning before discharge from the hospital to a specialized diabetes clinic or to the family doctor, as GeorgeAnn Eaks, CDE, notes in a 2007 AADE published newsletter.

It is beneficial to share with the patients the plans for their care. They should be told what to expect before, during, and after surgery, unless they wish otherwise. Such procedures, the frequency of blood sampling, meal times, insulin administration, and how the insulin will be covered with glucose if the patient is receiving intravenous fluids should be discussed.

Presurgical patients with diabetes need preparation specific to the surgical procedures they are to receive. Friends may have to be restricted from bringing in food of any kind. Food likes and dislikes must be noted so that dietary compliance will be more stable.

Seamless bridging to outpatient care is vital but is often not "seamless" when inpatient care is provided only by the surgeon or the new method—the Hospitalist. The primary care physician or the endocrinologist is frequently not notified of the hospitalization, included in the care, or notified of changes in management. They often find out about these things from the patient at the next scheduled checkup, proving a surprise to the physician or other health professional who must provide the long-term care. This is a problem that must be addressed by the health care system.

Immediate Postoperative Period

The health professionals in surgery and in the postoperative recovery room must be familiar with the fact that the patient has diabetes mellitus. They must know the signs of hypoglycemia, expected and desired blood glucose levels and other laboratory values, and be constantly observant of the possibility of hypoglycemia with the administration of insulin or some other medications.

Signs and symptoms that require action are diaphoresis, increased restlessness, rapid, strong pulse, and an increase or drop in blood pressure, which could be the only significant indication of hypoglycemia in the patient who is semiconscious or drowsy. Convulsions observed during this time in most instances are a sign of hypoglycemia. The standard treatment of 50% glucose is administered intravenously using various amounts depending on the size of the person (i.e., as a starting dose, 10 ml for a small child, 15–20 ml for an adolescent, and 20–50 ml for an adult).

During the semiconscious state postoperatively, blood samples should be obtained every hour (i.e., if on an insulin pump or intravenous infusion) to 6 hr (if on regular insulin subcutaneously). Careful recording of body fluid loss, through bleeding, emesis, and urinary output, is essential. With fluid loss, there is also an electrolyte loss. Thus, a patient with insulin-controlled diabetes may develop hyperglycemia quickly, osmotic diuresis follows, and increased urinary output results. Replacement of fluids, electrolytes, and insulin is as directed by the laboratory results. Monitoring of vital signs, intake and output, and testing of blood for glucose and urine or blood for ketones is mandatory especially when the patient has Type 1 diabetes mellitus (T1DM).

Maintenance of Blood Glucose Levels

The convenient method for maintaining control of diabetes is the testing of blood for glucose levels on a predetermined pattern. In most cases, it is desirable for the person with diabetes to also have blood glucose levels in the range of 110–140 mg/dl (6.1–7.8 mmol) during this postoperative period. With these parameters, there is less possibility that hypoglycemia will occur and serious hyperglycemia is prevented.

Some physicians prefer the Van den Berghe criteria for control of blood glucose levels of 80–110 mg/dl (4.4–6.1 mmol) in the postoperative period. This level of control is very difficult to attain and maintain in surgical patients that have diabetes. It should be remembered that the Van den Berghe protocol was not designed for surgical patients but was designed for patients of post-myocardial infarction, many of whom were not even known to have diabetes prior to the myocardial infarction. These patients had T2DM that was much easier to control than insulin-dependent T1DM or even patients with insulin-requiring T2DM.

If there are ketones in the urine or blood, the cause must be determined immediately. Laboratory values for blood glucose and carbon dioxide content should be obtained to rule out the presence of ketoacidosis. In the presence of diabetic ketoacidosis, increased regular crystalline or rapid-acting insulin and a possible increase in fluids should be quickly administered.

During the period in which healing is occurring, the insulin-controlled patient may have a drastically reduced need for insulin with the decrease of physiologic stress (i.e., as pain and fever decrease, blood glucose levels usually decrease). Careful observation for hypoglycemia is needed. Early morning diaphoresis can be a sign of too large a dose of insulin at bedtime and must be differentiated from diaphoresis secondary to fever. In the morning or throughout the day, confusion or headache or other behavioral changes are also important indications of hypoglycemia. In the older patients, who might have a history of fluctuating in their behavior and compliance, a blood glucose value may clarify whether the response is due to mental-processing problems or to exacerbations in blood glucose levels.

The patient with infection will require a more careful observation for hyperglycemia or hypoglycemia during the postoperative course of the hospital stay. The patient who did not require insulin before hospitalization and surgery (T2DM) might remain hyperglycemic as the surgical stress declines. Otherwise, after some healing has occurred, these patients usually return to the prehospital regimen. Discharge preparation of these individuals may include the need for improved control, the return to an oral agent regimen, and/or the possible reduction or discontinuance of insulin.

Maintenance of blood glucose levels within acceptable parameters is necessary to promote healing, decrease infection, and prevent secondary diabetes-related complications. The rainbow coverage, or sliding scale, must not be used because sliding scale use will result in treating the patient retroactively. If one chooses to use the sliding scale, they may note, when omitting insulin prior to a meal due to hypoglycemic values, there is no insulin coverage for the meal so the physiologic response is for the blood glucose levels to rise.

There are many reasons for not using sliding scale insulin treatment that are well covered elsewhere. With modern technologies, sliding scales in hospitals today should be considered obsolete and possibly malpractice because so many better management techniques are available.

A better method is to calculate the total daily dose, divide it proportionally and adjust the total daily dose based on the last 24-hr blood glucose profile. The insulin dose can then be increased or decreased on a daily basis, with the proportions remaining relatively the same during the 24-hr period, rather than being changed every 4–6 hr as is done with the traditional sliding scale. At least with a basal insulin present, this may not be as much of a problem, but still watch for rebound or hypoglycemia occurring a few hours after the correction dose is given.

Care During the Postoperative Period

The patient with diabetes is more susceptible to infection than the patient without diabetes. This is especially true of the patient with poorly controlled diabetes. Postoperative care should include:

a Scrupulous care of the wound,
b Careful observation and recording of the patient's temperature,
c Inspection of the wound daily to note the healing process, and
d Recording and reporting of any signs of inflammation and/or increased discomfort.

Generally, wound healing is not adversely affected by the presence of diabetes mellitus, providing optimal control is maintained (Schaberg & Norwood, 2002). Persistent hyperglycemia can prolong the healing time of the incision and facilitate infection. Healing time will be increased if wounds are dirty and if the circulation to the affected part is diminished. Meticulous care of the incision is indicated.

Preventive Health Care and Diabetes Teaching

Several surgical problems that bring the patient to the hospital should alert health professionals to include health teaching in the patient's care. Frequently, foot problems, such as ulcers, are a result of lack of education and/or personal observation. Knowing the guidelines for daily care is one thing. Following those guidelines is more difficult. Continuing education and support during each clinic visit help to maintain a prevention focus on self-care.

The signs and symptoms of infection (which include both visual signs, such as redness and edema, and sensory signs, such as pain and heat) must be explained. Emphasis is placed on the visual signs, because a patient with a long-standing neurologic and vascular deprivation in the lower extremities may observe changes during the intervals between clinic appointments. These should be reported promptly.

Continued observation and care of the surgical incision should be explained before discharge. Appointments to the physician's office or clinic must be made and the importance of follow-up care emphasized.

Summary

Normalization of blood glucose levels before, during, and after surgery supports healing. Precounseling and a thorough preassessment and education assist in the adjustment to the surgical procedure. Time must be considered for the pre-preparation prior to surgery and adequate support given afterward for any invasive procedure to ensure the best outcome for the person who has diabetes.

References

American Diabetes Association. (2008). Diabetes care in specific settings. In Standards of medical care in diabetes—2008. *Diabetes Care, 31*(Suppl. 1), S37–S41.

Aviles-Santo, L., & Raskin, P. (1998). Surgery and anesthesia. In H. Lebovitz (Ed.), *Therapy for diabetes mellitus and related disorders* (pp. 224–233). Alexandria, VA: American Diabetes Association.

Eaks, G. A. (2007). The Bridge Clinic: A win-win situation. *AADE in Practice, 1*(2), 2.

English, S., & Young, S. (2005). Diabetes care in the hospital—surgery. In B. Childs, M. Cypress, & G. Spollett (Eds.), *Complete nurse's guide to diabetes care* (pp. 356–357). Alexandria, VA: American Diabetes Association.

Funary, A. P., Zerr, K. J., Grunkeineier, G. L., & Starr, A. (1999). Continuous intravenous insulin infusion reduces the incidence of deep sternal wound infection in diabetic patients after cardiac surgery procedure. *Annals of Thoracic Surgery, 67*(2), 352–362.

Keith, K. S., & Pieper, H. (1989). Perioperative blood glucose levels: A study to determine the effect of surgery. *Journal of the Association of Operating Room Nurses, 50*(1), 103–104.

Krinsley, J. S. (2003). Association between hyperglycemia and increased hospital mortality in a heterogeneous population of critically ill patients. *Mayo Clinic Proceedings, 78*(12), 1471–1478.

Lober, D. L. (1995). Surgical management of the patient with diabetes. Part I: Overview, pre-admission assessment and preoperative care. *Practical Diabetology, 14*(4), 2–9.

Maser, R. E., Eller, J. M., & DeCherney, G. S. (1996). Glucose monitoring of patients with diabetes mellitus receiving general anesthesia: A study of the practices of anesthesia providers in a large community hospital. *American Association of Nurse Anesthetists' Journal, 64*(4), 357–361.

Peaston, R. T. (1998). Blood glucose: Point of care testing in the intensive care unit. *Care of the Critically Ill, 14*(1), 14, 16–18.

Pomposelli, J. J., Baxter, J. K., III, Babineau, L., Pomfret, E. A., Driscoll, D. F., Forse, R. A., et al. (1998). Early post operative glucose control predicts nosocomial infection rate in diabetic patients. *Journal of Parenteral and Enteral Nutrition, 22*(2), 77–81.

Schaberg, D. S., & Norwood, J. M. (2002). Case study: Infections in diabetes mellitus. *Diabetes Spectrum, 26,* 27–40.

Tao, L. S., Mackenzie, C. R., & Charlson, M. E. (2008). Predictors of postoperative complications in the patient with diabetes mellitus. *Journal of Diabetes Complications, 22*(1), 24–28.

Umpierrez, G. E., Isaacs, S. D., Bazargan, N., You, X., Thaler, L. M., & Kitabchi, A. E.(2002). Hyperglycemia: An independent marker of in-hospital mortality in patients with undiagnosed diabetes. *Journal of Clinical Endocrinology and Metabolism, 87*(3), 978–982.

Van den Berghe, G., Wilmer, A., Hermans, G., Meersseman, W., Wouters, P. J., Milants, I., et al. (2006). Intensive insulin therapy in the medical ICU. *New England Journal of Medicine, 354*(5), 449–461.

Van den Berghe, G., Wouters, P., Weekers, F., Verwaest, C., Bruyninckx, F., Schetz, M., et al. (2001). Intensive insulin therapy in the critically ill patient. *New England Journal of Medicine, 345*(19), 1359–1367.

Wilson, M., Weinreb, J., & Hoo, G. W. (2007). Intensive insulin therapy in critical care: A review of 12 protocols. *Diabetes Care, 30*(4), 1005–1011.

Wright, P. D., & Johnson, I. D. (1973). Insulin secretion and glucose intolerance during and after surgical operations. *British Journal of Surgery, 60,* 309.

Zerr, K. J., Funary, A. P., Grunkemeier, G. L., Bookin, S., Kanhere, V., & Starr, A. (1997). Glucose control lowers the risk of wound infection in diabetics after open heart operations. *Annals of Thoracic Surgery, 63*(2), 356–361.

26

Dental Problems and General Hygiene

Care of dental problems and general oral hygiene practices by the individual with diabetes are even more important than in the general population. High blood glucose levels promote the possibility of more frequent dental infections (Bakhshandeh, Murtomaa, Vehkalahti, Mofid, & Suomalainen, 2008). This susceptibility may also be accompanied by decreased circulation, abnormalities in immunologic responses, glycosylation of immunoglobulins, poor white blood cell activity in the presence of high glucose concentrations, and perhaps other factors such as "burning mouth syndrome" associated with Type 1 diabetes (T1DM) and patients who also have peripheral neuropathy (Moore, Guggenheimer, & Orchard, 2007). For those with Type 2 diabetes (T2DM), there was a correlation between insulin resistance and local dental inflammation (Schulze, Schonauer, & Busse, 2007). Consequently, the person with diabetes should be instructed in the general area of hygiene and infection prevention, paying particular attention to dental and foot care.

Care of the Teeth

People with diabetes mellitus, especially T2DM, are at increased risk for periodontal disease, with being a smoker as the leading risk factor and having an elevated HbA1c as the second risk factor (Jansson, Lindholm, Lindh, Groop, & Bratthall, 2006). Even children, adolescents, and adults with T1DM are not immune to this fact.

Periodontal disease is not the only problem to which people with diabetes are subject. According to Comroe, Collin, and Crane (1946), in a classic paper, these oral manifestations include the following:

1. Dryness of the mouth and thirst.
2. A deep red color of the mucous membrane.
3. Gingivitis: swollen, highly inflamed, dark-red gums, frequently detached from the teeth; universal among patients with poorly controlled diabetes.
4. Pus (pyorrhea) readily expressed from periodontal pockets and gum papillae.
5. Denture problems: some patients may have difficulty in wearing dentures because of pressure pain.
6. Loose teeth happen frequently and may seem to occur almost overnight.
7. Increased sensitivity about the necks of the teeth.
8. Ready bleeding from the gums on slight trauma.
9. Frequent formation of salivary calculus.
10. At times, an enlarged, thick, fissured, raw, ham-colored tongue.
11. Frequent occurrence of dry sockets.
12. Presence of acetone on the breath when the diabetes is not under control.

This paper goes on to give guidelines for recommended dental care that remain as true today as then:

1. The person with diabetes should be examined by a dentist at least every 3 or 4 months (every 2 months in children)—with well-controlled diabetes, every 6 months is acceptable.
2. A clinician should carefully control the diabetes status to successfully treat local conditions within the mouth.
3. Rigid oral hygiene must be carried out, with the frequent removal of accumulated calcareous deposits.
4. Establish diabetes control. The outcome may be the tightening of loose teeth.
5. Complete mouth roentgen ray should be performed yearly.
6. All tissues should be handled very gently with a minimum of trauma.
7. Any extensive work should be divided into several stages.
8. Treat apical abscess that may result at the site of a loose tooth.
9. No dental work should be undertaken without the full consent of the medical consultant.
10. Teeth with periapical infection should be removed, and root canal treatment should be attempted.
11. Extensive infiltration with local anesthesia should be avoided if possible.
12. Great care must be taken in the construction of the dentures.
13. Surgical asepsis must be employed in extractions, as the person with diabetes is very susceptible to infection. Epithelial ulceration and bony necrosis are not infrequent in people who have poorly controlled diabetes.

14. If an anesthetic is required, local anesthesia is the first choice. If nitrous oxide is used, the greatest of care must be exercised. Epinephrine should not be used in large amounts, as this substance tends to raise blood glucose. Ether should be avoided in persons with diabetes, because it may reduce the liver glycogen.
15. Remove abscessed teeth, which are a distinct liability. This may improve not only the general health, but also carbohydrate tolerance.

Periodontal disease appears to be interdependent with the general health of the body. If blood glucose levels are elevated, gingivitis is expected. If blood sugars remain elevated, then periodontal disease is more apt to occur.

Dental Surgery

If oral surgery is required, it is generally performed in the early morning. If the person with diabetes is receiving insulin therapy and the procedure is of short duration and performed the first thing in the morning, the patient should not take a rapid-acting insulin, might take a partial dose of insulin before the procedure if on an intermediate- or short-acting insulin, or, if taking a long-acting insulin, give as usual or, if on a pump (continuous subcutaneous insulin infusion [CSII]), stay on basal during the procedure. Bolus insulin or rapid-acting insulin would be given after the procedure, depending on the person's ability to eat after the surgery and the person's blood glucose level.

In the postoperative period of dental surgery, it is important that the blood glucose levels are tested a minimum of 4 or more times daily, and that a health professional be consulted should increased glucosemia develop. After oral surgery, sugar-containing fluids, such as soda or juice, may be given. Solids are often not tolerated. This is especially important when insulin is taken because lack of food may result in hypoglycemia.

If the person is on an insulin secretagogue, a hepatic glucose blocker, or an alpha-glucosidase inhibitor, this person should be cautioned to not take this medication prior to the surgical procedure. The decision to take or not take a thiazolidinedione should be made on an individual basis.

Antibiotic therapy is often begun after tooth extraction to help prevent the possibility of infection. It is often started 2–3 days before oral surgery. No dental surgery should be performed until the health professional states that blood glucose levels are under adequate control. The reasons for restricting surgery are as follows:

1. Increased infection is observed with poorly controlled diabetes.
2. The healing process is slower with increased glucose levels.
3. Diabetic ketoacidosis is possible if infection does develop.

Dental care for the person with diabetes is most important to prevent the progression from gingivitis to periodontal disease (Kiran, Arpak, Unsal, & Erdogan, 2005). It is obvious that any infectious site, such as the teeth and gums, will challenge blood glucose levels. Appropriate dental management must include control of blood glucose levels (McKenna, 2006) and frequent prophylaxis (Taylor et al., 2005).

Care of the Skin

Persons with diabetes are more prone to attack by staphylococci, beta-hemolytic streptococci, and fungi. *Helicobacter pylori* is also noted to be a problem especially if there is lack of vascularization as found in atherosclerosis and ischemic cardiovascular stroke (Hamed et al., 2008).

Furuncles and carbuncles are usually less common, but may require an increase in diabetes medication with the full-blown infection. The infecting organism should always be cultured and antibiotic therapy instituted. Infections that are associated with fever and leukocytosis result in hyperglycemia and often necessitate an increase in insulin or other diabetes medication.

Several specific types of lesions of the skin are more often observed in people with diabetes. One of the most common skin lesions, *diabetes dermopathy,* occurs in individuals with diabetes after age 30. It is commonly observed as a result of localized trauma and is most prominent on the shins. Diabetic dermopathy may appear as hyperpigmented areas, usually tan in color. They are not painful but are cosmetically unattractive. There currently is no treatment for this type of lesion.

Another lesion observed most frequently on the lower extremity is *necrobiosis lipoidica diabeticorum.* It is not a common disorder and may occur in subjects who do not have diabetes, but it is considered symptomatic of diabetes. The lesion is seen more commonly among women before age 40. It starts much like an area of dermopathy, enlarges to form a plaque, and may cover the entire lower leg. It is often a result of trauma, and ulcerations may be located within the area because in these areas the skin is very thin with a poor blood supply. Treatment may include injection of steroids around the periphery of the lesions, but this treatment is painful, and remission tends to be temporary. Two more recently introduced treatments have been found to have some success (in the past, little if any treatment has helped). Photodynamic therapy (Heidenheiss & Jemec, 2006) and another approach using a protease-modulating dressing (Stewart, 2006) have resulted in these areas looking less "angry." Patients often report that the areas look angrier when their blood glucose levels are elevated above normal.

Another lesion of the skin occasionally observed is *xanthoma diabeticorum.* With this condition, the patient has marked hyperlipemia when blood glucose levels have remained elevated for a long period. The lesion appears as firm nodules in scattered papules, which are pinkish yellow in color. The papules are predominantly located on the buttocks, extensor surfaces, palms of the hands, and soles of the feet, and are not painful. Treatment of xanthoma diabeticorum consists of lowering blood glucose levels, which in turn reduces the serum lipid levels. Antilipid drugs may also be needed.

One of the most common infections observed in women with diabetes is *candidiasis* (moniliasis). The presence of vaginal candidiasis should prompt investigation for diabetes mellitus. Candida organisms are normally present in the vaginal mucosa, and with the increased concentrations of glucose in the body, the candida multiply rapidly, causing vulvovaginitis in combination with severe pruritus. The labia may become swollen and red, and a cheesy-white discharge is often present. Candidiasis may also appear in the oral mucous membranes, under the arms, and under pendulous breasts. Treatment of candidiasis includes the use of topical powders, vaginal suppositories, and oral antifungal medication. The best treatment is the control of blood glucose levels and careful daily washing of the areas with soap and water.

Care of the Feet

The most important aspect of foot care for the person with diabetes is the prevention of serious problems. Standards of Medical Care state, "All patients must be educated about the risk and prevention of foot problems" (American Diabetes Association, 2004). The feet of the person with diabetes are prone to vascular insufficiency (in particular, small-vessel disease), neuropathy, and infection secondary to trauma. "The diabetic foot," as Dr. Marvin Levin refers to it (Levin, O'Neal, & Bowker, 1993, p.1), ". . . is not much different from the foot of any other person with advanced vascular disease, except for one outstanding feature—diabetic neuropathy, which interferes with the perception of trauma or pressure." Preventive foot care is based on knowledge of these possible complications of diabetes and on two other aspects: hygiene and other means of active prevention and the avoidance of trauma.

The insensate foot must be examined at least every three months and sensate feet evaluated thoroughly at least once a year. This includes, but is not limited to, the use of a 10-g monofilament placed on the middle of the top of the foot and held at a slight bend. Other sites of the feet to be examined in this manner are the first, third, and fifth toe and metatarsals, the inner and outer aspect of the arch, and the heel (Armstrong, 2000). Booth and Young (2000) report some differences in the 10-g filament, but also recognized that these differences may be due to technique. There is also the question whether the other weight filaments should be used. Once the 10-g (5.07) filament is not felt, moderate neuropathy should be suspected (mild neuropathy if the 4.17 cannot be felt, and severe neuropathy if the 6.10 filament cannot be felt). Nather et al. (2008) found that the Pin Prick Test was as good or better, if the person had diabetes of less than 5 years' duration. They felt this test was simple, less expensive, and still gave adequate screening results when compared with the Semmes–Weinstein monofilament and the Rapid Current Perception Threshold test using a neurometer.

Other parts of the foot exam are observation for clawing of the toes, hammertoes, calluses, and possible ulcers, or Charcot's joint (Brandy et al., 2001). Temperature would be felt and vibratory sense would be noted with the use of a tuning fork (Kalter-Leibovici, Yosipovitch, Gabbay, Yarnitsky, & Karp, 2001). The dorsalis pedis and the posterior tibial pulses should also be palpated and further evaluation of these pulses should be carried out by Doppler.

Foot Hygiene

People with diabetes should wash their feet daily. Lukewarm water should be used for this purpose. Because the temperature receptors in the lower extremities of the person with diabetes may be impaired, the water should always be tested with the wrist or elbow or by another family member. Mild hand soaps are best, but those with an antibacterial agent added give extra protection against infection. Particular care should be taken to pat the feet dry gently but thoroughly and to dry well between the toes. A bland foot powder can then be applied if the feet tend to perspire. If dryness is noted, lanolin, baby oil, foot cream, or even corn oil or Vaseline can be rubbed gently into the skin. Applying powder or lotion routinely also provides an opportunity for a more frequent inspection of the feet.

If athlete's foot is a problem, over-the-counter products may be used. If a shower is the usual way of bathing, be sure the patient is instructed to spray the shower after every use with a 10% solution of Clorox water or a product for that purpose purchased from the store.

Toenail fungus may be another problem. Use of various medications or over-the-counter treatments may be used: from a couple of capfuls of Clorox in a pan of water used 2 to 3 times a day to Tea Tree oil or Vicks VapoRub to prescription-needed Penlac (nail polish type treatment), or pills (Diflucan or Sporanox). Whatever the treatment, it usually takes three or more months to see any improvement.

Toenails, Corns, and Calluses

Immediately after washing is the best time to cut toenails or to care for corns or calluses because the warm water aids in softening them. Patients should be instructed to cut toenails along the top of the toe, without digging into the corners and without cutting below the end of the toe, unless there are thickened folds of skin on either side of the nail. (Ideally, at this point, the podiatrist should be involved because the manner of toenail cutting may be quite different for each individual with diabetes.) Nail scissors or clippers should be used in preference to a knife or other sharp object, which may slip and injure the foot. If the patient cannot see well or if the nails are extremely hard, a podiatrist should perform the job. Calluses or corns should be soaked and then rubbed gently with a soft towel or pumice stone. These areas should never be treated with corn remedies, which are usually harsh, or cut with a knife, scissors, or razor blade. A podiatrist can usually provide the best treatment for these problems. Remind patients that the podiatrist should be informed about them having diabetes.

Daily Inspection of the Feet

The person with diabetes should be instructed to carefully inspect the feet daily. This may be difficult to do because without sensation or with no indication of a problem (i.e., pain), this process might seldom be accomplished. Daily hygiene provides a regular time for this examination, which should include the tops and the soles of the feet, the heels, and the areas between the toes. If the patient cannot see well enough to do this himself, another person in the family should make the inspection or a metal camping mirror, placed on the floor, should be made available for checking the bottom of the feet. Even a minor injury or a change in the feet, such as a small reddened area, should be checked by the health professional. Many serious complications can be avoided if slowly healing wounds or other problem areas are reported early, that is, before they develop into an ulcer. Ulcerations can evolve rapidly; therefore, no foot problem should be taken lightly. The person with diabetes and peripheral neuropathy cannot rely on pain or discomfort as a clue to injury because of possible impaired sensation. Thus, daily examination is imperative in preventing the possible development of diabetic foot ulcers (Santos & Carline, 2000).

Proper Shoes and Socks

Clean socks or stockings and properly fitting shoes should be worn every day and changed frequently. Inspection of the feet can reveal areas that may be irritated or pressured by the shoes being worn. New shoes should be broken in carefully and slowly, and old shoes and slippers should be checked periodically to ensure that they are intact and still fit well. Shoes should not be worn without hose or socks, and the socks should be free of holes or darns. Even a curled thread in a sock can cause an irritation if unnoticed. If indicated, bunions, hammertoes, and pressure points should be protected by insoles to avoid pressure sores. Lamb's wool can be used between toes that rub or overlap. Special shoes may be fitted by a podiatric specialist. This is especially true if added depth is needed in the shoe.

Improving Circulation to the Feet and Legs

Active prevention of foot and leg problems should include measures to improve the circulation in the lower extremities. Buerger's exercises offer one method of stimulating circulation to the legs. These exercises consist of alternately:

a. Lowering of the feet below heart level and leaving them until the veins fill, and then
b. Elevating the feet to slightly above heart level to support the flow of the blood out of the feet, and
c. Circling the feet to the right and left and up and down ten times once or more times a day, on a daily basis.

Walking slowly can be a form of Buerger's exercise if the vein valves work properly. Muscle contraction forces blood up the deep veins, venous pressure decreases as the muscles relax, and the high arterial pressure produced by gravity fills the veins. Walking slowly should be strongly encouraged, especially in patients with occlusive arterial disease. If the patient has intermittent claudication, periods of rest can be alternated with walks, along with the taking of appropriate medication such as cilostazol (Pletal) or pentoxifylline (Trental). The person with venous insufficiency may require bed rest or at least elevating the extremities several times a day.

In addition to walking, abstinence from the use of tobacco helps support of peripheral circulation and prevention of vasoconstriction found when a person smokes.

Avoiding Trauma to the Foot

Trauma to the foot can lead to infection, and infection requires both an increased blood supply and increased insulin, both of which the person with diabetes may be lacking. The easiest way to avoid setting up this vicious cycle is to prevent trauma.

The possible impairment to sensation, because of neuropathy, should be kept in mind. Temperature sense, vibration sense, and proprioception may all be impaired in individuals with diabetes. These persons should avoid heat from hot water, heating pads, hot-water bottles, and other temperature-altered devices. They should also keep their feet away from open fires or stoves. Dry heat is dangerous because the person with diabetes may lack sensation and be afflicted with vasculopathy. Because blood acts as the body's cooling agent, decreased blood flow owing to vasculopathy may lead to overheating and a severe burn might be the outcome. The patient should be encouraged to use warm socks and extra covers if he or she has difficulty keeping warm. Frostbite may occur if the patient's circulation is poor, or the humidity is high and the temperature is 40°F or less. The body tends to conserve warmth by decreasing circulation to the extremities when the trunk is cold. The health professional should question the patient carefully about heating methods employed at home, because hot-water bottles, plastic bottles filled with hot water, or even hot bricks have been used.

The feet should be protected at all times from cuts, bruises, introduction of foreign objects, and fractures. Such protection can usually be accomplished if the person with diabetes wears shoes or well-fitted slippers that are sturdy and closed in at all times. Many amputations have resulted from the entry of an object, such as a staple, into the foot, without the person noticing it. It is not uncommon for minor fractures to go unheeded by the individual with neuropathy. Instead of protecting the injured foot, the person with decreased sensation will continue to use it for weight bearing, which leads to further deterioration, multiple fractures, and even Charcot's joint. The person with diabetes should never go barefoot, even around the house.

Socks or stockings should be worn in such a way that adequate circulation is maintained. Tight-fitting socks or stockings may lead to minute trauma, or mechanically cause a process of pathology. Tight elastic bands, circular garters, or twisted hose should never be used. Crossing the legs at the knees for long periods will also decrease circulation to the lower extremities.

Minor cuts should be kept clean and dry. The use of alcohol is not recommended as all harsh antiseptics and chemicals should be avoided. For instance, iodine, Merthiolate, Mercurochrome, or liniment should not be used on the feet. Corn pads and corn plasters can lead to ulcerations and should be considered taboo. Home remedies for cuts and scratches can be extremely dangerous. If in doubt, the patient should consult the medical team before any such first-aid measures are instituted.

The integrity of the skin on the feet should never be broken purposely in caring for toenails, corns, or calluses. Ingrown toenails should be promptly treated by a podiatrist, as should fungal infections of the nails. Fungus on the skin also requires medical attention. Athlete's foot should not be taken lightly, because if left untreated, it can lead to ulceration; fungus under the toenails can lead to loss of the toenail.

Avoidance of trauma should be of special consideration when a localized amputation, as of a single toe, has already been performed. In this case, the remainder of the extremity may be off balance and subject to changes in pressure of other areas of the foot. Shoes and padding must be carefully selected.

Treatment of Trauma and Lesions of the Feet

Conservative treatment of trauma to the foot of the person with diabetes has met with increasing success, particularly when problems are detected early and when vasculopathy is not advanced. The patient and the health care professionals must be compulsive in carrying out the therapy indicated. Frequent cleansing of the affected foot is usually ordered. High doses of antibiotics are generally prescribed for foot lesions, as are dry, sterile dressings. Resting the affected part is probably the most important element of treatment and must be strictly enforced. More recent treatment involves casting, which allows the person to continue daily activity; debridement, with or without the use of enzymes; or the use of platelet growth factors such as becaplermin (Regranex) to stimulate growth of healthy tissue.

Debridement of a lesion with a bland solution or use of an enzyme may be carried out, even on an outpatient basis, if treatment is begun early, and circulation is fairly good. Betadine solutions are drying and may cause cracking of the skin, and should be avoided. Various foot products may be helpful, but the patient should check with a health professional before using the product.

Amputation is usually indicated when wet gangrene has set in, infection is uncontrollable, pain is unrelenting, tissue has been destroyed, the infection has entered the bone, or an ulcer will not heal with the normalization of blood glucose levels. Amputations can range from a single toe to an entire limb. With proper rehabilitation therapy, amputation can often restore the patient to a more productive life.

Assessment of the Feet

Despite the serious consequences that can result from improper foot care, this area of therapy is frequently overlooked by health professionals during history taking, examination, and teaching. Health professionals seem to shy away from the first, quickest, and easiest step—inspection of the patient's feet. Teaching preventive foot care is often delayed, because it is not perceived to be as immediate a need as the taking or administering of a medication. Since people with diabetes are at high risk for amputation, assessment of the feet and patient education result in reducing the chance of this occurrence.

Demonstration and actual participation in the education process, especially regarding foot care, appear to increase knowledge more than just through lecture alone (Kruger & Guthrie, 1992). The result is that adequate foot care, education, and treatment lead to cost savings and a decrease in morbidity.

The program should begin with an assessment of what the patient is currently doing in terms of foot care. Inspection of the feet should be frequent and include the following considerations:

1. What is the condition of the shoes?
2. How well do the shoes fit?
3. Is the patient wearing socks or stockings? Are they clean? In good repair? Fit well?
4. Is the patient using circular garters? Twisting hose? Wearing tight elastic bands?

5. Are the feet clean? Are the feet warm to the touch? Do the feet have good color?
6. Is there hair growing on the toes (a usual indication of good circulation)? Is there any edema in the feet and ankles?
7. What is the condition of the toenails (is toenail fungus present)? How are they cut (too short; too long)?
8. Are there any corns, calluses, or bunions?
9. Are there any cuts? Fissures? Bruises? Ulcerations? (In examining for fissures, one gently separates the toes, because it is possible to create fissures between the toes in the examination process.) If so, does the tissue appear ischemic or gangrenous?
10. What is the general condition of the skin? Is it dry? Any rashes? The heels? The soles? Are there any apparent pressure points? Do the toes overlap?
11. Can the peripheral pulses be palpated? Are they strong (dorsalis pedis and posterior tibial)?
12. Does the patient have sensation to pain? Vibration? (One can test with a pin or tuning fork, or with standardized filaments.)
13. Are the leg muscles atrophied? Is there any abnormality in gait?

Observation of the foot-care routine with the patient's own equipment is the ideal way to assess the usual procedure for hygiene. Sending in a home health nurse is ideal. This person can gain the most information by going into the patient's residence, where he or she can assess the home facilities for bathing and on-site foot care. Watching the patient actually carry out the foot-care regimen is far more revealing than simply having patients state what they do.

Interviewing regarding foot-care practices can begin with general questions:

a. What has the patient already been told about proper foot care?
b. Why is foot care important for the person with diabetes?
c. What self-care practices are being carried out (if any)?

Eliciting information about symptoms can pinpoint potential foot-care problems. For instance, the health care provider might consider such a question as, "Is there pain when the foot is dangling, in a prone position, or both?"

Teaching About Foot Care

A thorough assessment of the foot-care regimen helps to gain a focus on the areas for which education is needed. The first step in instruction must be the rationale for good foot care. The do's and don'ts of foot care make sense to patients once they understand how complications of diabetes can affect the feet (see Table 26.1). Health care personnel often forget to emphasize the "why" when instructions are given.

If demonstration and practice with the individual is not feasible, many audiovisual aids are available and provide good education on proper foot care. Pictures of various foot problems also aid the patients in examination of their

26.1 — Instructions for the Do's and Don'ts of Foot Care

Do's	Don'ts
Examine feet daily – tops, soles, heels, and between toes.	Do not use hot water to wash feet or bathe in.
Wash feet every day with mild hand soap and warm water – check temperature with wrist or elbow.	Do not leave feet wet or dry them roughly.
Pat feet thoroughly dry – especially between the toes.	Do not cut toenails short or dig into the corners unless directed to do so; file corners.
Apply bland powder if feet perspire.	Do not use a knife to cut nails.
Apply lanolin, oil, or bland lotion to dry feet.	Do not use corn pads or corn plasters.
Cut toenails after washing – straight across in line with the top of the toe with clippers or scissors. Smooth with an emery board.	Do not cut corns or calluses.
Rub corns or calluses gently with a soft towel after washing: Consult the podiatrist if they persist.	Do not wear round garters or twist-top hose.
Wear clean socks or nonbinding pantyhose every day.	Do not wear socks or stockings with holes or loose threads.
Wear shoes all the time, inside and outside the house.	Do not walk barefoot.
Treat minor cuts or bruises with gentle cleansing, using water or normal saline.	Do not use iodine or other abrasive antiseptics on cuts.
Use warm socks and extra covers for cold feet.	Do not use heating or freezing products on the feet.

own feet and detection of potential trouble. But, the more hands-on teaching, the better the knowledge (Kruger & Guthrie, 1992).

Written do's and don'ts of foot care (see Table 26.1) give the patient a handy list to refer to when a question is encountered at home. A list of positive steps to take in daily hygiene and in treating injuries, as well as a list of situations to avoid, should be included in such a guide.

Bloomgarden (2008) has written an excellent review article on the diabetic foot covering what has been noted and even more. Another finding is that there is a higher correlation between depressive symptoms and lack of wound healing in a foot, although the correlation was stronger when the person was a smoker; the HbA1c was next (Monami et al., 2008).

The International Working Group on the Diabetic Foot has determined that there should be some alteration and updating of classifications related to peripheral neuropathy. In their review of the literature, overall, they found more complications as the risk group increased (ulcerations, infections, amputations, hospitalizations). They also found there were more complications in the patients with peripheral arterial occlusion disease than expected. These complications involved foot deformity, neuropathy, and amputations. In fact, there were enough differences in the comparisons to call for a need to reclassify diabetes foot problems (Lavery et al., 2008).

Summary

The most important idea to leave with a person with diabetes is that any hygiene problem, such as a dental, skin, or foot problem, can become a serious situation. The health professional's responsibility does not stop at checking the skin, teeth, and patient's feet, and imparting information about good hygiene. Health professionals often have the opportunity to assess the procedures, materials, and facilities available to patients for adequate hygiene care, and should guide them in using or altering these items within their means. Preventive care is essential if the person with diabetes mellitus is to avoid serious health problems (Albright, 2006).

References

Albright, A. L. (2006). Reducing risks. In C. Mensing (Ed.), *The art and science of diabetes self-management education: A desk reference for healthcare professionals* (pp. 771–789). Chicago: American Association of Diabetes Educators.

American Diabetes Association. (2004). Preventive foot care in diabetes. *Diabetes Care, 27*(Suppl. 1), S63–S64.

Armstrong, D. G. (2000). The 10-g monofilament: The diagnostic diving rod for the diabetic foot? *Diabetes Care, 23*(7), 887.

Bakhshandeh, S., Murtomaa, H., Vehkalahti, M. M., Mofid, R., & Suomalainen, K. (2008). Dental findings in diabetes adults. *Caries Research, 42*(1), 14–18.

Bloomgarden, Z. T. (2008). The diabetic foot. *Diabetes Care, 31*(2), 372–376.

Booth, J., & Young, M. J. (2000). Differences in the performance of commercially available 10g monofilaments. *Diabetes Care, 23*(7), 984–988.

Brandy, C., Bumbalough, M., Case, J., DeHart, A., Smith, L., & Weingartner, M. (2001). Charcot's foot in diabetes. *Nurse Practitioner, 26*(3), 85–86.

Comroe, A. B., Collin, L. H., Jr., & Crane, M. P. (1946). *Internal medicine in dental practice*. Philadelphia: Lea & Febiger.

Hamed, S. A., Amine, N. F., Galul, G. M., Helal, S. R., Tag El-Din, L. M., et al. (2008). Vascular risks and complications in diabetes mellitus: The role of *Helicobacter pylori* infection. *Journal of Stroke and Cerebrovascular Disease, 17*(2), 86–94.

Heidenheim, M., & Jemec, G. B. (2006). Successful treatment of necrobiosis lipoidica diabeticorum with photodynamic therapy. *Archives of Dermatology, 142*(12), 1548–1550.

Jansson, H., Lindholm, E., Lindh, C., Groop, L., & Bratthall, G. (2006). Type 2 diabetes and risk for periodontal disease: A role for dental health awareness. *Journal of Clinical Peridontology, 33*(6), 408–414.

Kalter-Leibovici, O., Yosipovitch, G., Gabbay, U., Yarnitsky, D., & Karp, M. (2001). Factor analysis of thermal and vibration thresholds in young patients with Type 1 diabetes mellitus. *Diabetic Medicine, 18*(3), 213–317.

Kiran, M., Arpak, N., Unsal, E., & Erdogan, M. F. (2005). The effect of improved periodontal health on metabolic control in type 2 diabetes mellitus. *Journal of Clinical Periodontology, 32*(3), 266–272.

Kruger, S., & Guthrie, D. W. (1992). Foot care: Knowledge retention and self-care practices. *The Diabetes Educator, 18*(6), 487–490.

Lavery, L. A., Peters, E. J., Williams, J. R., Murdock, D. P., Hudson, A., & Lavery, D. C.; International Working Group on the Diabetic Foot. (2008). Reevaluating the way we classify the diabetic foot risk classification system of the International Working Group on the Diabetic Foot. *Diabetes, 31*(1), 154–156.

Levin, M. E., O'Neal, L. W., & Bowker, J. H. (Eds.). (1993). *The diabetic foot* (5th ed.). St. Louis: C.V. Mosby.

McKenna, S. J. (2006). Dental management of patients with diabetes. *Dental Clinics of North America, 50*(4), 591–606.

Monami, M., Longo, R., Desideri, C. M., Masotti, G., Marchionni, N., & Mannucci, F. (2008). The diabetic person beyond a foot ulcer: Healing, recurrence, and depressive symptoms. *Journal of the American Podiatry Medical Association, 98*(2), 130–136.

Moore, P. A., Guggenheimer, J., & Orchard, T. (2007). Burning mouth syndrome and peripheral neuropathy in patients with type 1 diabetes mellitus. *Journal of Diabetes Complications, 21*(6), 397–402.

Nather, A., Neo, S. H., Chionh, S. B., Liew, S. C., Sim, E. Y., & Chew, J. L. (2008). Assessment of sensory neuropathy in diabetic patients without diabetic foot problems. *Diabetes Complications, 22*(2), 126–131.

Santos, D., & Carline, T. (2000). Examination of the lower limb in high-risk patients. *Journal of Tissue Viability, 10*(3), 97–105.

Schulze, A., Schonauer, M., & Busse, M. (2007). Sudden improvement of insulin sensitivity related to an endodontic treatment. *Journal of Periodontology, 78*(12), 2380–2384.

Stewart, E. (2006). Using a protease modulating dressing to treat necrobiosis lipoidica diabeticorum. *Journal of Wound Care, 15*(2), 74–77.

Taylor, G. W., Pritzel, S. J., Manz, M. C., Borgnakke, W. S., Eber, R. M., & Bouman, P. D. (2005). Frequency of dental prophylaxis and glycemic control in type 2 diabetes. *Journal of Dental Hygiene, 79*(4), 1–2.

Chronic Complications

VI

27

Cardiac, Cerebral, and Peripheral Vascular Disease

Since the advent of insulin in 1922, the incidence of death resulting from diabetic ketoacidosis has decreased markedly, although unfortunately it has not disappeared. Now, vascular disease and disease involving the nerves have become the leading causes of death among persons with diabetes. Vascular disease in diabetes affects all vessels of the body and can be divided into two categories: large-vessel disease (macrovascular disease or macroangiopathy) and small-vessel disease (microvascular disease or microangiopathy). Each of these problems and diabetic neuropathy will be discussed in this and the following chapters. The good news, as a result of the Diabetes Control and Complications Trial (DCCT) (1993), is the approximate risk reduction in retinopathy (76%), neuropathy (60%), and nephropathy (50%) by improved blood glucose control. The large-blood-vessel disease portion of the DCCT is still being studied, but to date there appears to be a 42% risk reduction associated with improved diabetes control (Strowig & Raskin, 1995; U.K. Prospective Diabetes Study, 1998) even though, at the time of the 1993 reporting, it was not considered statistically significant. A link between macroangiopathy and blood glucose control is hard to prove because of the many risk factors (smoking, lipid levels, genetics, lifestyle, and so on) that are intertwined in the development of cardiovascular disease.

What is becoming of concern is cardiovascular risk factors and occurrences in Type 2 diabetes mellitus (T2DM) in children. Vaughan, Ovalle, and Moreland (2007) reviewed the state of the art of vascular disease in children with T2DM. They felt there was a notable lack of consensus on a variety of factors along with the unavailability of approved medications to treat this population.

When attempting to predict Type 1 diabetes mellitus (T1DM) in children, family history had the predictive potential and appeared related to the cardiovascular risk factors. In the SEARCH for Diabetes in Youth study, Gilliam et al. (2007) assessed fasting C-peptide results against family history and its relation to potential cardiovascular disease. Such things as above-normal body mass index and abnormal lipid profiles were significant in a subgroup of the autoimmune population studied. This again emphasizes the need for prevention and early detection of diabetes in children as well as adults.

Large-Vessel Disease

The primary concern of adults with the non-insulin-dependent form of diabetes, T2DM, is disease of the large blood vessels, macrovascular disease. Macrovascular disease is increasing in people with T1DM as well. Macrovascular disease is an acceleration of the aging process, leading to early heart attacks and stroke. The causes of this complication are partially known and are multiple. No matter how many risk factors for macrovascular disease are present, the addition of diabetes increases the risk significantly. Improving diabetes control will at least slow the progression of disease (American Diabetes Association [ADA] Consensus Statement on Coronary Artery Disease, 2007b).

The World Health Organization notes that a person with the characteristics of obesity, fasting blood glucose levels higher than 100 mg/dl (5.5 mmol), a high triglyceride/high-density lipoprotein ratio, microalbuminuria over 30, a C-reactive protein more than 3.0, and hypertension are at high risk for cardiovascular disease. The American Diabetes Association Position Statement (2005) describes "diabetes-associated" metabolic syndrome, its care and expectations. Contributing factors and management guidelines are also found in position statements on smoking (ADA, 2004c), aspirin therapy (ADA, 2004b), dyslipidemia management (ADA, 2004a), and in consensus statements on waist circumference and cardiometabolic risk (ADA, 2007a), management of dyslipidemia in children and adolescents (ADA, 2003a), and peripheral arterial disease (ADA, 2003b). Case studies are presented by Balasubramanyam, Hinnen, and Polonsky (2006) to aid in translating therapeutic approaches into actual practice.

New studies are questioning the level of diabetic control for the prevention of cardiovascular disease. Diabetes control for the prevention of microvascular disease is no longer questioned (Dluhy & McMahon, 2008). The prevention of macrovascular disease is more difficult to tie to blood glucose control because of the multiple risk factors in this disease. After all, people without diabetes never develop diabetic-type retinopathy or nephropathy, but most people with macrovascular problems do not even have diabetes. This has led to clinical trials to prove whether intensive control of blood glucose will prevent macrovascular disease, specifically myocardial infarction and stroke.

The Action to Control Cardiovascular Risk in Diabetes (ACCORD) trial (Gerstein et al., 2008) and the Action in Diabetes and Vascular Disease: Preterax and Diamicron Release Controlled Evaluation (ADVANCE) trial (Patel et al., 2008) were designed to settle this issue. They did not do so. The ACCORD trial demonstrated an increase in cardiovascular mortality in the group of people in the intensive control arm of the study where the goal was to decrease A1c to 6%. Because of the increased mortality, this arm of the study was discontinued. The ADVANCE trial did not demonstrate prevention of cardiovascular disease with intensive control (their goal was an A1c less than 7%) but neither did it demonstrate the increased risk found in the ACCORD trial. An analysis of the differences and results of these two studies and the inferences for the future are contained in an editorial in the *New England Journal of Medicine* (Dluhy & McMahon, 2008). The relationship of blood glucose control to macrovascular complications in persons with diabetes mellitus is far from settled, yet we must strive for the best control possible until the final answer is in. We owe it to our patients to give them the benefit of the doubt.

Macrovascular Disease

The chief vessels affected by large-vessel disease are those to the heart, the brain, and the periphery, principally in the legs and feet. Disease of the large vessels of the body (cerebral, carotid, coronary, and peripheral) occurs through the process of arteriosclerosis. Arteriosclerosis occurs in most people, especially in the United States, as part of the aging process. It may also be associated with decubiti occurrences in the older individuals who also have diabetes (the Braden Scale is useful for predicting pressure sore risk—Braden & Bergstrom, 1989). The problem occurs at an earlier age and accelerates faster in persons with diabetes. Diabetes also obliterates the female protection to arteriosclerosis usually seen in women before menopause. The etiology of large-vessel disease is a multifactorial problem with interaction between age, genetics, diet, including lipid intake and lipid (particularly cholesterol) levels, blood glucose levels, obesity, smoking, hypertension, and perhaps many other factors (Calder & Alexander, 2000). The etiology of large-vessel disease is discussed in more detail in Chapter 4.

Cardiac Disease

Cardiovascular disease, such as coronary artery disease (CAD), is the leading cause of death in diabetes (ADA Consensus Statement, 2007b). Many persons with T1DM die of their renal disease first, but if they survive renal disease (by dialysis or transplant) or are fortunate enough to not develop renal disease, most of them will develop and die of coronary artery disease. Insufficiency of blood flow to the heart causing pain (angina) or blockage (myocardial infarction [MI]) may result from CAD.

These conditions can be reversed with medication, rest, or surgery (coronary artery bypass, stent placement, or balloon angioplasty). The patient may recover from angina or a heart attack and lead a near-normal life. Drugs such as beta blockers, calcium channel blockers, and aspirin have greatly enhanced survival. Intravascular enzymes or plasminogen-activating enzymes to dissolve the clots, proper monitoring, and cardiac support have greatly enhanced survival after an MI.

Special observations and interventions are needed for the person who has had an acute coronary event. Rigorous monitoring of all comorbidities and appropriate treatment can aid in decreasing the potential increase in mortality after such an event (Donahoe et al., 2007).

Another consideration is the occurrence of congestive heart failure. Not only do certain medications need to be stopped (thiazolidinediones [TZDs]), but also the careful use of diuretics (accompanied by antihypertensive medication as needed) should be instituted. A useful article in this field is by Giles and Sander (2004) who relate the background and treatment of such a problem in a person who also has diabetes.

Cerebral Disease

Cerebrovascular disease (CVD) may be manifest by the rupture of a cerebral artery with the escape of blood into the brain tissue. Such a cerebral hemorrhage may come without warning. Some of the preliminary symptoms may include dizziness, headaches, disturbances of speech, anxiety, or numbness of one side of the body. With cerebral hemorrhage, the patient usually loses consciousness and may have convulsions at the onset. Paralysis occurs on the side of the body opposite the hemorrhage. Aphasia may be experienced if the paralysis occurs on the right side. This problem is most commonly seen in persons who are hypertensive, a common problem found concurrently with the diagnosis of diabetes.

Cerebral thrombosis is another manifestation of CVD. Symptoms of large-vessel occlusion are the same as those for cerebral hemorrhage, but they may not be as profound. If the occlusion is of a small blood vessel, loss of consciousness does not usually develop. There may be symptoms of mental confusion, headache, and vertigo. Magnetic resonance imaging of the brain will usually differentiate hemorrhage from occlusion. It is important to make this differentiation because occlusion can be treated by anticoagulants or lytic enzymes, both of which are contraindicated in hemorrhage.

The carotid arteries, the large arteries leading from the aorta to the head, are subject to arteriosclerosis just as other arteries are. The blockage can occur anywhere in the vessel but is most likely to be at the bifurcation where the most turbulence occurs. Blockage of these arteries causes decreased blood flow to the brain. The most common problem with carotid artery disease is periods of lightheadedness or even fainting (transient ischemic attacks).

Treatment is controversial; vasodilators, calcium channel blockers, beta blockers, and other medications may help. Carotid endarterectomy has been shown to be the most effective treatment for long-term prevention but is not frequently performed because it carries a high risk of CVA.

Peripheral Vascular Disease

The major problems of peripheral blood supply are at least partially the result of evolution. Walking upright places a tremendous burden on the peripheral blood flow and increases susceptibility to arteriosclerosis in these areas. Law (2008) has documented that peripheral artery disease is on the rise.

Arteriosclerosis results in decreased circulation so that a cut or traumatized area with decreased blood supply may easily develop infection. Tissue necrosis and gangrene may result. Peripheral vascular disease can involve almost any artery in the lower extremities. Most commonly the sclerotic areas are at areas of turbulence such as the bifurcation of the vessels. Symptoms will depend on how high the obstruction occurs.

Sclerosis at the bifurcation of the aorta will decrease blood supply to one or both legs. This kind of high obstruction causes decreased blood flow to the entire leg or legs and causes severe pain with exercise or intermittent claudication. Pain occurs with walking and is relieved by rest. There will be poor or absent pulses in the lower extremities. Obstruction lower down occurs most commonly in the femoral arteries, although other smaller arteries, such as the popliteal arteries, can be involved. Multiple lesions are not uncommon. Decreased pulses peripheral to the obstruction are the most common finding. Small areas of gangrene can develop distal to the lesion if complete obstruction occurs.

Vascular bypass, balloon, laser angioplasty, and artificial grafts are used as treatments of choice. With the broad-spectrum antibiotics available and, more important, with education of the person who has diabetes regarding proper foot care and the modern techniques of bypass surgery and angioplasty, an amputation is seldom the choice of treatment. If intermittent claudication is experienced, treatment with Trental or Pletal once or twice a day often brings relief.

Cardiac catheterization, angiography of the neck and cerebral arteries, and angiography of the arteries for the pelvis and legs should be performed, especially including the assessment of cardiovascular autonomic neuropathy (Winters & Jernigan, 2000; Ziegler, 1999). Faulkner, Hathaway, Milstead, and Burghen (2001) found heart rate variability in adolescents and adults with T1DM was associated with atherosclerosis. Early intervention prevents loss of life. If an obstruction is found, appropriate bypass surgery or angioplasty is usually performed. With blood glucose controlled, the outcome of such surgery should be as good as in comparable individuals who do not have diabetes.

Summary

Early screening and appropriate interventions are adjunct to preventing complications from chronic hyperglycemia. Even adolescents with chronic hyperglycemia along with adults may need to be screened for heart rate variability (Faulkner et al., 2001). Even female children and adolescents with T1DM have earlier changes documented by echocardiographic testing (Suys et al., 2004). The earlier the abnormalities are caught, the earlier the interventions may be put in place, the better the potential outcome for that individual.

Various stress tests and electrocardiogram tests are useful, but their results may be normal even when there is pathology present. Blood tests, such as for C-reactive protein, may be the indicator that more aggressive and possibly invasive testing is needed. C-reactive protein is produced in the liver when inflammation is present in the body. A number of papers (Nesto, 2004; Ridker, 2006; Xu & Whitmer, 2006) have researched the testing results of C-reactive protein (>3.0) and concur with the correlation of inflammation findings and the cardiovascular risk potential. Other tests that may predict heart disease are homocysteine (an amino acid test potentially useful for a person with a family history of heart disease who does not smoke or have hypertension), elevated fibrinogen levels which may be a precursor to blood-clotting problems, and an enzyme in the white blood cells called myeloperoxidase that also may be linked to cardiovascular disease.

New interventions are constantly being sought to prevent CVD. One intervention that was found to have an association with a decrease in cardiovascular risk markers was the use of a meglitinide along with basal insulin (Wysham, Lush, Zhang, Maier, & Wilheim, 2008). Whether this improvement was due to the basal insulin alone, whether it was due to the addition of a meglitinide, or whether use of a basal insulin with a meglitinide had a synergistic effect, they agreed, was yet to be determined.

"Diabetes Guidelines" (2008) lists the updated recommendations of the American Diabetes Association to include testing of overweight adults, promoting lifestyle changes, and initiating earlier intervention with medication. For selected individuals, the A1c goal may need to be less than 6% to prevent macrovascular disease. A low CHO/low-fat diet is recommended for weight loss with a close monitoring of lipid profiles and kidney function; and, for children older than 10 with T1DM, failure on diet and lifestyle changes to control lipids should be followed by use of a statin. Also, Goede, Llund-Andersen, Parving, and Pedersen (2008) found that an intensive multifactored intervention with patients having T2DM had better cardiovascular outcomes.

Monitoring blood glucose levels (especially postprandial blood sugars [Glucomark], Ceriello, 2005) and hemoglobin A1c guide management approaches especially when weighed with the values obtained from yearly screening of the lipid profile, the metabolic profile, for microalbuminuria, for cardiovascular functioning, and peripheral vascular functioning (foot exam). There is a Framingham risk score assessment available from the National Institutes of Health (NIH) (2002, Publication 02-5215) as a tool for physicians to determine the 10-year risk of coronary heart disease (death and nonfatal myocardial infarction).

Dietary intervention, such as needed with weight loss, lipid or sodium restriction, and/or glucose control, may be found to aid in the development of individually prescribed meal plans. Various dietary approaches may be found in the list and descriptions given by Guthrie (2007), or the use of the well-documented DASH diet (Douglas et al., 2003)—composed of whole grains, vegetables, fruits, low-fat or fat-free dairy food, lean meats, poultry, and fish, nuts, seeds, and beans, reduced fat and oil intake, and limited sweets—may be used.

The NIH recommendations, from the Obesity Education Initiative, for weight loss are 500 to 1,000 kcal/day decrease in intake, activity for 30 min or more a day, behavior therapy, pharmacotherapy if problems with sleep apnea and diabetes with a body mass index (BMI) at or greater than 27, and weight loss surgery with a failed effort and a BMI at or greater than 35 if comorbid conditions are present, or the BMI is at or greater than 40.

New medications are constantly coming on the market. An abnormal endocannabinoid system control is associated with obesity and other abnormal cardiometabolic risk factors. Medications to control this system are being tested. Niskanene, Turpeinen, Penttila, and Uusitupa (1998) put into perspective the need for such interventions. For a meta-analysis of randomized trials since that year, refer to Stettler et al. (2006) and the findings of the control of blood glucose levels and cardiovascular disease for both T1DM and T2DM.

Self-care and self-management play an important role in attaining and maintaining a high degree of glucose control. According to Childs (2007), there are still unanswered questions as to how complications and comorbidities affect diabetes self-care behaviors. Even with these unanswered questions, it is the professional's responsibility to use what is available and to search out and develop potentially the most effective ways of assisting people in their health goals and in their needs and perceptions of a quality of life.

References

American Diabetes Association Consensus Statement. (2003a). Management of dyslipidemia in children and adolescents with diabetes. *Diabetes Care, 26,* 2194–2197.

American Diabetes Association Consensus Statement. (2003b). Peripheral arterial disease in people with diabetes. *Diabetes Care, 26,* 3333–3341.

American Diabetes Association Consensus Statement. (2007a). Waist circumference and cardiometabolic risk: A consensus statement from Shaping America's Health Association for Weight Management and Obesity Prevention; NAASO, The Obesity Society, the American Society for Nutrition, and the American Diabetes Association. *Diabetes Care, 30,* 1647–1652.

American Diabetes Association Consensus Statement. (2007b). Screening for coronary artery disease in patients with diabetes. *Diabetes Care, 30,* 2729–2736.

American Diabetes Association Position Statement. (2004a). Dyslipidemia management in adults with diabetes. *Diabetes Care, 27*(Suppl. 1), S68–S71.

American Diabetes Association Position Statement. (2004b). Aspirin therapy in diabetes. *Diabetes Care, 27*(Suppl. 1), S72–S73.

American Diabetes Association Position Statement. (2004c). Smoking and diabetes. *Diabetes Care, 27*(Suppl. 1), S76–S78.

American Diabetes Association Position Statement. (2005). Metabolic syndrome. *Diabetes Care, 28,* 2289.

Balasubramanyam, A., Hinnen, D., & Polonsky, W. (2006). Cardiovascular event prevention in the person with type 2 diabetes. *The Diabetes Educator, 32*(Suppl. 5), 163S–172S.

Braden, B. J., & Bergstrom, N. (1989). Clinical utility of the Braden Scale for predicting pressure sore risk. *Decubitus, 2,* 44–51.

Calder, R. A., & Alexander, C. M. (2000). Cardiovascular disease in people with diabetes mellitus. *Practical Diabetology, 19*(4), 7–10, 12–14, 16–18.

Ceriello, A. (2005). Postprandial hyperglycemia and diabetes complications: Is it time to treat? *Diabetes, 54,* 1–7.

Childs, B. (2007). Complications and comorbidities: Effects on diabetes self-care. *American Journal of Nursing, 107*(6), 55–59.

Diabetes Control and Complications Trial Research Group. (1993). The effect of intensive treatment of diabetes on the development and progression of long-term complications in insulin-dependent diabetes mellitus. *The New England Journal of Medicine, 329*(14), 977–985.

Diabetes guidelines: Screen more people earlier. (2008). *American Medical News, 51*(3), 1.

Dluhy, R. G., & McMahon, G. T. (2008) Intensive glycemic control in the ACCORD and ADVANCE trials. *The New England Journal of Medicine, 358*(24), 2630–2633.

Donahoe, S. M., Stewart, G. C., McCabe, C. H., Mohanavelu, S., Murphy, S. A., Cannon, C. P., et al. (2007). Diabetes and mortality following acute coronary syndromes. *Journal of the American Medical Association, 298*(7), 765–775.

Douglas, J. G., Bakris, G. L., Epstein, M., Ferdinand, K. C., Ferrario, C., Flack, J. M., et al.: Hypertension in African Americans Working Group of the International Society on Hypertension in Blacks. (2003). Management of high blood pressure in African Americans: Consensus statement of the Hypertension in African American Working Group of the International

Society on Hypertension in Blacks (recommendations on DASH—Dietary Approaches to Stop Hypertension). *Archives of Internal Medicine, 163*(5), 525–541.

Faulkner, M. S., Hathaway, D. K., Milstead, E. J., & Burghen, G. A. (2001). Heart rate variability in adolescents and adults with Type 1 diabetes. *Nursing Research, 50*(2), 95–104.

Gerstein, H. C., Miller, M. E., Byington, R. P., Goff, D. C., Jr., Bigger, J. T., Buse, J. B., et al. (2008). The Action to Control Cardiovascular Risk in Diabetes Study Group. Effects of intensive glucose lowering in type 2 diabetes. *New England Journal of Medicine, 358*(24), 2454–2559.

Giles, T. D., & Sander, G. E. (2004). Diabetes mellitus and heart failure: Basic mechanisms, clinical features, and therapeutic considerations. *Cardiology Clinics, 22*(4), 553–568.

Gilliam, L. K., Liese, A. D., Block, C. A., Davis, S., Snively, B. M., Curb, D., et al.; SEARCH for Diabetes in Youth Study Group. (2007). Family history of diabetes, autoimmunity, and risk factors for cardiovascular disease among children with diabetes in the SEARCH for Diabetes in Youth Study. *Pediatric Diabetes, 8*(6), 354–361.

Goede, P., Llund-Andersen, H., Parving, H. H., & Pedersen, O. (2008). Effect of a multifactorial intervention on mortality in type 2 diabetes. *New England Journal of Medicine, 24*(1), 580–591.

Guthrie, D. W. (2007). *Diabetes self-management's hidden secrets of natural healing* (pp. 129–140). New York: Diabetes Self-Management Books.

Law, B. M. (2008, January). Peripheral artery disease on the rise. *Diabetes, Obesity, Cardiovascular News, 7*.

National Institutes of Health. (2002). *Expert Panel final report of the third report of the National Cholesterol Education Program (NCEP) expert panel on detection, evaluation, and treatment of high blood cholesterol in adults*. NIH publication 02-5215.

Nesto, R. (2004). C-reactive protein, its role in inflammation, type 2 diabetes and cardiovascular disease, and the effects of insulin-sensitizing treatment with thiazolidinediones. *Diabetic Medicine, 21*(8), 810–817.

Niskanene, L., Turpeinen, A., Penttila, I., & Uusitupa, M. I. (1998). Hyperglycaemia and compositional lipoprotein abnormalities as predictors of cardiovascular mortality in type 2 diabetes: A 16 year follow-up from the time of diagnosis. *Diabetes Care, 21*, 1861–1869.

Patel, A., MacMahon, S., Chalmers, J., Neal, B., Billot, L., Heller, S., et al. (2008). The ADVANCE Collaborative Group. Intensive blood glucose control and vascular outcomes in patients with type 2 diabetes. *New England Journal of Medicine, 358*(24), 2560–2572.

Ridker, P. M. (2006, June). CRP level is highly predictive of cardiovascular risk. *Cardiovascular Risk Reduction Strategies, 4*–5.

Stettler, C., Allemann, S., Juni, P., Cull, C. A., Holman, R. R., Egger, M., et al. (2006). Glycemic control and macrovascular disease in types 1 and 2 diabetes mellitus: Meta-analysis of randomized trials. *American Heart Journal, 152*(1), 27–38.

Strowig, S. M., & Raskin, P. (1995). Glycemic control and the complications of diabetes: After the DCCT. *Diabetes Reviews, 3*(2), 237–257.

Suys, B. E., Katier, N., Rooman, R. P. A., Matthys, D., DeBeeck, L. O., DuCaju, M. V. L., et al. (2004). Female children and adolescents with type 1 diabetes have more pronounced early echocardiographic signs of diabetic cardiomyopathy. *Diabetes Care, 27*(8), 1947–1953.

U.K. Prospective Diabetes Study Group. (1998). Intensive blood glucose control with sulphonylureas or insulin compared with conventional treatment and risk of complications in patients with type 2 diabetes. *Lancet, 352*, 837–853.

Vaughan, T. B., Ovalle, F., & Moreland, E. (2007). Vascular disease in pediatric type 2 diabetes: The state of the art. *Diabetes Vascular Disease Research, 4*(4), 297–304.

Winters, S., & Jernigan, V. (2000). Vascular disease risk markers in diabetes: Monitoring and intervention. *Nurse Practice, 25*(6), 40, 43–46, 49, 65–67.

Wysham, C., Lush, C., Zhang, B., Maier, H., & Wilheim, K. (2008). Effect of pramlintide as an adjunct to basal insulin on markers of cardiovascular risk in patients with type 2 diabetes. *Current Medical Research Opinion, 24*(1), 79–85.

Xu, B. Y., & Whitmer, K. (2006). C-reactive protein and cardiovascular disease in people with diabetes. *American Journal of Nursing, 106*(8), 66–72.

Ziegler, D. (1999). Cardiovascular autonomic neuropathy: Clinical manifestations and measurement. *Diabetes Reviews, 7*(4), 300–314.

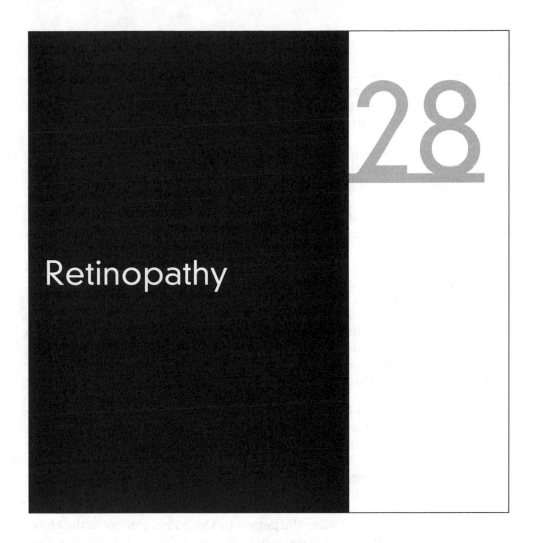

28

Retinopathy

Retinopathy is one of the small-vessel diseases. Microangiopathy involves the small blood vessels (capillaries) all over the body, but the clinical manifestations of microangiopathy occur for certain in only two organs: the kidney and the eye. Another condition, called cardiomyopathy, a too common problem in the person who has diabetes, may also be due to microvascular disease. Cardiomyopathy, as a disease of the heart, involves diffuse loss of heart muscle (myocardium) resulting in ineffective pumping and congestive heart failure. The diffuse loss of myocardium may be caused by disease in the myocardial blood supply, owing to disease and obstruction of the small blood vessels.

Retinopathy

The person with diabetes is subject to several changes occurring in the eye and early treatment accompanied by normalization of blood glucose levels and/or, as needed, early pan laser treatment of the retina appears to stabilize the eye (American Diabetes Association [ADA] Position Statement on Retinopathy, 2004). It is critical to assess eyes early, even in childhood, in the course of diagnosis and treatment (Lueder & Silverstein, 2005), recognizing there may be differences in severity related to long-standing hyperglycemia (Simmons, Clover, & Hope, 2007). The macula is the area most affected by diabetes and the area most important to preserve, because vision is largely dependent on its health.

Certain findings relate to the severity of this disease: Mild nonproliferative diabetic retinopathy is diagnosed when there are only microaneurysms. Moderate nonproliferative diabetic retinopathy is more than mild, but less than severe damage. Severe nonproliferative retinopathy is diagnosed when there are more than 20 intraretinal hemorrhages in each of 4 quadrants, venous bleeding in 2 or more quadrants, prominent microvascular abnormalities in one or more quadrants, but no signs of proliferative retinopathy. Proliferative diabetic retinopathy is diagnosed when neovascularization and/or vitreous/preretinal hemorrhage is documented (Aiello, 2005). The pathophysiology of basement membrane thickening that leads to retinopathy can be found in Chapter 5.

The three stages of retinopathy are (a) microaneurysm, (b) hemorrhage and exudates, and (c) retinitis proliferans. A microaneurysm, or small dilatation of a blood vessel that forms a sac, is caused by pressure exerted by the blood flow on a weakened blood vessel wall. This weakened blood vessel wall is one of the results of poor diabetes control. Microaneurysms can be visualized with the ophthalmoscope, and they usually appear as small red dots.

A hemorrhage results from a microaneurysm that breaks and then bleeds into the retina and/or the vitreous fluid of the eye. This occurrence may result in temporary or permanent blindness. After the hemorrhages are present for several weeks or months, they form waxy deposits called exudates. Through the ophthalmoscope, they appear as waxy areas, yellowish in color. Exudates are in essence scars from areas of infarction of the retina. Exudates may also be found as a yellowish deposit parallel to the blood vessels of the retina. This occurrence would be found when the person has high lipid content in the blood. Cotton wool spots are a result of damage to the nerve tissue and appear whiter and have more undefined edges.

Retinitis proliferans is a process of neovascularization. When there is hemorrhaging into the eye (which occurs in about 25% of the young adults with poorly controlled diabetes), new blood vessel growth (neovascularization) occurs primarily at the site of the disc. Small blood vessels extend out from the disc in an effort to nourish the tissue with a new blood supply. These small blood vessels are fragile, subject to hemorrhage. Moreover, these small vessels may compound the problem by growing into the vitreous and then contracting, thus causing retinal detachment, the primary cause of blindness in diabetes. Swelling of the macular area (macular edema) is a frequent concomitant of proliferative retinopathy but may occur early in the course of the eye disease.

Initial Assessment

The initial assessment, in the primary care office, should include a history and physical exam. An ocular history as well as a family history regarding eye diseases follows. A complete eye exam with a dilated pupil should be done annually.

This exam should include corrected visual acuity, intraocular pressure, slit lamp examination, and dilated fundus examination. Because even early diabetic retinopathy can be missed with a slit lamp and, more than likely, the average physician will not have a slit lamp as part of his or her equipment, it is preferred that this yearly exam be done by an ocular specialist. Any health professional should perform as much of an exam as possible when a specialist is not readily available. Optometrists are capable of completing a significant part of this examination, even including fundus photography, but a retinologist or ophthalmologist is recommended for final evaluation and treatment, especially if the person has Type 1 diabetes mellitus (T1DM).

More intense evaluation is completed with the use of fluorescein angiography or optical coherence tomography (OCT). The OCT is useful in showing cystic macular edema (CME), if present. Proliferative diabetic retinopathy is a risk indicator for a myocardial infarction, for the development of diabetic nephropathy, and also for amputation. Thus, examination of the eye, where the blood vessels can be seen, is a good screening tool for vascular disease in other organs where the vessels cannot be seen. Macular edema is frequently noted when a person has diabetic retinopathy (Nguyen et al., 2006). Macular edema is also considered the leading cause of legal blindness in patients with Type 2 diabetes mellitus (T2DM). Early detection of retinal abnormalities, such as macular edema, assist in delaying or preventing further progression of problems that can interfere with visual acuity.

Treatment

Early treatment for retinopathy included hypophysectomy, or removal of the pituitary gland, which resulted in improvement in the retinopathy but severe side effects due to loss of all pituitary hormones. The treatment worked because the hypophysectomy destroyed the ability of the pituitary gland to produce growth hormone that was responsible for the growth of new blood vessels in the eye to replace the occluded vessels in order to nourish the retina. These new vessels (neovascularization) are very fragile and break easily, causing retinal hemorrhage. This treatment is now obsolete. Newer treatment for retinopathy being performed throughout the country includes photocoagulation (pan lasering), individual vessel lasering, the scleral buckling procedure, vitrectomy, and lens replacement. Treatment should also include control of hypertension and dyslipidemia as one or both of these are frequent comorbidities that may exacerbate diabetic retinopathy.

Photocoagulation

Photocoagulation is used in the treatment of diabetic retinopathy to prevent macular edema, fibrovascular ingrowth into the vitreous, vitreous hemorrhage, and retinal detachment. The first instrument developed for photocoagulation was the Zeiss xenon arc photocoagulator. It is used most effectively at the origin of the hemorrhage. If the hemorrhage has resulted in neovascularization into the disc (proliferative diabetic retinopathy), then the argon laser is used to destroy these new vessels. This puts a stop to neovascularization and the potential resultant retinal detachment. Laser treatment is also used to stabilize macular edema. Laser photocoagulation may be of individual vessels or may be more extensive. Increased sophistication of the equipment and the operators has led to less pan-retinal photocoagulation and more precise photocoagulation at the points of need. Photocoagulation has been a major contributor, along with early and frequent screening, to the preservation of vision in people with diabetes in the last several years.

Scleral Buckling Procedure

The scleral buckling procedure has been useful for treating retinal detachment. The procedure is to place a band around the eye, narrowing it, and thus buckling the sclera forward into the detached area resulting in the retina reattaching. This procedure has been less needed in recent years than in the past because of earlier screening and improvements in photocoagulation.

Vitrectomy

Vitrectomy is another form of therapy for diabetic retinopathy resulting from hemorrhage into the vitreous. A single injection of bevacizumab (a monoclonal antivascular growth factor used most commonly to limit blood vessel growth into cancer tissue) was noted to clear vitreous hemorrhage clouding and thereby improve visual acuity (Spaide & Fisher, 2006). Vitrectomy is performed when conventional methods have failed or the hemorrhage has not absorbed in 5–6 months. In the procedures of vitrectomy, the vitreous of the eye is removed by an instrument called the vitreous-infusion-suction-cutter. After the vitreous is removed, the vacant cavity is filled with 60% air and 40% sulfur hexafluoride or saline solution. The hemorrhage and scar tissue are removed along with the vitreous fluid.

Macular Edema

Macular edema may now be treated with a variety of interventions (Ferris, 2006). These include the inhibition of growth hormone (vascular endothelial growth factor inhibitors), the use of a vitrectomy, the use of anti-inflammatory treatment, and what are called protein kinase C-beta (PKC-beta) inhibitors. Both the PKC-beta inhibitors and the vascular endothelial growth factor inhibitors have shown benefit in treating such a condition. Photocoagulation has also been found helpful especially since the new computer-guided laser equipment has become available. The newer laser equipment allows for precise photocoagulation near the macula without damage to the macula, the most important part of the retina needed for central vision.

A variety of new therapies, including aldose-reductase inhibitors and non-hormonal anti-inflammatory agents, and others, are rapidly being developed (Furlani et al., 2007). This should result in a better outcome for those suffering from macular edema.

In General

Prevention is best, but if some level of retinopathy is diagnosed, besides the on-site treatment, meticulous care must be given to blood pressure, lipids, hematocrit values, blood glucose levels controlled without any undue hypoglycemia occurring, and other health care issues, such as congestive heart failure (Gardner, 2005). In the EURODIAB Prospective Complications Study, it was demonstrated that there is an increased risk for mortality and cardiovascular disease when nonproliferative or proliferative retinopathy is diagnosed (Van Hecke et al., 2005). Because lipid elevations are known precursors to cardiovascular events, they must be normalized (Leiter, 2005). These findings add further impetus to the need to control blood glucose levels, blood pressure, and blood lipids and to treat diabetic retinopathy as early as possible.

Lens

Because the lens of the eye has no blood supply for nourishment, its nourishment depends on the aqueous humor. Thus, the lens reflects changes in the aqueous humor, such as changes in the glucose levels. Glucose levels of the aqueous humor are, in turn, reflections of the blood glucose levels. Changes within the lens cells result in cataracts, which can occur in anyone but are more frequent and occur earlier in people with poorly controlled diabetes.

Blurred Vision

The individual with diabetes may experience sudden changes in refraction and accommodation. Such changes are most often associated with osmotic changes in the lens. The person will complain of blurred vision, which is corrected when the blood glucose level becomes normal and stays normal for a period of time. Individuals should not have their eyes examined for glasses until blood glucose levels have been relatively normal for 4–6 weeks.

Summary

Individuals with a diagnosis of T2DM should have their eyes examined at diagnosis and then yearly. Those in whom T1DM is diagnosed should also have their eyes examined. Most of the literature states that this should be done 5 years after diagnosis, but after age 30, that ophthalmologic examination should start at the time of diagnosis. In light of a possible diagnosis of retinopathy and the institution of early treatment, others recommend a baseline intensive evaluation shortly after diagnosis. If pregnancy is planned, an exam should be given before conception and at 3-month intervals, beginning in the first trimester.

Many individuals are initially monitored by an optometrist. Although ophthalmologists and retinologists are needed for treatment and follow-up, a need was felt to improve the communication between the professions. Jones and Nichols (2007) researched and updated the American Optometric Association's form (which can be found at www.ooa.org), called the Diabetic Eye Examination Report (DEER), which can be filled out and sent to the referring physician. They felt information transfer on this form could also be used in the process of comanagement.

Photocoagulation, scleral buckling, and vitrectomy are now well-established procedures. Persons with diabetes should be informed of the availability of these procedures and referred to a capable ophthalmologist or retinologist even before retinopathy is present. Pan lasering, when needed, stabilizes the retina and usually prevents blindness by leading to a more stabilized retina. The full result of any eye surgery is not known until about 4–6 months after the lasering is performed. The good news is that whether retinopathy or other microvascular problems occur, the risk is less when intensive blood glucose management is maintained (Barr, 2001).

For a full review of information on diabetic retinopathy, refer to the article by Wilkinson-Berka and Miller (2008). The good news is that the progression of retinopathy can be slowed (or prevented) if care is taken to control blood glucose levels, hypertension, and hypercholesterolemia (Higgins, Khan, & Pearce, 2007).

References

Aiello, L. P. (2005). Molecular biology and natural history of diabetes retinopathy. *Advanced Studies in Ophthalmology, 291,* 8–13.

American Diabetes Association Position Statement. (2004). Retinopathy in diabetes. *Diabetes Care, 27*(Suppl. 1), S84–S87.

Barr, C. C. (2001). Retinopathy and nephropathy in patients with type 1 diabetes four years after a trial of intensive insulin therapy. The Diabetes Control and Complications Trial/Epidemiology of Diabetes Interventions and Complications Research Group. *New England Journal of Medicine, 342,* 381–389.

Ferris, F. L. (2006). Focus on diabetic macular edema. *Advanced Studies in Ophthalmology, 3*(1), 18–22.

Furlani, B. A., Meyer, C. H., Rodrigues, E. B., Maia, M., Farah, M. E., Penha, F. M., et al. (2007). Emerging pharmacotherapies for diabetic macular edema. *Expert Opinion on Emergency Drugs, 12*(4), 591–603.

Gardner, T. W. (2005). Current strategies and challenges in the management of diabetic retinopathy. *Advanced Studies in Ophthalmology, 3,* 10, 14–19.

Higgins, G. T., Khan, J., & Pearce, I. A. (2007). Glycemic control and control of risk factors in diabetes patients in an ophthalmology clinic: What lessons have we learned from the UKPDS and DCCT studies? *Acta Ophthalmologica Scandinavica, 85*(7), 772–776.

Jones, S. L., & Nichols, K. K. (2007). Diabetic eye examination report. *Optometry, 13*(5), 588–595.

Leiter, L. (2005). *Diabetes Research and Clnical Practice, 68*(Suppl. 2), S5–S14.

Lueder, G. T., & Silverstein, J. (2005). Screening for retinopathy in the pediatric patient with type 1 diabetes mellitus. *Pediatrics, 116*(1), 270–273.

Nguyen, S., Tatlipinar, S., Shah, J., Haller, E., Quinlan, J., Sung, I., et al. (2006). Vascular endothelial growth factor Is a critical stimulus for diabetic macular edema. *American Journal of Ophthalmology, 142*(6), 961–969.

Simmons, D., Clover, G., & Hope, C. (2007). Ethnic differences in diabetic retinopathy. *Diabetic Medicine, 24*(10), 1093–1098.

Spaide, R. F., & Fisher, Y. L. (2006). Intravitreal bevacizumab treatment of proliferative diabetic retinopathy complicated by vitreous hemorrhage. *Retina, 26,* 275–278.

Van Hecke, M. V., Dekker, J. M., Stehouwer, C. D. A., Polak, B. C. P., Fuller, J. H., Sjolie, A. K., et al. (2005). Diabetic retinopathy is associated with mortality and cardiovascular disease incidence: The EURODIAB Prospective Complications Study. *Diabetes Care, 28*(6), 1383–1389.

Wilkinson-Berka, J. L., & Miller, A. G. (2008). Update on the treatment of diabetic retinopathy. *Scientific World Journal, 8,* 98–120.

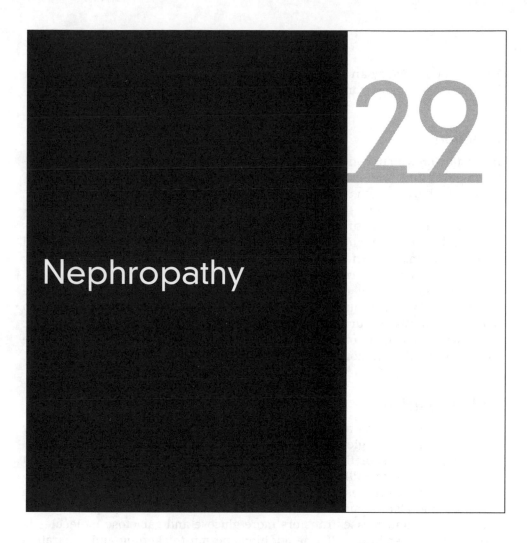

29

Nephropathy

Nephropathy classically was associated with foamy urine, hypertension, and renal edema formation or the triad caused by sodium retention and hyperglycemia. Yee (2008) reports that 30%–40% of "diabetic kidney disease (DKD)" will occur in people who have diabetes with about a third of these individuals developing end-stage renal disease.

End-stage renal disease (ESRD) is but one of the major problems that can occur with poor control of blood glucose levels. The cost for dialysis as an intermediary step to prevent this final process is expensive in both time and money. With poor blood glucose control, the kidneys are more susceptible to infection that can also damage these delicate tissues. So the two major problems related to the kidneys are infection and nephropathy and both need to be prevented or treated as early in the stage of the disease as possible (ADA: Nephropathy in Diabetes, 2004; Barr, 2001). The National Kidney Foundation recommends a yearly microalbuminuria test for those with Type 2 diabetes mellitus (T2DM) who are younger than age 70 and for others with Type 1 diabetes mellitus (T1DM) who are older than age 12. The American Diabetes Association recommends annual testing once T2DM is diagnosed, and for those with T1DM, annual testing should start 5 years after diagnosis. The goal? The microalbuminuria below

20 mg/L or 30 mg/day, an albumin/creatinine ratio less than 30 mg/g (Pagana & Pagana, 2006), or an estimated glomerulofiltration rate >60 ml/min.

Infection

In the person with uncontrolled diabetes, infection may invade the bladder, resulting in cystitis, or the kidneys, resulting in pyelonephritis. The common complaints are burning with urination, frequency of urination, and lower back pain. The level of blood glucose control should be investigated. If proper drug therapy is not promptly instituted for cystitis, the infection may ascend the ureters to the kidney tissue, resulting in pyelonephritis and potential damage to renal tissue, which may in turn lead to decreased kidney function. Pyelonephritis may also occur from bloodborne infection.

As another outcome of poor control, neuropathic changes in nerves to the bladder because of frequent infections or autonomic neuropathy can lead to bladder paralysis and urinary retention. In patients with any type of diabetic neuropathy, symptoms of any type of urinary or kidney infection should be treated promptly and monitored.

Pathophysiology

To review: The kidneys are composed of an intricate network of microscopic blood vessels, called glomeruli, that filter waste materials from the blood. The glomeruli are sensitive to changes caused by thickening of the basement membrane of their capillaries. The basement membrane consists of concentric, tightly packed circles of glycoproteins, which are infrequently tagged with galactose and glucose molecules. When insulin levels are inadequate, an enzyme, glucosyltransferase, transfers more glucose and galactose molecules to the basement membranes. These additions permit thickening and separation of the concentric circles of basement membrane material, allowing larger molecular weight substances such as proteins to pass through the more porous membrane. This condition may result in edema, hypertension, proteinuria, uremia, and death. There also appears to be damage to the mesangial cells of the kidney, increasing glomerular pressure and decreasing glomerular blood flow. This means that a person could have nephropathy from damage caused by elevated blood glucose levels and/or glomerulonephropathy from frequent infections or hypertension or both.

The kidneys normally excrete insulin through the urine. As kidney damage increases, insulin dosage and the dosage of various oral agents used to treat T2DM must be decreased to prevent hypoglycemia. For example, a patient who requires 48 Units of insulin at age 30 might require as little as 6–8 Units at age 68. Many patients may feel that their diabetes is improving, but it might be a result of renal failure. Also, if a person is taking a sulfonylurea and kidney damage is noted, the oral agent must be discontinued for this same reason. Biguanides are also not to be prescribed if kidney damage has occurred. Biguanides (metformin) should be discontinued in anyone with a serum creatinine greater than 1.4 mg/dl and in women with a creatinine greater than 1.3 mg/dl.

Normalized blood glucose levels and blood pressure, most of the time, continue to be the only way to prevent complications in the kidney in T1DM

(Zerbini, Gabellini, Maestroni, & Maestroni, 2007). This appears to be true also in T2DM emphasizing the fact that early detection of problems associated with kidney function should be important (Sego, 2007). Eknoyan (2007) emphasizes again that the two major causes of kidney disease are hypertension and diabetes in the obese population. He shares that obesity, even without known diabetes, is associated with filtration problems of the kidney, but these are reversed with weight loss.

Detection and Diagnosis

Diabetic nephropathy may become clinically manifest as micro and gross proteinuria, hypertension, and progressive renal failure, with a rising blood urea nitrogen and creatinine and potential concomitant uremic poisoning.

Another manifestation of diabetic renal disease is the nephrotic syndrome (albuminuria >300/24 hr, proteinuria >500 mg/24 hr, hypertension, and declining glomerular filtration rate [GFR]). In this condition proteinuria is severe, and the serum proteins drop to very low levels. The low serum protein levels result in loss of the osmotic gradient and loss of fluid into the tissue causing severe edema (anasarca). Serum lipids will be elevated in an attempt to regain osmotic pressure.

The first sign of diabetic renal disease is microalbumin in the urine. According to the Royal College of Physicians of Edinburgh Diabetes Register Group (2000), such findings can also predict progression into diabetic nephropathy. On the other hand, if a person smokes, has T2DM, and diabetic nephropathy, the progression to a more deteriorating state is faster even with the use of angiotensin-converting enzyme inhibitors (ACEIs) (Chuahirun & Wesson, 2002).

Using a dip stick for determining gross proteinuria was found to be inadequate screening (Mainous & Gill, 2001). Documenting microalbuminuria or calculating the albumin/creatinine ratio, and the therapy for either, along with tightening blood glucose control, is considered an important part of the total management program. Most proponents of intervention at the point that microalbuminuria is above 30 mg intervene with lower protein recommendations in the meal plan and the start of an ACEI (Microvascular Complications Round Table, 2000). A question was, should all patients use ACEIs prophylactically? In the past, the answer was no because of cost. Most ACEIs are now generic, so cost is no longer an issue. More widespread or earlier use of ACEIs may prevent or slow much renal damage.

The various stages in the decline of kidney function should be reviewed (see Table 29.1).

With no intervening factors, the continuum path starts from the early risk factors such as diabetes and/or hypertension. This progresses to endothelial dysfunction, microalbuminuria to macroalbuminuria to diabetic nephropathy followed by end-stage renal disease (ESRD) and death.

Early diagnosis of albuminuria may be obtained from a timed collection (µg/min), a spot collection (µg/g Cr), or a 24-hr collection (mg/24 hr) (ADA, 2004). Normal protein excretion is <20 µg in the timed collection and <30 in the other two types of collection. Microalbuminuria is a protein excretion from 20 to 199 mg/min in a timed collection and 30–199 mg/min in the other two types of collection. Macroalbuminuria is at or greater than 200 in the timed specimen

29.1 Stages of Nephropathy

Stage I	Is proteinuria with a normal or increased glomerulofiltration rate (GFR >90)
Stage II	Involves a mild decrease in GFR, i.e., 89–60
Stage III	Involves a moderate decrease in GFR, i.e., 59–30
Stage IV	Involves a severe decrease in GFR, i.e., 29–15
Stage V	Is considered kidney failure with a GFR of <15

and at or greater than 300 in the other collections. The most recommended test today (2008) is the spot collection to obtain an albumin/creatinine ratio and the estimated glomerular filtration rate or eGFR. If the GFR (not the eGFR) is more than 140 ml/min then there is a positive prediction that 63% of the time it will correlate with proteinuria; if less than 140, there is a 94% prediction. The normal GFR is 100–125 ml/min. Normal eGFR is usually reported only as greater than 60 with a correction factor for African Americans. The normal loss of GFR is 0.5–0.75 ml·min^{-1}·year^{-1}. A person with diabetic nephropathy may lose 2–20 ml·min^{-1}·year^{-1}. For an albumin/creatinine ratio, divide the milligrams per deciliter of protein by the grams per deciliter of creatinine.

Costacou, Ellis, Fried, and Orchard (2007) studied the use of eGFR compared with the standardized microalbumin measurements. In the prospective cohort study, completed concurrently with the Pittsburgh Epidemiology of Diabetes Complications Study, it was found that a creatinine clearance of less than 60–200 µg/min correlated with a low eGFR. The group also found that in some patients the low eGFR might precede the albuminuria. The eGFR has been accepted as the best overall measure for renal function. The eGFR is calculated by the following formula. This formula is not used if the GFR is greater than 60 ml/min (Ossman, 2006).

$$eGFR \ (ml \ urine·min^{-1}·1.73 \ m^{-2}) =$$

$$186 \times [serum \ creatinine \ (µmol/L) \times 0.0113] - 1.154 \times age \ (in \ years) - 0.203$$

$$(\times 0.742 \ if \ female)$$

The National Kidney Foundation classifies chronic kidney disease by stages (see Table 29.1).

The ADA recommends screening annually by measuring serum creatinne for eGFR calculation in all adults with diabetes with less than 30 as normal (µg albumin/µg/mg creatinine); microalbuminuria 30–299; and macroalbuminuria >300. The blood pressure target should be less than 127/75 if protein is present in the urine (>1.0 g per 24 hr) or the creatinine is abnormal.

Treatment

Treatment of diabetic renal disease may include diuretics, hypertensive medications (Baskar, Kamalakannan, Holland, & Singh, 2002), and infusion of serum albumin when anasarca (generalized swelling or peripheral edema) is present. Overall, treatment of diabetic nephropathy consists of control of the blood glucose, which early on may reverse some pathology or may slow the progression of nephropathy. Once diabetic nephropathy starts, blood glucose control may slow but will not stop or reverse the process. Control of hypertension also aids in slowing the progression of nephropathy.

Diabetes specialists are recommending the use of an ACEI as a preventive due to its action of promoting vasodilatation of the blood vessels going out of the kidneys. ACEIs are effective blood pressure-lowering agents but may cause a chronic cough. There are also angiotensin-II receptor antagonists (ARBS) specific to block vasoconstriction and to reduce aldosterone secretion. ARBS are effective in lowering blood pressure with a low incidence of the cough and angioedema seen with ACEIs. The goal is for the blood pressure control to be less than 130/80 (ADA, 2004). With proteinuria of 1 g/24 hr or the diagnosis of diabetic kidney disease, the blood pressure goal should be 125/75 or less. This may require two or more antihypertensive medications to be prescribed. A guideline to go by is if the blood pressure is 20/10 mmHg above goal, add a second agent.

A calcium channel blocker might be added or used in place of ACEI (if an ACEI is not tolerated) and to aid in dilating the blood vessels going into the kidney. A calcium channel blocker might also be used along with an ACEI when more blood pressure control or more kidney function is desired.

Protein restriction in diabetes has been controversial unless a person has developed kidney disease. Robertson, Waugh, and Robertson (2000) found that such a decrease in protein intake did slow progression of nephropathy but not significantly so. They concluded that different types of protein intake need to be researched because of patient variability in absorption and processing. If an abnormal eGFR is obtained, or if there is protein in the urine without any explanation other than diabetes, the target of daily protein intake should be lowered but not less than 0.8 kg/body weight. The point to be considered is that a protein-restricted diet (0.3–0.8 g/kg) seems to slow down the progression of frank diabetic nephropathy (Waugh & Robertson, 2006). Compliance with such a diet is difficult.

The possibility of hypoalbuminemia by severe protein restriction could occur and, so, is another concern. Such a restricted diet might also mean a greater need for the monitoring of phosphorus, sodium, calcium, and potassium which is also a concern if a person has diabetic nephropathy. A balance or a combination of foods to prevent hypertension, control blood glucose levels, and, as needed, a modest weight reduction is considered the best approach for dietary management (Franz, 2006).

Renal dialysis has progressed rapidly in recent years and is now a much simpler and more efficient procedure than in years past. Dialysis may be by hemodialysis or peritoneal dialysis. Hemodialysis may be performed in the hospital or at a dialysis center, or now, by portable home dialysis units. Peritoneal dialysis is an excellent alternative because the insulin can be put in the dialysis fluid and infused intraperitoneally. The insulin is then absorbed into the portal system and into the liver as in the nondiabetic state. Excellent control of diabetes can be achieved. There is a high incidence of peritoneal infection with peritoneal dialysis. There is also infection, and clotting, as frequent occurrences at the shunt site in patients on hemodialysis. Surprisingly, those patients on dialysis were in relatively good mental health despite the low rating they gave on their physical health (Sorensen et al., 2007).

For those with early albuminuria, a fenofibrate (over a three-year period) was found to reduce the progression of albumin excretion (Ansquer, Foucher, Rattier, Taskinen, & Steiner, 2005). This appeared to be independent of improved lipid levels and creatinine levels. In conclusion, though, the improvement of albumin excretion was correlated with improvement in the lipid profiles.

Dialysis is usually discussed when the person's kidney function is down to 20% or less. Their choices are a kidney transplant, peritoneal dialysis, or hemodialysis (an access arteriovenous fistula in place). There is more of a chance of hypoglycemia with hemodialysis vs. peritoneal dialysis which has a high concentration of glucose, held in the abdomen overnight, to create an ultrafiltration of excess fluid.

A kidney transplant is usually considered the last option. More often now, a pancreas transplant is placed in the decision-making process slightly before or when end-stage kidney disease occurs. Coppelli et al. (2005) found that a successful pancreas transplant, rather than a kidney transplant, improved diabetic nephropathy in the patients they followed. The creatinine concentrations or clearances did not differ from before the transplant of the pancreas, but the urinary protein excretion decreased. The waiting list for renal transplant is long, and patients on the list should be told that the availability of kidneys for transplant is limited. If they can find a living related donor, they will receive a kidney much sooner than if they must wait for a cadaver donor.

Summary

Renal transplantation now has a good prognosis, with improved surgical technologies, better tissue matching via a national computerized network, and new immunosuppression drugs. The use of better tissue match, presurgical transfusion, splenectomy, cyclosporin, and newer monoclonal antibodies to immune cells has resulted in a more than 90% successful transplantation rate in some programs. The outcome appears to be even better if a pancreas and kidney are transplanted at the same time.

Basi and Lewis (2007) reviewed the literature on microalbuminuria and again found evidence that its presence predisposed to the comorbidities of cardiovascular disease and nephropathy. The literature emphasized the findings that if microalbuminuria is controlled, cardiovascular and kidney functions also improved.

To review: For the person with diabetic nephropathy, the blood pressure goal is less than 125/75 (WHO, <130/80); if blood pressure is elevated, use an ACEI and add an ARB or calcium channel blocker and/or diuretic as needed; hemoglobin A1c should be reduced to 6.5%; no NSAIDS/COX-2 inhibitors should be used (acetaminophen or narcotics for pain); and referral to a nephrologist when any of the following occur: there is hematuria; the blood pressure is out of control; there is greater than 500 mg/protein in the urine; the creatinine is above the normal limits, 2.0 or higher; and/or the creatinine clearance is less than 60 ml/min. The overriding goal is to prevent the occurrence and/or the progression of diabetic nephropathy, and an ACEI (or ARB) should be started as soon as any microalbuminuria is determined to be present (Hall, 2006).

References

American Diabetes Association Position Statements. (2004). Nephropathy in diabetes. *Diabetes Care, 27*(Suppl. 1), S79–S83.

Ansquer, J., Foucher, C., Rattier, S., Taskinen, M., & Steiner, G. (2005). Fenofibrate reduces progression to microalbuminuria over 3 years in a placebo-controlled study in type 2 diabetes: Results from the Diabetes Atherosclerosis Intervention Study (DAIS). *American Journal of Kidney Diseases, 45*(3), 485–493.

Barr, C. C. (2001). Retinopathy and nephropathy in patients with type 1 diabetes four years after a trial of intensive insulin therapy. The Diabetes Control and Complications Trial/Epidemiology of Diabetes Interventions and Complications Research Group. *New England Journal of Medicine, 342,* 381–389.

Basi, S., & Lewis, J. B. (2007, December). Microalbuminuria as a target to improve cardiovascular and renal outcomes in diabetic patients. *Current Diabetes Reports, 7*(6), 439–442.

Baskar, V., Kamalakannan, D., Holland, M. E., & Singh, B. M. (2002). The prevalence of hypertension and utilization of antihypertensive therapy in a district diabetes population. *Diabetes Care, 25*(11), 2107–2108.

Chuahirun, T., & Wesson, D. L. (2002). Cigarette smoking predicts faster progression of type 2 established diabetic nephropathy despite ACE inhibitors. *American Journal of Kidney Diseases, 39*(2, Suppl. 1), 376–382.

Coppelli, A., Giannarelli, R., Vistoli, F., Del Prato, S., Rizzo, G., Mosca, F., et al. (2005). The beneficial effects of pancreas transplant alone on diabetic nephropathy. *Diabetes Care, 28*(6), 1366–1370.

Costacou, T., Ellis, D., Fried, L., & Orchard, T. J. (2007). Sequence of progression of albuminuria and decreased GFR in person with type 1 diabetes: A cohort study. *American Journal of Kidney Disease, 50*(5), 721–732.

Eknoyan, G. (2007). Obesity, diabetes, and chronic kidney disease. *Current Diabetes Reports, 7*(6), 449–453.

Franz, M. J. (2006). Medical nutrition therapy for hypertension and albuminuria. *Diabetes Spectrum, 19*(1), 32–38.

Hall, P. M. (2006). Prevention of progression in diabetic nephropathy. *Diabetes Spectrum, 19*(1), 18–24.

Levey, A. S., Bosch, R. P., Lewis, J. B., Greene, T., Rogers, N., & Roth, D. (1999). A more accurate method to estimate glomerular filtration rate from serum creatinine: A new prediction equation. Modification of Diet in Renal Disease Study Group. *Annals of Internal Medicine, 130,* 461–470.

Mainous, A. G., III, & Gill, J. M. (2001). The lack of screening for diabetic nephropathy: Evidence from a privately insured population. *Family Medicine, 33*(2), 115–119.

Microvascular complications of diabetes: The role of angiotensin converting enzyme inhibitors: Proceedings of a round table meeting, June 1999, San Diego, CA. (2000). *Practical Diabetology International, 17*(8, Suppl.), 1–12.

Ossman, S. S. (2006). Diabetic nephropathy: Where we have been and where we are going. *Diabetes Spectrum, 19*(3), 153–156.

Pagana, K., & Pagana, T. (2006). *Mosby's manual of diagnostic and laboratory tests* (3rd ed.). St. Louis: Mosby/Elsevier.

Robertson, L., Waugh, N., & Robertson, A. (2007, October). Protein restriction for diabetic renal disease. *Cochrane Database System Review, 17*(4), CD002181.

Royal College of Physicians of Edinburgh Diabetes Register Group. (2000). Near-normal urinary albumin concentrations predict progression to diabetic nephropathy in Type 1 diabetes mellitus. *Diabetic Medicine, 17*(11), 782–791.

Sego, S. (2007). Pathophysiology of diabetic nephropathy. *Nephrology Nursing Journal, 34*(94), 631–633.

Sorensen, V. R., Mathiesen, E. R., Watt, T., Bjorner, J. B., Andersen, M. V., & Feldt-Rasmussen, B. (2007). Diabetic patients treated with dialysis: Complications and quality of life. *Diabetologia, 50*(11), 2254–2262.

Waugh, N. R., & Robertson, A. M. (2006). Protein restriction for diabetic renal disease. *The Cochrane Library, 1*, CD002181.

Yee, J. (2008). Diabetic kidney disease: Chronic kidney disease and diabetes. *Diabetes Spectrum, 21*(1), 8–10.

Zerbini, G., Gabellini, D., Maestroni, S., & Maestroni, A. (2007). Early renal dysfunctions in type 1 diabetes and pathogenesis of diabetic nephropathy. *Journal of Nephrology, 20*(Suppl. 12), S19–S22.

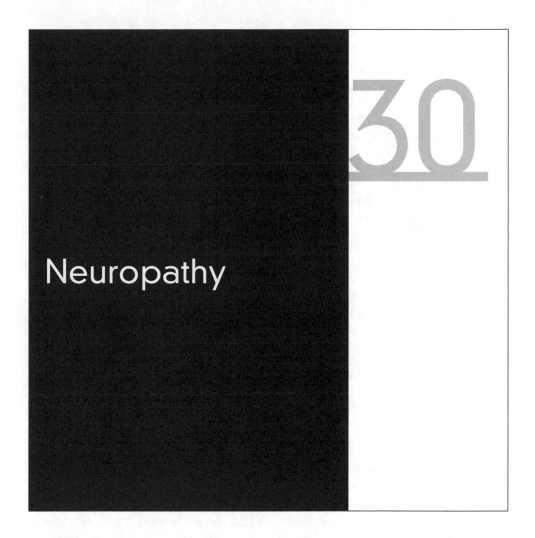

Neuropathy

30

A problem too often observed in the adult with diabetes is neuropathy. Diabetic neuropathy may have many manifestations. A single nerve or multiple nerves may be affected. Damage may occur to sensory and/or motor nerves. Nerves of the autonomic nervous system, especially the parasympathetic nerves, may also be damaged. If circulation is poor, there will be less nutrition to the nerves and neuropathy can develop. If neuropathy has developed, poor circulation to that area of the body as well as direct damage to the nerves from high blood glucose levels needs to be suspected.

Diabetic sensory neuropathy is manifested by aching pain and burning of the lower extremities and ultimately loss of sensation and numbness. Loss of autonomic nerve function may cause bladder paralysis, stomach paralysis (gastroparesis), diarrhea, and impotence. Motor neuropathy can cause muscular paralysis and atrophy. Neuropathy is most often associated with increased blood glucose levels. The pain usually subsides after lower blood glucose levels are established. Strangely enough, the pain of diabetic neuropathy usually worsens at night while the patient is at rest, and many patients with peripheral sensory neuropathy say that they cannot tolerate the slightest stimuli to their feet—not even bedclothes.

After the individual has had diabetes for 10–20 years accompanied with poor control of blood glucose levels much of the time, painless neuropathy or numbness may develop. The ability to feel painful stimuli is decreased, which may result in an injury that the person with diabetes does not perceive. For example, the person may, in walking barefoot, step on a tack and not find it until taking a bath later that evening. This type of neuropathy, combined with large- and small-vessel disease, can result in serious damage to the feet and requires constant vigilance.

Diabetic neuropathy can involve one or more large nerves (mononeuropathy or mononeuropathy multiplex), small nerves (ocular neuropathy), sensory nerves or motor nerves, and the autonomic nervous system (ANS). The ANS may, in turn, involve the cardiovascular, gastrointestinal, genitourinary systems, or hypoglycemia unawareness. Various mechanisms may be involved, but large- and small-nerve disease does appear to be related to diabetes control. The mechanism of diabetic neuropathy in these nerves appears to be the polyol pathway previously mentioned in Chapter 5. Sorbitol or fructose accumulation in the Schwann cells of the nerve tissue results in damage to these cells, leading to decreased myelin production. Without their myelin sheaths, nerves do not function adequately, and the clinical manifestations of neuropathy develop. Damage can also occur to axonal cells, resulting in decreased nerve repolarization and thus decreased nerve action. These and other types of diabetic neuropathies will be discussed.

Distal Symmetrical Polyneuropathy

Large-nerve disease may cause loss of function of muscle groups, with manifestations such as foot drop or ocular muscle paralysis. Neuropathy may also cause hyperesthesia (pain) or hypoesthesia (decreased sensation). The hypoesthesia especially is a problem because decreased sensation leads to decreased perception of injury. Foot ulcers in the person who has diabetes are both neuropathic and vascular in origin with foot infections the "single most common cause of hospitalization and lower extremity amputation" (Andersen & Roukis, 2007). Pressure is not perceived; therefore, the individual will stand, keeping pressure on that part of the foot longer than usual, leading to pressure ischemia and ulcer formation. There may also be motor nerve loss with atrophy of the interosseous muscles and breakdown of the arch integrity of the foot, changing the pressure points. Joint stiffness may be noted in ankle and knees in the late phases of the disease (Williams, Brunt, & Tannenberg, 2007).

Distal symmetrical polyneuropathy (DSP), also termed diabetic peripheral neuropathy (DPN), is associated with tingling and numbness of the feet. Adequate control of diabetes influences this neuropathy. Symptoms subside and eventually disappear in most cases when early intervention is instituted and blood glucose levels are normalized. Patients may need to be warned that the resulting regrowth of nerve fibers may be uncomfortable, but such discomfort should resolve in six months to a year if normalization of blood sugars is maintained as much as possible.

One form of DSP that does not have as good a prognosis is neuroarthropathy (Charcot's foot), but if caught in its early stages, it may be stabilized. Charcot's foot is less frequently observed today than in the past, but it is still present

(Levine, Kaplun, Shavelson, & Poretsky, 2006). It appears in the joints of the ankles and feet when there is both sensory and motor neuropathy and inadequate circulation to the extremities. The person with the following should be suspected of having Charcot's foot: the foot (usually the ankle) is warm, swollen, and erythematous. X-ray would reveal collapse of one or more of the following joints: the calceneo-cuboid joint, the talo-navicular joint, Charcot's joint, the first metatarso-cuneiform joint, the first metatarso-phalangeal joint of the hallux, and/or the ankle joint. Osteomyelitis is to be ruled out. The atrophic phase comes first; the destructive or coalescence process comes next; and the reconstruction or deformity is the last. Diabetes control and foot centering (stabilizing the foot and ankle with an orthotic) is the first approach; amputation only if all else fails.

Another neurologically associated problem is carpel tunnel syndrome. This may be surgically treated by enlarging the opening through which the nerves to the hand are found. The surgery is especially useful when numbness and loss of finger/grip control has occurred. Nerve entrapment in the elbow should be suspected if all the fingers are numb.

Some supplements have been studied for neuropathy, but are still in need of further analysis. The most evidenced-based studies have been completed on alpha-lipoic acid and capsaicin, which have been found to be effective in some patients. Individual response differences and some untoward side effects have been noted. Evening primrose oil was found only possibly to be effective with people who had very mild neuropathy (Halat & Denneby, 2003).

If a diabetic foot ulcer is present because of DSP, the chances of reversal become less when both infection and ischemia are present with grade 3 wound (the wound penetrating to bone or joint; grade 2, penetrating to tendon or capsule; grade 1, not involving tendon capsule or bone). Aggressive treatment with blood glucose control and the use of Regranex (becaplermin) or platelet growth factors has been successful even with severe ulcers, but side effects may occur. Hollister and Li (2007) review the use of becaplermin in chronic wound care. Pergabalin as well as other seizure medications and SSRIs has been found to be safe and efficacious in the treatment of painful diabetic peripheral neuropathy but will have no effect on the healing of ulcerative disease or the insensate foot (Freeman, Durso-Decruz, & Emir, 2008). Sugar or honey in the wound has also been used successfully to cause regranulation of diabetic foot ulcers. Wallace (2007) noted that patient education and surgical debridement of the infected site should be accompanied with intensive diabetes control and appropriate antibiotic therapy.

Increasing circulation and decreasing pain in the extremities are the potential outcome with the use of anodyne therapy. This therapy involves the use of monochromatic infrared photo energy with highly efficient light-emitting diodes (LEDs) placed in direct skin contact (Leonard, Farooqi, & Myers, 2004). This technique was reviewed by Goldberg (2005) as he assessed the literature that included the study of more than 1,200 subjects studied using this intervention. Collectively, he found that these treatments were associated with improved foot sensation. There are an increasing number of these centers available throughout the country.

Early and ongoing screening, along with meticulous diabetes control, has been shown to be the most effective way to prevent or reverse early neuropathic changes (Vinik, 2006b).

Autonomic Neuropathy

This type of neuropathy involves nerves that work independently of conscious control, such as those nerves that control bladder muscles, the heart, and intestinal tract function, that is, the sympathetic and parasympathetic nervous systems. Problems associated with this form of neuropathy include impotence, vaginal dryness, dizziness while standing (postural hypotension), diarrhea (especially at night), gastric retention (gastroparesis), loss of the usual sweat response, and vasomotor disturbances. Control of blood glucose levels has not been found to be a factor in improving this type of neuropathy over short periods of time but does seem to play a part in preventing the autonomic neuropathy or improving it over longer periods of time (Prendergast, 2001a [pathology], 2001b [treatment]). Screening, with the use of autonomic nerve testing, has been determined to be an adjunct to the institution of early intervention (Maguire et al., 2007).

Key observations of cardiovascular involvement include a resting heart rate of 90–100 bpm, orthostatic hypotension, fatigue with little exertion, or a fixed heart rate on exertion. Orthostatic hypotension is often a great problem because the same patients often also have hypertension. Treatment of the hypertension will make the orthostatic hypotension worse. These individuals have difficulty standing up and maintaining balance. Treatment is with support hose, mineralocorticoids, and midodrine.

Cardiac autonomic neuropathy (CAN) signs were found in children ages 10–19 years of age (Boysen, Lewin, Hecker, Leichter, & Uhlemann, 2007) indicating a need to screen for such signs at an earlier age. They found that the heart rate variability and baroreflex were more sensitive to picking up early signs than the testing of cardiorespiratory reflexes.

Neurogenic bladder is an especially serious complication. Urinary retention leads to overflow obstruction with overflow incontinence, and also to chronic cystitis and pyelonephritis. Glucosuria contributes to pyelonephritis, which may become chronic, leading to renal destruction and uremia. Neurogenic bladder can be diagnosed by radiographic and cystometric studies that are able to measure the urine flow, pressure, and volume as well as residual urine. A suprapubic tap with transabdominal needle insertion into the bladder can also be used to measure pressure, strength of contraction, and sphincter tone of the bladder.

Individuals with urinary retention from a neurogenic bladder should be taught to void frequently, to keep fluid intake to low/normal levels, and to use Crede's maneuver (i.e., pushing down on the bladder behind the symphisis pubis) during and after urination. Valsalva's maneuver during urination may also be helpful in emptying the bladder, but this procedure should not be used if the person is hypertensive or has retinopathy as it may cause stroke or a retinal bleed. Bladder neck resection has occasionally been used. Sexual dysfunction is an important problem of diabetic neuropathy in the diabetic adult and is discussed in Chapter 24.

Gastrointestinal or diabetic gastropathy neuropathy may be manifest as chronic constipation, fecal incontinence, chronic diarrhea, or gastroparesis diabeticorum (stomach is dilated and hypotonic). Gastroparesis is recognized by the history of nausea, vomiting, bloating, and a feeling of fullness. The delayed gastric emptying can cause great difficulty in blood glucose control because of the difficulty in timing food with insulin. There can be severe vomiting, with great weight loss and even death. Severe disease may require the placement of an intestinal feeding tube.

Gastroparesis can be demonstrated by radionuclide gastric-emptying time studies or by abdominal magnetic resonance imaging (MRI) studies. Treatment is with oral or IV metoclopramide or erythromycin (domperidine and oral cisapride, at this time, are only available on a research basis); or with small, frequent feeding (low fat; low fiber), with enteral feedings, or with gastric electrical stimulation.

Gastroesophageal reflux was found to have approximately the same percentage of occurrence in persons with diabetes as in control subjects, but on further questioning of the subjects with diabetes, it was found that they had a significantly higher body mass index (BMI), and had more diabetes-related complications (Kase et al., 2007). Their recommended focus for this population was blood sugar control and decreased weight.

Diabetic diarrhea is not as common as gastroparesis, but it is a problem when it occurs. It is usually worse at night, disrupting sleep. Dehydration and malnutrition can occur. Treatment is very difficult and is usually unsatisfactory. Stool thickeners, bowel paralytics, and antibiotics are often used. Surgical intervention for the placement of a colostomy has also been of assistance.

Sudomotor autonomic neuropathy will cause sweating of the face with eating (gustatory sweating) or anhidrosis with compensatory sweating on the trunk of the body and the face. These individuals are at risk for heatstroke and hyperthermia when anhidrosis is present. Treatment for gustatory sweating is the avoidance of spicy or hot foods and the use of scopolamine patches or glycopyrrolate (a drug specific for this response).

Hypoglycemia unawareness is more common in Type 1 diabetes. These individuals may report mental dullness, cognitive dysfunction, visual disturbances, even seizures and coma. As noted in Chapter 33, Blood Glucose Awareness Training is the first approach to altering this type of dysfunction. Allowing the blood glucose level to remain at slightly hyperglycemic levels with no hypoglycemia can sometimes restore the sympathetic reserve and restore hypoglycemia awareness. The hyperglycemia must be of a fairly short time (not more than 3–6 months), however, or other complications related to hyperglycemia may become worse.

Cardiovascular autonomic nerve damage has, as yet, no specific treatment other than the normalization of blood glucose levels over time. Alpha lipoic acid has been used to nourish the nerves and as an attempt to assist in their healing when early signs of autonomic neuropathy are found related to cardiovascular functioning.

Focal and Multifocal Neuropathies

Proximal Motor Neuropathy

In proximal motor neuropathy (PMN), nerves to the muscles are damaged, resulting in weak and shrinking muscle fibers (i.e., atrophy). The skin may become abnormally sensitive with this type of neuropathy. Pain may be mild but is often described as a deep, burning pain as sensory nerves are usually concurrently involved. Recovery of the sensory component is usually seen in

6–18 months. The motor component, especially if there is motor atrophy, is usually permanent. This form of neuropathy commonly affects the hands and inner aspect of the thighs. It is called amyotrophy.

Cranial Mononeuropathy

This type of neuropathy usually involves the muscles around the eyes resulting in the inability to move the eyes in concert. Double vision will then occur. One or both eyelids may droop. Pain may or may not be present. Cranial mononeuropathy is usually a self-limited disease. Recovery is usually 2 weeks to 4 months. This is the most common type of diabetic neuropathy seen in children and usually follows a relatively short period of poor control. Although pressure neuropathies (compression neuropathies such as carpel tunnel syndrome) are not listed as a separate group, they may accompany or be indirectly associated with other types of neuropathies.

Treatment

Families should be instructed to assist the persons involved if pain or numbness is experienced. Areas such as wrists, ankles, and elbows should be watched. The person should be kept off their feet, if appropriate, and provided with softer and less irritating clothes, blankets, and shoes.

Painful neuropathy has been treated in a variety of ways. The most frequently used medications have been the tricyclic antidepressants (desipramine or Norpramin and nortriptyline or Pamelor) and the anticonvulsants (carbamazepine or Tegretol and topiramate or Topamax). Opioids and serotonin-noradrenaline reuptake inhibitors have also been used. The new medications, Cymbalta (duloxetine: an antidepressant selective serotonin reuptake inhibitor/antipain) and Lyrica (pregabalin: an anticonvulsant), have found an important place in the treatment of peripheral neuropathy. In a European study, pregabalin was effective, only exhibiting mild to moderate untoward responses in the subjects in the study (Tolle, Freynhagen, Versavel, Trostmann, & Young, 2008).

If foot ulcers are present, then treatment with a Uniboot, total foot contact casting, or platelet growth factor, initially obtained from the person's serum or in a synthesized form, are applied to the site. Pain and burning of the feet may be treated with over-the-counter counterirritant creams such as capsaicin. These creams, made from the active ingredient of jalapeno peppers, are available in various concentrations. The patient is instructed to use the lowest concentration for a week, five to seven times a day, and to increase to the next higher concentration the next week if desired results have not been achieved. Once the desired effects have been obtained, the person can change to using the treatment two to three times a day. Patients should be told that burning most likely will be experienced on use of the product, but the burning should subside once the therapeutic level of use is achieved.

McKeage (2007) and Boulton (2008) list a number of medical and physical treatments to aid in the symptomatic relief of painful neuropathy. They also found that the natural history of the disease may be altered with "stable near-normoglycemia." On Boulton's list of interventions is alpha-lipoic acid and various neurotropic agents and inhibitors. Managing neuropathic pain has come a long way, but there is still much to consider. Most of these topical agents and oral medications relieve pain locally or centrally but do not cure the neuropathy. The neuropathy can progress then without symptoms to the painless state with the danger of pressure ulcers without awareness of the patient. The only known prevention for this progression is careful control of blood glucose levels. All these patients should be trained in careful foot care.

The resources available to assist in the diagnosis and treatment of complications related to the nerves are increasing. Education for early recognition and management and prompt treatment will aid in stabilizing or restoring function to the parts affected.

Summary

Neuropathies may be more or less related to blood glucose control, but whatever the association, it is better to give the person the benefit of the doubt and maintain normal blood glucose levels as much of the time as safely possible. Neuropathies have even been noted in children and adolescents, especially in the developing countries (Vinik, 2006a). The time to start normalization of blood glucose levels as safely as possible is at the time of diagnosis.

Ziegler (2007) reported that about 50 new drugs for the treatment of neuropathy are being studied. He noted that more controlled trials are needed to document what and how diet and exercise may improve distal nerve function for short periods of time in people with prediabetes. He believes that treatment should safely aim for normal blood sugars, target the pathogenetic mechanisms for treatment, and relieve the symptoms of discomfort.

The reclassification system of the diabetic foot is in process through the work of the International Working Group on the Diabetic Foot (Lavery et al., 2008). Their assessment of people with diabetes, new available therapies, methods of prevention, and the recognition of those at greater risk points to a need to change the present classification.

The risk of developing complications associated with diabetes mellitus is considered preventable by a high degree of metabolic control of the diabetes (Diabetes Control and Complications Trial, 1993). Great effort should be made to accomplish this goal (HbA1c <7.0% [ADA]; <6.5% [International Diabetes Federation; American Association of Clinical Endocrinologists]) and prevent the destructive complications of the disease.

Again, prevention is best. Involving high-risk patients, whether they have had a history of foot ulcer or not, to daily self-assess by observation, by using the 5.07 (10 Gm) filament (sensate), and/or by using a temperature monitor has been demonstrated to be useful (Chao et al., 2007; Lavery et al., 2007). Note again if a 4.17 filament is not felt, mild neuropathy is the possible diagnosis; if a 5.07 filament is not felt, moderate neuropathy is the possible diagnosis, and the foot is classified as insensate; and if the 6.10 filament is not felt, severe neuropathy is usually present.

Refer to the American Diabetes Association's position statement on neuropathy (2005).

References

American Diabetes Association Position Statement. (2005). Neuropathy. *Diabetes Care, 28,* S256.

Andersen, C. A., & Roukis, T. S. (2007). The diabetic foot. *The Surgical Clinics of North America, 87*(5), 1149–1177.

Boulton, A. J. (2008). The diabetic foot grand overview, epidemiology and pathogenesis. *Diabetes Metabolism Research Review, 24*(Suppl. 1), S3–S6.

Boysen, A., Lewin, M. A., Hecker, W., Leichter, H. E., & Uhlemann, F. (2007). Autonomic function testing in children and adolescents with diabetes mellitus. *Pediatric Diabetes, 8*(5), 261–264.

Chao, C. C., Hsieh, S. C., Yang, W. S., Lin, Y. H., Lin, W. M., Tai, T. Y., et al. (2007). Glycemic control is related to the severity of impaired thermal sensations in type 2 diabetes. *Diabetes and Metabolism Research Reviews, 23*(8), 612–620.

Diabetes Control and Complications Trial Research Group. (1993). The effect of intensive treatment of diabetes on the development and profession of long-term complications in insulin dependent diabetes mellitus. *New England Journal of Medicine, 329*(14), 957–985.

Freeman, R., Durso-Decruz, E., & Emir, B. (2008). Efficacy, safety, and tolerability of pregabalin treatment for painful diabetic peripheral neuropathy: Findings from seven randomized, controlled trials across a range of doses. *Diabetes Care, 31*(7), 1448–1454.

Goldberg, N. (2005, March/April). Monochromatic infrared photo energy and diabetic peripheral neuropathy. *Diabetic Microvascular Complications Today,* 30–32.

Halat, K. M., & Denneby, C. E. (2003). Botanicals and dietary supplements in diabetic peripheral neuropathy. *Journal of the American Board of Family Practice, 16,* 47–57.

Hollister, C., & Li, V. W. (2007). Using angiogenesis in chronic wound care with becaplermin and oxidized regenerated cellulose/collagen. *Nursing Clinics of North America, 42*(3), 457–465.

Kase, H., Hattori, Y., Sato, N., Banba, N., & Kasai, K. (2007). Symptoms of gastroesophageal reflux in diabetes patients. *Diabetes Research in Clinical Practice, 79*(2), 6–7.

Lavery, L. A., Higgins, K. R., Lanctot, D. R., Constantinides, G. P., Zamorano, R. G., Athanasiou, K. A., et al. (2007). Preventing diabetic foot ulcer recurrence in high-risk patients: Use of temperature monitoring as a self-assessment tool. *Diabetes Care, 30*(1), 14–20.

Lavery, L. A., Peters, E. J., Williams, J. R., Murdoch, D. P., Hudson, A., Lavery, D. C., International Working Group on the Diabetic Foot (2008). Reevaluating the way we classify the diabetic foot: Restructuring the diabetic foot risk classification system of the International Working Group on the Diabetic Foot. *Diabetes Care, 31*(1), 154–156.

Leonard, D. R., Farooqi, H., & Myers, S. (2004). Restoration of sensation, reduced pain, and improved balance in subjects with diabetic peripheral neuropathy: A randomized, double blind, placebo controlled study. *Diabetes Care, 27,* 168–172.

Levine, P., Kaplun, J., Shavelson, D., & Poretsky, L. (2006). The pre-Charcot foot: A new clinical entity to prevent Charcot joint disease. *Practical Diabetology, 25*(3), 24–28.

Maguire, A. M., Craig, M. E., Craighead, A., Chan, A. K. F., Cusumano, J. M., Hing, S. J., et al. (2007). Autonomic nerve testing predicts the development of complications: A 23 year follow-up study. *Diabetes Care, 30*(1), 77–82.

McKeage, K. (2007). Treatment options for the management of diabetic painful neuropathy: Best current evidence. *Current Opinions in Neurology, 20*(5), 553–557.

Prendergast, J. J. (2001a). Diabetic autonomic neuropathy: Pathophysiology (Pt. 1). *Practical Diabetology, 20*(1), 7–15.

Prendergast, J. J. (2001b). Diabetic autonomic neuropathy: Treatment (Pt. 2). *Practical Diabetology, 20*(2), 30–33, 36.

Tolle, T., Freynhagen, R., Versavel, M., Trostmann, U., & Young, J. P., Jr. (2008). Pregabalin for relief of neuropathic pain associated with diabetic neuropathy: A randomized, double-blind study. *European Journal of Pain, 12*(2), 203–213.

Vinik, A. I. (2006a). Neuropathies in children and adolescents with diabetes: The tip of the iceberg. *Pediatric Diabetes, 7*(6), 301–304.

Vinik, A. I. (2006b). Optimizing the management of diabetic neuropathy. *American Diabetes Association's Physician's Weekly: Diabetes Roundtable,* 8–10.

Wallace, G. F. (2007). Debridement of invasive diabetic foot infections. *Clinical Plastic Surgery, 34*(4), 731–734.

Williams, D. S., III, Brunt, D., & Tannenberg, R. J. (2007). Diabetic neuropathy is related to joint stiffness during late stance phase. *Journal of Applied Biomechanics, 23*(4), 251–260.

Ziegler, D. (2007). Management of painful diabetic neuropathy: What is new or in the pipeline for 2007? *Current Diabetes Report, 7*(6), 409–415.

VII

Special Subjects

31

Self-Management Education

Self-management education has become an integral part of diabetes management. Even before the discovery of insulin almost 70 years ago, persons with diabetes calculated and weighed their food—a task that required knowledge about a dietary regimen. Self-care tasks require education and repeated evaluation. Self-management, to have the normalization of blood glucose levels most of the time, not only requires self-care but also the knowledge and ability to safely alter medication in relation to food intake and activity or exercise level.

Current scientific data indicate that both acute and chronic complications can be prevented or at least delayed if the individuals maintain good control of their diabetes the majority of the time (Diabetes Control and Complications Trial, 1993; U.K. Prospective Diabetes Study Group, 1998). Part of this good control may be the result of rapid advances in technology. However, control is best influenced by the actions of the individuals involved or their caregivers, as noted by Brown (1992) in his classic meta-analysis paper.

Education is a dynamic process. Health professionals should continually attempt to improve teaching programs in terms of timeliness, relevance, effectiveness, efficiency, and innovation. More individuals with the disease are living longer. If long-term complications occur, expenses rise because hospitalization may be required, and consumers are becoming more vocal in their demands on the health care system. Finally, there is an increasing recognition by health professionals as well as individuals with diabetes of the need and potential benefits that could be derived from participating in a teaching program. All of these factors have contributed to the increased development of diabetes education programs all over the world.

Whenever possible, diabetes education requires a team approach. The team ideally includes a diabetes educator to assist the patients in the acquisition of knowledge and a positive attitude toward health. Other members of importance are the physician, dietitian, counselor/psychologist, and social worker because they each play a part in assisting the individual with the behavior change needed to improve diabetes control and, thereby, decrease health care costs. As with any team, there is the leader—and we all step back to acknowledge that without the patient being this leader (individual needs relating to professional decisions), little if anything would be attained other than immediate control.

The American Association of Diabetes Educators (AADE), the American Diabetes Association (ADA), the American Dietetic Association, the Centers for Disease Control and Prevention (CDC), the American Association of Clinical Endocrinologists, and the National Diabetes Advisory Board (NDAB) all have an interest in and are involved in patient and professional education. As a result of efforts by the ADA, the NDAB, and the CDC, many insurance carriers are currently reimbursing diabetes outpatient education programs in the United States. To meet the standards required for third-party payers to acknowledge payment for such programs, the AADE developed The Scope and Practice, Standards of Practice, and Standards of Professional Performance for Diabetes Educators as reported in *The Diabetes Educator* (2005a). The ADA continues to update the National Standards for Diabetes Self-Management Education (2008b) (also reported in *The Diabetes Educator*, 2007a), the ADA Standards of Medical Care (2008c), and third-party reimbursement for diabetes care (2008a). The American Association of Clinical Endocrinologists (AACE) has also developed guidelines for diabetes management (2007a, 2007b). Medicare (2000) joined this endeavor with expanded coverage for supplies and coverage for basic education (10 hr of basic education plus 2 hr a year for ongoing education).

Note: It requires the development of a personal follow-up plan for ongoing self-management support. Funnel (2007) reviews what this and other standards mean for the provider.

In addition, the numbers of reimbursed diabetes teaching programs have increased along with the numbers of diabetes specialists. Both of these groups have been influenced by the ADA recognition programs (patient education program and provider recognition program).

The certification program for diabetes educators, originally developed by the AADE and now overseen by the National Board of Certified Diabetes Educators (NBCDE), ensures a sound knowledge base in diabetes education and teaching methods for the diabetes educator. The Advanced Practitioner needs were first reported by Nettles and Kreitzer (1994). Advanced practice not only includes master's-prepared nurses, but also dietitians and pharmacists, with the American Nurses Credentialing Center (ANCC) offering an examination for board certification in advanced diabetes management.

The Need for Patient Education

Health professionals realize that random, haphazard teaching can be incomplete, ineffective, and dangerous. There is no place for haphazard teaching. In the hospital or community setting, patient teaching must be prioritized and focused on content that will meet the immediate needs of the person and his or her family. In addition, the increased acuity of people who have diabetes significantly impacts readiness to learn and must be addressed in program content areas and regimen development. Intensive control cannot be achieved safely unless self-management education has been involved. Education is an important part in the safe management of the diabetes regimen. Knowing how to proceed prevents the loss of valuable time (Funnell & Mensing, 2005).

Various national organizations that establish policies for the U.S. health care system have all philosophized about the extreme importance of both patient and family health education. These groups include the American Hospital Association (AHA), the Joint Commission on the Accreditation of Health Care Organization (JCAHCO), the American Nurses Association (ANA), the American Medical Association (AMA), and health maintenance organizations (HMOs), to name a few. Education is important, but cost effectiveness is also sought. One classic study demonstrated that cost-effective measures affected the outcome when a diabetes team was involved, that is, the length of stay was lowest in those patients who had access to the skills and direction of a diabetes team (Levetan, Salas, Wilets, & Zumoff, 1995).

There are several reasons for education assisting cost savings, which, as of 2008 is now, we repeat, officially $174 billion a year as reported by the ADA Diabetes Caucus (www.diabetes.org/costs). There is a national focus on health, prevention of illness, and prevention of disease-related complications in chronic diseases such as diabetes. There is no doubt that the influence of consumerism has played an important role in this movement. There is also an existing philosophy among health care providers that patients have a responsibility to resume an active role in the treatment of diabetes and in the prevention of its complications. To accomplish this, patients must be educated in the essential aspects of the disease and, as stated previously, a team approach is needed.

Patients have the right to have knowledge about their disease in understandable terms. The prevention of complications of diabetes and the resultant savings in health care costs have been the motivation for third-party reimbursement for patient education, even though fewer full diabetes education programs are available as part of an inpatient stay and more are available on an outpatient basis.

Worldwide, international groups and individuals work to find ways to enhance the health of people with diabetes. One example is a nurse, Jean Suren, KRN, BSC, CDE (Past President of AADE, working in Kenya for over 20 years), who has developed a Diabetes Education Trust to fund a proposal for boarding/secondary schools to be contracted by the foundation to accept children with diabetes. Individual AADE chapters and other organizations are urged to "adopt" one or more of these children to cover the cost of supplies, health care, and personnel to be certified to teach self-care and self-management (Diabetes Education Trust, P.O. Box 35181 00200, Nairobi, Kenya).

In one state, a program has been developed to assist students with diabetes to succeed through the use of a diabetes primer, an action plan, tools for effective diabetes management, and education about school responsibilities under law (Section 504 of the Rehabilitation Act of 1973, American With Disabilities Act of 1990, Individuals With Disabilities Education Act 1994). The action plan calls for a preset quick-reference emergency plan, individual meal plan guidance, treatment of hypo- and hyperglycemia education as needed, treatment of the student with the respect afforded any other student in the school, and communication with nursing or other personnel when there are concerns about individual students.

Developing a Program

Most inpatient or "after diagnosis in the clinic setting" education is focused on survival skills (SS), the basic knowledge or skills needed by the patient for initial safe care at home (how to take a medication/injection; how to test for blood glucose levels; how to eat; and how to call for help when help is needed, e.g., hypoglycemia). These people (or family members) should then be referred to and attend a diabetes education program where there is more time to focus on having their questions answered and what to do when, that is, self-management guidelines; ketone testing when appropriate; risk factors vs. complications; and so on. The basic Home Management Skills usually take a day and a half; (i.e., 10 hr). Self-management education requires an extra 8 hr or so (most insurance companies at least cover the Home Management Skills, whereas there is about 80% coverage for the total self-management program).

Long-term follow-up education should also be considered, at least 2 hr a year. This could include education received at an office visit or at a diabetes meeting or at a preset diabetes education workshop.

Occasionally, patients are discharged without learning basic (survival) skills either because they were too ill, not ready to learn, or an educator was not available. This makes outpatient education even more critical. When the patient is homebound and requires the services of a home health nurse, the home nurse may initiate selected teaching subjects depending on the person's emotional and physical limitations.

The following are the steps generally applicable in developing an education program:

1. Assess program and patient needs.
2. Obtain administrative and professional support (develop an advisory board).
3. Determine potential clients, sources of referral, and subsequent follow-up.
4. Plan program content, to include all or part of the recommended subjects, with a small interdisciplinary team (committee).
5. Determine program goals, behavioral objectives, desired outcomes, and evaluation methods.
6. Select learning strategies.
7. Determine and use available resources.
8. Recruit, motivate, train, and cross-train teaching personnel.

9. Implement the program.
10. Document teaching.
11. Follow-up—ideally in one week, one month, three months, then six months.
12. Evaluate teaching and program effectiveness.
13. Revise program as needed.
14. Update personnel education.

These steps are offered as a general outline for developing a program for clients with diabetes in a variety of settings. Much of the following information can be applied or adapted. The success or failure of a program depends on several important factors: staff time, interested personnel, teaching materials, space, patient referrals, administrative support, professional support, and funding.

Organizing a Program

Teaching programs are now a way of life. Offices want the convenience of offering added services to their clients. Competition can improve the quality of the teaching program regardless of whether it is designed for inpatients, outpatients, or both. In fact, it can be used to advantage when requesting funding for various aspects of the teaching program (e.g., staff time, materials, and space). There are a number of models from which to choose, but the model should be chosen as most financially sustainable and most effective in diabetes self-management training.

One model focused on metabolic control and looked at Education and Counseling (Gallegos, Ovalle-Berumen, & Gomez-Meza, 2006). Another model looked at the overall picture of chronic care. Siminerio et al. (2006) assessed the Chronic Care Model as facilitating educational needs when considering the development of a program (involvement and consideration of the health system, the community, decision support, self-management support, clinical information system available, and the system of delivery system design). Another evidenced-based approach for patient education has been the AADE 7 Diabetes Self-Care Behaviors program (ADA, 2007; Mulcahy et al., 2003; Mulcahy & Lumber, 2004; AADE, 2007a). The seven behaviors are: (1) being active, physical activity (exercise), (2) eating, (3) medication taking, (4) monitoring blood glucose, (5) problem solving especially for blood glucose: high and low levels, and sick days, (6) reducing risks of diabetes complications, and (7) living with diabetes (psychosocial adaptation). This approach to education has tools developed to achieve behavior changes, to assess effectiveness of the program when used, to compare with benchmarks already assessed, and to contribute to the diabetes self-management education in overall diabetes care.

Determining a Need for the Program

In an effort to justify the development of a program, it is necessary to research the need for a program for diabetes patient education. This assessment may be accomplished through questionnaires or interviews with health professionals and patients and local community members. With proper authority, medical records may be assessed for the impact of the diabetes on the hospital, the clinic, and/or various community health agencies (such as home health nursing, community health nursing, or through the local or state diabetes associations).

Assessing the need for the program is different from assessing patient learning needs, which should also be done to determine program content and techniques used in teaching that content. This may be done by determining outcomes. Behaviorally oriented objectives need to be focused on outcomes. They need to be realistic, feasible, and relevant for the individual learner and his or her family. In addition, most will follow the critical pathways that will assist professionals and people with diabetes to meet both long-term and short-term goals. A useful method is to contract with the patient for the achievement of selected outcomes once the patient expresses his or her desires related to the education process. A client contract based on behavioral change can be as simple or as complex as one wishes to make it. Traditionally, the health professional learns what the level of confidence is that the patient is able to provide certain information, that is, such as the results of blood glucose testing, or the professional agrees to teach a skill while the patient agrees to practice and perform the skill. Written contracts are usually more effective than verbal contracts. Providing rewards for successfully reaching a goal will provide feedback and an incentive for future changes in behavior. The most important aspect of contracting is that the contract must be mutually agreeable.

Another way is to ask the person, on a scale of 1–10, how confident they feel they are to complete an agreed upon task. If patients are demanded to agree to some task, they are not as likely to comply unless they feel empowered to be part of the decision-making process.

Stating behavioral goals is a method of contracting that has the person identify two or three behaviors they will focus on changing over the following designated period of time. There is no other expectation of the professional than the education, direction, and support given.

Obtaining Education Materials

Teaching materials do not necessarily have to cost a lot, but some materials (and methodologies) are more cost-effective than others. Classically, the three most cost-effective methods for education are the use of support groups, small discussion groups, and large discussion groups (Funnel, Donnelly, Anderson, Johnson, & Oh, 1992). Videotapes and PowerPoint slides were disclosed as being the more educationally effective materials, whereas audiotapes were found to be the least effective.

Good, basic, professionally prepared teaching materials and other literature can be obtained without cost from the various pharmaceutical companies that manufacture diabetes-related products. Other resources include county agricultural extension services, dairy councils, local, city, and state departments of health, and companies that produce or distribute dietetic or diabetes products. Food labels become teaching tools within themselves. Local and state diabetes associations have a wealth of teaching materials. The National Diabetes

Information Clearinghouse (NDIC) has materials for specific purposes (e.g., low literacy, various language, or special subject pamphlets and booklets).

In general, a superabundance of material is available. One should be cautious and discriminating in choosing such materials. It is far better to have a few quality items than too many of a mediocre quality. Printed materials serve to complement the teaching program, not to replace it. Materials should be chosen carefully and with respect to the patient's vision, reading level, socioeconomic level, and culture, that is, the language most frequently spoken in the home. The effectiveness of teaching aids can be totally negated if the person does not read, cannot see well enough to read, cannot understand the medical terms, or does not understand or read English. This problem can be avoided if an adequate patient assessment is completed before the first education session begins. The educator's responsibility is to ensure that all subjects appropriate for that population are covered and that these subjects are completed in an accurate manner. Whatever the materials used, which could also include games and discussion maps, patient-led discussion that is professionally monitored has the potential for better understanding along with the fun of participation.

Determining Cost

If your materials or program is unique or innovative, you may want to consider funding sources outside of your own institution. Grants are available for this purpose from the Diabetes Research and Education Foundation (DREF), the AADE local chapters, the American Heart Association, health departments, and diabetes-related food and pharmaceutical companies. Funding for the program may or may not be a problem, depending on the institution's commitment, capability, and interest in client health education.

The following items should be included in the budget if or when a proposal is written: direct costs (salaries and other administrative costs, space, instructional materials, and food, i.e., an allowance for food should be made if a meal or snack is provided as a part of the educational process or during the day's education session) and indirect costs (rent, heating, lighting, photocopying, etc.).

It is certainly not beyond the realm of possibility to conduct a program with little or no apparent outside funding if space and utilities are donated. Personnel and their time will constitute the greatest portion of the budget. The other most expensive budget item is audiovisual equipment. All the possible offerings on the market should be examined, and selection should be based on the type of program, age of the patients, capabilities of the educator, and equipment already available. One should be aware that equipment that has limited software could quickly become outdated.

Logical sources of funding include grants, gifts, or donations from former patients, service clubs, or hospital auxiliaries, and class fees. The local diabetes association should be contacted for interactive support, or perhaps to possibly initiate a collaborative effort.

Personnel to Be Involved

The following personnel should be considered as teachers for the program: family or specialist physician, nurse, dietitian, podiatrist, pharmacist, counselor or psychologist, social worker, dentist, physiotherapist, and knowledgeable persons with diabetes. It is more important to have the best possible teacher than a poor teacher with the proper credentials. The one or two health professionals organizing the program should be certified as diabetes educators to be able to meet one of the standards when applying for program recognition.

Consider the following when selecting teaching personnel:

1. If the same person or the same team members teach a topic or the course, the continuity in the learning process will be better.
2. If a member of a specific discipline, that is, a specialist in eye care, is selected, it should be verified that the person has the ability to teach. Occasionally professionals will be found who are willing and eager but cannot teach. If a diplomatic solution cannot be found to discharge that "teacher," one could temporarily eliminate the topic or, better yet, shift the content to another teacher's presentation and notify the former teacher, expressing appreciation for the time and effort previously given.
3. Although teachers are willing to volunteer their time, it has been noted that if some reimbursement is given for teaching, there is a stronger, long-term commitment to the program and therefore less teacher absenteeism.

All health professionals involved should agree to participate in personal education and reeducation to improve their effectiveness in teaching patients. This includes not only core content but also how to teach. With recognition of the scope of practice for diabetes educators (AADE, 2005a, 2005b) and the trends in advanced nursing practice, the quality and quantity of knowledge will be challenged when the professional's credentials are up for renewal—either through retaking an exam or through continuing education.

Program Planning

The most successful program planning is accomplished by a committee composed of the various disciplines that are related to the program. The committee can be used in many ways, including assessing the need for a program, brainstorming for ideas, and devising, supporting, and finalizing the plans. It saves time to prepare in advance for the first meeting and to have available statistics supporting the need for the program, the various resources (personnel and materials) that are potentially available for the program, an outline of course content, and a list of the needs of the program.

Referring to the requirements addressed in the ADA's Self-Management Recognition process makes it easier to complete the application when the program is ready. Refer to Maryniuk (2006) for this and other ideas to be considered when planning a program.

An advisory committee can help to maintain the program's dynamism through a yearly review of statistics and their relevance to the needs of the target population. Because of our mobile society and shifting job markets, the target population of a community can change rather quickly. The influx of certain ethnic groups, for example, might drastically change a community and its educational needs.

A yearly review of the facilities and evaluation of the program keeps the committee involved and enthusiastic. Monetary and administrative support may also be facilitated by a review of the statistics (e.g., the program has outgrown its resources and space). See Appendix M for suggestions on course content, remembering that this information needs to be tailored to the needs and abilities related to the class or the individual. Appendix N gives a sample of a teaching record.

Program Implementation

The program should only be implemented after the course outline has been developed (see Appendix M for topics that might be integrated into the course, depending on the patients' needs) and approved by the appropriate personnel, the funding determined, the teaching personnel recruited and trained, a patient referral system developed, and teaching materials selected. Delay in implementation because of few patients or other reasons can quickly lead to a decrease in interest and enthusiasm for the program.

Publicity or marketing is important in implementing the program. Information about the program should be circulated approximately a month in advance of its commencement to allow for an adequate response. Numerous methods are available for disseminating information. In general, these include announcements in e-mails, Web sites, newspapers, radio and television, posters, brochures, fliers, and letters. If a public relations person is available, he or she should be well informed about the program, especially in the period immediately before the program begins. The choice of media to advertise or to announce the program will probably be determined by the type of community in which the institution is located (urban or rural), its population mix, socio-economic and cultural backgrounds of the clients, and timing. Regardless of the medium, the announcement should include the intended audience, place, time, frequency, length, and cost of the program and a method for obtaining more information, such as a telephone number, e-mail address, or Web site. Other suggestions for implementation and maintaining an ADA patient education recognition program are given in Maryniuk, Bronzini, and Lorenzi's article in 2004 and in Lorenzi's AADE book chapter in 2006.

Perhaps the most difficult thing for those conducting an inpatient clinic or outpatient education program is to understand that a pretest and posttest, or a return demonstration during the program, is not a guarantee that a change in behavior has occurred. Learning involves behavior change. This does not occur spontaneously. It is extremely important to realize that changing a person's behavior takes time.

The matter of evaluation is clarified if the outcome objectives for the patient are written properly. These outcomes should be realistic. Can they be accomplished within a reasonable amount of time with the majority of patients and/or their families? Are the outcomes clearly stated? If the outcomes are well written, they will provide a guide for planning and an idea of what the learner should be able to accomplish by the end of the program. These outcomes also serve as a basis for evaluation of the quality of the program. Although the outcomes are well written and realistic, it is important to understand that the patient still has the choice to decide for or against the acceptance of the goals. The health professional should not be frustrated as long as he or she has provided the person with the necessary facts and skills training to function adequately and to make intelligent, safe decisions.

Although there are obviously methods for evaluating or measuring learned knowledge (the cognitive domain) with an oral or written quiz before or after the program, demonstrating a skill such as blood glucose testing or interpreting the meaning of the results of those tests discloses only short-term outcomes. For example, individuals may be able to explain, in a written test, the reasons for monitoring blood glucose levels and describe the appropriate action to be taken if the results are positive. They may also demonstrate the correct method of testing. However, the skill and knowledge demonstrated in writing or return demonstration may not be adapted to the home situation.

Again, acquisition of knowledge and skills does not mean a change in behavior has occurred. Long-term effectiveness of learning, which is extremely important in terms of the patient's health, is more complex and not always convenient, especially if the patient may never be seen again.

Program Documentation

In view of the current status of health education, documentation is important. Points to be documented on the hospital chart, or education or clinic record, should include an assessment of the person's knowledge and skills before the program, the plan for teaching, what teaching was actually accomplished, barriers to learning, the person's individual response, barriers to care, and areas for reinforcement and follow-up. Some programs incorporate this information in a computerized program developed for that particular purpose. Peyrot, Peeples, Tomky, Charron-Prochownik, and Weaver (2007) participated in developing and testing such a tool that could be used for documentation as well as assessment.

Occasionally a checklist for teaching is convenient for documentation, but a checklist does not usually allow for recording observed behavior responses to teaching. A compromise would be comprehensive documentation with a checklist having sufficient space for comments and observations.

Because education is an ongoing process, a copy of the documentation, with the patient's permission, is sent to the patient's health care provider or clinic. It is also beneficial to give the client a copy of specific instructions (such as activity, a medication dosage and time of administration, and meal plan guidelines) or what we call a "Take Home Sheet"—a self-carboned form (refer to Appendix I) on which we place discussed needs, concerns, and recommendations. Patients have reported that the Take Home Sheet is useful in helping them to remember what was said during their clinic visit. This particular sheet has a self-carbon copy so that it might be scanned for the paperless office or kept in the patient's chart.

Communication between inpatient, outpatient, or office is extremely important and helpful to the patient and to the health educator or health care provider. The nature of diabetes with its ever-changing technologies requires ongoing education for patients as well as their health care providers. Be sure that documentation of any changes and what has been taught or reviewed is included in some form (see Appendix N) and whether the person has achieved preset objective outcomes (see Appendix O). Weighing and comparing these outcomes should give guidance as to the safety and efficacy of any diabetes education program.

Both program revision, from past evaluations completed by the participants, and the updating of the knowledge of the educators, through CMEs or CEUs, are crucial and must be completed on a predetermined schedule. If either is omitted, the program and its optimal benefits to the patients will be lost.

Ensuring the Program's Success

Several factors are necessary to ensure that the program will be successful once it is started. These are administrative support, professional support, and space.

Support from the administration, whether from a clinic, a hospital, or a physician, is essential to both the short- and long-term success of the program. Because of the increasing financial demands being made on health care facilities in terms of services, plus the effects of inflation, providing patient health education may be viewed initially as a potential for added cost with little apparent benefit. With increasing support of third-party payers, these programs can generate some revenue, which should gain some administrative support. A nonincome benefit, yet a significant one, is the public relations effect in the community.

Health professional support is important to the success of the program. The referral of clients to the program will depend on whether the health care provider thinks that the program is worthwhile and a valuable part of the diabetes treatment regimen. In the past, there was resistance by health care professionals because they were wary of the program content and concerned that their patients might become "too educated." Involving the family's health care professional in the planning of the program and addressing his or her concerns early in the planning stages will diminish such resistance.

The availability of space in which to teach can pose either a real or imaginary problem in the implementation of a teaching program. If the program is group centered rather than on a one-to-one basis, a classroom-type setting would be needed. In a hospital or clinic, such a classroom would ideally be located in relation to patient rooms or exam rooms. If the person is to be seen in his or her room or in a clinic room on a one-to-one basis, the cost-effectiveness of doing this must be considered. Ideally, in the hospital setting, a classroom would be located entirely within a specialty area such as a diabetes center.

Providing a relaxed atmosphere conducive to learning is not exclusively dependent on space but on the personality and attitude of the teaching personnel. If the interest in developing a program is genuine, any area may be adapted for use. If either administrative or professional support is questionable or weak, a space problem can easily become an excuse for delaying the implementation of the program whether it is in a hospital or in a clinic setting. In problem situations, a suggested approach might be to find an area that could be used for group teaching, find furniture and equipment that is not in use, and work out the details regarding the day and time of use.

To review: the program package, including the "who, what, where, when, and why" should be presented to the appropriate personnel or committee for approval. If possible, any and all questions and roadblocks should be prepared for in advance of implementing the program.

Third-Party Reimbursement

Just as the organization of diabetes education programs has been in the forefront of the health education efforts, so has third-party reimbursement for diabetes programs. Diabetes education programs have developed faster than for any other chronic illness. Historically, the 1974 White Paper on Patient Health Education, developed by the Blue Cross Association, defined diabetes education as a reimbursement cost based on its potential for cost savings (Simonds, 1974). It is important to realize, however, that the Blue Cross Association on a national scale is composed of individual local and state plans that may or may not totally agree with this concept of reimbursement.

An initial check with a particular insurer might be made by phone. If diabetes education is not covered, a proposal might be written and submitted to the individual insurers to obtain reimbursement. In this case, it is especially important to know the language and key phrases to use in your proposal. It is a good idea to meet personally with representatives from a particular insurance company before submitting any written proposal.

Evidence of cost savings would be key information for all insurers. Many insurers now respect the Self-Recognition Program of the ADA as a measure of effectiveness and have stated their willingness to reimburse programs that have achieved such recognition. Recognition is not a guarantee for reimbursement, but it is highly desirable both in terms of reimbursement and for the program's credibility. If your program has not become involved in the Self-Recognition Program, it should be considered and determined from the Web site information (ADA: www.diabetes.org), whether the particular program meets the preset standards.

The Importance of Individual Assessment

Assessment of individuals with diabetes is a necessary adjunct to management and to preparing for diabetes education. When beginning to teach persons with diabetes, one should know when to teach, what to teach, how to teach, who in the family needs to be taught, and how soon to allow the people involved to be on their own. It is highly important that the education process be driven by the individual or group's age, ability, and cultural needs. Nurses, dietitians, physicians, and others involved in the care and education of patients find that they need a method of gathering the kind of information that will assist them in the patient's education and management. Applied to the person who has diabetes, assessment is a method of identifying physical, social, and emotional needs that may influence educational abilities and long-term management of the disease (Clark et al., 2001).

The use of a guide to assess needs will aid in establishing priorities and eliminate the needless repetition of material, both for the program or for the person (family). Such material is available through the ADA National Standards for Diabetes Self-Management Education (2008b; ADA, *The Diabetes Educator*, 2007). Although repetition may be used as a teaching tool, much time can be wasted in teaching patients something they already know. Conversely, some concepts need to be emphasized and reemphasized to be learned. Assessment and reassessment is then needed to determine the material to be taught, material to be retaught, and material to be eliminated as part of the individualized needs in the learning process.

A person's attitude in relation to what is taught and how it is taught is just as much a part of this assessment process. Rossing and his group (2001) found that this was also true for the professionals. Having a sense of peoples' attitudes should be a concern when assessing a population to be educated.

The information the assessment gives to the educator can also be used to individualize the patient-teaching program. It may be obvious from the initial assessment that certain materials would be too complex for the patient and more simplified ones should be used. Certain information, such as adjustment of insulin dosage, may be inappropriate for some patients and should be deleted from their teaching program. Perhaps the individual does not have the coping strategies, the mental capability, or the social support to follow through on what is being requested as part of the diabetes regimen. The information the assessment gives to the educator helps to direct ways to motivate the participant toward the desired result. The idea of listing the goals and objectives of the teaching program and telling the patient how to reach the goals may be quite foreign to the usual way for that patient to learn.

Determining the risk-taking activities of a person (smoking, seatbelt use, carrying hypoglycemia treatment) along with the individual needs should prepare the health professional for potential barriers in teaching, monitoring, and following up. Making such determinations will save much time and money in the long run. When the problems are anticipated, greater efficiency on the part of the professional and greater motivation on the part of the patient are often the outcome.

The question professionals need to ask themselves is, "Why should patients do what we ask them to do?" They should also ask, "Does the person (family) have adequate coping skills?" When the person applies self-management practices on a lifelong basis, assessment must reveal whether the person has the desire for learning as well as the ability for self-care, let alone self-management. This assessment should not only be a one-time assessment, but should be redone on a regular basis.

Is the person ready to learn or where is the person in line with readiness to learn? This is the most important part of the assessment process. Is he or she in the precontemplative stage (no intention of taking action in the foreseeable future), the contemplative stage (intends to take action in the foreseeable future), the preparation stage (intends to take action in the immediate future), the action stage (recently changed overt behavior to goal level), or the maintenance stage (changed overt behavior to goal level). Guidelines are given by Prochaska and Velicer (1997). For further reading about the application of the transtheoretical model, refer to Highstein, O'Toole, Shetty, Brownson, and Fisher (2007) or the book *Changing for Good* (Prochaska, Norcross, & DiClemente, 1994).

Patient empowerment has long been recognized to support the person's desire to attain and maintain better self-care. The framework of empowerment in the education process provides knowledge and skills and also the responsibility to effectively change behavior. In the classic report of the randomized, controlled trial, Anderson and colleagues concluded that empowerment was an effective approach to developing educational interventions focused on the psychosocial aspects of living with diabetes and for improvement of blood glucose control (Anderson, 2007; Anderson et al., 1995; Anderson & Funnell, 2005).

There is also a need for the family of the individual to be involved in the teaching program. Early assessment will reveal what form the involvement of the family should take. Family members will usually be responsible for assisting the patient in the home and monitoring (when appropriate) of the patient's progress. Family (or significant others) will often aid the individual who has diabetes toward increased self-care and safer self-management if the aid is given appropriately.

When to Assess

A variety of situations and settings direct the professional to assess the person's needs as soon as first contact is made. Patients should be assessed when they first enter the hospital, once they are fully conscious, or in the outpatient clinic to determine the current status. Assessment also needs to be done near the end of any hospitalization or clinic visit to reassess the involved person's understanding of the changes in management that might have occurred as a result of the education or recommendations. Assessment can be performed in the home by the visiting nurse and in the physician's office during follow-up visits. In other words, any time the person with diabetes is seen by a health professional, some type of assessment or reassessment of needs and practices should be carried out.

Assessment of patients' understanding of their disease can be used in several ways. Although an evaluation that deals entirely with diabetes management practices is not applicable to the person with newly diagnosed diabetes, this type of assessment certainly is helpful for the newly admitted patient with previously diagnosed diabetes. In this midwestern center's practice, we have found that patients with previous diagnoses need almost as much teaching as individuals with new diagnoses. The use of an initial assessment identifies these patients and also their individual and family knowledge deficits.

In addition to determining the patient's past management practices, it is just as important to identify the physical, social, and emotional needs of the patient at each contact. It is possible that a person has experienced vision or hearing loss. Perhaps a close relative has died. All of these factors—physical problems, social needs, and emotional responses—need to be identified at each renewed contact. However, many times, because of an absence of a formal assessment guideline, these factors are either overlooked or ignored.

Methods of Assessment

There are various methods of assessment, including use of questionnaires (written or verbal), demonstrations, and interviews. A combination of these three types of assessment is the most useful (unless the patient does not read or write). Ideally, the evaluation should also have a built-in mechanism for teaching the patients as well as gathering information about them.

The questionnaire should obviously include the client's name, address, phone number, present date, birth date, and school or employment status. It should include details regarding the present regimen, along with methods of self-medication, monitoring, meal planning, exercising, hygiene, emergency care, and the desire to participate or to determine the safety in participation in self-management.

A questionnaire form for individual assessment might include a detailed social history, information about how the patient has managed the diabetes in the past, some general knowledge questions about diabetes, and some questions to indicate learning ability. Patients can fill this out at their leisure but preferably before admission into the program. If they are unable to read, someone can ask them the questions. The questionnaire saves much time for the instructor, especially when the instructor is working with a large number of patients at one time (see Appendix P for an example).

The person with diabetes or an appropriate family member or friend should always have an opportunity to demonstrate and return-demonstrate that they can perform the various tasks they will have to do at home. Professional comments should accompany the observations of these demonstrations. The use of the diabetes self-management education tool (Peyrot et al., 2007) is helpful in an assessment that what has been desired has been achieved. This reassessment process should be promoted as what the staff needs to know to help them to find the reasons for any problems associated with less-than-adequate control of the diabetes and, thereby, to reduce the stress associated with living with diabetes.

In the classroom, conduct an entrance-and-exit discussion or question-and-answer session to gain further information about incorrect knowledge. For example, the educator may find that a topic or answer has been misinterpreted. This is the time to correct misconceptions. In addition, an individual interview gives the educator the opportunity to assess emotional status and gain information about the patient's family, work, habits, and activities that may require referral to various outside resources.

Some programs may consider a full history and physical as part of the total assessment. Histories and physicals should be focused on the specific problems and needs of the person with diabetes.

If intellectual capability for reading and writing is sought, a shortened version of the Wide Range Achievement Test (WRAT) (Sullivan & Hawkins, 1995) could be used or develop your own, that is, ask the person to complete two- and three-column addition and subtraction as well as one-, two-, and three-column division and multiplication. Ask them to use two- and three-syllable words in a sentence. This information will assist you in recognizing whether the person has the skills to participate in a group education setting or needs more one-to-one support (read Wysocki et al. [1996] for in-depth information).

Emotional adjustment can be revealed through such simple screening tools as the Zung Depression Index (Zung, Magruder-Habib, Velez, & Ailing, 1990) and other wellness indexes. Just circling the items on a list can aid the educator in describing the present emotional state that is presently being experienced: anger, anxiousness, belligerence, fear, hostility, hyperactivity, confusion, disorientation, embarrassment, euphoria, withdrawal, sadness, or happiness.

If there is observable conflict in the family, or with a spouse, obtaining background information or obtaining the completion of the Myers-Briggs personality type indicator (Briggs-Myers & McCaulley, 1985) can give some indication of the interaction problems that might be occurring in the home (e.g., the male is very rigid and judgmental but the female is laid back and relaxed). The children's version of the Myers-Briggs Scale (Murphy-Meisgeier Type Indicator for Children [Meisgeier & Murphy, 1987]) includes the assessment of learning styles based on the dominant personality type. These could be administered feedback by a psychologist or a certified therapist.

Determining the quality of life can give some indication of the personal meaning of diabetes and its management, especially for the youth (Ingersoll & Marrero, 1991). Asking the person his or her purpose in attending the course will also reveal the present level of acceptance.

In-depth knowledge assessment can be gained through self-made or available questionnaires. Unless the professional is motivated to develop and administer the tests, obtain permission to use those tools that have already been validated and found reliable. Contacting the National Diabetes Information Clearing House would be good places to start.

Finally, there are times to refrain from an initial assessment. For example, a woman with newly diagnosed diabetes has an uncle with diabetes who had an amputation as the result of diabetes-related arteriosclerosis. The patient is terrified that the same thing will happen to her and is therefore unable to concentrate and learn. Once determining this fear, time needs to be given for counseling. Counseling and having someone available to answer her questions are needed immediately. Real learning has to wait.

Assessment of the Program

The program assessment should be divided into two parts: the process measures and the outcome measures. The process measures include the program objectives, the target population, the actual participants themselves, and the qualifications of the instructors and core content. These measures should also include acceptable methods of referral, both into and after the program has been completed. The outcome measures allow the professional to know the quality of the program. Is it being kept up to date? Where does it need to be improved? The four key components guide you: knowledge, skills, behavior, and attitudes. If one of these four key components is missing, the program is not of the quality desired.

Other measures to determine the indications of health status and attitude are the number of diabetes-related hospitalizations, diabetes-related emergency room visits because of hypoglycemia or hyperglycemia, and, when appropriate, perinatal problems. One reported method to determine patient satisfaction with a diabetes education program has been the use of the Mastery of Stress instrument (Stamler, Patrick, Cole, & Lafreniere, 2006), even though the conclusion that more research was needed before the generalized support of such an instrument could be recommended.

To document that the program itself is contributing to change, read the suggestions by Boucher and VanWormer (2006) on other ways to evaluate programs and outcomes from a diabetes contact or education session, including the Peyrot et al. (2007) assessment report tool.

Programs should also assess the specifics of content. Well-written lesson plans include behavioral outcomes expected, a course outline (see Appendix M), and a method of evaluation to determine whether outcome criteria have been met. Comments should include the percentage of the criteria met or problems encountered in learning or teaching a topic. The patients' signatures indicate that they (legally) agree with the educator's notations. A copy of this sheet should not only become part of the permanent record, but also be given to the person or family member responsible for care. As noted earlier, a copy should be sent to the referring physician or other referring professional.

Follow-Up of the People Involved

Assessment should never end with discharge from the hospital or a clinic visit. It should also occur in the home where patients will be managing their diabetes. It is in the home where assessment should continue.

It would be ideal if every person with diabetes could be visited by a home health nurse within the first month after discharge and periodically thereafter. In practice, home visits are difficult to schedule because of the lack of personnel, but there are many patients who do receive home visits and many times astonishing facts are discovered.

Garay-Sevilla et al. (1995) carried out a study that involved 200 patients. They disclosed that adherence was associated with social support (Spirito, Coustan, McGarvey, & Low, 1993) and willingness to comply with treatment associated with perceived or actual obstacles. They were listed as negative emotions, resisting temptation, eating out, feeling deprived, time pressure, temptation to relapse, poor planning, competing priorities, social events, family support, dislikes of certain foods, and friends' support. Their assessment of an adolescent population found similar obstacles plus the added obstacles of peer pressure, food cravings, loneliness, and boredom.

Although further studies have been performed with patients in other settings, the studies in these settings indicated the difficulty in achieving patient compliance in the home, even while under close medical supervision. (Note: Rather than compliance, adherence—rather than adherence, empowerment.) Interaction and support from group-based education have been found to be an effective aid in empowerment (Smaldone & Weinger, 2005). Our program finds that the most success in patients feeling empowered is with a combination of both group and individual contact, as have others (Tibbetts, 2006).

Perhaps early and ongoing assessment is the way to identify needs and problems early on so that patients will have the full benefit of educational programs better tailored to the needs of each individual.

Other Assessment Considerations

Use of interdisciplinary conferences, teaching flow charts, and clinic visits will aid in communicating the needs of the person. Questions to be asked are: Is the group or individual learning at the expected rate? Are there certain limitations or intermediaries that have affected the person either physically, intellectually, or emotionally?

No method of assessment is perfect and any method should be adjusted as situations change. Some of the following guidelines, however, can be helpful to anyone setting up criteria for assessment:

1. The assessment should begin during the initial contact with the patient. (It is very discouraging to find out the day of discharge or months later that the patient's vision is so poor that he or she cannot see the markings on the syringe and that poor vision may be the reason for the poor control that brought the patient to the hospital or clinic visit in the first place.)
2. Physical, social, and emotional needs as well as the current diabetes orientation should be assessed. (If the patient's wife does the cooking, she should be involved in the education process, too. Or the patient who recently had a death in the family may be too emotionally upset to learn at this time.)
3. Use more than one method of assessment: question-and-answer sessions, questionnaire, demonstration, or interview. (The patient may be able to verbalize exactly how to do the blood test but may not actually be doing the test correctly on a demonstration.)
4. Assessment should continue throughout the education process and afterward. (A review is needed each time the patient returns to the health professional's office. Further teaching or reinforcement of earlier teaching will help to remind the patient of the responsibilities of self-management and/or self-care.)
5. A copy of the assessment should be available for the health professional's office, home health or community nurse, and the client.
6. There is a well-written and documented booklet on Continuous Quality Improvement (2005). This should be a part of all diabetes education libraries. This guide is most beneficial in assisting the professional(s) in the need to reevaluate and make up-to-date changes in their program.

Summary

Assessment of a patient's knowledge, ability to understand, emotional responses, and needs is an important part of patient education and management. Assessment should initially be performed repeatedly as part of the education process and repeated after basic education is completed.

Reassessment should be performed on various aspects of patient knowledge, skills, and emotional adjustment at each follow-up visit. Having patients and families looking to the positive may assist with the psychosocial adjustment. It is difficult to have any chronic disease, but discussion in a group or individually has brought up such topics as having a support group, learning more about themselves, being healthier, becoming more spiritually aware, and so forth. Subscribing to patient-oriented journals has also helped individuals to see the broader picture. It also keeps them hopeful, especially when ongoing on-site education is not present: *Diabetes Forecast, Self-Management of Diabetes, Diabetes Health, Diabetes Health Monitor*, and *Diabetes Living*. A number of these magazines are both online and in print.

Empowerment is the up-to-date term (Anderson, 2007). Compliance (Mertig, 2007) is not what health professionals should be seeking, even though they might think that is what is desired. Adherence to a regimen (Garay-Sevilla et al., 1995) gets closer to empowerment, but it still relates to "do as I say" rather than "what do you think you are able to do." New technology and updated education do help, but the behaviors (Highstein et al., 2007) and problem solving (Glasgow, Fisher, Skaff, Mullan, & Toobert, 2007), taking into consideration the stages of change (Jones et al., 2003) of the individual and/or family, lead to the best possible outcomes (Boucher & Van Wormer, 2006).

As further work is done with computer-assisted interventions to improve self-management outcomes (Williams, Lynch, & Glasgow, 2007) and cellular phone use in improving glycemic control (Yoon & Kim, 2008), the potential for safe and effective management becomes less of a dream and more of a reality. Anderson and Funnell (2008) conclude that the evidence and the tools exist but they question whether there is the willingness for the educators to follow through, assess, and document their abilities to establish a therapeutic alliance with patients. In their search of the medical literature, they found science and health behavior for the science; respect and social values for the art of diabetes education. For the art of nursing they found compassion and empathy with the most hits. They expressed that "... compassionate, patient-centered diabetes (health professionals) are both unique and fundamental to the success of (diabetes education)."

We trust that the preceding information has given practical suggestions and approaches that may be used in developing a teaching program and aiding the patient to attain the best quality of health care possible (see Appendix Q for lab test information and Appendix R for other useful resources). This information is intended to be a springboard for further planning, study, and research.

References

American Association of Clinical Endocrinologists. (2007a). *Clinical guidelines*. Retrieved March 31, 2008, from www.aace.org

American Association of Clinical Endocrinologists. (2007b). Medical guidelines for clinical practice for the management of diabetes mellitus. *Endocrine Practice, 13*(Suppl. 1), 3–68.

American Association of Diabetes Educators. Martin, C., Daly, A., McWharter, L. S., Shewide-Slavin, C., & Kushion, W. (2005a). The scope of practice, standards of practice and standards of professional performance for diabetes educators. *The Diabetes Educator, 31*(4), 487–488, 490, 492.

American Association of Diabetes Educators. (2005b). The scope of practice for diabetes educators and the standards of practice for diabetes educators. *The Diabetes Educator, 26*(1), 25–31.

American Diabetes Association. (2007a). *AADE 7 self-care behaviors: Measurable behavior change is the desired outcome of diabetes education*. Retrieved March 31, 2008, from www.diabeteseducators.org

American Diabetes Association. (2007b). National standards for diabetes self-management education. *The Diabetes Educator, 33*(4), 599–615.

American Diabetes Association. (2008a). Third-party reimbursement for diabetes care, self management education, and supplies. *Diabetes Care, 31*(Suppl. 1), S95–S96.

American Diabetes Association. (2008b). National standards for diabetes self-management education. *Diabetes, 31*(Suppl. 1), S97–S104.

American Diabetes Association. (2008c). Standards of medical care in diabetes. *Diabetes Care, 31*(Suppl. 1), S12–S54.

Anderson, B. (2007). Taking diabetes self-management education to the next level. *Diabetes Spectrum, 20*(4), 202–203.

Anderson, B., & Funnell, M. (2005). Putting empowerment into practice. In C. Mensing (Ed.), *The art of empowerment* (2nd ed., pp. 221–250). Alexandria, VA: American Diabetes Association.

Anderson, R. M., & Funnell, M. M. (2008). The art and science of diabetes education: A culture out of balance. *The Diabetes Educator, 34*(1), 109–117.

Anderson, R. M., Funnell, M. M., Butler, P. M., Arnold, M. S., Fitzgerald, J. T., & Feste, C. C. (1995). Patient empowerment. Results of a randomized controlled trial. *Diabetes Care, 18*(7), 943–949.

Boucher, I. S., & VanWormer, J. J. (2006). Evaluating and documenting outcomes. In C. Mensing (Ed.), *The art and science of diabetes self-management education* (pp. 633–649). Chicago: American Association of Diabetes Educators.

Briggs-Myers, I., & McCaulley, M. H. (1985). *A guide to the development and use of the Myers-Briggs type indicator.* Palo Alto, CA: Consulting Psychologists Press.

Brown, S. A. (1992). Meta-analysis of diabetes patient education research: Variations in intervention effects across studies. *Research Nursing Health, 15*(6), 409–419.

Clark, C. M., Jr., Fradkin, J. E., Hiss, R. G., Lorenz, R. A., Vinicor, F., & Warren-Boulton, E. (2001). The national diabetes education program, changing the way diabetes is treated: Comprehensive diabetes care. *Diabetes Care, 24*(4), 617–618.

Continuous Quality Improvement. (2005). The CQI process. In *A step by step guide for quality improvement in diabetes education* (pp. 17–45). Chicago: American Association of Diabetes Educators.

Diabetes Control and Complications Trial Research Group (1993). The effect of intensive treatment of diabetes on the development and progression of long-term complications in insulin-dependent diabetes mellitus. *New England Journal of Medicine, 329*(14), 977–986.

Funnell, M. M. (2007). National standards for diabetes self-management education: What do they mean for providers? *Review of Endocrinology, 1*(4), 51–53.

Funnell, M. M., Donnelly, M. B., Anderson, R. M., Johnson, P. D., & Oh, M. S. (1992). Perceived effectiveness, cost, and availability of patient education methods and materials. *The Diabetes Educator, 18*(2), 139–145.

Funnell, M. M., & Mensing, C. R. (2005). Diabetes education in the management of diabetes. In B. P. Childs, M. Cypress, & G. Spollett, *Complete nurse's guide to diabetes care* (pp. 188–198). Alexandria, VA: American Diabetes Association.

Gallegos, E. C., Ovalle-Berumen, F. A., & Gomez-Meza, M. V. (2006). Metabolic control of adults with type 2 diabetes mellitus through education and counseling. *Journal of Nursing Scholarship, 38*(4), 344–351.

Garay-Sevilla, M. E., Nava, L. E., Malacara, J. M., Huerta, R., Diaz-de-Leon, J., Mena, A., et al. (1995). Adherence to treatment and social support in patients with noninsulin dependent diabetes mellitus. *Journal of Diabetes Complications, 9*(2), 81–86.

Glasgow, R. E., Fisher, L., Skaff, M., Mullan, J., & Toobert, D. J. (2007). Problem solving and diabetes self-management: Investigation in a large, multiracial sample. *Diabetes Care, 30*(1), 33–37.

Highstein, G. R., O'Toole, M. L., Shetty, G., Brownson, C. A., & Fisher, E. B. (2007). Use of the transtheoretical model to enhance resources and supports for diabetes self-management: Lesions from the Robert Wood Johnson Foundation Diabetes Initiative. *The Diabetes Educator, 33*(Suppl. 6), 1935–2005.

Ingersoll, G. M., & Marrero, D. (1991). A modified quality-of-life measure for youths: Psychometric properties. *The Diabetes Educator, 17*(2), 114–118.

Jones, H., Edwards, L., Vallis, T. M., Ruggiero, L., Rossi, S. R., Greene, G., et al.: Diabetes Stages of Change (DiSC) Study. (2003). Changes in diabetes self-care behaviors make a difference in glycemic control; The Diabetes Stages of Changes study. *Diabetes Care, 26*(3), 732–737.

Levetan, C. S., Salas, J. R., Wilets, I. F., & Zumoff, B. (1995). Impact of endocrine and diabetes team consultation on hospital length of stay for patients with diabetes. *The American Journal of Medicine, 99*(7), 22–28.

Lorenzi, G. M. (2006). Implementation of diabetes education. In C. Mensing (Ed.), *The art and science of diabetes self-management education* (pp. 615–632). Chicago: American Association of Diabetes Educators.

Maryniuk, M. D. (2006). Developing the plan for education. In C. Mensing (Ed.), *The art and science of diabetes self-management education* (pp. 597–614). Chicago: American Association of Diabetes Educators.

Maryniuk, M. D., Bronzini, B. M., & Lorenzi, G. M. (2004). Quality diabetes self-management education: Achieving and maintaining ADA education program recognition. *Diabetes Educator, 30*(3), 467–475.

Medicare News: Medicare program; expanded coverage of self-management training and diabetes outcome measurements for outpatient diabetics. (2000). *Press release and fact sheet information, December 28, 2000.* Retrieved from http://www.hcfa.gov/nubaffr.htm

Meisgeier, C., & Murphy, E. (1987). *Murphy-Meisgeier type indicator for children manual.* Palo Alto: CA: Consulting Psychologists Press.

Mertig, R. G. (2007). Client noncompliance. In R. G. Mertig (Ed.), *Teaching diabetes self-management* (pp. 143–158). New York: Springer Publishing Company.

Mulcahy, K., & Lumber, T. (2004). Ongoing diabetes self-management education (DSME). In K. Mulcahy (Ed.), *The diabetes ready reference for health professionals* (2nd ed., pp. 49–50). Alexandria, VA: American Diabetes Association.

Mulcahy, K., Maryniuk, M., Peeples, M., Peyrot, M., Tomky, D., Weaver, T., et al. (2003). Technical review: Diabetes self-management education core outcomes measures. *The Diabetes Educator, 29*(5), 1–25.

Nettles, A. T., & Kreitzer, M. J. (1994). Trends in advanced nursing practice and implications for care of diabetes patients. *Diabetes Spectrum, 7*(6), 344–349.

Peyrot, M., Peeples, M., Tomky, D., Charron-Prochownik, D., & Weaver, T. (2007). Development of the American Association of Diabetes Educators' diabetes self-management assessment report tool. *The Diabetes Educator, 33*(4), 818–827.

Prochaska, J. O., Norcross, J. C., & DiClemente, C. C. (1994). *Changing for good.* New York: William Morrow.

Prochaska, J. O., & Velicer, W. F. (1997). The transtheoretical model of health behavior. *American Journal of Health Promotion, 12,* 38–48.

Rossing, P. J., Andersen, H., Hesselholdt, L., Thorsteinsson, B., Reimers., Binder, C., et al. (2001). Attitudes towards diabetes and its care: Evaluation before, immediately post-course for diabetes teams or equal to 1 year after a practical, international inter-disciplinary course for diabetes teams. *Practical Diabetes International, 18*(2), 39–44.

Siminerio, L. M., Piatt, G. A., Emerson, S., Ruppert, K., Saul, M., Solano, F., et al. (2006). *The Diabetes Educator, 32*(2), 253–260.

Simonds, S. K. (1974). Current issues in patient education. *American Association of Medical Clinics.* New York: Core Communication in Health, Inc.

Smaldone, A., & Weinger, K. (2005). Review: Group based education in self management strategies improves outcomes in type 2 diabetes mellitus. *Evidence Based Nursing, 8*(4), 111–113.

Spirito, A., Coustan, D., McGarvey, S. T., & Low, K. G. (1993). Self-reported compliance with diabetes self management during pregnancy. *International Journal of Psychiatric Medicine, 23*(2), 195–207.

Stamler, L. L., Patrick, L. J., Cole, M. M., & Lafreniere, K. (2006). Patient perceptions of satisfaction following diabetes education: Use of the Mastery of Stress Instrument. *The Diabetes Educator, 32*(5), 770–776.

Sullivan, T. E., & Hawkins, K. A. (1995). Support for the abbreviation of the Wide Range Achievement Test. Revised spelling subtest in neuropsychological assessments. *Journal of Clinical Psychology, 51,* 552–554.

Tibbetts, C. J. (2006). Diabetes self-management education: A saga of angels and demons. *Diabetes Spectrum, 19*(1), 54–57.

U.K. Prospective Diabetes Study Group. (1998). Intensive blood glucose control with sulfonylureas or insulin compared with conventional treatment and risk of complications in patients with type 2 diabetes. *Lancet, 352,* 837–853.

Williams, G. C., Lynch, M., & Glasgow, R. E. (2007). Computer-assisted intervention improves patient-centered diabetes care by increasing autonomy support. *Health Psychology, 26*(6), 728–734.

Wysocki, T., Taylor, A., Hough, B. S., Linscheid, T. R., Yeates, K. O., & Naglien, J. A. (1996). Deviation from developmentally appropriate self-care autonomy association with diabetes outcomes. *Diabetes Care, 19*(2), 119–125.

Yoon, K. H., & Kim, H. S. (2008). A short message service by cellular phone in type 2 diabetic patients for 12 months. *Diabetes Research in Clinical Practice, 79*(2), 256–261.

Zung, W. W., Magruder-Habib, K., Velez, R., & Ailing, W. (1990). The co-morbidity of anxiety and depression in general medical patients: A longitudinal study. *Journal of Clinical Psychiatry, 51,* 77–81.

32

Stress Management and Diabetes

The Chinese word for crises, which is often described as stress, is represented by the combination of the symbols standing for danger and opportunity. Stress, even though often accompanied by uncomfortable symptoms and perhaps danger, offers the strength and opportunity for fight or flight.

Stress is a part of everyday life, but if adequate coping mechanisms are lacking, blood glucose levels may be adversely affected. To avoid stress one would have to do and think nothing, in fact, not exist. The word stress denotes something negative when in reality stress is not always bad. It is part of excitement, adventure, and achievement. Some level of stress is considered appropriate for everyone. The balance of stress is what all people should try to achieve. Too much or too little stress can result in physical or mental illness. For the factory assembly worker who might experience too little stress or the executive who may experience too much, there should be a balance that can be achievable. If such a balance, as a goal, is not attempted, stress-related illness is likely to be the result.

Stress responses aggravate health problems such as diabetes (Carter, Gonder-Frederick, Cox, Clarke, & Scott, 1985; Delamater & Cox, 1994). Stress may bring about vascular problems, immunologic problems, and infections.

Stress affects the emotional response and is affected by the emotional adjustment. There is a need for coherence, for trust, and a sense of quality of life for each person (Delgardo, 2007). It is also known that stress management is related to blood glucose level control, especially in Type 2 diabetes mellitus (T2DM; Surwit et al., 2002).

Many diseases are attributed to inappropriate human interaction with the stress and strain of everyday living. In diabetes mellitus, the physical response to stressors (environmental stimuli, perceptions, and fears) can be a part of the multifactorial process that results in the development of metabolic intolerance to carbohydrates. The physiologic responses to stressors include several responses that parallel the physiologic changes that accompany diabetes. Two of these are loss of appetite (which would occur in the latter stages of diabetic ketoacidosis) and loss or gain of weight, with increasing symptoms of anxiety. There may also be enlargement of the adrenal glands, shrinkage of the lymph system, and an occurrence of ulcers in the stomach and intestine. This disease process was simplified by Selye (1974) in a three-phase stress process called the general adaptation syndrome. This process includes alarm, resistance followed by some adaptation, and exhaustion. The final phase can continue or increase until the body becomes utterly exhausted. In its extreme or ultimate form, stress may result in death.

In applying this simple model to the field of diabetes, the alarm or acute stress phase could be described as the initial emotional response at the time of the diagnosis of the disease or complication. It could be the occurrence of diabetic ketoacidosis or hypoglycemia. The resistance phase could represent the chronicity in the choice of nonadherence to self-care, or the lack of adjustment to the initial diagnosis or diagnosis of a complication. The exhaustion phase might be the development of a complication or the complete denial of the disease, represented by the frequency of diabetic ketoacidosis or hypoglycemia. This simplified approach does not consider the myriad effects, genetics of the person, or impact of the environment on the total person. To recognize such effects, one must consider the responses of the body to stress.

Physiologic Response to Stressors

The physiologic response to stress in both the individual with diabetes and the person without diabetes can result in changes in blood glucose levels. When stress occurs, the hypothalamus directly stimulates the medulla of the adrenal gland to secrete epinephrine, which in turn causes the liver to release stored glucose (glycogenolysis). Epinephrine secretion results in an increased circulatory rate, increased cardiac output, increased mobilization of glucose and fats for energy, constriction of peripheral blood vessels, and dilatation of gastrointestinal tract blood vessels.

The hypothalamus may also stimulate the anterior pituitary gland, causing it to secrete adrenocorticotropic hormone, which stimulates the cortex of the adrenal gland to release glucocorticoids. Glucocorticoids stimulate the liver to convert amino acids to glucose (gluconeogenesis). The stimulation of the pituitary gland, as a physiologic response to a stressor, may also cause the secretion of thyroid-stimulating hormone, which causes the release of thyroxine from the thyroid gland. Thyroxine can stimulate an increased rate of uptake of glucose from the intestines. The stimulation of the pituitary gland also results in a release of growth hormone, which, in this instance, is not responsible for growth but for the mobilization of fats rather than glucose for energy. Again, this is a normal physiologic response. All of these effects result in more available glucose to the brain and other parts of the body. It prepares the body for fight or flight, and, if not in overload, for clearer thinking. The main difference between the individual with diabetes and the individual without diabetes is the availability of insulin to control the glucose levels, should those levels become elevated.

In all, stress results in "enhanced peripheral glucose uptake and utilization, hyperlactatemia, increased glucose production, depressed glycogenesis, glucose intolerance, and insulin resistance" (Mizock, 1995).

Techniques to Alter Stress Responses

Many adaptations may be used to balance the acute effects of stress or to help the person cope with the immediate and long-term effects of stress. Some of these follow.

Assertiveness Training

Anyone that has diabetes needs to be assertive at some point in their life. Whether it is questioning the waiter as to the method of preparation of an item of food or saying the right thing at the right time in the right way to prevent the possibility of any future emergencies, people with diabetes should learn to work on a Win–Win basis. In this way, the person with diabetes is best able to take care of health needs or the family member.

Biofeedback

Biofeedback training is usually accomplished over an 8- to 10-week period (kids usually can be trained in 6 to 8 weeks) (Guthrie, Moeller, & Guthrie, 1983). Learning to relax with the feedback of muscle relaxation or peripheral temperature rising is enhanced when sound or sight, that is, a graph, helps to demonstrate when a person is relaxed or not. The galvanic skin response also demonstrates what happens physiologically when the person is in a certain relaxed physical position or frame of mind. These responses are then trained to change the physiology to a new frame of reference.

Blood Glucose Awareness Training, or BGAT

BGAT is a system that trains the learner who has lost the physical signals that blood glucose levels are too low or even too high. Because the adrenergic response may be blunted when a person is insulin dependent on the average of five years, hypoglycemia unawareness may occur (Cox et al., 2006). Through a series of feedback information and training, the individual learns to identify other parameters that indicate low blood sugars. This program is now also available online (http://www.bgat.com)

Breathing Techniques

These techniques date back to early times. When a person breathes shallowly, he or she does not adequately use the oxygen efficiently and often requires more oxygen to do the same mental processing. Abdominal breathing occurs when the breathing is "so deep" that the abdomen goes out on an inhale and in on an exhale without the chest or shoulder moving. Three deep breaths help bring back short-term memory. A sequence of 10 to 12 deep breaths bring about relaxation, or as Dr. Herbert Benson calls it, "The Relaxation Response," when a person breathes correctly while thinking a repeating thought and passively handling intrusive thoughts. Blood pressure lowers, pulse rate lowers, and oxygen is used more efficiently.

Coping Skills Training

Coping Skills Training goes hand in hand with Assertiveness Training. Assertiveness Training is one of the coping skills a person can use. Other skills are Conflict Resolution and Negotiation Training even though a coping skill might be anything that permits the person to go forward without frantically raising blood glucose levels or personal physiologic responses.

Dance

Dancing is fun and good exercise. One patient who tried dancing returned to the clinic after a month wearing brighter clothes and having a neater appearance. She wondered why dancing was not thought of as an exercise before. When told to try it, because she felt uncomfortable walking in her neighborhood, she found dancing both enjoyable and helpful to her diabetes health. Her average blood sugars lowered to the extent that she needed to cut her medications a third (she had also lost four pounds).

Drumming

Men might not care for the dancing alone at home, but they might be interested in drumming or responding to drum sounds (women don't need to be left out either). There are retreats that use and/or teach drumming. There are drum beats for fun and laughter and drum beats for sorrow. Various sounds might be made on the drum that accentuate other feelings and concerns. Such an activity might be a basis or outlet for lowering blood glucose levels or handling feelings of frustration or anger or both.

Exercise Techniques: Including Qigong, Tai Chi, and Yoga

Much more information can be found in Chapters 11 and 19. In regard to stress management, exercise increases the feeling of well-being and decreases depression. In the Asian therapies, those exercises listed above and others join the ranks of focusing on something other than problems of the day. So these activities not only assist in improving balance, but they also aid in modulating the pulse rate and respiration rate along with lowering blood pressure responses.

Guided Imagery

This process has been used for many purposes. It has been especially helpful in individuals who are suffering from cancer. For those who have diabetes, it is a tool to soothe the individual as they purposefully focus on a place of calm or complete a body scan to see whether their body has any tight muscles or hot spots of possible infection. Imagery may use visual scenes of a pleasant nature for problem solving or resolution. Imagery may be filled with nonassociated symbolism (such as a beautiful scenic view) or with specific symbolism (a ship in a stormy ocean representing a person in the clutches of potentially overwhelming stress). It may be directed by a guide who opens the setting with verbal descriptions or nondirected by a guide who sets the stage but allows the individuals involved to fill in the setting with individualized meaningful thoughts, scenes, or people. In general, it is used to tell a healing story or just to have a peaceful moment.

Journaling

This technique has long been known to help a person process concerns and feelings. Writing at times of concern or just keeping a daily diary has aided many people in handling fears and anxieties related to having diabetes. Thinking through the process of the day's happenings by writing them down often brings relief as the person comes to an understanding of what is going on in his or her mind.

Meditation

This ancient practice is becoming more common. Again, meditation is activity that focuses the person's mind off the problems of the day. Meditation slows the pulse rate, decreases the release of epinephrine, and promotes a general feeling of well-being. Meditation may be centered on a sound, picture (visual or mental), a thought, or a prayer. Daily meditation, as with other modalities, may aid in modulating physiologic responses that might result in challenges to blood glucose levels.

Nutrition: Vitamins, Minerals, and Herbs

Choosing appropriate healthy foods and ingesting adequate fluid lead to a healthier outcome. Vitamins and minerals help to fill the gap even if healthy food choices are frequently made. Herbs might take the place of some medications or be used along with present prescriptions if appropriate for that person and if safe from interacting with other medications in an untoward way. Upset stomachs do not lead to any sort of relaxation. Frequent illnesses continue to be hard on managing blood sugars. Adequate nutrition through foods and liquids forms a basis of a better immune system and a decreased need for added medications.

Personal Counseling

Just talking to someone is useful. Cognitive behavioral therapy has been found to be even more effective (Golden, 2007). The chapters concerning psychological responses (Chapters 13 and 21) go into this process and others in more detail. Problems that just fester in the mind have a definite affect on the mind and the body. Encouraging people to talk out their problems or concerns helps them to clarify their thoughts and to make decisions more appropriately in relation to desired outcomes.

Refuting Irrational Ideas

People can think irrationally. Often the worst irrational thought is about injecting insulin. Because a relative died or had to have an amputation after starting on insulin, the person might conclude that such is going to happen to him or her once started on insulin. As a person learns to talk out these uncorrect or irrational ideas, the easier it is to put those ideas to rest. Education is one of the best ways to refute these ideas that have developed through history or through incorrect thinking.

Relaxation

Autogenic therapy and progressive relaxation are effective tools to use to combat the devastating effects of stress and diabetes control (Lammers, Nailboff, & Straatmeyer, 1984). Relaxation, in its specialized meaning, is a structured mechanism by which a person trains the self to be more in control. One relaxation format requires a number of weeks of practice (usually a shorter time for children and adolescents and a longer time for adults). Various techniques such as progressive relaxation (sequentially tensing and relaxing groups of muscles starting from the toes and working upward in the body) or autogenic therapy (making self-statements in regard to breathing deeply or feeling heavy and warm; related to various parts or all of the body) may be used.

The combined process of progressive relaxation, or autogenic therapy, and biofeedback assists the participant to identify a cue (e.g., the way the muscles feel or some visualization of a pleasant place) that is eventually used to transfer the relaxation responses to the social environment.

Self-Hypnosis

Hypnosis, the actual or learned ability to concentrate, assists people to relax by focusing on the decrease of fear and anxieties and the stress of just having diabetes (Diment, 1991). This is a learned process in which the therapist only acts as a guide. Often people think that hypnosis is a mind-control activity rather than a way to learn how to handle pain, fears, problems, and other negative thoughts, emotions, or physiologic functions. It is easier for some people to learn to relax or to use the other techniques than it is for others. No matter what the ability to learn self-hypnosis, anyone who has the ability to concentrate can learn this technique.

Therapeutic Massage

More and more articles are written in refereed journals about the ability of a massage to lower blood glucose levels. Therapeutic massage is useful for relaxation and it is useful for lowering blood glucose levels. Even infants and children having a variety of health and environmental problems, including diabetes, can benefit in their clinical course from the use of massage. One type of massage might be more pleasing than another type to a particular person. Finding the right one, whether Swedish or Thai or Shiatsu or a sports massage or a deep fascia massage or craniospinal therapy, might take a little time, but the exploration, time, and money would be worth it (just check blood glucose levels before and after treatment).

Thought Stopping

Thought stopping is a simple technique that is often difficult to do. Being able to stop thinking negative thoughts is often too hard. Learning how to turn off the mind from an unpleasant thought to a pleasant one is a task in itself, but once learned becomes very effective in preventing sleep deprivation problems.

Other Considerations

Many people use other mechanisms to decrease stress. Some might participate in a stress management training course. Others read or daydream to take their minds off the present or unpleasant experience. Others use either loud, overwhelming music or soft, pleasantly stimulating music, depending on their preferences. Others may do work around the house or yard, or they may work out in a gym or just bend a piece of coat hanger wire until all the energy that is developed by the stressful situation is diffused. Each person usually develops some methods that soothe and thereby relieve the tension of too high or too low a level of stress.

Effect of Stress on Blood Glucose Levels

There has been some controversy about the effect of stress on blood glucose control. Bruce, Chisholm, Storlien, Smythe, and Kragen (1988) reported that people with T2DM did not respond to psychologic stress with elevated blood glucose levels. Then later, Goetsch, VanDorsten, Pbert, Ullrich, and Yeater (1993) concluded that some stressors can have a hyperglycemic effect in T2DM, but they felt that further research was needed to see whether these findings could be found in the natural environment. Despite these findings, Surwit and Feinglos (1983) have demonstrated that relaxation practice can be beneficial in lowering blood glucose levels in individuals with T2DM, and later (1992), along with Schneider, found this was also true for people with Type 1 diabetes mellitus (T1DM).

There is more controversy surrounding those people who have T1DM. Feinglos, Hastedt, and Surwit (1987) concluded that people with T1DM do not respond to relaxation training (using only electromyography). They assumed this was because of a lack of counterregulatory response lost or blunted about 5 years after diagnosis.

Guthrie et al. (1983) in a pilot study found that Type 1 individuals do respond to relaxation training, based on the need to lower insulin dosages as the relaxation training during the study period progressed. This study could be flawed because of the small size of the population, although findings demonstrated significant changes (the study's major difference from Feinglos et al. was the use of temperature training along with electromyography training). Later, Bailey, Good, and McGrady (1990) reported similar findings, noting that average blood glucose levels dropped, "allowing a reduction in insulin dosage." McGrady, Bailey, and Good (1991) replicated the findings without changing insulin dosages by observing subjects progress from a greater hyperglycemic state to a lesser hyperglycemic state.

Although some people respond better than others to relaxation training, it appears that whatever the mechanism of focus, when the participant gets his or her mind off problems the body is allowed to drift into a relaxed state (i.e., temperature increase; electromyographic results decrease; galvanic skin responses or pulse rate decrease). It is now assumed that stress management training is beneficial and safe for any person so long as alterations are made in diabetes medications to prevent hypoglycemic events.

Stress Management Education

Stress management education can be given in a variety of settings and in a variety of methodologies. Whether in a classroom, at a retreat center, or hooked up to biofeedback equipment, the results of increased relaxation and thereby decreased stress levels are possible. The person who "tries to relax" will have as much difficulty as the person who "tries to go to sleep." Just the opposite will occur: The person will usually become tenser. Therefore, there are a number of considerations to having a complete relaxation program along with the age of the people involved (Hains, Davies, Parton, Totka, & Amoroso-Camarata, 2000) and, in T2DM, possibly related to the individual's personality (Lane, McCaskill, Ross, Feinglos, & Surwit, 2000).

In order to be able to participate in a full stress management program, there are a number of things to consider. If any one of the parts of a stress management program is omitted, the possibility for a sense of decreased stress responses will be smaller. The program that will be described has been in effect for more than 10 years. Both adults and children with T1DM and T2DM and parents of children who have diabetes have participated.

Assessment

First, an assessment of the individual's needs may be obtained in a variety of ways. Holmes and Rahe's (1967) Social Readjustment Rating Scale reveals the chance of developing a stress-related illness. This is a relatively less stable statistical instrument that has some predictive values, that is, if the total score is 150 or less, after summing up the ranked episodes perceived as most stressful (score of 10) to least stressful (score of 1), have a less than 33% chance of developing a stress-related illness in the next two years; if the scores fall between 150 and 300, there is a 50% chance of becoming seriously ill during this same period; if the person scores over 300 points, there is a 90% chance of this occurring. The test takes about 10 min to administer.

Another tool is the Stress Map (Orioli, Jaffe, & Scott, 1991). This instrument is self-administered and identifies a state of stress level at the time the test is completed. It also includes suggestions for interventions to correct the stressful state. The person taking the test responds to a Likert-like scale to situations and responses, which are summed and then plotted on a shaded graph. The highest scores indicate the severest stress (or burnout). It usually takes little more than 30 min to complete all the questions.

The Parenting Stress Index (Abidin, 1995) is a tool used to determine the stressors leading to dysfunction in the family. Special scoring sheets are needed for this test and domain profiles need to be purchased. Child domain scores indicate percentile ranks related to adaptability, acceptability, demandingness, mood, distractibility, and reinforcement (or manipulation) of parents. The parent domain score reveals depression, level of attachment, perceived restriction of the parent role, sense of competence, level of social isolation, relationship with spouse, and general perception of parent health. It has the capability to document, among others, the permissive parent and the abusive parent. A life scale is included through interpretation of the scores. This test has 101 (possibly 120 if life stress score is desired) items and is Likert based. It requires at least 30 min to complete.

The Berkeley Stress and Coping Project's Daily Hassles Scale reveals to what extent daily irritants or hassles serve as stress indicators. It is available in a combined form (including an uplift scale as well as a hassles scale). This test has 117 items to grade whether the item did or did not occur as an extremely severe hassle. The test can be completed in 20–30 min (Delongis, Coyne, Dakof, Folkman, & Lazarus, 1982).

Refer to the October 2007 issue of the *Journal of Pediatric Psychology* for the Blount et al. article on an evidence-based assessment of coping and stress in pediatric psychology for children. Children that experience the stressor of a chronic illness potentially respond with erratic self-care behaviors and physiologic responses.

There is an apparent need for an approach that includes stress management as one of its components. The following is offered.

The PARENT Program

The PARENT Program is an approach to participating in a total stress management program. It goes by the acronym, PARENT—this word is both a reminder that the components of the program are important not only while parenting a child, but also in parenting oneself. Each of these letters stands for a part of the program. P stands for positive thinking, A for assertiveness, R for relaxation, E for exercise, N for nutrition, and T for touch.

Positive thinking can be achieved through behavioral conditioning such as the use of positive affirmation statements, laughter, prayer, meditation, or reframing. Saying positive things makes a person feel more positive about themselves, that is, more self-confident. Some people who have a chronic illness, such as diabetes, sometimes feel that they and their family need permission to laugh. Reframing is as it says: taking a negative thought and turning it around 180 degrees. P may also stand for pattern—the recognition that self-management is made easier by responding to the patterns of blood glucose levels in relation to the patterned lifestyle either as a result of interactive responses or by observing patterns of blood glucose in relation to responses to food eaten.

Assertiveness is a social response that can be used at home, at work, in the school setting, and in other social settings. If people are not assertive, they have a tendency to feel neglected, have their feelings hurt, feel angry, and feel pushed around—all of which result in physiologically stressful responses by the body. Being able to negotiate needs and to caringly confront puts fewer physical demands on the mind and therefore the body. This component should also include the person's attitude and the recognition if an attitude affects self-care.

Relaxation training develops a skill that may be used at any time or place. (Note: A change in medication may be necessary if the blood glucose levels become too low during the time of training or afterward at the time of use. Blood glucose monitoring is a must.) The choice of relaxation training depends on the interest of the learner.

Exercise sessions should be at least 30 min long 3 times a week or 20 min long 4–6 times a week. They should include low-impact aerobic activity such as walking, bike riding, swimming, or floor exercises. Isometric exercise should only be included if appropriate for that individual. Isometric exercises may increase pressure to the vascular system because they are performed against stable resistance.

Nutrition involves following a well-balanced meal plan that includes high fiber, low fat, and decreased concentrated sweets. Food should be appropriately distributed throughout the day to best meet activity needs and the actions of the diabetes medication.

Touch should include a minimum of four hugs a day plus self-nurturing, spiritual nurturing, and self-esteem-building activities. It also includes, for the person who has diabetes, giving a shot, checking blood glucose levels, and checking for ketones if the blood glucose levels are >240 mg/dl (13 mmol/L).

Whatever the program chosen, stress management becomes an effective tool to assist in the total balance of the person—to provide a sense of wholeness despite diabetes' powerful effects.

Summary

Something other than just eating, medication, and activity causes blood glucose levels to rise and fall in people with diabetes. Something is occurring that results in the majority of people raising their hand, when asked, "Do your blood sugars go up or down when you are highly stressed?" (Note: Some people become more agitated when stressed and their blood glucose levels go down rather than up.) A known response is reliable within individual patients but cannot be generalized to include all people.

A number of educational booklets are available through various pharmaceutical companies that may give assistance to individuals who want or need to cope with the stressors in their life. The study of mindfulness (becoming a popular approach to work through pain and depression) and stress reduction training (www.umassmed.edu/cfm.org) can be obtained from an Internet course, or through reading the literature, such as John Kabat-Zinn's article in *Clinical Psychology: Science and Practice* (2003) or through research studies, such as the pilot study on improving glycemia control in people with T2DM (Rosenzweig, Reibel, Greeson, Edman, & Jasser, 2007).

Stress has different meanings for different people. An effort should be made for individuals to give a personal definition of stress and then to guide them to identify mechanisms by which their kind of stress may play a key role in their lifestyle. Stress should then be identified on the continuum from extremely unpleasant (excess of stress) to extremely pleasant. Mechanisms for intervention, to maintain the balance and to promote the best physical, emotional, and mental health, should then be discussed.

Recommended Reading

Seward, B. L. (2004). *Managing stress: Principles and strategies for health and well-being* (4th ed.). Boston: Jones and Bartlett Publishers.

References

Abidin, R. R. (1995). *Parenting Stress Index* (3rd ed.). Odessa, FL: Psychological Assessment Resources.

Bailey, B. K., Good, M., & McGrady, A. (1990). Clinical observations on behavioral treatment of a patient with insulin-dependent diabetes mellitus. *Biofeedback and Self Regulation, 15*(1), 7–13.

Blount, R., Simons, L. E., Devine, R. A., Taaniste, T., Psychol, M., Cohen, L. L., et al. (2007). Evidence-based assessment of coping and stress in pediatric psychology. *Journal of Pediatric Psychology, 32*(9), 1099–1110.

Bruce, D. G., Chisholm, D. J., Storlien, L. H., Smythe, G. A., & Kragen, E. W. (1988). Acute psychological stress does not cause hyperglycemia in non-insulin dependent diabetes mellitus despite an increased sensitivity to sympathomimetic agents. *The Diabetes Educator, 14,* 229.

Carter, W. R., Gonder-Frederick, L. A., Cox, D. J., Clarke, W. L., & Scott, D. (1985). Effects of stress on blood glucose in IDDM. *Diabetes Care, 8,* 411–412.

Cox, D. M., Gonder-Frederick, L., Ritterband, L., Patel, K., Schachinger, H., Fehm-Wolfsdorf, G., et al. (2006). Blood glucose awareness training: What is it, where is it, and where is it going? *Diabetes Spectrum, 19*(1), 43–49.

Delamater, A. M., & Cox, D. J. (Eds.). (1994). Psychological stress, coping, and diabetes. *Diabetes Spectrum, 7*(1), 17–49.

Delgardo, C. (2007). Sense of cohesion, spirituality, trust, and quality of life in chronic illness. *Journal of Nursing Scholarship, 39*(3), 229–234.

Delongis, A., Coyne, J. C., Dakof, G., Folkman, S., & Lazarus, R. S. (1982). Relationship of daily hassles, uplifts, and major life events to health states. *Health Psychology, 1,* 119–136.

Diment, A. D. (1991). Uses of hypnosis in diabetes related stress management counseling. *Australian Journal of Clinical and Experimental Hypnosis, 19*(2), 97–101.

Feinglos, M. N., Hastedt, P., & Surwit, R. S. (1987). Effects of relaxation therapy on patients with type I diabetes mellitus. *Diabetes Care, 10,* 72–75.

Goetsch, V. L., VanDorsten, B., Pbert, L. A., Ullrich, I. H., & Yeater, R. A. (1993). Acute effects of laboratory stress on blood glucose in non-insulin dependent diabetics. *Psychosomatic Medicine, 55*(6), 492–496.

Golden, S. H. (2007). A review of the evidence for a neuroendocrine link between stress, depression, and diabetes mellitus. *Current Diabetes Reviews, 3*(4), 252–259.

Guthrie, D. W., Moeller, T., & Guthrie, R. A. (1983). Biofeedback and its application to the stabilization and control of diabetes mellitus. *American Journal of Clinical Biofeedback, 6,* 82–87.

Hains, A. A., Davies, W. H., Parton, E., Totka, J. & Amoroso-Camarata, J. (2000). A stress management intervention for adolescents with type 1 diabetes. *The Diabetes Educator, 26*(3), 417–424.

Holmes, T. H., & Rahe, R. H. (1967). The social readjustment rating scale. *Psychosomatic Research, 11,* 213–118.

Kabat-Zinn, J. (2003). Mindfulness-based interventions in context: Past, present, and future. *Clinical Psychology: Science and Practice, 10*(2), 144–156.

Lammers, C. A., Nailboff, B. D., & Straatmeyer, A. J. (1984). The effects of progression relaxation on stress and diabetes control. *Behavior Research and Therapy, 22,* 641–650.

Lane, J. D., McCaskill, C. C., Ross, S. L., Feinglos, M. N., & Surwit, R. D. (2000). Relaxation training for NIDDM: Predicting who may benefit. *Diabetes Care, 16*(8), 1087–1094.

McGrady, A., Bailey, B. K., & Good, M. P. (1991). Controlled study of biofeedback-assisted relaxation in type I diabetes. *Diabetes Care, 14*(5), 360–365.

Mizock, B. A. (1995). Alteration in carbohydrate metabolism during stress: A review of the literature. *The American Journal of Medicine, 98,* 75–84.

Orioli, E. M., Jaffe, E. M., & Scott, C. D. (1991). *Stress map.* New York: Newmarket Press.

Rosenzweig, S., Reibel, D. K., Greeson, J. M., Edman, J. S., & Jasser, S. A. (2007). Mindfulness-based stress reduction is associated with improved glycemic control in type 2 diabetes mellitus: A pilot study. *Alternative Therapies, 13*(5), 36–38.

Selye, H. (1974). *Stress without distress* (pp. 19, 20, 148). New York: New American Library.

Surwit, R. S., & Feinglos, M. (1983). The effects of relaxation on glucose tolerance in non-insulin dependent diabetes mellitus. *Diabetes Care, 6,* 176–179.

Surwit, R. S., Schneider, M. S., & Feinglos, M. N. (1992). Stress and diabetes mellitus. *Diabetes Care, 15*(10), 1413–1422.

Surwit, R. S., vanTilburg, M. A. L., Zucker, N., McCaskill, C. C., Parekh, P., Feinglos, M. N., et al. (2002). Stress management improves long-term glycemic control in type 2 diabetes. *Diabetes Care, 25*(1), 20–24.

33

Complementary and Alternative Medicine Therapies, Medications, and Drugs

Almost 50% of people will use a variety of complementary and alternative medicine (CAM) practices, including various therapies, vitamins, minerals, and herbs, during a lifetime (Eisenberg et al., 1998). The practices might be used in place of needed therapy (alternative) or may actually enhance the therapy (complementary) directed by the traditional health professionals. The amount or type of CAM practices using vitamins, mineral, or herbs may be helpful or harmful. In addition, many medical drugs can cause untoward responses in people who have diabetes, which can indirectly result in other diseases (side effects of vitamins, minerals, and herbs are minimal, but can be very serious). For example, the use of antibiotics to treat viral infections can result in a severe superinfection because the antibiotics may also kill good or saprophytic bacteria, allowing overgrowth of pathologic bacteria. An example of adverse drug interaction is St. John's Wort. This neutraceutical has been used extensively for depression. It has now been shown to interact and modify the action of anticoagulants and this interaction has caused death.

Hard evidence is still lacking about using specific herbs or supplements for diabetes. The ones that appear to warrant further study, as of 2003, are American ginseng, chromium, Gymnema sylvestre, vanadium, nopal, alpha lipoic acid, and aloe vera (Yeh, Eisenberg, Kaptchuk, & Phillips, 2003). Panax ginseng use, in a well-controlled study (Vuksan et al., 2008), resulted in improved plasma glucose and plasma insulin regulation. American ginseng was found to reduce postprandial blood glucose levels in healthy individuals (Dascalu et al., 2007). Chromium picolinate was shown to have no effect in one population (Kleefstra et al., 2007), but to improve glucose metabolism when used in combination with biotin in an overweight population (Albarracin, Fuqua, Evans, & Goldfine, 2008). Gymnema sylvestre is being used more frequently in the United States. Leach (2007) completed a review of the literature to determine whether there is help or harm in using this herb for those with Type 2 diabetes mellitus (T2DM). His conclusion related to supplementation or early use, finding that more blood glucose level control is noted in the papers from India than in the papers published in this country. Vanadium was found to have an adipogenic effect by Shukla and Bhonde (2008) in their population of people with T2DM. There is nothing in the U.S. reviewed literature on Nopal (cactus derivative), but two papers in the Spanish literature (in 1989 and 1992) cautioned its use in therapeutic doses, even though they found a glucose response. Alpha lipoic acid, besides chromium, has been one of the more frequently studied supplements. Alpha lipoic acid is now available in a controlled-release form. It has been found to be functional as an antioxidant and to have a beneficial effect on total body glucose metabolism (Evans, Heymann, Goldfine, & Gavin, 2002). It is especially useful in the treatment of neuropathic pain in the feet. Aloe vera was noted to be helpful in treating wounds, edema, and pain (1988). Cinnamon use is supported in one study with subjects that had diabetes (Pham, Kourlas, & Pham, 2007), but not in others (Kleefstra et al., 2007; Solomon & Blannin, 2007). Glucosamine did not have a significant effect on glycemic control or lipid levels in a two-week study (Albert et al., 2007).

If used incorrectly, vitamins, minerals, herbs, or even medications may also interact adversely. In evaluating the effect of botanicals (e.g., fenugreek, Gymnema sylvestre, cayenne) or neutraceuticals (e.g., vitamins, chromium, alpha lipoic acid) or medicines in persons with diabetes, all of the precautions regarding drugs and drug interactions in general must be understood. Persons with diabetes frequently require a variety of other medicines to treat associated diseases such as hypertension, neuropathy, cardiovascular disease, and others. Failure to adequately record the present history of the use of vitamins, minerals, and herbs, including alcohol, tobacco, or other social drugs may lead to problems with other medicines prescribed or to ethical problems when a CAM therapy is chosen over a traditional therapy (Thorne, Best, Balonk, Kelner, & Rickhy, 2002). This article also focuses on the fine line and the definitions used between curing and healing. Choices are possible, but the wrong, uneducated choice might have disastrous outcome.

CAM and Its Uses

Eisenberg and his group (1998) studied the use of CAM therapies in the general population. They found that such use has increased in frequency, despite out-of-pocket expense, over a 7-year period. Because some of the CAM practices may have some effect on blood glucose control, it is important to be aware of this and take the information into consideration when educating a person or family and when the person is monitored in the clinic setting (recognize that CAM therapies include more than just nutritional supplements—but nutritional supplements are a major focus of this chapter even though other CAM therapies are addressed).

If unsure of or wanting more CAM information, contact the clearinghouse for database literature through www.nccam.nih.gov. This National Center for Complementary and Alternative Medicine (NCCAM) has divided such practices into:

1. Alternative Medical Systems (e.g., naturopathy, traditional Chinese medicine, homeopathy, Ayurveda);
2. Mind–Body Interventions (e.g., art therapy, dance, hypnosis, meditation, prayer);
3. Biologically-Based Therapies (e.g., biologicals [bee pollen, and so forth], diets [Atkins, Ornish, Pritikin, and Weil], herbal, orthomolecular [e.g., magnesium, megavitamins]);
4. Manipulative and Body-Based Methods (e.g., chiropractic, osteopathic manipulation, reflexology); and
5. Energy Therapies (e.g., biofield therapy [reiki, qigong, therapeutic touch] and bioelectromagnetic field therapy [magnetic fields, pulsed fields, direct or alternating fields])

Nationally funded research studies are being carried out in more than 10 university-based centers. For example, acupuncture and reiki have been or are being studied in relation to their therapeutic value in pain control for those that have neuropathy. Other centers are studying various botanicals and neutraceuticals and acupuncture.

Complementary practices, such as exercise, may be quite harmless, may be therapeutic, or may be overdone. Exercise could also be an alternative intervention, such as its therapeutic value for people with mild depression. Massage, another complementary practice, may aid in lowering blood glucose levels (Giffany et al., 1997), and even more so when someone is on a hypoglycemic agent or is on insulin. This same blood glucose-lowering potential could also occur when biofeedback-enhanced relaxation therapy is taught (Guthrie, 1999), or if therapeutic touch or reiki or any other of the healing energy therapies are part of a person's chosen regimen. Any of these practices might be used and might be quite successful (Guthrie, 2007).

Some herbs are known to lower or raise blood sugars (Guthrie, 2000). Without appropriate knowledge, supervision, or self-management education, again, hypoglycemia could occur.

If such practices of massage therapy, exercise, good or not-so-good food choices, vitamins, minerals, herbs, medical or social drugs, have been a part of the lifestyle of the individual before diabetes was diagnosed, they might interfere with the expected outcome if not taken into consideration when the diabetes regimen is developed. Other environmental factors, such as one's home or community environment or finances, play a large part in the choice to abstain from using, continuing to use, or beginning the use of CAM. CAM may be medically inappropriate.

Just the process of the use of aromatherapy and its potential to soothe or stimulate may lower or raise blood glucose levels. Some examples are lavadula angustifolia, which is known as a calming agent, but other types of lavender can be used to keep one awake.

Extra caution is needed regarding changes in the diabetes medications when treatment with other medication is instituted, altered, or discontinued.

CAM/Drug Action

Physiologically, the body may respond to CAM/drugs in a variety of ways that may affect diabetes control. Some medications may increase the rate of circulation. This could allow more glucose to be available to the cells, which may or may not be able to handle the load. Medical drugs such as the adrenal or other hormonal-blocking agents are used frequently. Examples are agents that have beta adrenergic blocking agent properties. Drugs used in cardiac disease and hypertension are called beta blockers. These drugs may decrease the ability of the body to regulate blood glucose by the release of catecholamines for glycogenolysis and thus block the ability to perceive low blood glucose levels. Some CAM drugs can also have beta-blocking properties. Certain drugs frequently prescribed may decrease the mobility or absorption capacity of the intestinal tract, thus decreasing glucose uptake. There are many drugs and herbs that, if taken in large enough quantities, may cause hypoglycemic effects from the chemical action or cause diarrhea or other negative responses. Some CAM/drugs that reduce stress may cause a rapidly dropping need for insulin when what is being taken is accomplishing its specific purpose.

Resources

There are a variety of resources to assist the professional in the findings and possible problems related to giving a CAM/drug to a person with diabetes. Description of specific herbs and vitamins and minerals does not always include information on a possible response of blood glucose levels. Even the *Physicians' Desk Reference* ([PDR] 2008) does not usually caution that a nondiabetes treatment medication may alter blood glucose levels. The PDR for Herbal Medicines (2007), the PDR for Nutritional Supplements (2008) and the PDR for Non-Prescription Drugs, Dietary Supplements, & Herbs (2009) are all useful companions to the basic knowledge and interactions of many CAM herbal and nutritional therapies.

The Food and Drug Administration (FDA) issues a drug bulletin monthly that refers to glucose interaction when new drugs or findings on old drugs are reported (FDA, 2008). One should report an adverse herb/drug reaction that has not been listed in at least one of the preceding resources, especially the PDR. This confidential information should be addressed to the Assistant to the Director for Medical Communications, Bureau of Drugs, BD-40, FDA, 5600 Fishers Lane, Rockville, MD 20852, or file a complaint at https://rn.ftc.gov/pls/dod.

Special consideration should always be given to new herbs/drugs as to whether an herb/drug has been tested and considered safe for pregnant women and children. Special training for a more in-depth understanding of the

CAM field may be obtained through a variety of programs such as the Complementary and Alternative Health Care Certificate Program of the University of Southern Indiana and the Residency and Fellowship program at the University of Arizona at Tucson.

CAM/Drug Interactions

CAM therapies that affect glucose control are more likely to cause hyperglycemia than hypoglycemia. It is not possible to list here all the herbs that affect blood glucose levels, but some of the common ones will be discussed.

CAM Therapies and Hormones Inducing Hypoglycemia

A variety of herbs can knowingly or not (if not researched) result in untoward responses. One of the earliest problems was discovered when individuals took ginkgo biloba and were already taking an anticoagulant. This combination was found to alter the clotting and augment the anticoagulant effect. Ginseng and herbs that contain cardiac glycosides in combination with insulin and hypoglycemic agents affect glucose levels. Excessive sedation is seen when valerian is used with barbiturates. Hypertension is noted when yohimbe and monoaminoxidase inhibitors are combined. If you use an anticonvulsant along with evening primrose oil, a lowering of the seizure threshold will occur. This is why herbs need to be used carefully.

A position statement (American Diabetes Association [ADA], 2004) gives guidelines for unproven therapies. Consideration should be addressed as related to the following categories: (1) approved by the FDA; (2) accepted by two or more articles in reviewed journals; (3) recommended by a credible organization that supports the use (of a specific herb, vitamin, mineral, or modality) for people with diabetes; or (4) endorsed or recommended by the American Diabetes Association Professional Practice Committee (ADAPPC). The ADA notes the therapy as (I) clearly effective, (II) somewhat/sometimes effective, or (III) effective for certain categories of patients, (IV) unknown/unproven but possibly promising, or (V) clearly ineffective.

Two things must be considered to begin dialogue as to whether the person is safely using an alternative or complementary practice:

a. Ask whether such practices are used, and
b. Find out how they interact with the present state and medication used.

Recognition of Hypoglycemia-Inducing CAM

Insulin is the only regulatory hormone known to lower blood glucose levels. Some herbs that lower blood glucose levels are Gymnema sylvestre, bitter melon, fenugreek, carob, ginseng roots, prickly pear, psyllium, reisi mushrooms, and spinach leaves. This blood glucose–lowering effect might be quite mild, as in the use of Gymnema sylvestre or because of the fiber content, as found in the use of fenugreek, or related to increased activity or energy level that is associated with the use of ginseng.

Other Medications

Many medicines may cause moderate reductions in blood glucose levels, but few if any will cause sufficient reductions to be of therapeutic value. It has been known since the nineteenth century that aspirin and other salicylates will lower blood glucose levels. The dosage required for the hypoglycemic effect, however, is so great that toxic side effects result before therapeutic value is attained. Other compounds are currently being tested for hypoglycemic effects.

From another standpoint, a high-protein diet may result in lowered blood glucose levels, but it should be noted that calcium is the major mineral lost when involved in such a program. Calcium loss might accompany the need for a greater fluid intake so that azotemia (protein-in-the-blood condition) might not be experienced.

CAM Therapies and Hormones Increasing Hyperglycemia

In contrast with the preceding discussion, there are more drugs and hormones that will increase blood glucose levels. Some of these drugs are naturally occurring drugs and some are synthetically produced. Much caution must be used in prescribing drugs to persons with diabetes because of the glucose-elevating effect of so many medications. The herbs that may raise blood sugar levels are cocoa seeds, coffee seeds, mahuang plant, or rosemary leaves, to name a few. The mechanisms of action in elevating blood glucose levels in individuals who have or who do not have diabetes may be different with different herbs. Some herbs or medications inhibit the secretion of insulin (e.g., catecholamine, thiazides, and adrenergic blocking agents). Some herbs, vitamins, minerals, or medications cause glycogenolysis or inhibit glycogenesis (e.g., catecholamine, glucagon, and perhaps growth hormone). Some cause increased gluconeogenesis (glucocorticoids), and some medications may have peripheral effects that inhibit glucose uptake by tissues.

Catecholamines

Catecholamines are epinephrine and norepinephrine. Many synthetic derivatives of these drugs are used for a variety of purposes. Oral and topical decongestants, such as those found in many cold and allergy preparations and nose drops, belong to this category of drugs, as do many of the drugs given as bronchodilators for persons with asthma, such as ephedrine. Appetite suppressants such as dextroamphetamine (Dexedrine), which is no longer used for that purpose, and phenylpropanolamine (Propadrine), which used to be found in over-the-counter diet preparations, also contained catecholamines that can stimulate blood glucose elevation and vasoconstriction leading to increased blood pressure. Catecholamines work to elevate blood glucose levels by suppressing insulin secretion in persons with intact beta cells (T2DM), and increasing liver glycogenolysis in both Type 1 diabetes mellitus (T1DM) and T2DM.

The hormones of the sympathetic nervous system, including epinephrine and norepinephrine, act through the stimulation of alpha and beta adrenergic receptor sites on cell membranes. Various drugs have been developed to block the receptors and prevent the effect of catecholamines. The beta blockers are especially popular in the treatment of cardiac disease, including angina pectoris and arrhythmias, and in treating hypertension. Because catecholamine-induced glycogenolysis is an important counterregulatory mechanism to maintain blood glucose levels and because beta adrenergic blockers may block this effect, an important counterregulatory mechanism to prevent hypoglycemia in insulin-dependent diabetes may be lost. This hazard has been emphasized in the literature, but from our experience the hazard may have been overemphasized. Many patients taking the commonly used beta blocker propranolol (Inderal) report symptoms of hypoglycemia no different than those before they began taking the medicine. The newer cardiospecific beta blockers, such as metoprolol tartrate (Lopressor and other similar medications), have less effect on blocking peripheral adrenergic effects.

Thiazide Diuretics

Thiazide diuretics elevate blood glucose levels by suppressing insulin secretion. They are a problem only in persons with T2DM or in persons with T1DM that still have some ability to secrete insulin. The thiazide diuretics are frequently used in the treatment of hypertension or fluid retention, which is more commonly found in T2DM. Thus the glucose-elevating effect of these drugs may thwart the effort to reduce blood glucose levels through diet or diet and medication. It is suggested that other diuretics, such as furosemide or, even less challenging to the blood glucose levels, imipramide, be used to treat hypertension or fluid retention. When used in low doses, this blood glucose level elevation does not seem to have as much hyperglycemic effect as when used in large doses. If thiazide doses are kept at 25 mg/day or less, they have little effect on the blood glucose level.

Steroidal Medications

Adrenocortical steroids may be divided into two groups: mineralocorticoids and glucocorticoids. Mineralocorticoids affect salt metabolism and blood pressure, but have little effect on blood glucose. Glucocorticoids, conversely, have a profound effect on blood glucose. This effect is similar whether the hormones are produced internally by stress or given as synthetic compounds. The blood glucose–elevating effect of steroids occurs because of stimulation of gluconeogenesis by the liver. This effect can occur regardless of the route of administration. It is too frequently forgotten that steroids by any route, including skin creams for dermatitis, inhalers for asthma, or injections into joint spaces for various kinds of arthritis or bursitis, can cause profound, persistent effects on blood glucose levels for up to several weeks. Insulin requirements have been known to double and sometimes triple for a few weeks after a single injection of cortisone into a joint space.

Other Medications

The interactions of some other medications should be noted. For example, insulin drives potassium into the cell, and thiazides cause potassium loss in the kidney. Persons with diabetes who take diuretics should therefore receive potassium supplements or at least have their serum potassium levels monitored. Many times, newly referred patients come to the doctor with a grocery bag or shoe box full of drugs they are taking. Many of these people do not feel good because of the adverse interactions among these drugs. Often these individuals go from one health professional to another with their various complaints. Busy health professionals may fail to take complete histories and simply prescribe a drug. Soon the person is taking many drugs that may themselves be the cause of the symptoms for which the patient is doctor shopping to find relief.

In General

Careful histories should include the taking of vitamins, minerals, and/or herbs along with medications as well as the history of diabetes therapy. We now have the advantage of having pharmacies connected to a computer network that lists drug/drug/herb interactions so that errors may be caught and any necessary changes made. An example would be the use of TagametHB if used with Glucophage resulting in too rapid an excretion of the drug before the desired action of the medication can be achieved.

Social Drugs

Alcohol

Alcohol is a common social drug with a variety of effects on diabetes. Too much alcohol at one time causes enzyme inhibition. Chronic alcoholism causes enzyme stimulation and fibrosis of the pancreas and liver. Both of these actions can have adverse prolonged physical effects and can cause instability of the diabetes. Excessive alcohol ingestion can exacerbate these complications.

Alcohol-induced hypoglycemia in people without diabetes usually requires 2–3 days of fasting from food to occur, but alcohol consumption after an overnight fast in a person with diabetes can result in a decreased availability of glucose from the liver.

Alcohol affects the body in many ways that are similar to the antidiabetic agents. Too much of a social drug, an herb, or a medication may result in nausea, vomiting, and diarrhea. Both diabetes and alcohol ingestion can result in frequency of urination and damage to the liver, heart, and blood vessels. There are similarities between alcohol and diabetic ketoacidosis (DKA) such as fruity smelling breath, flushed face, irritability, staggering gait, drowsiness, and coma. In one study, ketones present in blood and urine were not noted to alter the breathalyzer test by more than 0.01% (Brick, 1992).

There are also similarities between alcohol ingestion and low blood glucose levels (hypoglycemia), for example, staggering gait, coma, and drowsiness. Responses to DKA, hypoglycemia, or excess alcohol consumption can also be similar to a stroke, head injury, hemorrhage, and certain responses to epilepsy. If a person who has diabetes also drinks, the confusing symptoms should not cause treatment to be delayed or omitted.

If there is any reason to believe the person is hypoglycemic, treatment for hypoglycemia should begin immediately. If the person is unconscious, a finger stick blood sugar test will tell the difference between hypoglycemia, DKA, or alcohol-induced unconsciousness. But, if in doubt, treat for low blood sugar. A 50 mg/dl (2.7 mmol/L) change from 20 mg/dl (1.1 mmol/L) to 70 mg/dl (3.8 mmol/L) can save brain cells, while a transient 400 mg/dl to 450 mg/dl (22.2 to 25 mmol/L) change will not make that much difference.

In the past 10 years, an important finding has been made. Even though there is carbohydrate content in most alcoholic beverages, there is little significant change in the blood glucose level after ingestion of alcohol after some food intake when only a modest amount is ingested. With a large dose of alcoholic beverages, there may be a 20%–50% rise in the blood glucose level of the person who has recently eaten or the person without alcoholism who is inebriated. If the person is an alcoholic or habitual alcohol user, the rise in blood glucose levels after alcohol is consumed is not observed and hypoglycemia is more common. Hypoglycemia in the person with diabetes who has consumed alcohol may be the result of the inhibition of hepatic gluconeogenesis (Richardson, Weiss, Thomas, & Kerr, 2005). Insufficiency of hypothalamic-pituitary-adrenal release of adrenal hormones may contribute to the hypoglycemia.

Heavy alcohol consumption is associated with a peripheral neuropathy similar to that seen in diabetes. The alcoholic neuropathy, however, is thought to be a result of vitamin deficiency, whereas diabetic neuropathy results from circulatory and nutritional deficit mechanisms. In general, the use of alcohol in persons with diabetes mellitus is discouraged.

Other Social Drugs

Other social drugs (other than alcohol) are classed as depressants, stimulants, and hallucinogens. Each of these categories has an impact on diabetes directly or indirectly and requires consideration. Drug abuse may be recognized by inappropriate behavior, twitching movements, bloodshot eyes with consistent extremes in pupil size (dilated or constricted), poor skin turgor accompanied by general physical deterioration, extremes in emotional lability, appetite variations (usually extremes), drowsiness, poor mental and moral responses, and infections (such as boils) at the site of injections. Many of these indications of drug abuse sound vaguely familiar to a person experiencing the extremes of diabetes.

Depressants

Depressants include barbiturates and heroin. Barbiturates have a variety of slang names, such as stumblers, downers, or goofballs. These may be given by the oral or injectable route. The depressants are most often found in capsules, which have slang names of their own: blue heavens are amobarbital (Amytal), rainbows are amobarbital with secobarbital (Tuinal), yellow jackets are pentobarbital (Nembutal), and red devils are secobarbital (Seconal). Names of street drugs may vary from time to time and place to place. Anyone working with potential drug abusers or persons with diabetes who may be drug abusers should be aware of the names used in their area at any point in time.

Central nervous system depression caused by depressants will be indicated by dilation of pupils, drowsiness, uncoordinated movement, and slurred speech. Because one of the physiologic responses to depressants is increased metabolism of drugs (barbiturates stimulate enzymes of the liver), the result could be an altered effectiveness of oral hypoglycemic agents. Action of depressants on the central nervous system could and does interfere with self-care by the person with diabetes because they reduce motivation and self-image. As with other social drugs, depressants may cause memory to be impaired, resulting in missed meals or medications, thus interfering with diabetes control.

Heroin is called by a variety of names, such as smack, dope, junk, joy powder, horse, and white stuff. Heroin may be taken orally or injected subcutaneously or intravenously (most commonly the latter). Because this drug is also a central nervous system depressant, taking it will result in drowsiness that may be accompanied by confusion or a staggering gait. As with barbiturates, heroin also has a depressing effect on appetite. It causes the skin to be pallid in appearance, and in contrast to barbiturates, the pupils constrict rather than dilate. In some instances, there may be a craving for sweets and liquids. New, highly pure, and very potent forms of heroin are currently on the street. These drugs are frequently fatal. A new fad among teenagers is the use of dextromethorphine, a drug commonly found in cough medicines. Cough medicines with dextromethorphine are available over the counter and are relatively inexpensive. In the usual doses, they are harmless, but in large doses (kids will drink several bottles of the cough medicine or take 30–40 tablets at a time) the drug can be and has been fatal.

Stimulants

Stimulants are a category of drugs that include amphetamines and cocaine. Amphetamines, like barbiturates, come in pills, capsules, or intravenous injections (methamphetamines). Amphetamine sulfate (Benzedrine) and dextroamphetamine sulfate (Dexedrine) come in tablets or capsules. Street names are speed, meth, or uppers. The white tablets are called bennies or whites. The green or pink, heart- or diamond-shaped tablets are called hearts. There are green, white, orange, or yellow capsules called dixies. There is a new form of methamphetamine called ice, which can be smoked. Cheap and easy to produce, it is highly addicting. In contrast to the depressants, the stimulants cause an increase in pulse, blood pressure, body motility, and speech. Inhibitions are released, resulting in socially unacceptable behavior. Confusion and violence may occur. Metabolism and energy levels are increased. Pupils may be noticeably dilated. Because metabolism occurs at a faster rate, glucose will be used at an increased rate. This would result in a lowered blood glucose level.

Cocaine is also a stimulant. Besides being taken orally, cocaine may be sniffed, smoked, or injected, which may enhance the physical and mental effect of the drug. When combined, cocaine and heroin are called speedballs. Toot, snow, coke, or crack are street names for cocaine, the intake of which results in loss of appetite. Insulin reactions could easily occur if insulin is not decreased in the individual who uses cocaine.

Cocaine deserves some special consideration because it is the most commonly used social drug after alcohol and tobacco. It has long been used therapeutically as a local anesthetic to the mucous membranes and as a vasoconstrictor to reduce bleeding. It is commonly used in oral and vasopharyngeal surgery. As a social drug, it has been known for a long time and was legal until recent years. It was prescribed by such leaders of psychiatry as Sigmund Freud and others. When the drug again became popular in the 1970s and 1980s, it was initially thought to be relatively safe and nonaddicting. With the development of purer and more potent forms of the drug, it has become evident that the drug is indeed addicting and frequently lethal.

One form of the drug is crack, a crystalline form of the drug made by heating cocaine powder with bicarbonate of soda. The effect of the drug is to stimulate the receptors of the pleasure center of the brain producing an instant high. As soon as it is over (a few hours with powdered cocaine, a few minutes with crack and more recently ice), there is a strong desire to have it again. This and the increasing doses required to produce the high result in the addiction to the drug.

All of the stimulants directly or indirectly result in weight loss, which is a result of a loss of appetite or an altered sensorium that causes the person to forget to eat or to take medication.

Hallucinogens

Hallucinogens, including lysergic acid diethylamide (LSD), phencyclidine (PCP), marijuana, and others, have in the past been the most destructive of the street drugs. Methamphetamine holds that "honor" today. After the initial effect of the hallucinogen wears off, many flashbacks can occur. Acid, or LSD, can result in brain tissue damage as well as in chromosomal changes. Marijuana has been found to contribute to abnormal results on electroencephalograms, a decrease in maturity of behavior, lowered sperm counts in men, and a shortened luteal phase of the menstrual cycle in women. Other drugs in the hallucinogen category are called dimethoxymethylamphetamine, dimethyltriptamine (the businessman's special), STP, peyote, mescaline, and angel dust, to name a few. LSD may be purchased as a liquid, capsule, sugar cube, or pill. Dimethyltriptamine is usually found in a powder but could be put in a capsule. STP and peyote are usually found in a capsule. Flashbacks, bummers, or freakouts are the terms given to a psychologically negative and usually frightening retrogression experience often seen with the hallucinogens. Because many of these drugs can be easily synthesized in basement laboratories, it is difficult to control them.

Marijuana, called grass, pot, weed, or tea, may also be referred to as reefers or joints. Marijuana may be smoked; eaten, as in pudding, cakes, and cookies; or brewed into tea. In the form called hashish, which is a resin, gum, or powder, it may be smoked, chewed, or sniffed. As a liquid, it may be injected. In this form, marijuana is most deadly because it is made from a resin of the marijuana plant, hashish, and is 10 times stronger than the leaf form.

Hallucinogens, especially marijuana, are appetite stimulants. The munchies often accompany the use of marijuana. Although marijuana may produce a craving for sweets and liquids, there may also be difficulty in swallowing. The tendency of marijuana users is to eat or snack (the munchies), which may raise the blood glucose levels and increase weight in the person with diabetes. If the person eats in varied amounts and/or forgets to eat, anything from hyperglycemia to hypoglycemia to weight gain or loss could occur.

The hallucinogens can cause a psychologic dependence, and smoking them can irritate the respiratory tract. Marijuana intoxication results in nausea, vomiting, possible high fever, shock, and coma, which can mimic or hide diabetic ketoacidosis.

Other Drugs

Although codeine is considered a stimulant and morphine a depressant, they are both found in the group named narcotics. They are addicting drugs. The withdrawal from narcotics is usually most intense. The effect of addiction or withdrawal on diabetes management may also be most intense.

Tobacco use has not been mentioned, but it too can affect diabetes, although usually indirectly. Because nicotine is a peripheral vasoconstrictor, blood vessels damaged by diabetes may be further damaged by nicotine, thus decreasing their ability to bring adequate nutrition to the extremities. Irritation to the lungs from smoking can lead to the increased chance of infection—especially in those who have elevated blood glucose values. Tobacco use therefore compounds the adverse cardiovascular effects of diabetes and should be strongly discouraged.

Summary

There can be no doubt that pharmacology has been a boon to medicine. CAM therapies of vitamins, minerals, herbs, and various modalities, along with new medications, have and are greatly changing the way medicine is practiced. Their use has cured some diseases, controlled others, and benefited many people. Vitamins, minerals, herbs, and medications, when properly used, can be of value.

The information presented about some of the more accepted herbs, in the first part of this chapter, indicates that there is still controversy, and longer-term studies need to be completed before some final decisions are made about specific supplements.

All CAM/drugs have side effects, however, and the more potent or the larger the dose of the herb, the medication, or the social drug, the greater the potential for more severe side effects. This is multiplied in patients with diabetes, especially if they have the vascular complications of the disease. Therefore, individuals should always beware of drug–drug interactions as they should be aware of herb–drug interactions especially when multiple CAM/drugs are used.

Persons with diabetes should be discouraged from using social drugs and encouraged to use therapeutic or CAM therapies and prescribed medications wisely, judiciously, and thoughtfully (Thorne et al., 2002). Patients then have a greater possibility of benefiting from the positive value of either or both CAM oral therapies and traditional medication, but care must be taken to not substitute one proven therapy with CAM.

References

Albarracin, C. A., Fuqua, B. C., Evans, J. L., & Goldfine, I. D. (2008). Chromium picolinate and biotin combination improves glucose metabolism in treated, uncontrolled overweight to obese patients with type 2 diabetes. *Diabetes Metabolic Research Reviews, 24*(1), 41–51.

Albert, S. G., Oiknine, R. F., Parseghian, S., Mooradian, A. D., Haas, M. J., & McPherson, T. (2007). The effect of glucosamine on serum HDL, cholesterol and apolipoprotein A1 levels in people with diabetes. *Diabetes Care, 30*(11), 2800–2893.

American Diabetes Association. (2004). Position statement for unproven therapies. *Diabetes Care, 27*(Suppl. 1), S135.

Brick, J. (1992). *Diabetes, breath acetone and breathalyzer accuracy: A case study.* Santa Monica, CA: International Symposium: Alcohol, Drugs, and Transportation.

Dascalu, A., Sievenpiper, J. L., Jenkins, A. L., Stavro, M. P., Laiter, L. A., Amason, J. T., et al. (2007). Five batches representative of Ontario grown American ginseng root produce comparable reduction of post prandial glycemia in healthy individuals. *Canadian Journal of Physiology and Pharmacology, 85*(9), 856–864.

Eisenberg, D., Davis, R., Ettner, S., Appel, S., Kilkey, S., Van Pompay, M., et al. (1998). Alternative medicine use in the United States 1990–1997. *Journal of the American Medical Association, 280*(18), 1569–1575.

Evans, J. L., Heymann, C. J., Goldfine, I. D., & Gavin, L. A. (2002). Pharmacokinetics, tolerability, and fructosamine-lowering effect of a novel, controlled release formulation of alpha lipoic acid. *Endocrinology Practice, 8,* 29–35.

Food and Drug Administration. (2001). *FDA drug bulletin.* Rockville, MD: U.S. Department of Health and Human Services.

Giffany, R., Hernandez-Reif, M., LaGreca, A., Shaw, K., Schanberg, S., & Kuhn, C. (1997). Massage therapy lowers blood glucose levels in children. *Diabetes Spectrum, 10*(3), 237–239.

Guthrie, D. W. (1999). Holistic health and diabetes. *Diabetes Spectrum, 12*(1), 49–51.

Guthrie, D. W. (2000). *Alternative and complementary diabetes care.* New York: John Wiley & Sons.

Guthrie, D.W. (2007). *Diabetes self-management's hidden secrets of natural healing: Using foods, supplements, and more to slow or even reverse the complications of diabetes.* New York: Diabetes Self-Management Books.

Kleefstra, N., Houweling, S. T., Bakker, S. J., Verhoenven, S., Gans, R. O., Meyboom-de Jong, B., et al. (2007). Chromium treatment has no effect in patients with type 2 diabetes in a western population: A random, double-blind, placebo controlled trial. *Diabetes Care, 30*(5), 1092–1096.

Leach, M. J. (2007). Gymnema sylvestre for diabetes mellitus: A systematic review. *Journal of Alternative and Complementary Medicine, 13*(9), 977–983.

Pham, A. O., Kourlas, H., & Pham, D. O. (2007). Chromium supplement in patients with type 2 diabetes mellitus. *Pharmacotherapy, 27*(4), 595–599.

Physicians' Desk Reference. (2008). Montvale, NJ: Thompson PDR.

Physicians' Desk Reference for Herbal Medicines (4th ed.). (2007). Montvale, NJ: Thompson PDR.

Physicians' Desk Reference for Non-Prescription Drugs, Dietary Supplements & Herbs: A definitive guide to over the counter medications (28th ed.). (2009). Montvale, NJ: Thompson PDR.

Physicians' Desk Reference of Nutritional Supplements. (2001). Montvale, NJ: Thompson PDR.

Richardson, T., Weiss, M., Thomas, P., & Kerr, D. (2nd ed.). (2008). Day after the night before: Influence of evening alcohol on risk of hypoglycemia in patients with type 1 diabetes. *Diabetes Care, 28*(7), 1801–1802.

Shukla, R., & Bhonde, R. R. (2008). Adipogenic action of vanadium: A new diversion in treating diabetes. *Biometals, 21*(2), 205–210.

Solomon, T. P., & Blannin, A. K. (2007). Effects of short-term cinnamon ingestion on in vivo glucose tolerance. *Diabetes and Obesity Metabolism, 9*(6), 895–901.

Thorne, S., Best, A., Balonk J., Kelner, M., & Rickhy, B. (2002). Ethical dimensions in the borderland between conventional and complementary/alternative medicine. *The Journal of Alternative and Complementary Medicine, 8,* 907–915.

Vuksan, V., Sung, M. K., Sievenpiper, J. L., Stavro, P. M., Jenkins, A. L., Di Buono, M., et al. (2008). Korean red ginseng (Panax ginseng) improves glucose and insulin regulation in well-controlled, type 2 diabetes: Results of a randomized, double-blind, placebo-controlled study of efficacy and safety. *Nutritional Metabolism and Cardiovascular Disease, 18*(1), 46–56.

Yeh, G. Y., Eisenberg, D. M., Kaptchuk, J. J., & Phillips, R. S. (2003). Systematic review of herbs and dietary supplements for glycemic control in diabetes. *Diabetes Care, 26,* 1277–1294.

34

Disaster
Preparedness

Even with the stress of day-to-day happenings, we must always be prepared for a variety of disasters that could affect a person with diabetes. Prevention, if possible, is the best policy but being prepared is next best. Some key principles may be applied for any type of disaster so this chapter will try to address as many as possible. Some information may be repeated, but as it fits the situation it will be useful in remembering about what to educate patients concerning their preparedness.

First, here are the possible disasters that could happen: a fire in the home, a flood in the home, an earthquake, a tornado (a cyclone, depending in which part of the world one lives), a hurricane, a tsunami, or a man-made disaster.

Second, certain supplies should always be quickly available whatever the disaster. A three to five days' supply of medication should be kept in a fireproof box accompanied by the supplies needed to administer such medication. If the medication is best kept under refrigeration, this fireproof box might even be placed in a corner of a refrigerator. This box should also include some method and supplies for checking blood glucose levels, some method for checking for ketones whether in the blood or urine (especially for those with Type 1 diabetes), and some method of treating low blood sugar.

Third, a supply of food whether in nutrition bars or packets that are easy to grab and most portable. These nutritious snacks could be kept inside the fireproof box or just next to it. So, medication, needles/syringes, monitor and their supplies, hypoglycemia treatment, and food complete the listing of five groups of items to be placed in that box. If the person is taking an oral medication, then next is the need for some sort of fluid. This fluid is best sugar-free so that it might be used both for hydration and as a vehicle for taking the oral medication. If insulin or oral medication is needed and unavailable, fluid intake, for a short period of time, will at least dilute the rising blood sugars in the individual.

Home Fire

The response, if not known before, is, "stop, drop, and roll," if on fire; "stop, drop, and crawl" if getting away from a fire. For those with diabetes, there is one additional item that is needed in the second situation. If it is safe, grab (the fireproof box) then, "stop, drop, and crawl" in the process of getting out of a burning building.

Having the predetermined meeting place for family members is also on the list of being prepared. So, emergency supplies, keeping close to the floor when getting out of the building, and meeting in a prearranged location outside of the building are the basic parts of the preparedness plan.

If there is time to call 911 from the house, do it—if no time, get out and go to a neighbor's house and call. It may be possible to retrieve the fireproof box after the blaze is controlled, in case there wasn't time to do so beforehand.

Ideally, having a fire extinguisher and knowing how to use it might prevent any other calamities by just quickly dousing the fire.

Flood

If a flood has occurred, the first thing is to "Call for Help"—if not immediately needed, a person should grab the fireproof (leak-proof) box before leaving the residence unless the person lives in an area of a greater potential for flooding, such as below a dam or in a low-lying area of the country. Again, if possible, taking some snacks and a bottle of water can fill the gap until other supplies are obtained.

Earthquake

Heading for a doorway brace or away from a building(s) is the first recommendation. Instruction could be given for a person to have a backpack or fireproof box placed near the refrigerator so that snacks and a bottle of water could be easily carried to the place of safety. Expect one or more aftershocks and, when returning to a residence, open doors carefully because items might have been moved directly behind such areas. Without carefully noticing this, a person might get hit with unexpected items on opening those doors.

Tornado (Cyclone)

In the case of bad weather, it is important to receive warning information. There should be a battery-operated weather radio available in case the electric power is interrupted. Have a shelter identified at all times and go there when there is a warning. If the persons involved cannot get to a shelter, instruct them to get to the lowest and innermost spot in the building with, hopefully, something to hold onto. In the house or other building, being away from windows is good; being under some heavy furniture is better; and being in a bathtub with a mattress pulled on top is best—if a storm shelter is not available. If there is a storm shelter, it should already have some emergency supplies available. Because these shelters are usually underground, a fireproof and leak-proof box should contain some insulin and syringes or other diabetes medications. Because these shelters maintain a relatively constant temperature year round, the insulin or other medication(s) to control blood glucose levels should be safe. An unopened bottle of insulin in a cool place is usually good for the shelf life of the bottle. Other supplies for sleeping and daily maintenance should be stored in that location.

Hurricane (and Tsunami)

A hurricane will cause flooding as well as building and infrastructure damage. Always heed a warning to go to higher ground or to buildings that were built to withstand stronger winds or are away from the site that has the greatest potential for destruction. Instruct people never to try to "ride out the storm." Before leaving the house, have people take the prearranged emergency box, the snacks, and the fluid. Taking some funds and a change of clothes might come in handy. In most cases, only one suitcase per person is reasonable. One sleeping bag and pillow might also be recommended depending on the time allowed to leave the premises. Identification for medical needs and an address indicating ownership or rental of a particular property would aid in allaying potential future problems.

Tsunamis can follow hurricanes or can occur because of ocean floor earthquakes. Warning systems are in place to warn people to go to high ground. If the person lives in a potential tsunami area, they should always have emergency supplies ready to go in case of warning.

Man-Made Disaster

It is a shame to have to include such possibilities, but, in this day and age, it is only realistic to be prepared for the worst and hope for the best. A warning may be given or this might be a sudden occurrence such as occurred on 9/11. If a warning is possible, move quickly to a shelter. In any case, the emergency box should be the first thing to go with the person along with the food and water. Having supplies to last three to five days is recommended.

In times of war or disaster, triage will be carried out and people with chronic diseases are down the line to receive attention especially if they are not wounded. Suffering from a complication concurrently with their chronic condition will not give priority in the triage system. Also, supplies for treating people with diabetes or other chronic conditions might not be readily available. Supportive care might be the only care available to them. Having some emergency supplies available in their emergency pack might be the only way they would receive help until the disaster has stabilized and/or some outside supplies have been delivered.

An important part of pre-preparations to teach families, according to the American Red Cross, is a designated out-of-town contact. They should have these numbers available at home, at work, and at school if they have children. E-mail often gets through when phone lines are jammed, so whenever possible have them include such information. Instruct them to choose a meeting place away from home (that also includes pets) and keep a disaster supply in an easily carried container. This container should include special needs (from diapers to medications), a change of clothing for every person, sleeping bags or bed roll, extra batteries for the flashlight, laptop computers, and radio, some food (lightweight dried foods, peanut butter and crackers, honey [for treating lows], powdered or canned milk are useful in most situations), and water plus water treatment tablets, if possible. Tools, such as a hammer, wrench, and screwdrivers, are also items that are helpful to have. Also, tell them to keep copies of their prescriptions, licenses, passports or birth certificates, insurance policy, power of attorney, and will(s) in that container. In fact, ask them to get a set of copies of their documents to another family member or friend. Cash also may become a necessity since infrastructure for credit cards, checks, and electronic transfer of funds may be destroyed. And, if there are children in the family, find out the school's emergency plan.

If people are instructed to go to a shelter in their home, they are to close and lock all windows and doors, close the fireplace damper, and turn off all fans and heating and air-conditioning systems. The best place for them is to go to an interior room without windows, taking with them their radio and disaster container of supplies and information. If this is a chemical threat, an above-ground location is better. If such is suspected or known, people should seal all cracks (i.e., around doors and windows) with duct tape. They are to stay there until instructed through the use of a battery-powered radio, cell phone, or other form of announcement.

Overall Considerations

Strongly encourage families to have some sort of communication device, especially a shortwave radio. This will help to keep the person(s) up-to-date as to help being available, how long that help might take to arrive, and/or where to go for help. The key need is for the person to know that as adults with diabetes or parents of a child with diabetes, they need to contact the Red Cross or other designated agency as soon as possible. Specific needs for medication and food and water must be relayed to such an agency so that lifesaving items will go to those as soon as they are obtained.

For those with diabetes, the stressors experienced when a natural or man-made disaster occurs will result in the body responding as if having an illness or infection. If the person happens to become more active than usual, it is possible that the blood glucose levels will go lower and hypoglycemia treatment will need to be initiated. In most cases the blood glucose levels will go higher. These higher glucose levels should be treated as if the person has an illness that needs the administration of more, rather than less, diabetes medication. If blood glucose levels should be elevated, the first course of action is to push fluids. If adequate fluids are not available or blood sugars or symptoms/signs indicate otherwise, then changes in medication should be considered.

For those on oral medications, supplemental insulin might be needed. For those on insulin, supplemental doses of insulin of 10% (or 20% if ketones are present) of the total daily dose given four times a day at the time of usual administration or at a meal time or 0.05 (0.1 if ketones are present) of a unit per kilogram body weight of regular insulin (given in the muscle) or rapid-acting insulin (given subcutaneously) if the blood sugar is 250 mg/dl or more. If the person is very sensitive to insulin or if new to insulin (the oral agents are not holding the blood sugars down), 0.025 or ¼ of a unit per kilogram body weight could be the choice. These doses could be given on a one- or every two-hour basis to control the blood sugars until they are stabilized at under 250 mg/dl or lower.

If there is a need to stay in a disaster shelter, people should seek out a health professional and share the information about their diabetes condition. They should also maintain an awareness of the location of their supplies, maintain a sharps container, and, after the disaster, seek psychosocial help if talking about what happened or profound feelings and reactions continue to be present.

Resources

The American Diabetes Association (2006) offers *The Disaster Preparedness Guide for People With Diabetes*. One copy should be in the home of every person who has diabetes. It includes a list of basic emergency supplies for everyone plus those of extra need when the person has diabetes. It recommends foods to keep on hand that are easily packed and that have a long shelf life. The pamphlet systematically states what to do if there is an actual emergency from the person identifying that he or she has diabetes to sticking with the individual testing and medication program as much as possible. Highly useful is a list of 800 phone numbers for insulin, glucose meter, and pump manufacturers, along with the phone numbers of emergency preparedness organizations. This is a useful booklet whether the person has any type of diabetes.

The American Red Cross (2001) has a booklet on its disaster services, *Terrorism: Preparing for the Unexpected* (2001). We all hope this never happens, but being prepared does blunt the impact of such a catastrophe.

There are also a variety of articles, such as "Preparing for the Perfect Storm: Disaster Planning for Older Adults," by K. K. Moon (2007). Becton Dickinson has a booklet, *Planning Your Diabetes Care: During Disaster Conditions* (2002), available in both English and Spanish. The February 2006 issue of *Diabetes Forecast* had a number of articles on disaster planning.

On the Web, go to www.cdc.gov/docs/hurricanes.html (Centers for Disease Control and Prevention, 2007) (information retrieved March 22, 2008) or www.diabeteshealth.com/read/2008/03/22/5484.html, for more information on managing your diabetes during a natural disaster. The *ADA: Professional Section Quarterly*, summer of 2007, also had a message from the President of Health Care and Education on preparing for emergencies (Albright, 2007). The American Nurses Association had a dedicated and informative conference on "Life, Death and Disaster" (DeDonder, Feldman, & Hamlin, 2007). All of these and more are resources available online or in bookstores.

Summary

The Boy Scouts' rule is quoted here, "Always be Prepared!" This is certainly true for any person with a chronic condition and especially true for the person who has diabetes mellitus. If any disaster strikes, follow the recommendations of the Red Cross: Remain calm and be patient; follow the advice of local emergency officials, but also tell them about the person with the chronic illness needs; listen to the radio for the latest information; check for injuries and give first aid as needed; check for damage (use a flashlight, not a candle or lighted match); sniff for gas leaks; turn off any main valves; call (cell phone) or e-mail your contact; and check on your neighbor. If you have to evacuate, if possible, wear long-sleeved shirts, long pants, and sturdy shoes. Take your disaster container and your pets. Lock your home and follow the directions for the routes you are to use for evacuation. Watch for and avoid downed power lines.

Advise the family to check with the American Red Cross for first aid training: to control bleeding, care for shock, care for burns, care for body injuries, reduce any other health care risks, and be aware of biologic or radiologic exposure. The families and individuals can get more information on preparedness by viewing the Web site www.redcross.org/services/disaster/beprepared or you can request brochures from the American Red Cross or use other contacts for information such as the Centers for Disease Control and Prevention (www.bt.cdc.gov), the U.S. Department of Energy (www.energy.gov), the U.S. Department of Health and Human Services (www.hhs.gov), the Federal Emergency Management Agency (www.rris.fema.gov), the Environmental Protection Agency (www.epa.gov/swercepp), or the U.S. Department of Homeland Security (www.ready.gov).

Disasters happen. Being prepared aids in blocking further problems by knowing what to expect or how to take action (ADA Workgroup Report, 2007; DeDonder et al., 2007). Being prepared assists in keeping the outcome of a disaster from becoming worse.

References

Albright, A. (2007, Summer). Preparing for emergencies. *ADA: Professional Section Quarterly,* 1–2.

American Diabetes Association. (2006). *The disaster preparedness guide for people with diabetes.* Alexandria, VA: Author.

American Diabetes Association Workgroup Report. (2007). ADA statement on emergency and disaster preparedness: A report of the Disaster Response Task Force. *Diabetes Care, 30*(9), 2395–2398.

American Red Cross Disaster Services. (2001). *Terrorism: Preparing for the unexpected.* Washington, DC: American Red Cross.

Becton Dickinson. (2002). *Planning your diabetes care: During disaster conditions.* Or online at www.bddiabetes.com. Franklin Lakes, NJ: BD Consumer Healthcare.

Centers for Disease Control and Prevention. (2007). *Help for people with diabetes affected by hurricanes.* Retrieved March 22, 2008, from www.cdc.gov/diabetes/news/docs/hurricanes.hte

DeDonder, J., Feldman, J., & Hamlin, L. (2007). A report from ANA's 2007 Quadrennial Policy Conference Nursing Care in Life, Death, and Disaster. *Kansas Nurse, 82*(6), 3–6.

Moon, K. K. (2007). Preparing for the perfect storm: Disaster planning for older adults. *Advance for Nurse Practitioners, 15*(10), 88–90.

VIII

View of the Whole Person

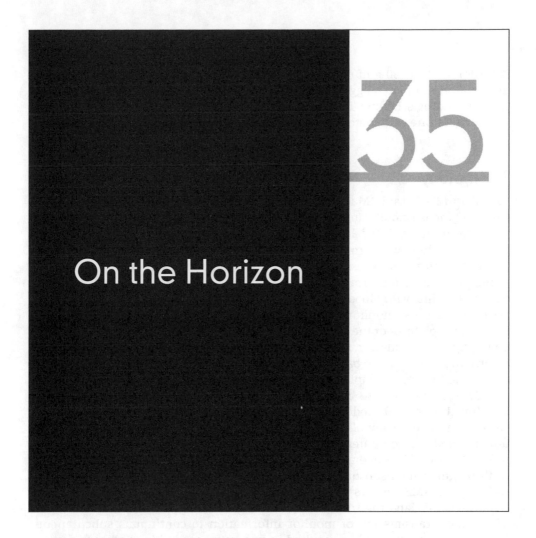

On the Horizon

Research is continually needed. In patient care alone, there are factors over and above the "clinical, socioeconomic, psychosocial, and behavioral factors" (Selby et al., 2007) that are associated with the control of blood glucose levels. Maintaining a level of hope for individuals with diabetes assists them in continuing from day to day, with the recognition that a better quality of life and better health may be just around the corner.

Technology and new drugs in diabetes therapy are the most active research areas other than the prevention of diabetes in the first place. The goal of research is that participating in self-care practices by the patients will be quicker, less cumbersome, and yet control blood glucose levels better and safer. With the increase in childhood obesity, further problems are envisioned. Shin et al. (2008) found that children with obesity have higher C-reactive proteins and lower adiponectin—indicating an inflammatory problem exists that might lead to early cardiovascular compromise. Other studies reported in this chapter demonstrate the state of the art and eventually the science of diabetes prevention and/or treatment.

At least we are not back in the dark ages, where the *Journal of the American Medical Association* (*50,* 861–865, 1908) reported the use of the Van

Noorden diet of 250 g of oatmeal, 250–300 g of butter, and 100 g of some vegetable albumin (6 to 8 eggs or their whites may be substituted) with an every-2-hour feeding schedule. This does point to the fact that nutritional food intake is a cornerstone of diabetes management even today.

Technology

Kowalski (2007) said, "Machines will make it happen." He is certain that continuous glucose monitoring will be utilized as part of expected therapy with the recognition that a closed-loop artificial pancreas is near. Monitoring of diabetes has come a long way. From urine testing to blood glucose monitors, we have made significant progress and revolutionized diabetes monitoring. Fingers, palm, earlobe, or forearm can only be pricked so many times, and there is a certain lag time with blood obtained from one site (arms) versus other sites. Intermittent glucose monitoring by finger stick or off-site monitoring only gives a few instant pictures of the blood glucose level. Blood glucose is a dynamic, ever-changing event, and even four or eight instant pictures a day gives us very little information on which to base major changes in medication. Newer technologies are needed for our receipt and utilization of information.

Continuous glucose monitoring (CGMS) was developed several years ago, but the original models were not as accurate as desired and the sensors were short lived. They also could not be read in real time but needed to be downloaded to a computer every 3 days. This had to be done at the physician's office. New CGMS systems have been and are being developed (we are now to third-generation sensors) that can be read out in real time and can last up to 7 days. CGMS sensors can now be programmed to indicate hypoglycemia, hyperglycemia, and the trend in the blood glucose movement, that is, the rate of change. Transmission of monitor information to continuous subcutaneous insulin infusion pumps has resulted in improvement of blood glucose control, but so have insulin analogs given by injection.

The goal is for the treatment to mimic the body as much as possible so the artificial pancreas or closed-loop system is believed to be the technical answer. With the funding and support of the Food and Drug Administration, the Juvenile Diabetes Research Foundation (JDRF), technology companies, private capital, and the National Institutes of Health (NIH), the closed-loop artificial pancreas is well on its way. It must be remembered though that many problems remain. Present-day continuous glucose sensors have a time delay between blood glucose levels and readout times. This time delay is not usually a problem and can be compensated by setting alarms at levels that give more time for the people to react. In a closed-loop system, the time delay may be a problem, especially during times of immediate crisis. Another problem with a closed-loop system is counterregulation. The islet cell not only produces insulin but also produces amylin, glucagon, somatostatin, pancreatic polypeptide, and perhaps other hormones that interact with insulin secretion to maintain minute-to-minute blood glucose control. At the present time, technologies do not exist to mimic this minute-to-minute control and counterregulation. Future research may make it possible to more closely mimic normal insulin and associated hormone secretion.

Children with Type 1 diabetes mellitus (T1DM) have a longer time in a lifetime to have diabetes, and the introduction of newer technologies has the potential to lead to safer and more effective care. Recurrent episodes of severe hyperglycemia and severe hypoglycemia can result in cognitive dysfunction and hypoglycemia unawareness could result in the intensive management becoming more harmful than helpful. Widely fluctuating blood glucose levels may also increase the cardiac risk by enhancing oxidative stress, which is the factor that links all the mechanisms of vascular damage in people with diabetes (Brownlee, 2005; Monnier et al., 2006). Advances in the administration of insulin, the monitoring of blood glucose levels, and telemedicine have the potential for safely reaching the goal of normalizing blood sugars (Shalitin & Phillip, 2007).

Other Technologies

A new technology is available for the visually impaired. It is the Kurzweil-National Federation of the Blind Reader. You just point at the site to be read and it vocally reads the text aloud.

Cardiovascular disease is one of the chronic complications that is too often associated with diabetes control. The desire is to have early intervention before the painful or not so painful blockage occurs. One of the advances is the CardioNet Ambulatory Monitor. It is similar to a Holter monitor crossed with a Palm Pilot and a cell phone. This wireless sensor relays information that allows the doctors to capture arrhythmic events (for up to 21 days) by cellular technology (www.cardionet.com).

Similar telemedicine technologies using wireless or telephone systems are being developed for monitoring glucose control especially from distant and rural areas with few health care professionals.

Transplantation

Beta cells are the entire problem in T1DM, but only part of the problem in Type 2 diabetes mellitus (T2DM). The question is, "Is it feasible to protect pancreatic beta cells?" Beta cell dysfunction has already been observed in patients with prediabetes (Bonora, 2008). Bonora also notes that the focus on protection of these beta cells could be as simple as a reduction in "glucotoxicity, lipotoxicity, insulin resistance, inflammation, oxidative stress, and/or apoptosis" to name a few. It has been found that some medications appear to have an effect on the beta cell in a positive manner. Incretin-mimetics and peroxisome-proliferator-activated receptor gamma (PPAR-gamma) agonists and inhibitors of the renin-angiotensin process seem to have an effect on functions or increase numbers and/or life of the beta cells. As the mechanism of beta cell loss is ascertained, new drugs will be developed to preserve them. In T1DM, monoclonal antibodies to CD4 cells are being tested as agents to prevent immune system damage to beta cells. Other monoclonal antibodies are being developed to attack leukokines and other parts of the immune system for the same purpose. Some of these tests are being done by private companies and some as part of TrialNet, a national research network developed by and supported by the NIH. These trials are under way, and to date little information is available in human subjects. Animal studies have been positive, but many animal studies have not translated to humans. Many therapies are effective in preventing diabetes in the NOD mouse, a model of T1DM, but have not been effective in preventing diabetes in humans.

Transplantation of the pancreas or islet cells has come a long way. The outcome, with a whole pancreas or islet cell transplant (from 15% to 60% nonrejection after 1 year; Fiorina & Secchi, 2007), has been the normalizing of blood glucose levels wholly or in part without significant hypoglycemia occurring. From the islet cell perspective, centers have reported up to 80% insulin independence at 1 year after transplantation, but within 5 years, this insulin independence lasts in only 10% of the patients (Onaca et al., 2007).

Side effects of the surgical operation when a whole pancreas is put into place are more than just the transplant of islet cells themselves. More immunosuppression medications are needed for the whole versus just the islet cell transplants and have their own untoward responses. "Although recent advances have led to an increased rate of obtaining insulin-independence following islet transplantation, further developments are needed to improve the long-term viability . . ." (Meloche, 2007).

The good news is that the onset of posttransplantation diabetes and the redevelopment of diabetes have been halved over the past decade possibly because of the use of lower doses of steroids and changes in immunosuppressive medications (Valderhaug et al., 2007). The surgical transplantation of both pancreas and kidney at the same time continues to result in less rejection than just the pancreas transplant itself (Lipshutz & Wilkinson, 2007). Islet cell transplantation is now considered an option if a person has unstable T1DM and hypoglycemic unawareness or intractable neuropathy. A treatment drug (alpha-galactosylceramide) has been found to prevent the loss of transplanted islet cells in animals (Yasunami et al., 2005). Safety and efficacy for this and other drugs have not yet been established. The final answer for islet cell transplant is that immunosuppression will not be needed. Several answers to this problem are under research such as retraining the immune system so it will not recognize the transplanted cells as foreign bodies. There are several approaches to this problem being tried across the world, but none has been successful as yet. Few human trials have been done and none completed but this remains a viable area of research for now and the future.

Another problem with islet cell and pancreas transplant is supply. Cadaver pancreas is needed. For islet cell transplant two pancreases are needed. Too few are harvested each year to make transplant a viable option for everyone. There are several possible solutions to this problem. One solution is stem cells. Stem cell research will be discussed below. Another approach for the future is stem cells or fetal pancreatic ductal tissue from pigs. Pig insulin is almost identical to human insulin so this would be a good source of cells. The problem in the past has been the presence of many viruses in pigs that are dangerous to humans. Efforts are being made to raise pigs in sterile environments to eliminate these viruses. Several generations of pigs are needed to accomplish this, but work is under way.

Another approach to the problem of the supply of beta cells is to unlock the secret of beta cell synthesis in the embryo. There is a gene in the embryo that turns on the development of islet cells from pancreatic ductal tissue. This gene turns off after birth. If this gene can be identified and a way found to turn it back on or the enzyme formed by the action of the gene found and given, the body could make new islets all the time from adult ductal tissue in vivo or in vitro for an endless supply. Research is in progress in several centers on this problem.

Current obstacles for transplantation remain availability, cost, and improved immunosuppression therapy (Hogan, Pileggi, & Ricordi, 2008).

Stem Cell Therapy

Stem cell therapy may be the final answer for the need of immunosuppression medications, but social, political, and cultural problems exist. Lu et al. (2007) found in their review of the literature that stem cells from the pancreas, liver, spleen, bone marrow, umbilical cord blood, and peripheral blood could become insulin-producing cells. Whether grown in or out of the human body, the research shows conflicting results (Palma, Lindeman, & Tuch, 2008). So far, embryonic stem cells have shown the greatest chance of producing insulin in research completed in Pakistan (Hingorjo, Syed, Qureshi, & Kumar, 2007). The older the stem cell (embryonic is the youngest, adult marrow or peripheral blood is the oldest) the less effective it is to produce large enough numbers of long-lasting adult cells.

There is a report announcing a study that demonstrated E1-INT—epidermal (injectable) 1-islet neogenesis therapy (TM; von Herrath, 2005). TM therapy can stimulate the regeneration of human islet cells transplanted into animals. The number of human insulin-producing cells had increased in the mice more than 10 times than in the placebo group with the use of E1-INT (TM) therapy. Much further testing is needed (in Phase IIa), but this looks promising (information retrieved from diabetesincontrol.com on April 3, 2008). If human islets can be made to grow in animals, then removed and transplanted back into humans, the supply of islets could be increased. Also, it raises the question addressed above—if human islets can be made to grow in animals, can animal islets be made to grow in humans?

Genetics

There are many types of genes related to T1DM or to T2DM. Identifying these genes is the first step in determining ways to intervene and possibly prevent the development of the diagnosis of the disease. The environmental influence on the genetics must also be manipulated to prevent further damage. Francis Collins, MD, the director of the National Human Genome Research Institute, reported, during the 67th Scientific Sessions of the American Diabetes Association (2007), an international research consortium has now linked seven genes to T2DM and three others had previously been found. These 10 genes account for approximately 80% of the risk of T2DM in their findings of more than 32,000 people representing 4 population groups (Zeggini et al., 2008). Knowing this information and breaking this information into subtypes increase the possibility of more specific targeting in the use of the variety of medications available now and in the future.

Refer to the *Journal of the American Medical Association*, issue of March 19, 2008, for the review and ideas for translation of genomic medicine to patient care. Another resource is the Web site www.diabetesincontrol.com. One report from this site indicated that hemoglobin A1c values may be affected by factors other than blood glucose level averages, resulting in inaccurate measurements especially in some ethnic minority groups.

Other Studies

The National Diabetes Information Clearinghouse released an information booklet on diabetes entitled *Diabetes Overview*. Go to www.diabetes.niddk.nih. gov or call 1-800-860-8747 to request a copy. *Diabetes Overview* reports definitions and studies related to further research on a variety of diabetes-related topics. For example, the 2006 booklet describes the TODAY (Treatment Options for Type 2 Diabetes in Adolescents and Youth) study, TEDDY (The Environmental Determinants of Diabetes in the Young), the Type 1 Diabetes TrialNet, and an update on the Diabetes Prevention Program study started in 1996. Patients or their family members may meet the criteria for participating in some of these studies and may wish to participate.

There is a Phase II randomized trial on bevacizumab for the treatment of diabetic macular edema that seems promising for "some eyes" (Diabetic Retinopathy Clinical Research Network, 2007).

Inhaled insulin has come and gone. The Phase III studies continued to look into the safety and feasibility of this approach. Finding subjects for this phase and the lack of interest by consumers and endocrinologists, once it was placed on the market, led to the decision to remove this product "from the shelves." Inhaling a protein into the lungs on a long-term basis is still in question. The primary problems with this product were expense, calculating doses in milligrams, efficiency (only 25% of the insulin is used), bulky equipment, and the need for pulmonary function studies. Three companies have withdrawn inhaled insulin. One company is continuing to research inhaled insulin.

Oral insulin has been the subject of research for many years. Insulin is a protein and cannot be given orally because it is digested in the intestinal tract just as any protein would be. Coating the insulin with various chemicals to prevent digestion in the upper intestinal tract and removal of the coating in the lower tract has been tried with limited success. The problem with this method of administering insulin is timing—getting the coating to dissolve at the right time to get the insulin into the bloodstream when it is needed to cover the food. A new method of administering oral insulin is being tried. The insulin is put into a solution and sprayed into the cheek or under the tongue. The insulin is then absorbed through the mucosa of the mouth and never enters the intestinal tract. This insulin, call Ora-Lyn, is currently being marketed in India and Ecuador and is being tested in the United States, Canada, and Europe.

Insulin administered by patch has also been tried by several companies with very limited success because of the size of the molecule.

ADVANCE (Action in Diabetes and Vascular Disease) found in their study of 11,140 high-risk patients with T2DM no evidence of increased death risk by intensive normalizing of blood glucose levels. A previous report by the ACCORD (Action to Control Cardiovascular Risk in Diabetes) trial stated that, in their results, which represented twice as much data, intensive control increased the death rate. The conclusion is that the present study does not provide enough evidence to counter the ACCORD trial because the studies were not identical. It should be noted that in the ACCORD trial, most of the patients with diabetes studied also had preexisting heart disease and the level of control desired was an HbA1c of less than 6.0%. These patients were thus susceptible to cardiac events with hypoglycemia. The cause of the high death rate in ACCORD has not yet been determined, but the low goal for A1c certainly raises the possibility of hypoglycemic precipitation of cardiac events. What this study may really tell us is that in patients at high risk we may have to aim for higher A1c goals than in patients without high-risk indicators, not that we should aim higher in all patients. The ADA is awaiting the full reports from ACCORD and ADVANCE (Dluhy & McMahon, 2008) along with the results of a third trial, the VA Diabetes Trial (Duckworth, McCarren, & Abraira, 2001).

Long-term use of fenofibrates has been found useful in preventing the progression of diabetic retinopathy by reducing oxidative stress and thereby decreasing the need for laser treatment in people with T2DM (Keech et al., 2007). Fenofibrates are activators of PPAR-alpha-activated enzymes in the liver and thus reduce triglycerides. Triglycerides have been found to cause activation of the inflammation via the oxidative stress reaction and are thus a causative factor in vascular damage.

Grape skins could prevent cellular damage leading to vascular disease in people with diabetes. Resveratrol is the chemical found in grape skins, in peanuts, and in red wine. It assists cells in preventing leaks resulting in the circulation of free radicals linked to elevated glucose levels (Lu, Bambang, Armstrong, & Whiteman, 2008).

Another finding is that hypoglycemia may be prevented for those with T1DM by giving a low-dose of glucagon by injection at bedtime. An extended-release injectable formulation of low-dose glucagon is being developed (www.diobex.com) in effective dosages of 2 and 4 $ng·kg^{-1}·min^{-1}$. The outcomes did not appreciably raise blood glucose levels (were about 150 mg/dl) with the 8 ng/kg dosage demonstrating over 200 mg/dl (reported by Edelman, 2007).

Obesity, diagnosis, treatment, and diabetes control continue to be a problem. Adipose tissue is more than a storage place. It plays a role in appetite, insulin resistance, and the homeostasis of energy. Billyard, McTernan, and Kumar (2007) reviewed the data and identified leptin, adiponectin, obestatin, cytokines, peptide YY, and other hormones (at least 12 chemicals that affect metabolism—good or bad have been found) as having an effect on glucose metabolism directly or indirectly. Their further research plans to focus on the four peptides (leptin, adiponectin, obestatin, and peptide YY).

The diabetes epidemic has stimulated research by many pharmaceutical companies to look for new drugs to treat diabetes particularly in T2DM. This has brought forth the TZD class of drugs as well as incretins, DPP-4 inhibitors, and others. Many drugs in these classes, as well as new classes of drugs for the treatment of T2DM, are under study. As we understand the mechanisms of insulin production by the beta cell, the reasons for beta cell death, and the mechanisms of insulin signaling in the peripheral cell, we can look forward to many more new drugs that are specifically targeted to defects we find in these cells. A discussion of all the drugs being looked at is impractical here. Suffice it to say many are on the way. This will make life much more difficult for caregivers, who must know all the drugs and treatments available and how to apply them to an individual patient. It will, however, make life much better for the individual with diabetes, and that, after all, is what it is all about.

Summary

Research is important not only for general knowledge but to give hope to people who have diabetes. For the present, normalization of glucose level as much as can be safely tolerated is the goal. The resources to accomplish this task in the most updated fashion can be found in the first supplement of the year published in *Diabetes Care* by the American Diabetes Association and in any updates of the guidelines as made available through the American Association of Clinical Endocrinologists.

This is an exciting time for diabetes research. Only a small number of recent research findings are cited here. Whole volumes could be filled with an update on recent research and research under way. Space allows us to cite only a few areas that are of practical use today or may come into use in the very near future. Other research can be found by going to a variety of Web sites such as the NIDDK, NIH, TrialNet, CDC, Diabetes in Control, ADA, JDRF, AACE, the Endocrine Society, and many others. Diabetes mellitus is a terrible disease and a heavy burden for patients, health care providers, and the health care system. The past was bleak. The future, however, is bright. More research is being done today than ever before, though much more is needed. People with diabetes need to know the consequences of poor control, the innovations of care we have made, and the prospects of the future so they will have hope for a better life and do their part to maintain themselves so that they can benefit from the improvements and perhaps breakthroughs of the future.

References

Billyard, T., McTernan, P., & Kumar, S. (2007). Potential therapies based on antidiabetic peptides. *Best Practices in Clinical Endocrinology and Metabolism, 21*(4), 641–655.

Bonora, E. (2008). Protection of pancreatic beta-cells: Is it feasible? *Nutrition, Metabolism, & Cardiovascular Disease, 18*(1), 74–83.

Brownlee, M. (2005). The pathophysiology of diabetic complications: A unifying mechanism. *Diabetes, 54,* 1615–1625.

Collins, F. (2007). Presentation at the 67th Annual Scientific Sessions of the American Diabetes Association, Washington, DC.

Diabetes in Control. (2008). Retrieved April 3, 2008, from www.diabetesincontrol.com

Diabetic Retinopathy Clinical Research Network; Scott, I. U., Edwards, A. R., Beck, R.W., Bressler, N. M., Chan, C. K., Elman, M. J., et al. (2007). A phase II randomized clinical trial of intravitreal bevacizumab for diabetic macular edema. *Ophthalmology, 114*(10), 1860–1867.

Dluhy, R. G., & McMahon, G. T. (2008). Intensive glycemic control in the ACCORD and ADVANCE trials. *New England Journal of Medicine, 358*(24), 2630–2633.

Duckworth, W. C., McCarren, M., & Abraira, C. (2001). Glucose control and cardiovascular complications: The VA Diabetes Trial. *Diabetes Care, 24*(5), 942–945.

Edelman, S. (2007). *Low-dose glucagon may prevent hypoglycemia*. Retrieved August 2007 from www.clinicalendocrinologynews.com

Fiorina, P., & Secchi, A. (2007). Pancreatic islet cell transplant for treatment of diabetes. *Endocrinology & Metabolism Clinics of North America, 36*(4), 999–1013.

Herrick, J. B. (2008). The oatmeal diet in the treatment of diabetes mellitus. *Journal of the American Medical Association, 299*(10), 1202.

Hingorjo, M. R., Syed, S., Qureshi, M. A., & Kumar, A. (2007). Current trends in type 1 diabetes mellitus: Stem cells and beyond. *Journal of Pakistan Medical Association, 57*(12), 603–606.

Hogan, A., Pileggi, A., & Ricordi, C. (2008). Transplantation: Current developments and future directions: The future of clinical islet transplantation as a cure for diabetes. *Frontiers in Bioscience, 13*(1), 1192–1205.

Keech, A. C., Mitchell, P., Summanen, P. A., O'Day, J., Davis, T. M., & Moffitt, M. S. (2007). Effect of fenofibrate on the need for laser treatment for diabetic retinopathy (FIELD study): A randomized controlled trial. *Lancet, 370*(9600), 1687–1697.

Kowalski, A. (2007). New technology and diabetes management. *American Journal of Nursing, 107*(6 Suppl.), 16–17.

Lipshutz, G. S., & Wilkinson, A. H. (2007). Pancreas-kidney and pancreas transplantation for the treatment of diabetes mellitus. *Endocrinology & Metabolism Clinics of North America, 36*(4), 1015–1038.

Lu, C., Bambang, I. F., Armstrong, J. S. & Whiteman, M. (2008). Resveratrol blocks high glucose-induced mitochondrial reactive oxygen species products in bovine aortic endothelial cells: Role of phase 2 enzyme induction? *Diabetes, Obesity, and Metabolism, 10*(4), 347–349.

Lu, P., Lie, F., Yan, L., Peng, T., Liu, T., Yao, Z., et al. (2007). Stem cell therapy for type 1 diabetes. *Diabetes Research & Clinical Practice, 78*(1), 1–7.

Meloche, R. M. (2007). Transplantation for the treatment of type 1 diabetes. *World Journal of Gastroenterology, 13*(47), 6347–6355.

Monnier, L., Mas, E., Ginet, C., Michel, F., Villon, L., Cristol, J-P., et al. (2006). Activation of oxidative stress by acute glucose fluctuations compared with sustained chronic hyperglycemia in patients with type 2 diabetes. *Journal of the American Medical Association, 295*(14), 1681–1687.

Onaca, N., Naziruddin, B., Matsumoto, S., Noguchi, H., Klintmalm, G. B., & Levy, M. F. (2007). Pancreatic islet cell transplantation: Update and new developments. *Nutrition in Clinical Practice, 22*(5), 485–493.

Palma, C. A., Lindeman, R., & Tuch, B. E. (2008). Blood into beta-cells: Can adult stem cells be used as a therapy for Type 1 diabetes? *Regenerative Medicine, 3*(1), 33–47.

Selby, J. V., Swain, B. E., Gerzoff, R. B., Karter, A. J., Waitzfelder, B. E., Brown, A. F., et al.: TRIAD Study Group. (2007). Understanding the gap between good processes of diabetes care and poor intermediate outcomes: Translating Research into Action for Diabetes (TRIAD). *Medical Care, 45*(12), 1144–1153.

Shalitin, S., & Phillip, M. (2007). The role of new technologies in treating children and adolescents with type 1 diabetes mellitus. *Pediatric Diabetes, 8*(Suppl. 6), 72–79.

Shin, J. Y., Lee, S. Y., Jeung, M. J., Eun, S. H., Woo, C. W., Yoon, S. Y., et al. ((2008). Serum adiponectin, C-reactive protein and TNF-alpha levels in obese Korean children. *Journal of Pediatric Endocrinology and Metabolism, 21*(1), 23–29.

Valderhaug, T. G., Hjelmesaeth, J., Rollag, H., Leivestad, T., Roislien, J., Jenssen, T., et al. (2007). Reduced incidence of new-onset post-transplantation diabetes mellitus during the last decade. *Transplantation, 84*(9), 1125–1130.

Von Herrath, M. (2005). E1-INT (Transition Therapeutics/Novo Nordisk). *Current Opinion of Investigated Drugs, 6*(10), 1037–1042.

Yasunami, Y., Kojo, S., Kitamura, H., Toyofuku, A., Satoh, M., Nakano, M., et al. (2005). V alpha 14 NK T cell-triggered IFN-gamma production by Gr1+ CD11b+ cells mediates early graft loss of syngeneic transplanted islets. *Journal of Experimental Medicine, 202*(7), 913–918.

Zeggini, E., Scott, L. J., Saxena, R., Voight, B. F., Marchini, J. L., Hu, T., et al. (2008). Meta-analysis of genome-wide association data and large-scale replications identified additional susceptibility loci for type 2 diabetes. *National Genetics, 40*(5), 638–645.

36

The Parents' and Patients' Perspective

In diabetes, patients care for themselves. Although they employ professionals to teach them and give advice, in many ways they serve as their own doctors. Daily they must inject their dosages of insulin, test their specimens of blood and urine, balance their diets, exercise their bodies, adjust their dosages, treat their reactions, and even determine whether and when they need medical assistance. How surprising that they are rarely consulted when a program is devised for their care. When asked why the patient's viewpoint was not included in his teaching, a medical school professor said that no literature was written by patients. Here, then, is a glimpse of the problems of diabetes, as perceived by those who live with it.

Most patients are troubled more by the emotional factors associated with diabetes than by its biomedical aspects. It is in the emotional area, however, that they are least likely to receive support and guidance. It is impossible to separate psyche from soma and treat only the ills of the body. Patients have an intense emotional involvement with their disease. It ranges from the stress caused by responsibility for a demanding daily regimen to the accumulated fears from anticipating disabling complications and the possibility of a premature death.

Persons with diabetes do not only think about the medical aspects of their disease. They are concerned about the concept of themselves as whole and healthy individuals. They want to retain their independence. They wonder if they will be able to keep their jobs and support their families. They worry about the long-term financial cost of this disease and whether they can obtain adequate medical and life insurance. They dread social discrimination. They hope they can marry despite the disease and that love will continue even if they become chronically disabled. They wonder whether they will be able to have children and whether their children will inherit the disease. They fear becoming dependent on those they love or even on public assistance.

Although these are not precisely medical concerns, they deserve your attention and that of every health care professional who deals with a person who has diabetes. Good diabetes management cannot be achieved without careful and constant monitoring by the patients themselves. Therefore, it is essential that they be in good emotional health to provide self-care, let alone self-management. Successful therapy must include consideration for the whole person. Jonathan Miller (1981) describes this consideration well when he says, "Man is not a machine with a bit of temperament thrown in; a robot who happens to blush." In fact, the same emotions that cause the temperament or blush may serve to unbalance your patient's hard-won glucose control.

Quite apart from externally imposed stress, diabetes includes a metabolic fluctuation that can precipitate mood and behavioral changes that are totally predictable. Anyone who has experienced the irrational anger or depression sometimes related to premenstrual tension will understand the frustration this can cause. Insulin reactions or sudden changes in blood glucose level can create such embarrassing behavior as weeping, fighting, or slurred speech. Think how it feels to live in dread of an attack that causes socially unacceptable behavior. Can you imagine cursing at your boss, weeping in the classroom, or being arrested for public drunkenness with no one knowing you were having an insulin reaction? To make matters worse, these people usually have no memories of these episodes. They must wait for others to tell them what physical or social damage they have caused. Often they do not receive the explanation, just the consequences.

Another observation has been that a person treats what he or she thinks is an insulin reaction but, without some blood glucose monitoring, were not actually having an insulin reaction at all. This may mean that the patients needed a better understanding of the physical sensations that warn of an impending reaction. More likely it reflects their great fear of experiencing the reaction. It is frightening to lose control of yourself. Many decide to be safe and treat any funny feeling by taking some sugar. After several years of diabetes, patients often find that their early warning signals change or disappear altogether. The resulting unpredictability is also a cause of considerable stress.

Diabetes demands an extraordinary amount of attention from the patient. We can appreciate the preoccupation with injections, pens, pumps, inhaled insulin, testing, diet, and exercise. It is not often perceived that people who live with diabetes must be constantly aware of their bodies. They cannot simply acknowledge a headache, fatigue, blurred vision, or sweating. They must immediately ask themselves "Why is this happening?" and decide what action to take.

They must wonder if they need food, fast-acting glucose, regular insulin, exercise, rest, or if instead they should quickly seek medical care. They may need to self-diagnose and make as many as a dozen of these urgent decisions in a single day. This awareness, often with attending apprehension, is stressful in itself, but it also has other emotional consequences. The patient with diabetes is forced to become very self-centered. In any relationship, this single priority can be a difficult one with which to live. The partner without diabetes often develops a kind of jealousy toward the diabetes, because its needs must always come first. Family counseling, in this instance, is good preventive medicine.

We hear a lot about the noncompliant patient, the patient who, for some unfathomable reason, refuses to follow instructions carefully and thus makes good therapy impossible. We do not, however, hear much about the priorities of patients. Diabetes is seldom the only thing that is going on in their lives. Few people lead lives that are compatible with optimal diabetes management. They are bound to be caught in a traffic jam or be closing an important business deal just when they ought to be eating their lunches. They find that testing is awkward almost anywhere but at home, and troublesome and boring even there. They may not have enough money to see their physicians. Life can be complicated by many things. One young mother described her dilemma of experiencing an insulin reaction just as her toddler had escaped the yard and was running toward the street. What was her priority?

The greatest contribution of the health professional would be to teach patients just how their bodies ought to work and how diabetes impairs that normal function. They then need to know the manner in which food and medication can be used to improve the problem. With this working knowledge in place of the usual checklist of rules, they will have the flexibility to adjust their care to meet the variables in their lives. No one seeks the role of martyr or outcast. Your patients now have more tools that will enable them to cope when the hostess serves dinner an hour later than planned or the college crowd goes out for beer and pizza at midnight. They need to know how to use them. They need to know how to cope with an attack of intestinal flu. These are the kind of daily problems that confound the individual and realistic solutions will automatically produce better compliance.

Take time to listen to your patients. They may need a little encouragement if they are awed, frightened, or inarticulate in a medical setting. It can be difficult for patients to raise a controversial issue with someone on whom their lives may depend. In the name of efficiency, it is tempting for you to do all of the talking, but listening may resolve some mysteries. One man retired from his job because he blacked out every afternoon. He accepted this as a normal consequence of diabetes, but he had not told his physician about it because the physician never asked. Children are often burdened with guilt when they believe diabetes is a punishment for some imagined wrong. This is seldom discovered and resolved because, again, no one thinks to ask. All patients hear frightening misinformation from friends and neighbors. Listening may help to correct these myths and resolve the fears. Patients who pay handsomely for care may still be reluctant to bother you with their questions. Assure them of your interest. If you give them better information, it will simplify your task.

Try to choose your words carefully. Their beta cells may be out of order, but that does not make your patients second-class citizens. They are often offended at being called by the name of their disease, a diabetic. They dislike being accused of cheating when they eat the same food as others. Words such as control and management are common currency, but they have an unpleasant connotation when it sounds like they refer to patients instead of the disease. Medical terminology such as ketoacidosis, glycosuria, and hypoglycemia can sound scary and threatening to them. Nothing about diabetes is so complex that it cannot be explained in basic English. Familiarity with your subject can lead to the use of jargon, but your patients may envision a hula dance if you tell them to rotate their injection sites. If you say, "Look at your feet every day," it is best to explain how, why, and for what, so patients will not just check to see if their feet are still there.

All diabetes care should be provided in a nonjudgmental manner. Children often feel they are being judged as good if their blood tests are in the normal range or their urine tests are negative and bad if their blood glucose levels are elevated. By this implication you not only damage their self-image but also encourage them to falsify their records to win your approval. Occasionally your patients will make poor nutritional choices. Rather than regard this as cheating, you can help them with a neutral statement such as, "This meal plan doesn't seem to suit you. Let's see how we can adjust it to fit your needs." They may be eating out of boredom or anxiety. They may not understand their meal plans. Conversely, perhaps they are taking too much insulin or too many pills or the timing is off. In either case they will be very hungry. To decide that they simply lack willpower will prevent you from identifying these problems. Such a judgment will also destroy your rapport.

Control of obesity is a major goal in treating most Type 2 patients with adult-onset diabetes. Here again is an example where the therapy is the responsibility of the patient. If you would truly help them, do not just send them home with a 1,200 cal diet and a stern admonition. Food, in our society, has many emotionally charged meanings. Food certainly represents sociability and hospitality. Can you imagine a party or holiday where food was not available in abundance? For some, food is a symbol of affluence. Most people learn as children to regard food as a sign of love and comfort. These feelings persist in times of pain or loneliness. Think how often a child is rewarded for good behavior with a sweet treat. Although withholding food can reduce the body, it can also create an anguish of denial for your patient.

Success in weight reduction depends on your skill and ability to deal simultaneously with the physical and emotional needs of your patients. Dietary requirements are easily determined, but emotional therapy and motivation must be tailored to suit the individual. First, see if you can get a feeling for what inclines your patient to overeat. Then, you can gently suggest better reasons that might tempt them to eat less or not eat the foods that are detrimental. Feeling better is only a motivation if your patient feels badly to begin with. Looking better does not work in the absence of personal pride. Most people are motivated to undertake a difficult task if they can learn "What's in it for me?" Perceive their personal goals and adjust your weight reduction program to meet them. Once they have embarked on this program, be lavish with your support. You will find that positive reinforcement in the form of compliments, encouragement, and praise will work better than any meal plan, or perhaps more accurately, the meal plan is not likely to work without your support.

There is a lonely quality to life with a chronic disease. I have often heard a patient say, "No one really understands what diabetes is doing to my life." As you read through this book, try making a list of the sentences that begin, "The patient should," as in, "The patient should wash, soak, and inspect the feet daily." Consider the time and effort involved in each simple instruction. No request is unreasonably demanding, but the accumulated total will amaze you. Include in your calculations the number of times a patient is referred to a different health care professional, such as the podiatrist, the dietitian, and the ophthalmologist. Consider the cost of these visits, and remember the time lost from work for appointments, travel, and dawdling in waiting rooms. Many of these providers will recommend that patients purchase equipment such as syringes, testing kits, or special foods. Include this additional cost and multiply it by a lifetime of use. Now total the time and expense and apply it to your own budget and busy schedule. How would you afford it? Where would you find time to fit it all in? Persons who live with diabetes are not blessed with additional time or money. It is no wonder they react with anger, frustration, and noncompliance when this load is laid on them. At a time when their health is poor and they fear for their future, the burden of this regimen may seem to be the last straw.

One diabetes health care team decided to follow the regimen they had been prescribing for one week. By the week's end their compliance score was shamefully low but their level of empathy had increased considerably. Caring for diabetes is a boring and frustrating job and one that can never be successfully completed. If you provide your patients with plenty of encouragement and practical advice, they will know you appreciate what they must deal with and that will make their task seem easier. Long-term patients need this reinforcement as much as the beginners.

Health professionals fill unique positions in the eyes of the patient. Patients are likely to view them as friends and confidants who also have medical knowledge. The nurse or psychologist may seem more approachable than the other health professionals and have more time to provide counseling on a broader range of concerns. In all, be sensitive and responsive to your patient's needs and do not be too concerned about evaluating your success. Do not be discouraged because you tried to persuade your patients to accept diabetes and they would not. They may never accept it. Why should they? It has no redeeming features. If they accept it, they give up, and they do not dare give up. They have to fight back every day. Your goal does not need to be their acceptance of diabetes, just their adjustment to it. If you can help them accomplish that, you will have made an important contribution indeed.

Let us back up for a minute and talk about the onset of diabetes and the attending patient education. Learning that you have diabetes is like being run over by a dump truck. The mind goes quite blank except for a blinking neon sign that keeps saying "Why me?" At that time no one is ready to sit down and absorb a crash course in diabetes management. Education does not work unless there is reception as well as transmission. One woman described the experience by saying, "The nurse came in and told me everything I needed to know, and when she left the room, all the information went right out the door with her." Often the instructor is busy telling how while that patient is still coping with why. It would be interesting to see an annotated teaching manual with the patients' reactions written in the margin. They would read something like this: "I couldn't possibly give myself an injection. Look at that needle. I know it's going to hurt." "What do you mean, test my urine for ketones? What a disgusting idea." "I can't eat at 5 P.M. My husband doesn't even get home until 7 P.M." "How on earth am I supposed to know what food is carbohydrate?" "They don't understand. My life is different than what they're describing."

What then should you do? After all, the diabetes exists, your patients are available, and their lives depend on the information you have to give them. How about starting with just survival information to get them through the first week or so until they can adjust to the idea of having diabetes? Granted, that is not the most efficient method, but it is likely to be more successful in the long run. Tell them there is a great deal to learn, but that you will be there to help them when they are ready. Then devote a bit of time to reassuring them. Right after they decide they do not want any part of diabetes comes the chilling fear that maybe they cannot handle it. You make the daily management sound easy, but they are still suspicious because they know that is your job. It would be a great comfort to talk with someone who has actually managed all these impossible tasks and still seems to live a happy and normal life. Perhaps you can arrange that for them.

Sex education, as it relates to diabetes, should be an essential part of all patient education courses. There is virtually no other source for this information. Your patient needs to be reminded that sex is exercise and requires the same extra food supplement one might take in preparation for a game of tennis. Sex has been known to heighten emotions, and blood sugar levels often go along for the ride. Peer group discussion can help provide answers to personal problems. In one group a lively conversation was sparked by the question, "Is it less romantic to spoil a tender moment by getting up for orange juice than to wait and go into reaction?"

Every young woman needs to understand how contraception will affect her diabetes. Medical care has now overcome many past threats to pregnancy in the women with diabetes and the survival rate for babies is approaching the norm. Some risk remains, however, and she must be able to decide whether the problems caused by the pregnancy are greater or less than those caused by preventing it. She must know that oral contraceptives can elevate her blood sugar levels and may require a medication adjustment, that an intrauterine device may precipitate an infection that would be difficult to control, and that contraception methods dependent on regular menstrual cycles may not be for her. She needs to know that her best chances of a successful pregnancy depend on optimal blood glucose control and careful medical supervision throughout her pregnancy, and she needs to know all of this well before conception.

Women of all ages with diabetes need sensitive medical care. Nearly every function characteristic of their sex makes diabetes management more difficult for them. From an often-delayed menarche through a moody menopause, the woman's unstable hormones complicate diabetes control and play havoc with her emotions. Recurring vaginal infections are uncomfortable and interfere with normal marital relations. Physical symptoms of menopause are difficult to distinguish from insulin reactions. Pregnancy is fraught with emotional pitfalls, and the gravid patient ought to receive personal and family counseling along with good physical care.

Every diabetic adolescent male is haunted by the specter of impotence. It is a subject rarely discussed, and you can count on him not to ask about it. Do him a favor and give him the facts. It is not exactly good news, but it is far better than he has been imagining. Because he represents a prime dropout in diabetes management, he may mend his ways on learning that high blood sugar levels can cause temporary impotence. Be sure he also understands that there can be correctable psychologic reasons for impotence unrelated to diabetic neuropathy. We know that 50%–60% of men with diabetes have sex-related complications. If the situation warrants it, you may want to recommend a discussion for sexual counseling for his partner and himself. The subject is often embarrassing for all concerned, but your tactful handling of it can prevent unnecessary personal tragedy.

Most people who live with diabetes are also members of families. Because of the nature of the disease, which demands carefully planned, but less precisely timed meals and includes insulin emergencies and occasional personality fluctuations, it is as important for family members to understand the disease as it is for the patient. This fact is often overlooked in education programs that focus on the patient alone. At least one family member should be invited to attend your classes, and a family conference is a good idea, especially if the patient is a child.

There are a few pitfalls to avoid when working with family members. Make sure everyone understands that the responsibility for daily management lies with the patient and that the role of the family is supportive. This avoids situations like the one in which a man sent his wife to the nutrition classes, reasoning that he did not need the information because she was the one who fed him. Sometimes family members play games with one another, so be perceptive of attitudes that may prove to be detrimental. Occasionally a family member will seize on the details of daily management as an arsenal of weapons with which to nag the patient. On the other hand, patients can rationalize their negligence because no one forced them to comply. An abstract discussion of these games can often thwart them before they begin.

All family members should understand that patients are expected to live a quite normal life and that there is no need to treat them as helpless invalids. The patients should be cautioned neither to use their disease to manipulate their families nor to obtain special privileges. A common reaction to the diagnosis of diabetes is for the family to cleanse the household of sweet foods and to restructure the family's routine to suit the patient's regimen. This is neither necessary nor advisable. It can breed resentment among discomfited family members, make the patient feel guilty for the inconvenience, and make it more difficult for them to adjust to living in a normal environment. These are subtle, but human, reactions that will require your prompt and sensitive attention.

The manner in which the family reacts to the disease is a crucial factor in the patient's adjustment to it. This is particularly true in the case of a child with diabetes and should be brought to the attention of the parents. Before you can expect the parents to provide a tranquil atmosphere for their child, however, you will have to help them resolve the struggle with their own emotional conflicts. Parents are usually devastated to learn that their child has contracted this chronic and menacing disease. They feel grief for the loss of their healthy child and their attending dreams and aspirations. They fear for their child's future and the ugly complications that may ensue. They are angry at this cruel fate and at the physician's inability to reverse it. They are afraid they cannot cope with the daily management and depressed because they feel so helpless. Obviously, you will not be able to dismiss these feelings with a wave of your wand. These feelings are as chronic as the disease itself. Your understanding, factual information, and thoughtful counseling will all help to improve the impact of this emotional crisis.

When counseling, encourage the parents to get away from time to time for a weekend vacation or even just a movie. You will find some parents become almost imprisoned by diabetes. They are afraid to leave their children for fear there will be an emergency. For the same reason, sitters and friends may be reluctant to assume the responsibility. Restorative periods of separation are necessary because the marital stresses are tremendous for parents of a chronically ill child. They cannot reveal their fears and frustrations to the child, so they take them out on each other. You might suggest that the parents exchange sitting care with the family of another child or send their child to one of the good diabetes summer camps for 2 weeks. This would allow the parents some freedom from the constant responsibility and help the child develop a feeling of independence.

The overprotective mother is frequently considered the person responsible for the emotional problems of the child who has diabetes, yet the parameters of this overprotection are never defined for her. She feels the obligation to keep her child alive and well and does not know when and how to relinquish that duty. Often the doctor encourages overprotection by holding her accountable for the child's poor management, even well into adolescence. Fathers of these children may seem removed from concern for their children's problems. This is unfairly considered indifference or even rejection. In fact, this remoteness should be attributed to the mother's traditional role of caring for sick children, as well as his unavailability for medical conferences. Eventually the mother becomes the expert, and he finds he has no role to play. It is important for all concerned that fathers be included in the counseling, teaching, and care as often as possible. Siblings sometimes respond with jealousy to the exceptional attention the child who has diabetes is receiving. They can also fear that something bad will happen to their brother or sister, and then worry that perhaps it will happen to them too. Obviously, there is much within the family that can have an impact on the emotional state of the child, and consequently on the child's ability to sustain good diabetes management.

Although this chapter is primarily about the feelings of patients and their families, medical professionals have human emotions too. Therefore you need to be aware of the ways in which you are affected by this incurable disease. Your honest response can benefit your patient as well as yourself. Basically you view yourselves as healers, yet diabetes cannot be cured. You do not know what causes it and you cannot prevent it. You do have a greater ability to help prevent many of its serious complications. That is the state of the art at this time. Often your best efforts will meet with disappointment. Diabetes care, like all medicine, is more of an art than an exact science. The goals are now more clearly defined. The roads are sometimes poorly marked. You commit yourselves to attaining normal blood glucose levels, yet if this could actually be achieved, it would mean the absence of diabetes. You are therefore forced to settle for something less. This should never be construed as failure. The only failure is not to try.

It is important that you share with your patients the truth about diabetes. Hope is an essential component in their daily battles, but false hope is cruel. Tell them of the tremendous progress that has been made in diabetes care since the days when diagnosis was little more than a death sentence. Tell them of the exciting developments in current diabetes research. Do not imply, however, that strict adherence to your prescribed therapy will assure them of a future free from complications. When they learn otherwise they will feel betrayed. If you tell them it is a gamble in which you can increase their odds and that you will work together to keep them feeling as well as possible, they will undoubtedly accept your offer. If eventually your patients must endure complications, you will have spared them unnecessary guilt and a sense of failure.

Too often healers, faced with an inability to heal, are inclined to turn the blame and responsibility back on the patient and his or her family A particularly tragic example of this involved the mother of a 27-year-old woman with diabetes. The daughter had eye, kidney, vascular, and neuropathic complications. When she suffered a serious stroke, the physician said to her mother, "You knew there was diabetes in your family. You should never have had this child. Because of your selfishness, she has had to live a miserable life and now she may die." Of course the mother found this insensitive statement to be devastating. The physician was purged of a feeling of failure but at a terrible cost. Although this physician may represent an extreme minority, many nurses have reported a prejudice against patients with diabetes in their hospitals. It seems the patients are perceived as being there through their own negligence.

Both patients and professionals need to be more realistic about the limitation of medical care. We do not have all the answers. Creating guilt and placing blame are never effective ways to achieve cooperation and resolve problems. Let us consider diabetes to be a no-fault disease. Then the patient, the patient's family, and the professionals can work together, using the best therapeutic tools now at hand. Instead of nonproductive recrimination, we can expend our energies working against our common enemy, which is diabetes.

Reference

Miller, J. (1981). *The body in question.* New York: Random House.

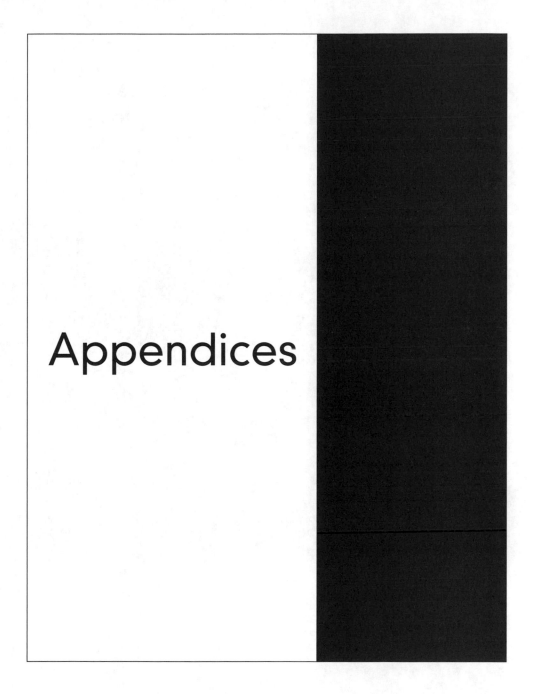

Appendices

Appendix A

HISTORY OF DIABETES MELLITUS

BCE 1552	Papyrus Ebers of Egypt, in the 3rd Dynasty—Hesy-Ra, physician, mentioned the passing of "too much urine (or polyuria)."
	Hindus in the Vedas—insects and flies attracted to urine that tasted sweet.
1000	Suruta, a Hindu, called the father of medicine in India, diagnosed diabetes mellitus.
	Celsus, a Greek, described diabetes.
	Aretaeus, a Greek, differentiated between diabetes mellitus and diabetes insipidus.
276	Demetria of Aparnea refined the diagnosis of diabetes.
230	Celium Aurelianus said that Apollonius of Memphis coined the term "diabetes" (to siphon through: 'dia' = through; 'betes' = to go), but Apollonius thought it was a form of dropsy.
	Paul of Aegina described diabetes as a weakness of the kidneys; excess moisture from the body, leading to dehydration. The remedy he prescribed was endive, lettuce, rock-fishes, juices of knotgrass, elecampane in dark-colored wine, and decoctions of dates and myrtle to drink in the first stages of the disease; followed by "cataplasms to the hypochondrium (over the kidneys)" consisting of vinegar, rose oil, and navel-wort. He warned against the use of diuretics, but venesection (cutting of veins) was permitted.
CE	First century Arateus described "the melting down of flesh and limbs into urine."
45–117	Aetius prescribed a "cooling diet, diluted wine, and cooling applications to the loins in the early stages." He used opiates and "mandragors" in the "late stages."
865–925	Rhazea, an Arabian writer, translated information about diabetes from the Hindus.

Information adapted from notes e-mailed by Judy Renwick; Benjamin Lee Gordon, MD; from a pamphlet released by BD/Lilly; and from the book, *Diabetes and Denmark*, C. Binder, T. Deckert, & J. Nerup (Eds.), Denmark: GAD Publishers, 2007.

900–1037	Avicenna prescribed emetics and sudorifics; suggested that all diuretic foods and drugs should be avoided; and recommended engaging in exercise (preferably on horseback) to "employ moderate friction" in the early stages. In the late stages he recommended tepid baths and fragrant wine.
	Haly Abbas, a Moslem, thought diabetes was caused by excessive heat within the viscus; he called it dysentery or the discrepancy.
	Diabetes commonly diagnosed by "water tasters"—who drank the urine of those suspected of having diabetes—"mellitus" the Latin word for honey, was then added to the name.
1257	Physicians prescribe purgative to counter the strain on the kidneys; astringents and remedies that made you feel cool.
1501–1576	Cardona concluded that people with diabetes lose more water than they take in by measuring input and output of fluids; he didn't know why.
	Paracelsus identified diabetes as a "serious disorder."
1622–1675	Hindu Dr. Susruta's works were rediscovered. Diabetes was said to be due to humoral changes and excessive drinking, therefore, astringents were prescribed as a remedy. It was theorized that diabetes was a blood disease.
1798	John Rollo tests and finds excess sugar in the blood.
	Early nineteenth century. First chemical tests developed to indicate and measure the presence of sugar in the urine.
1813–1878	Claude Bernard theorizes that diabetes was caused by the breakdown of glycogens stored in the liver.
1816–1876	L. Traube found a relationship between the intake of carbohydrates and the increase of glucose levels in the urine.
1866	Dr. Lancereaux differentiated between Type 1 and Type 2 diabetes mellitus (T1DM and T2DM).
1869	Paul Langerhans, as a German medical student, presented in his dissertation that the pancreas contains cells that secrete normal pancreatic juice and the other cells an unknown secretion. (Several years later, these cells are called, the "islets of Langerhans" in his honor.)
1870s	Bouchardat (French physician) formulated "starvation diets" noted from observations of the disappearance of glycosuria in his patients with diabetes during the rationing of food in Paris while under siege by Germany during the Franco-Prussian War;
	I. V. Pavlov, a Czech researcher, studied how the pancreas works and about the glycogen metabolism of the liver.
1889	Joseph von Mehring and Oskar Minkowski, of the University of Strasbourg, France, produced diabetes in dogs by removing their pancreas.

	Catoni, Italian diabetes specialist, isolated his patients under lock and key in order to get them to follow their diet of restricted food.
1908	Georg Zuelzer, a German scientist, developed the first injectible pancreatic extract to suppress glycosuria; however, there are untoward side effects of this treatment.
1910–1920	Frederick Madison Allen and Elliot P. Joslin emerged as the two leading diabetes specialists in the United States. Joslin described diabetes to be "the best of the chronic diseases" because it was "clean, seldom unsightly, not contagious, often painless, and susceptible to treatment."
1913	Dr. Allen, after 3 years of diabetes study, published his work concerning glycosuria and diabetes.
1915	Dr. Hans Christian Hagedorn, appointed to hospital; studied foods and the resulting response re glucose in the urine.
1920	Dr. Banting conceived of the idea of insulin after reading Moses Barron's article, published in the November issue of *Surgery, Gynecology, and Obstetrics*, on the relation of the islets of Langerhans to diabetes.
1921	Banting and Best, through the study of pancreatized dogs, find insulin is secreted from the islet cells of the pancreas.
1/23/1922	Leonard Thompson, a 14-year-old boy from Toronto, received the first human dose of insulin extract developed by Dr. Collip.
3/1923	Dr. Hagedorn, insulin produced in his home, gave himself an injection.
5/30/1923	Eli Lilly and Company and the University of Toronto enter a deal for the mass production of insulin in North America.
10/25/1923	Dr. Banting and his colleague, Professor Macleod, are awarded the Nobel prize in Physiology; Banting shares his award with Best; Macleod shares his award with Collip.
1920s–1930s	Harold P. Himsworth, MD, introduces the concept that many patients have insulin insensitivity (resistance) rather than absolute insulin deficiency.
	Becton Dickinson manufactured the first insulin syringe.
1930s	Dr. Joslin noted an increase in diabetes with obesity. Insulin+ Adrenalin Novo was marketed in Denmark for a few years.
1936	Dr. Hagedorn, Norman Jensen, and coworkers discovered protamine insulin but pH had to be neutralized before it was given—worked almost twice as long (became NPH or neutral protamine Hagedorn).
1938	Zinc Protamine Insulin Novo introduced to the Danish market.

1940s	Link is made between diabetes and long-term complications, that is, kidney and eye disease.
	Rachmiel Levine, MD, discovers that insulin "works like a key" transporting glucose into the cells.
	The American Diabetes Association and the International Diabetes Foundation are established.
1944	Standard insulin syringe is developed (for 40 Units/cc; later 80 Units/cc).
1950s	Discovery of the autoimmunity relation with diabetes.
1955	Oral drugs (sulfonylurea class) are introduced to lower blood glucose levels.
1957	Phenothyl-biguanide (DBI) introduced.
1958	Chlorpropamide (Diabinese) introduced.
1959	T1DM (insulin-dependent) and T2DM (non-insulin-dependent) are officially recognized.
1960s	Insulin purity is improved; home testing for sugar in urine increases ability to improve blood sugar control.
	First insulin syringe with a permanently attached needle launched by BD.
	Berson and Yalow—reported the immunoassay of insulin.
1964	Acetohexamide (Dymelor) introduced.
1965	Tolazamide (Tolinase) introduced.
1966	First pancreas transplant performed at the University of Manitoba.
1968	Steiner reported discovery of Pro Insulin.
1970s	Blood glucose meters and insulin pumps developed; laser therapy use in retina treatment; recognition that T1DM has an autoimmune basis.
	American Association of Diabetes Educators is founded; HbA1c test is introduced.
	First U100/1/2 cc syringe introduced.
1973	Somatostatin discovered by Roger Quillen.
1975	Banting Award Lecture on Glucagon given by Roger Unger.
1977	Rosalyn Yalow (received the Nobel Prize in Physiology for Medicine) and Solomon Berson discovered the radioimmunoassay for insulin.
	Pre Pro Insulin (8 extra amino acids) discovered.
1978	Insulin became the first human protein to be manufactured through biotechnology.

1980s	American Diabetes Association publishes a position statement recommending glycemic control.
	First examination is offered for certification of diabetes educators.
	The first National Diabetes Education Week is observed.
	First $3/10$ cc insulin syringe is introduced.
	First biosynthetic human insulin made with recombinant DNA technology is introduced: Dr. Richard Guthrie gave this first injection in the United States.
1985	NovoPen launched.
1986	Insulin delivery by "pen" is introduced.
1988	Dr. Gerald Reaven identified the collection of signs now called the metabolic syndrome (dysmetabolic syndrome).
1989	Novo and Nordisk merged.
1990s	Lilly launches the first rapid-acting analog insulin.
	Lilly and Takeda introduce a thiazolidinedione for the treatment of diabetes.
	Congress passes a bill that allows for Medicare coverage of education and diabetes supplies.
	The first Diabetes Education and Behavioral Research Summit is held.
1993	Diabetes Control and Complications Trial report is published—demonstrating scientifically that intensive therapy delays and/or prevents the onset of complications of diabetes.
1997	The Expert Committee on the Diagnosis and Classification of Diabetes Mellitus proposed a more accurate grouping of subclasses.
1999	NovoNordisk launched NovoRapid.
2000s	Insulin analogs (designer insulins) available in rapid- and long-acting forms.
	A synthetic amylin and associated treatments for diabetes are released; incretins released.
	The first Advanced Diabetes Management (BC-ADM) exam is offered. BD introduces the first blood glucose monitoring system that communicates with an insulin pump.
	American Association of Diabetes Educators launches the "7 Self-Care Behaviors" framework and completes the first comprehensive environmental scan of the diabetes educator profession.

Appendix B

ETIOLOGY CLASSIFICATION

I. Type 1 diabetes (beta cell destruction, usually leading to absolute insulin deficiency) (Patients with any form of diabetes may require insulin treatment at some stage of their disease. Such use of insulin does not, of itself, classify the patient.)

Immune mediated

Idiopathic

II. Type 2 diabetes (may range from predominantly insulin resistance with relative insulin deficiency to a predominantly secretory defect with insulin resistance)

III. Other specific types

A. Genetic defects of beta cell function
   1. Chromosome 12, HNF-1 alpha (formerly MODY 3)
   2. Chromosome 7, glucokinase (formerly MODY 2)
   3. Chromosome 20, HNF-4 alpha (formerly MODY 1)
   4. Chromosome 13, insulin promoter factor (IF-1; MODY 4)
   5. Chromosome 17, HNF-1 beta (MODY 5)
   6. Chromosome 2, NeuroD (MODY 6)
   7. Mitochondrial DNA
   8. Others

B. Genetic defects insulin action
   1. Type A insulin resistance
   2. Leprechaunism
   3. Rabson–Mendenhall syndrome
   4. Lipoatrophic diabetes
   5. Others

C. Diseases of the exocrine pancreas
   1. Pancreatitis
   2. Trauma/pancreatectomy
   3. Neoplasia
   4. Cystic fibrosis
   5. Hemochromatosis
   6. Fibrocalculus pancreatopathy
   7. Others

American Diabetes Association (2008). Etiologic classification of diabetes mellitus in "Diagnosis and Classification of Diabetes Mellitus," 2008, *Diabetes Care, 31*(Suppl. 1), p. S55–S60.

D. Endocrinopathies
1. Acromegaly
2. Cushing's syndrome
3. Glucagonoma
4. Pheochromocytoma
5. Hyperthyroidism
6. Somatostatinoma
7. Aldosteronoma
8. Others

E. Drug or chemical induced
1. Vacor
2. Pentamidine
3. Nicotinic acid
4. Glucocorticoids
5. Thyroid hormone
6. Diazoxide
7. Beta adrenergic agonists
8. Thiazides
9. Dilantin
10. Alpha interferon
11. Others

F. Infections
1. Congenital rubella
2. Cytomegalovirus
3. Others

G. Uncommon forms of immune-mediated diabetes
1. "Stiff-man" syndrome
2. Anti-insulin receptor antibodies
3. Others

H. Other genetic syndromes sometimes associated with diabetes
1. Down's syndrome
2. Klinefelter's syndrome
3. Turner's syndrome
4. Wolfram's syndrome
5. Friedreich's ataxia
6. Huntington's chorea
7. Lawrence Moon Beidel syndrome
8. Myotonic dystrophy
9. Porphyria
10. Prader–Willi syndrome
11. Others

IV. Gestational diabetes mellitus (GDM)

Appendix C

DIABETIC KETOACIDOSIS INTRAVENOUS INSULIN PROTOCOL

1. Test for urine ketones and blood glucose on admission (bedside monitoring of glucose is permissible unless the glucose value exceeds the limits of the bedside monitor).
2. Stat: complete blood count, multichemical profile-6 or -12 (electrolytes), blood urea nitrogen (BUN) and creatinine, and urinalysis. Call results. Bicarbonate level less than 10 mEq/L requires a critical care bed.
3. Repeat multichemical profile-6 every 2 hr × 2 and then every 4 hr × 2, then every 8 hr until the ketoacidosis has resolved. Call results.
4. Check urine samples with each voiding until negative for ketones.
5. Nothing by mouth. May have sips of sugar-containing clear liquids when blood sugar/electrolytes become stabilized and patient is without gastrointestinal distress (usually <300 ml/dl).
6. Start intravenous fluids of 1,000 cc normal saline @ ____ml/hr with potassium chloride of ___mEq or potassium phosphate ____mmol/L added.
7. If BS greater than 500, give ____Units human U100 regular insulin by intravenous push (0.1 Unit/kg) one time only. Recheck blood sugar in 30 min.
8. U100 human regular insulin, 50 Units to 50 ml of normal saline by an intravenous pump. Run @ ___Units/hr ($0.1\ Unit \cdot kg \cdot hr^{-1}$).
9. When blood sugar falls approximately to 250 mg/dl (13.89 mmol) or ½ of the admitting blood sugar, add 1,000 ml of D5-½ normal saline or D10 ½ normal saline at __/hr. Add KCl____ mEq or KPO_4____mmol/L to above solution.
10. Measure blood glucose level hourly, at bedside, or by lab if the value exceeds the limits of the bedside meter.
11. Blood glucose should fall by 50–100 mg/dl (2.8–5.6 mmol/L) hourly, and insulin may be titrated at nurse's discretion to maintain that rate of fall.
12. If blood glucose does not fall by 50 mg/dl (2.8 mmol/l)/hr, increase insulin infusion by 1 Unit greater per hr. If blood glucose falls more than 100 mg/dl (5.6 mmol/L) per hr, decrease insulin 1–2 Units less per hour.
13. Maintain blood glucose 100–200 mg/dl (5.6–11 mmol/L).
14. If blood glucose is less than 100 mg/dl (5.6 mmol/L), shut autosyringe off. Recheck blood glucose in a half-hour until blood sugar is more than 100 mg/dl (5.6 mmol/L) and then restart the insulin pump on a lower dosage. If the blood glucose becomes greater than 200 mg/dl (11.1 mmol/L),

restart insulin as needed. Physicians to be notified when blood glucose remains less than 100 mg/dl (5.6 mmol/L) for more than 2 hr.

15. Routine hypoglycemia orders.
16. Telemetry: Yes ___ No ___.
17. O$_2$ as needed per nurse's discretion (e.g., 2–3 L as needed).
18. Vital signs every 2 hr × 8 hr.

Appendix D

MODIFIED YALE INSULIN INFUSION MANAGEMENT

(Non-DKA Orders: Adult patients >40 kg)

- Complete blood cell count (CBC) and basic metabolic panel unless done in the last 24 hours.
- Vital signs hourly or as predetermined.
- IV fluid: 0.9% NaCl at ___ml/hr (when blood glucose < or = to 250 mg/dl [13.8 mmol] change IV fluid to D5/0.9% NaCl at the same rate).
- Human short-acting insulin 1 Unit/1 ml 0.9% NaCl (administer via infusion pump in increments of 0.5 Unit/hr).
- Starting insulin dose: 0.05 Unit/kg body weight per hour and adjust as needed.
- Goal: maintain blood glucose (BG) between 90 and 119 mg/dl (5–6.6 mmol).
- Monitoring: check BG every hour until stable (three consecutive values within target range) then checks can be reduced to every 2 hr × 4 checks; then every 4 hr if BG remains in desired range.
- Resume every-hour checks in BG monitoring if any change in insulin infusion rate occurs; if there are significant changes in clinical condition; if pressor or steroid therapy is initiated or stopped; if there is initiation or cessation of renal replacement therapy, i.e., hemodialysis, etc.; if there is initiation, cessation, or rate change of nutritional support (total parenteral nutrition, tube feedings, etc.).
- If continuous IV insulin therapy is ordered when the patient eats food by mouth, the health professional must start the transition plan to subcutaneous administration (see Appendix E).
- Subcutaneous insulin must be started in a timely manner before IV insulin is discontinued, otherwise there will be a gap in insulin coverage.
- If BG is lower than 50 mg/dl (2.7 mmol), discontinue infusion and give D50W 20 ml IV; recheck BG every 15 min; when BG ≥ 90 mg/dl (5 mmol), wait 1 hr, recheck BG; if still ≥ 90 mg/dl (5 mmol) then restart insulin infusion at 50% of the previous rate.
- If BG is 50–69 mg/dl (2.7–3.8 mmol), discontinue infusion—if symptomatic (or unable to assess) give D50W 50 mg IV (2.7 mmol); recheck BG every 15 min until BG is more than 100 mg/dl (5.5 mmol); if asymptomatic, give D50W 25 ml IV or 8 ounces of juice; recheck BG every 15 min until BG is more than 100 mg/dl (5.5 mmol); when BG is more than 90 mg/dl (5 mmol), wait 1 hr, recheck BG; if still more than 90 mg/dl (5 mmol), then restart infusion at 75% of previous rate.

■ If BG is more than 70 mg/dl (3.8 mmol), do the following: (1) determine the current BG level; (2) determine the hourly rate of change from the prior BG level and move to the right, referring to the table below, i.e., hourly rate of change in GB = change in BG divided by the number of hours between checks.

BG 70–89 (4–5 mmol)	BG 90–119 (5+–6 mmol)	BG 120–170 (6+–9 mmol)	BG ≥180 (10 mmol)	Change
		BG up by >40 mg/dl	BG up	IV 2×
	BG up by >20 mg/dl	BG up by 1–40 mg/dl	BG un-changed	IV 1×
		Or BG unchanged	Or BG down 41–80 mg/dl	
BG up	BG up by 1–20 mg/dl	BG down by 1–40 mg/dl	BG down by 41–80	No Chg
		BG unchanged or BG down 1–20 mg/dl		
BG un-changed or	BG down by 21–40	BG down by 41–80 mg/dl	BG down by 81–120 mg/dl	IV 1×
BG down by 1–20 mg/dl				
BG down >20 mg/dl	BG down by >40 mg/dl	BG down by 80 mg/dl	BG down >120 mg/dl	Hold[a]

Current Rate (units/hr)	1× Rate Change (units/hr)	2× Rate Change (units/hr)
<3	0.5	1
3–6	1	2
6.5–9.5	1.5	3
10–14.5	2	4
15–19.5	3	6
20–24.5	4	8
≥25	≥5	10 (consult MD)

[a]Discontinue insulin infusion: check BG every 30 min; when BG ≥ 90, restart infusion at 75% of most recent rate or 2× rate of change lower.

Appendix E

TRANSITION FROM INTRAVENOUS TO SUBCUTANEOUS INSULIN—GUIDELINES

General Guidelines

1. The half-life of IV insulin is 3–4 min; therefore, there must be subcutaneous insulin in place before the IV insulin is discontinued.
2. Regular insulin takes 1–2 hr to begin acting.
3. Rapid-acting insulin analogs (Novolog, Humalog, and Apidra) act in 5–15 min.
4. Neutral protamine Hagedorn (NPH) insulin acts in 1–2 hr.
5. Long-acting insulin analogs (Lantus and Levemir) act in 2 hr.
6. IV insulin infusion should be continuous until the patient is ready to leave the intensive care unit, or until the patient is ready to eat regular food and the subcutaneous insulin has begun to be absorbed.
7. Optimal treatment is with a long-acting insulin analog (Lantus or Levemir) given the night before the IV insulin is discontinued, then stop the IV infusion at a meal time and give a rapid-acting insulin with the meal.

Specific Guidelines

No Known Diabetes Prior to Admission

In persons with no known diabetes prior to admission, the diabetes may be stress induced and may disappear when the stressor is past. In this case, no insulin may be needed once the stressor is past. Blood glucose levels should be measured until there is proof that they are normal and stable. Many of these people, however, may be people with undiagnosed diabetes and may need continued treatment. An elevated HbA1c may clarify this issue. Even in people with stress diabetes that may remit, insulin should be given until blood glucose levels are normalized with no insulin. A good starting insulin dose is $0.5 \text{ Unit·kg}^{-1} \text{·day}^{-1}$.

Patients on Insulin Prior to Admission

There are several ways to calculate the subcutaneous insulin doses after IV insulin doses.

1. Use the patient's previous insulin doses or
2. Calculate a total daily dose based on body weight (usually $0.5 \text{ Unit·kg}^{-1}\text{·day}^{-1}$) or

3. Calculate the total amount of insulin given IV in the last 24 hr. This can be done by actual addition or by using the last 4 hr and multiplying by 6. This latter method is best because the IV dose usually comes down with time after the initial event (myocardial infarction, surgery, etc.). If the actual total amount given IV in the last 24 hr is used, then the total should be reduced by 20% to compensate for the decreasing requirement.

4. By whatever method used, calculate the total daily insulin dose (TDI) and divide as follows: 50% of the TDI is given as long-acting insulin (Lantus or Levemir) at bedtime, 20% of the TDI is given as rapid-acting insulin (Novolog, Humalog, or Apidra) with breakfast, 13% as rapid-acting insulin at lunch, and 17% at supper.

> Breakfast: 20% of TDI as rapid-acting insulin
> Lunch: 13% of TDI as rapid-acting insulin
> Supper: 17% of TDI as rapid-acting insulin
> Bedtime: 50% of TDI as long-acting insulin

Patients With Type 2 Diabetes on Oral Agent(s)

1. If the diabetes is well controlled prior to admission (check HbA1c) and the incidence of hospitalization mild, the oral agents may be resumed when the IV insulin is discontinued.

2. In most cases, the insulin should be continued and given as above, starting with a dose of 0.5 Unit·kg^{-1}·day^{-1}.

Patients on Enteral or Parenteral Feedings

1. Patients on parenteral feeding should be continued on IV insulin until an oral intake is established. Insulin put into the parenteral feeding bag is often precipitated on the bag in variable amounts (35%–65%) and leads to unstable management.

2. Patients on enteral feeding may be managed by IV insulin or by subcutaneous insulin.

3. Subcutaneous insulin may be given differently depending on the enteral feeding method. If the feeding is given by continuous feeding, the insulin management may be different than if the feeding is given by bolus.

   a. If the feeding is given by bolus, the insulin may be given as a long-acting insulin at bedtime and a bolus of insulin as regular or a short-acting analog with each bolus.

   b. If the feeding is given continuously, the insulin may be given as regular every 6 hr, a rapid-acting analog every 4 hr, or as a long-acting analog once per day with or without a rapid- or short-acting insulin.

4. Regular insulin every 6 hr may be calculated by any of the above methods if a previous dose is not known. The total daily dose is then divided into 4 equal doses. Blood glucose is measured every 6 hr before each insulin dose. BG call parameters are given to the nurses and if the value is outside the

call parameters the total daily dose is changed and redivided into 4 equal doses. Some long-acting insulin may be given once a day and this amount subtracted from the total before the q 6 hr regular dose is calculated.

Abbreviations

TDI = Total daily insulin dosage
RAI = Rapid-acting insulin = Novolog, Humalog, or Apidra
SAI = Short-acting insulin = regular insulin
IAI = Intermediate-acting insulin = NPH insulin
LAI = Long-acting insulin = Lantus or Levemir
BG = Blood glucose level
ISF = Insulin sensitivity factor

Correction Doses

Correction doses of insulin may be calculated by various means such as 10% of the TDI, or as 1 Unit for every 50 mg over target, but the recommended method is the 1,700 rule of Bode, Tamborlane, and Davidson (2002).

1,700 RULE:

1,700/TDI = the insulin sensitivity factor, or ISF
ISF = How many mg/dl 1 Unit of insulin will decrease BG levels
BG target/ISF = Units of insulin needed:
Example: TDI = 50 Units; BG 300; Target = 140 mg/dl (mmol)
1,700/50 = 34 – the ISF
300 – 140 = 160
160/34 = 4.7 Units (round off to 5 Units of insulin)

Note. Correction dose should be given at the time the BG is determined and, if recurrent, should be added to the preceding insulin dose. When a rapid-acting insulin is being used before meals, it is important to check the blood glucose levels 2 hr postprandial rather than premeal, because the effective duration of action of these insulins is 3–4 hr.

Reference

Bode, B. W., Tamborlane, W. V., & Davidson, P. C. (2002). Insulin pump therapy in the 21st century. Strategies for successful use in adults, adolescents, and children with diabetes. *Postgraduate Medicine, 111*(5), 69–77.

Appendix F

INSULIN DURING ENTERAL OR PARENTERAL FEEDINGS

Insulin for patients with diabetes on enteral feedings:

- Determine whether the enteral feeding is to be by continuous tube feeding or by intermittent bolus tube feeding.
- If by continuous feeding, the following methods may be used:
- IV insulin per the modified Yale protocol[1] (cardiac monitoring must be available) or
- 25% of the total daily insulin dose as regular insulin every 6 hr or
- Basal insulin alone as Lantus or Levemir or
- Basal insulin at 50% of the total daily insulin and the remainder as bolus insulin with short-acting insulin 6 hr or rapid-acting insulin every 4 hr.
- If feeding is given by bolus, give 50% of the total daily dose as basal insulin and the remainder as short- or rapid-acting insulin pre-bolus of feeding, that is, use short-acting insulin if 4 feedings per day or rapid-acting insulin if 6 feedings per day.
- If the volume or concentration of the feedings changes, the insulin must be recalculated accordingly.
- Blood glucose levels should be determined as per feeding protocol, that is, hourly for the modified Yale protocol and before each insulin dose for the other protocols.
- Based on the blood glucose level, the total daily insulin dose, not just the bolus dose, should be changed and the individual doses recalculated according to the formulas above.
- Sliding scale insulin is not appropriate for this therapy.

Insulin for patients with diabetes on total parenteral nutrition (TPN):

- Nothing by mouth.
- None or limited insulin in the TPN fluid.[2]
- Insulin may be given by any of the following methods:
- IV per the modified Yale protocol with the IV insulin "piggy-backed" on the IV fluid line or
- The patient's total daily insulin given as short-acting insulin subcutaneously (sub-Q)—25% of total daily insulin (TDI) every 6 hr or
- Basal insulin (50% of the TDI as Lantus or Levemir) every 24 hr and the remainder as rapid-acting insulin (17% of TDI) every 4 hr sub-Q.

473

- Blood glucose measurement should be performed hourly for IV insulin, and before each insulin dose for sub-Q insulin.
- For IV insulin, dosage of insulin should be modified by the Yale protocol.
- For sub-Q insulin, the 24-hr insulin dose should be modified by the BG level, then the every-6-hr doses or the every-4-hr doses divided by the appropriate percentage.
- Sliding scales are not appropriate for TPN use.

1. Modified Yale protocol—see Appendix D.
2. Studies have shown that variable amounts of insulin electrostatically cling to the bottle and tubing, so control of blood glucose levels cannot be tightly controlled by insulin in the TPN fluids. In addition, insulin in the TPN flows at the rate of the TPN fluid and thus cannot be controlled for the insulin sensitivity of the patient or renal excretion rate. Small amounts of insulin can be put in the TPN especially when sub-Q insulin is used but should not be relied on as the primary source of insulin for the patient.

Appendix G

INTERVAL HISTORY

PRIMARY CARE PHYSICIAN	PATIENT	
ADDRESS	ACCOUNT NO.	SEX
	DATE OF LAST VISIT	DATE OF BIRTH

PREV. HEIGHT in.	CURRENT HT. in.	PREV. WT. lbs.	CURRENT WT. lbs.	WT. CHG. lbs.	INSULIN			
B.P.	L.M.P.		E.D.C.		BRAND OF INSULIN	BRAND OF PUMP	PEN	DILUTION

DIABETES ONSET	CLASS DATE	PLACE OF ED	(C) COMPLETED (P) PARTIAL

TIME	DOSE	TYPE
A.M.		
NOON		
P.M.		
H.S.		
OTHER/BASAL RATES		

KEY PROBLEMS OR QUESTIONS

DIET

NO. CALORIES PER DAY	CALORIES CHANGED TO	NO. MEALS	NO. SNACKS

☐ EXCHANGES ☐ CHO ☐ POINTS ☐ CALORIES ☐ OTHER ☐ NO PLAN

FOOD: ☐ WEIGHED ☐ MEASURED ☐ ESTIMATED

TOTAL UNITS	COMMENTS

GLUCOSE MONITORING

BLOOD (AVERAGES)	NO. PER DAY	PER WEEK	☐ NO RECORDS
METHOD(S)			FASTING
PC BREAKFAST	AC LUNCH		PC LUNCH
AC SUPPER	PC SUPPER		HS
OTHER		OVERALL	

HYPOGLYCEMIA

NO. PER MONTH	UNCONSCIOUS SINCE LAST VISIT ☐ YES ☐ NO
USUAL TIME OF DAY	SEVERITY / SYMPTOMS

EXERCISE

TYPE / AMOUNT

URINE TESTING AVAILABLE
KETONES ☐ YES ☐ NO. BRAND:
COMMENTS:

MEDICATION

NAME OF MEDICATION / DOSAGE	D.C.	NAME OF MEDICATION / DOSAGE	D.C.

LAB RESULTS

URINE TEST				BLOOD TEST		TEST (TIME)	LAST FOOD (TIME)	LAST INSULIN (TIME)
GLUCOSE		PROTEIN	+	GLUCOSE	mg/dl	am/pm	am/pm	am/pm
KETONES	+	PH		RECHECK GLUCOSE	mg/dl	am/pm	_____ Hgb A1c/DATE	
OTHER				TREATMENT:			_____ CHOL/DATE	

FINDINGS & RECOMMENDATIONS

DATE OF LAST COMPLETE FOOT EXAM: _____ LAST DILATED EYE EXAM: _____

Review of History	Comments	Education/Review
Surgery/Illness/Hospitalization		Meter Technique Nutrition Review
Renal	Proteinuria _____ Alb/Cr Ratio: _____	Insulin Administration Med Review
Thyroid		Problem Solving
Neurological		Risk Reduction
Cardiovascular	Lipids: date _____ LDL _____ HDL _____ Trig _____ ASA Yes ____ No ____ Pulse _____ BP _____	
Growth/Development Nutritional Status		

Chief Complaint/Psychosocial/Concerns

Glucose Control

Assessment

Plan

_____ INSTRUCTIONS PROVIDED

DIAGNOSIS

☐ DM, Type 1   ☐ DM, Type 2
☐ C   ☐ UC   ☐ C   ☐ UC   ☐ GDM   ☐ PRE DIABETES   ☐ Other _____

COMPLICATIONS

☐ NEUROPATHY   ☐ NEPHROPATHY   ☐ RETINOPATHY   ☐ HYPERTENSION   ☐ CAD   ☐ PVD   ☐ HYPERLIPIDEMIA   ☐ HYPOTHYROIDISM

LAB ORDERED/RECOMMENDED:

☐ A_1C ☐ MCAB   ☐ T_4 ☐ LIVER ENZYMES   ☐ TSH   ☐ LIPID PROFILE   ☐ _____ CULTURE

☐ CBC   ☐ SMAC   ☐ FRUCTOSAMINE   ☐ 12/24 HR + TP/CC   ☐ OTHER _____

RETURN IN:
_____ WEEKS
_____ MONTHS

PHYSICIAN / PROVIDER SIGNATURE

_____   _____
R. A. GUTHRIE, M.D. / B. P. CHILDS, ARNP / D. W. GUTHRIE, ARNP   DIABETES EDUCATOR

Appendix H

SELF-CARE HISTORY
Mid-America Diabetes Associates, PA

NAME:	DATE:

What are your concerns you would like to discuss during today's visit?

Do you follow a meal plan for diabetes management? Please circle below:
Calories, Points, Carbs, Exchanges, Other_____ Do you have a calorie goal? _____

LIST THE FOODS/BEVERAGES THAT YOU TYPICALLY EAT IN A DAY AND YOUR INSULIN DOSES AND TIMES IF YOU TAKE INSULIN: (MEAL EXAMPLE: 1 c. 2% milk, 1 fried chicken thigh, 1/2 cup mashed potatoes)

First Meal: Usual Time _____ Insulin Dose(s): _____ Insulin type: _____
Food/Beverages:

Second Meal: Usual Time _____ Insulin Dose(s): _____ Insulin type: _____
Food/Beverages:

Third Meal: Usual Time _____ Insulin Dose(s): _____ Insulin type: _____
Food/Beverages:

Do you eat snacks? Yes ☐ No ☐ If so, what time of day? _____
Typical Food/Beverages:
If you are on insulin, do you take insulin with snacks? Yes ☐ No ☐ If Yes, what dose?

Morning basal insulin (i.e. Lantus/Levemir/ 70/30) insulin type _____ dose _____ time _____
Evening or Bedtime Insulin type: _____ dose: _____ usual time: _____

Pump Basal Rates: _____
Name of Insulin Pump: _____
If you are on insulin or insulin pump, what sites do you use? Circle: arms legs abdomen back hips other _____
Do you have lumps or dips where you give shots? Yes ☐ No ☐ Do your shots burn? Yes ☐ No ☐ Bleed? Yes ☐ No ☐

Brand of Glucose Meter | **Do you have control solution?**

Enter your ACTUAL average blood glucose from your downloaded meter or record book:
(Our medical assistant will be happy to assist you if needed)

Breakfast		Lunch		Supper		Bed-time	Other
Before	After	Before	After	Before	After		

Reaction/Blood Sugars below 60 (Number past month) _____

Any resulting in unconsciousness: ☐ Yes ☐ No How many? _____

How was the severe low treated? _____

PHYSICAL ASSESSMENT HISTORY

PLEASE ANSWER THE FOLLOWING QUESTIONS BY CHECKING THE CORRECT BOX OR FILLING IN THE UPDATE INFORMATION. INFORMATION SHOULD RELATE TO THE LAST FEW WEEKS UNLESS OTHERWISE INDICATED.

HEALTH QUESTIONS	YES	NO	COMMENTS
Any headaches?			
Any sore or bleeding gums?			
Do you wear dentures?			
Any unusual dryness of skin? Heel cracks?			
Any rash or unusual discoloration to the skin?			
Any feelings of being too hot or too cold?			
Any chest pain or feelings of chest tightness?			
Any numbness, tingling, burning, or pain in feet or hands?			
Any difficulty breathing or shortness of breath?			
Any dizziness when standing?			
Do you snore or have you been told you snore?			
Do you wake up tired after a full night's sleep?			
Any abdominal cramps, diarrhea, or constipation?			
For women, vaginal discharge?			
Women please list the date of your last menstrual period.			
Any pain or burning on urination?			
Any incontinence or loss of urine?			
Problems with sexual functioning			
Any muscle aches, pains, backache, leg cramps?			
Any joint aches or pains? Where?			
Do you have any vision changes?			
Do you wear glasses or contacts?			
Do you smoke or use other tobacco products? What and how much?			
Do you use alcohol? How much, how often?			
Date of last visit to the eye doctor?			
Date of last visit to dentist? Foot Doctor?			
Do you feel you are under stress? ☐ Mild ☐ Moderate ☐ A lot of pressure			
In the past month, have you been bothered by feeling down, depressed or hopeless? Yes ☐ No ☐			
Had little pleasure or interest in doing anything? Yes ☐ No ☐			
Do you participate in physical activity? Yes ☐ No ☐ What and how often?			

Please review your medication list and note any changes and/or prescriptions that need filled.

****

Appendix I

PATIENT RECOMMENDATIONS
(Take Home Sheet)

Name: _____ Date of Appointment: _____

Height: _____ Weight: _____ Weight Change: _____ Blood Glucose: _____ Urine Leukocytes: _____

Blood Pressure: _____ Urine Protein: _____ Urine Ketones: _____

	Time	Amount	Type
INSULIN:	Breakfast	_____ units	_____
	Lunch/Noon	_____ units	_____
	Dinner	_____ units	_____
	Bedtime	_____ units	_____

MEDICATION: _____

_____

POINTS: Breakfast _____ AM Snack _____ Lunch _____

Afternoon Snack _____ Dinner _____ Bedtime Snack _____

Follow-up with dietitian in _____ weeks. Total Calories: _____

GLUCOSE MONITORING: Do Blood Sugars _____ times per day.

_____ days per week.

Usual Times to Test: Fasting and 2 hours after each meal or before each meal and bedtime (4 times a day).
ALWAYS BRING YOUR GLUCOSE RECORDS TO YOUR APPOINTMENT.
If lab is done at another lab, please bring copies or have results faxed to us.

Call (316) 687-3100 or Fax (316) 687-4491 your blood sugars to _____ in _____ days.
Write your name and a phone number to call on your fax, please. Include your current diabetes medication.

EXERCISE: _____

ADDITIONAL COMMENTS: _____

GOALS FOR NEXT VISIT: _____

Please Remember:
1. Always bring blood sugar and food records.
2. 18 yrs. +: Foot check 2-4 times a year.
3. 18 yrs. +: Eye checks yearly.
4. Dentist: Every 6 months.
5. Aspirin if > 30 years old.
6. A yearly lipid screen.

_____
Physician/Diabetes Educator

Appendix J

NUTRITION ASSESSMENT

Date _____

Name _____ Date diabetes was diagnosed _____

Height _____ Weight _____ Age ____ Desired weight _____

What was your highest weight (nonpregnant)? _____ When _____

Has your weight changed in the past 6 months? _____
    Lbs lost or gained _____

How many meals do you eat daily? _____
    How many snacks daily? _____

Do you consider yourself sedentary _____ moderately active _____
    active _____

How many meals a week do you eat away from home at the following places:

fast food _____ cafeteria or restaurant _____ sack lunch_____

senior citizen center _____other (specify) _____

Who cooks at home? _____ Who shops for food? _____

Please check yes or no for the following

Yes	No	Do You:
___	___	Have a good appetite?
___	___	Have food allergies?
___	___	Have trouble chewing or swallowing?
___	___	Have constipation or diarrhea?
___	___	Have adequate funds for food?
___	___	Live alone?
___	___	Buy dietetic or health food?
___	___	Take vitamins or mineral pills?
___	___	Take laxatives?
___	___	Take herbs?
___	___	Are you on a special diet? If yes, what kind?

Daily calories _____ Do you use calorie points? _____

Exchanges _____ Carb counting _____

What medication(s) do you take? _____

Typical Daily Food Intake

Please write down everything you would eat or drink in a typical day, including snacks and beverages. Include sugar, salad dressing, butter, cream, and so forth.

What type of milk do you use? Skim ____ 2% ____ Whole ____

Three- to five-day food history: Please be specific about the types of foods and amounts you eat

Time   Food eaten   Amount

_____

_____

_____

_____

_____

_____

_____

_____

Appendix K

What Happens in Type 2 Diabetes?

The fuel your body runs on is glucose. Where does that come from? — the food eaten. The food begins to break down in the stomach and completes the break-down in the small intestine. From there, it is absorbed by the blood. So blood sugar goes up. If diabetes is not present, the increase in blood sugar triggers a release of insulin by the pancreas.

Insulin is the hormone that helps the fuel (glucose) to get into the muscle and fat cells of the body. These cells are like the engine of your car. They have to have fuel to run. In your car, you may have a tank full of gas, but you don't go anywhere until you get the fuel into the engine. You have to turn the key to get the fuel to the engine so the car can go. So, in your body, you have to have the key (insulin) to help get the glucose into the engine (muscle and fat cells).

The liver plays a role in diabetes as well. One of the liver's jobs is to be a big storage tank. You use some of the glucose from the food you eat shortly after the meal, but the glucose you don't need is stored as sugar in the liver. The liver is supposed to let little bits of sugar out into the bloodstream when you are not eating, as at night.

Now, we have learned in recent years that other hormones play a role in this process as well. The gut hormones have an impact on Type 2 diabetes mellitus (T2DM). The gut hormones' number 1 job is to nudge the pancreas to secrete the right amount of insulin at the right time. These "helper hormones" from the gut help all the steps to work better. They help the liver not overreact and dump in too much previously stored sugar, especially after a meal. They also help a person feel full.

What Changes When You Get T2DM?

Insulin resistance increases and the beta cells can't keep up. Insulin resistance is related to the liver. Remember, one of the liver's jobs is to store the extra sugar that you don't need after you eat a meal. In T2DM, instead of the liver letting a little bit of sugar out into the system when you aren't eating, the liver "dumps" sugar into the system. This happens after meals and especially at night. If your liver is dumping sugar into the system, especially at night, which blood sugars will be the highest? The answer is the fasting blood sugars, first thing in the morning. You can remember this by thinking of "leaky liver."

Another part of the insulin resistance story is related to the glucose trying to get into the cells. Insulin has to fit on to the outside of the cell. Think of a jigsaw puzzle piece. If you think of insulin as having that little notch, it has to fit onto the outside of the cell just right. If it fits *and* everything else inside the cell is working just right, the cell doors open and the glucose can get inside the cell. Then the muscle cells need energy to do their work. Now, if some of the insulin doesn't fit just right, or there isn't enough insulin, or the internal workings of the cell aren't up to speed, then the doors don't come open. Some of the cells don't get glucose and they are starving. What message do you think that sends to your brain? You're hungry . . . Please eat . . . No problem. So as you eat more, the food breaks down to glucose, the blood sugar levels go up, the message goes to the pancreas . . . "We need more insulin."

So, the pancreas is working double time. When the pancreas gets to the point it can't make enough insulin is when the beta cells begin dying and the diabetes is diagnosed.

In fact, before you get diabetes, the pancreas is putting out a lot more insulin than you would normally need. When the pancreas can't keep making insulin fast enough, and the beta cell begins to fail, that is when the diabetes is diagnosed. At the time you are diagnosed, you are down about 50% on your insulin-producing beta cells. Your insulin-producing beta cells die faster than they can reproduce.

Another bad actor in this story is fat. We used to think fat just sat there, being ugly, but not really causing any harm. Now we know that fat actually breaks down and causes destruction of the insulin-producing beta cells. It also can produce hormones that stimulate your appetite and cause you to want to eat more.

So we have several problems going on internally that make the sugars go up:

1. Leaky Liver, the liver is dumping glucose into the system after meals and at night, and
2. The "doors are locked" and the cells can't get the sugar inside because of insulin resistance, and
3. The pancreas is not making enough insulin, beta cells are down by about 50%, and
4. There are decreased levels of gut hormones.

We have learned that the gut hormones play a role in keeping the glucose levels in control. In T2DM, the gut hormones are diminished. Research tells us that the gut hormones help the other steps, which we just talked about, work better. So if your gut hormones aren't up to speed, your insulin may not be coming out at the right amounts after the meals, the liver may be dumping too much sugar into the bloodstream, especially after meals, the food may be leaving the stomach too fast, and you may be feeling hungry most of the time. Now we have discovered several other reasons that your system may be getting signals to eat. The extra pounds and the decrease in activity will make the insulin resistance worse.

So How Do We Tackle These Problems?

If you are making enough insulin internally, you may be able to control your blood sugars with diet and exercise for a while.

Stretching out the food throughout the day makes a big difference in the way your body can handle the calories. If your pancreas is making some insulin, you want to eat smaller amounts and maybe your pancreas can make enough insulin to keep up with a smaller amount of food. Often in America, we don't eat breakfast, we have a small lunch, but supper goes from 6 p.m. to 10 p.m. So we are hitting our bodies with the equivalent of Thanksgiving dinner every evening. No way can your pancreas keep up with that kind of eating. Modest-sized meals with a mix of protein, fat, and carbohydrate will help your pancreas have a chance to "keep up."

Exercise works like "invisible insulin." If your body doesn't have as much insulin as it used to, you want every bit of the insulin you still have to be able to work for you. Exercise helps the "doors open" at the level of the muscle and fat cells.

Now, if you eat less and exercise more, you may lose some weight. This will make a difference in your blood sugars as well. Ten pounds of weight loss is a great goal to get started.

Appendix L

HYPERGLYCEMIA MANAGEMENT FOR PREOPERATIVE PATIENTS

- Nothing by mouth.
- If on metformin, discontinue the day before surgery.
- Check early a.m. blood glucose (e.g., 05:30).
- If blood glucose is 150 mg/dl (8.3 mmol), notify surgeon for orders or request "Hyperglycemia Management for Preoperative Patients."
- For the person with known diabetes:

Determine the usual Total Daily Insulin 24-hr dosage (includes all insulin types).

- Divide 1,700 by the amount of total daily insulin to equal the Insulin Sensitivity Factor (ISF).
- Find the differences between the current blood glucose and 150.
- Divide this number by the ISF. This is the dose to give of subcutaneous rapid-acting insulin required.
- Monitor blood glucose every 30 min until patient's blood glucose is <150 mg/dl (8.3 mmol), and as needed until the patient goes into surgery.
- Notify attending surgeon if blood glucose is not decreasing.

Example: The patient's blood glucose is 300 mg/dl (16.6 mmol). Their usual daily insulin need is 50 Units. Take 1,700 ÷ 50 = 34 (the ISF); subtract 150 from 300 to equal the difference between actual and desired BG; 150 divided by the ISF (34) equals 4.4 Units (round to 4 Units) of rapid-acting insulin.

- Give initial rapid-acting insulin subcutaneously. If the dose is greater than 10 Units, check calculations with another health professional before giving.
- Document initial and succeeding blood glucose levels and interventions.
- Repeat dose correction calculation every hour until blood glucose is below 150 mg/dl (8.3 mmol) and document.

Appendix M

Topics That Might Be Questioned or Taught at Some Point

I. What is diabetes mellitus?

   A. Diabetes mellitus is a chronic disease in which there is an inadequate supply of insulin or a complete lack of insulin for the inside of the cell; thus, insulin is unable to assist in the body process of metabolizing or burning carbohydrates, protein, or fats.

   B. Basic information that makes diabetes such an important disease

   C. Proposed causes of diabetes

      1. Heredity

         (a) Genetic theories
         (b) Implications of genetics

      2. Infection of pancreas
      3. Tumor of pancreas
      4. Injury or removal of pancreas
      5. Use of stress medications (steroids)
      6. Other illness (pheochromocytoma, hemochromatosis)

   D. Diagnosis criteria and causes

      1. Overt diabetes: elevated fasting and/or 2 hr or random blood glucose level (abnormal results from oral glucose tolerance test as needed)

         (a) Type 1 diabetes: insulin dependent
         (b) Type 2 diabetes: insulin resistant or insulin requirement

      2. Prediabetes: fasting blood sugar 100 to 110 mg/dl (5.5–6.1 mmol); random blood sugar >140 mg/dl (7.7 mmol) or <200 mg/dl (11.1 mmol)
      3. Gestational diabetes: fasting blood sugar >110 mg/dl (6.1 mmol); 2 hr >149 mg/dl (7.7 mmol)
      4. Causes

II. Insulin and glucagon in the body

   A. Action of insulin

      1. Synthesis
      2. Release of insulin

3. Activity in circulation
4. Activity with the cell membrane

B. Action of glucagon

1. Cause of release
2. Response to release

III. Meal planning

A. Normal nutrition

1. Carbohydrates
2. Proteins
3. Fats
4. Vitamins and minerals
5. Calories

B. Nutrition choices—keeping track of basic needs

1. Exchange system
2. Points system
3. Carbohydrate counting
4. Calorie counting
5. Total available glucose system

C. Keeping food records

1. Following a system
2. Variation of a system
3. System during illness

D. Food and exercise

1. Increased exercise
2. Decreased exercise
3. Somogyi effect
4. Dawn phenomenon

E. Social events and travel

1. Dining out
2. Parties
3. Travel, including driving
4. Backpacking, hiking
5. Cultural differences
6. School/work

IV. Medications

A. Oral agents—use and action

1. Types of oral agents
2. Untoward effects
3. Use in the body

B. Insulin—use and action

1. Types of insulin (human: plain or designer)

(a) Rapid-acting insulin
(b) Short-acting insulin
(c) Intermediate-acting insulin
(d) Long-acting insulin
(e) Premixed insulin

2. Use in the body
3. Untoward effects

V. Insulin delivery systems and use

A. Syringes and needles (length and thickness)
B. Insulin pens (prefilled and cartridge filled)
C. Insulin pumps
D. Insulin aids (e.g., multiple doses through one diaphragm)
E. Injection procedures (including sites and angle of injection)
F. Mixing insulin in a syringe
G. Untoward effects

1. Hypertrophy
2. Atrophy
3. Allergic effects
4. Insulin resistance

H. How to care for supplies

1. Syringes
2. Pens
3. Infusion pumps

VI. Blood sugar/urine testing/monitoring procedures

A. Sticks
B. Monitoring

1. Home testing

(a) Glucose
(b) Ketones
(c) Cholesterol

2. Continuous testing
3. Hemoglobin A1c
4. Fructosamine test
5. Postmeal testing
6. Microalbumin
7. Metabolic profile
8. Lipid profile
9. Thyroid profile
10. Complete blood count
11. Estimated glomerular filtration rate

C. Test supplies and their care

VII. General hygiene

    A. Eye care (include routine check-up as well as check for retinopathy)
    B. Care of teeth
    C. Skin care

        1. General care
        2. Cuts and scratches
        3. Foot care

            (a) Observation—what to look for
            (b) Procedures—what to care for, equipment needed

VIII. Exercise

    A. Action of exercise

        1. Decreased exercise
        2. Increased exercise

    B. Food versus exercise
    C. Somogyi effect
    D. Types of exercise
    E. Developing an exercise program

IX. Recordkeeping

    A. What to record
    B. Why to record it
    C. Interpretation of recordings—what to do

        1. Blood glucose levels normal

            (a) Increased activity
            (b) Decreased activity
            (c) Increased hypoglycemia

        2. Patterned hyperglycemia same time of day

            (a) Decrease previous snack (or meal)
            (b) Increase previous snack and meal
            (c) Return food and increase insulin/or other medication as instructed
            (d) Expect to see decrease of glucose in blood/urine if exercise increased
            (e) When not to exercise

        3. Increased blood glucose levels

            (a) Increase of insulin or other diabetes medication
            (b) Decrease of food
            (c) Increase of exercise

        4. When to call the physician, nurse, dietitian, or other health professional

X. Psychologic adjustment

    A. Adjusting to a chronic illness
    B. Physical and mental changes caused by stress

        1. Symptoms of stress/depression
        2. Methods of handling stress

            (a) Relaxation
            (b) Meditation
            (c) Imagery
            (d) Biofeedback
            (e) Exercise

    C. Communicating with the family
    D. Human sexuality

XI. Illness

    A. Review of diet during illness

        1. Variations management
        2. Use of insulin
        3. Oral agents during illness

    B. When to notify the health professional

XII. Hypoglycemia

    A. Causes

        1. Glucose levels below 60 mg/dl (3.3 mmol)
        2. Blood glucose below accustomed levels
        3. Hypoglycemia unawareness

    B. Treatment

        1. Mild hypoglycemia: food
        2. Moderate hypoglycemia: simple sugar (20–40 calories)

            (a) Prepared products, tubed glucose, tablets
            (b) Household product—juice, table sugar, honey, other

        3. Severe hyperglycemia (seizure possibilities—keep airway open); glucagon

    C. Identification

        1. Bracelets
        2. Necklaces
        3. Cards
        4. School cards

    D. Prevention

XIII. Complications of diabetes

    A. Acute complications

        1. Diabetic ketoacidosis
        2. Hypoglycemia
        3. Hyperglycemic hyperosmolar nonketotic syndrome

    B. Intermediate complications

        1. Illness
        2. Pregnancy

            (a) Importance of prepregnancy planning
            (b) Emphasis on normal blood sugars during pregnancy

        3. Surgery
        4. Prolonged emotional crisis
        5. Dawn phenomenon
        6. Somogyi effect (rebound)

    C. Chronic complications

        1. Retinopathy
        2. Nephropathy
        3. Neuropathy
        4. Cardiomyopathy—macroangiopathy

XIV. Research

    A. Pancreatic replacement

        1. Islet/beta cell transplants
        2. Artificial pancreas

    B. New medications
    C. Genetic markers
    D. New instrumentation

XV. Review

    A. Return demonstration

        1. Meal plan
        2. Insulin procedure
        3. Urine test procedure
        4. Exercise plan
        5. Stress reduction plan
        6. Recordkeeping

    B. Description and treatment of:

        1. Hyperglycemia/hypoglycemia
        2. General discussion

      (a) Methods of communication

          i. Clinic
         ii. Phone
        iii. Letter
        iv. Record

      (b) Follow-up

          i. Clinic
         ii. American Diabetes Association
        iii. Continuing education
        iv. Other

      (c) When to call the health professional

XVI. Spirituality

  A. Preferences:

    1. General beliefs
    2. Concepts of self-worth
    3. Concept of self-efficacy
    4. Likes
    5. Dislikes
    6. Quiet-time practices
    7. Developing a quality of life

Appendix N

DOCUMENTATION OF TEACHING
COMPLETED OR IN PROGRESS

Patient Name: _____   Day—Evening—Gestational—Outreach

Special learning needs _____

Desired Health Outcomes:

Wt Loss ☒ Lower A1C ☒ Reduce Stress ☒ Keep BS 70–150 mg   Other _____

NA = Needs Assessment   PA = Post Assessment

TOPIC	NA	INSTRUCT DATE	RE-INSTRUCT	PA	NOTES/MATERIALS
OVERVIEW Type 1, 2, GDM Benefits/Risks of BS control					
GLUCOSE MONITORING					Meter type:
Schedule/Record Keeping					
Ketone Testing					
Other					
NUTRITION GUIDELINES					
Calorie Points/Carb Budgeting					
Lipid Management					
EXERCISE/ACTIVITY					
MEDICATIONS **INSULIN/ORAL AGENTS**					
Injection/Site Rotation					
Syringe/Pen/Pump					
HYPER/HYPOGLYCEMIA					
RELATIONSHIP of Nutrition, Meds, Exercise					
ILLNESS MANAGEMENT					
COMPLICATIONS/ **RISK REDUCTION**					
Hygiene Feet, Skin, Dental					
Travel/Alcohol/Drugs					
HOME PLAN					
PATTERN MANAGEMENT					
COMMUNITY RESOURCES					
STRESS-MANAGEMENT					
BEHAVIOR CHANGE/ **GOAL SETTING**					
Other					
PRECONCEPTION/PREGNANCY					
Other					
Intensive Insulin Tx Options					CSII FLOW SHEET
PUMP START					

S = safe: verbal understanding/return demo   L = limited understanding   N = needs more teaching/assistance   NIC = Not in Class

EDUCATORS: _____   _____   _____

497

Appendix O

JOINTLY DEVELOPED PATIENT OUTCOMES

Central objective: This is presented to assist the nurse or other health professional in supporting the patient to learn about themselves in relation to having diabetes, and the treatment, methods of communication, self-care, and (as appropriate) self-management, to live a safe, useful, and productive life.

Outcomes: On completion of this course/class/visit, the patient will (these are examples):

1. Define diabetes mellitus in a simplified way.
2. Describe the signs and symptoms of both hypoglycemia and hyperglycemia.
3. State how insulin helps their body.
4. Describe the problems related to glucose levels "out of control."
5. Describe treatments and actions, that is, call the office, for hypoglycemia and hyperglycemia.
6. Complete blood glucose monitoring as discussed in cooperation with recommendations.
7. Be able to or have a significant other know what to do in case of emergency.
8. State what an emergency might be.
9. Complete the process for testing blood glucose levels and ketone levels (as needed).
10. Correctly and safely administer medication by mouth and/or by injection.
11. Demonstrate blood sugar testing procedure(s) and describe an appropriate course of action for continued abnormal results.
12. Eat more nutritious meals in relation to content and amount.
13. Participate in increasing activity levels or participate in an exercise program.
14. List food intake variations for illness, travel, social events, and extra exercise.
15. Correctly take care of medication products and blood glucose supplies (and ketone test strips, if appropriate).
16. Describe and carry out good hygiene practices (e.g., brushing and flossing of teeth, checking feet frequently, and so on).

Appendix P

INDIVIDUAL ASSESSMENT QUESTIONNAIRE

Name _____ Interview date _____

Address _____

Birth Date _____ Phone no. _____

I. General appearance

    A. Color _____

    B. Mobility _____

    C. Communication _____

    D. Deformities _____

    E. Affect _____

    F. Obesity _____

II. Concept

    A. Concept of illness

        "Why are you here?"_____

        "What are you expecting at this time?"_____

    B. Concept of diabetes

        1. Diagnosed when _____

        2. "Do you recognize your reactions? yes ___ no___ ; treatment?"_____

        3. "Do you know when your blood sugars are high? yes___ no ___; treatment?"_____

        4. Testing, methods used and frequency:_____

        5. Previous class instruction: date _____ where ____

        6. "Are you or have you used a pen (yes ___ no ___) or a pump?" (yes___ no___)

        7. If on a pump—what are your basals? What is your range of boluses per meal and snack?

            _____

            _____

III. Physical history

   Temp _____ Pulse _____ Resp_____

   B/P_____ Height _____ Weight ___

A. Systems review

   1. Respiratory (smoker, SOB, and so forth) _____

   2. Circulatory (legs, edema, blood pressure problems) ____

   3. Sensory (blurry vision, ears, touch) _____

   4. GI (bowels, stomach, ulcers, elimination needs) ____

   5. GU (urinary, reproductive) _____

   6. Skin (feet, leg ulcers) _____

   7. Neuroskeletal (arthritis, neuritis, Parkinson's, CVA, Fx, and so forth) _____

   8. Metabolic (thyroid, diabetes) _____

B. Past hospitalizations and surgeries_____

   _____

C. Allergies (drug, food, cosmetics, tape, and so forth) _____

D. Medications (current); insulin (kinds and times) _____

E. Diet (Carb counting; exchanges; points); special needs; _____ snacks _____

F. Prosthesis

   1. Dentures (upper-lower, partial bridge) _____

   2. Glasses or contacts _____

   3. Other (limb, eyes; special equipment: walker, cane, and so forth) _____

IV. Personal data

A. Home life: who does the patient live with or near? ____

B. Social assistance (VNA, social welfare) _____

C. Spiritual needs: chaplain, pastor, priest, or rabbi to be notified?: Yes____ No____Contact: _____

V. Emotional state (check all that apply):

Alert	Confused	Fearful	Other
Angry	Critical	Hostile	
Answers questions readily	Demanding	Hyperactive	

Answers questions reluctantly   Disoriented   Tearful

Anxious   Embarrassed   Withdrawn

Belligerent   Euphoric

VI. Diabetes care

A. "Tell me what the doctor wants you to do about your blood (urine) test." _____

B. "What has been possible for you to do?"

   1. For blood sugar:

     Monitor name: _____

     Person tests ___times a day(s) _____/week

     Person does not test _____

     Demonstration outcome: _____

   2. For urine (blood) ketones:

     Person tests ___ times a day(s) _____/week

     Person does not test _____

     Demonstration outcome: _____

   3. Test correctly

     Yes_____ No_____

   4. Reads results correctly

     Yes_____ No_____

C. "Do you ever change the times you test your blood sugars?"

     Yes ___ No _____

     "Do you know when to test more frequently?"

     Yes _____ No _____

D. "Do you keep a written record?"_____

   1. "What do you include?"_____

   2. "Do you bring your record to the clinic?"_____

E. Insulin administration

   1. Injection sites:_____

   2. Demonstration outcome: _____

   3. Preparation of syringe (mixed and/or single dose) ____

     Or oral hypoglycemic agent _____

   4. Verbalized knowledge of uses, action, and appropriate administrative time

F. Diet management

1. Described diet management program exchanges, points, or carbohydrate

2. Notation of familiarity regarding: free foods, foods to avoid, and achieving and maintaining a desirable weight _____

3. Demonstrates knowledge of his/her meal plan: Yes ____ No____

4. Problems with meal planning _____

G. Concept of diabetes regulation

1. Explains causes, treatment, and prevention of hypoglycemia; recognizes symptoms _____

2. Explains causes, symptoms, treatment, and prevention of hyperglycemia _____

3. "What is the action of insulin?" _____

    (a) "What is your dosage?" _____

    (b) "When do you take it?" _____

    (c) "How does it work (timing)?"_____

4. "What is your exercise program?" _____

H. Complications

"Do you know the types (or names) of the complications associated with diabetes?"_____

I. Foot care

"What do you do to care for your feet?" _____

J. Illness

1. "What are you supposed to do during illness?" _____
    _____

2. "What are the signs and symptoms of ketoacidosis?"* _____
    _____

    * Note: Patient should indicate that illness, especially infection, vomiting, diarrhea, and uncontrolled stress levels, may precipitate ketoacidosis.

VII. Interviewer's comments

LABORATORY AND ASSESSMENT GUIDELINES FOR CARE*

	Ideal	Acceptable
Fasting and Preprandial	<100 (5.5 mmol)	80–120
Bedtime Glucose & post meal	<110 (6.1 mmol)	100–140
Plasma		
Fasting and Preprandial	<110 (6.1 mmol)	90–130
Bedtime Glucose & post meal	<120 (6.7 mmol)	110–150
Glycated hemoglobin (HbAlc)	<6% if safely done	<7%

For Lipid and Blood Pressure Goals

Cholesterol	<200	Systolic	<130
LDL-C	<100 (2.6 mmol); preferably <70	Diastolic	<80
(For children –	<110) (2.8 mmol)	(BP to age-adjusted 90th percentile)	
HDL-C	>45 for women and 35 men (1.15 mmol)		
Triglycerides	<150		

Key Tests/Exams

Glycated hemoglobin	Quarterly; 2 times/year if stable
Dilated eye exam	Yearly (10 yrs of age–3–5 years from diagnosis; all patients checked yearly after age 30)
Foot exam	Every regular visit; thorough every visit if insensate; or once a year if sensate
Lipid profile	Yearly (more frequently if abnormal or taking lipid-lowering medication – i.e., every 6 mo.)
Urinalysis	Yearly
Protein	Yearly microalbumin if negative for gross protein
	Preferably by albumin-creatinine ratio in a random, spot sample or 4 hr or overnight collection.
	If gross protein present, 24 hr collection with a simultaneous measurement for creatinine clearance or an eGFR (estimated glomerular filtration rate from a random sample)
Blood pressure	Every regular diabetes visit
Weight	Every regular diabetes visit
Height	Every regular diabetes visit until 18; yearly for age 55+

Nutritional Goals

Provide regular nutritional advice and guidelines	Every visit
Balance food intake with drug therapy and exercise	Assess every visit

Maintain reasonable weight by monitoring calorie consumption
- 10–20% of calories from protein
- 0% of calories from saturated fat
- <10% of calories from polyunsaturated fat
- <30% of calories from monounsaturated fat
- 60–70% of calories from carbohydrate
- <300 mg cholesterol per day

*Refer to *Diabetes Care*, Suppl. 1, every January for updated recommended changes.

Appendix R

OTHER RESOURCES

Catalogs/Supplies
1. American Association of Diabetes Educators:
   a. AADE 7 Diabetes Self-Care Behaviors: www.diabeteseducator.org/AADE7/index.shtml
   b. AADE's Educational Resources Catalog
2. American Diabetes Association:
   a. Essential Resources for Diabetes Health Professionals
   b. Resource Guide in *Diabetes Forecast*—January issue
3. Continuing Your Journey With Diabetes: Conversation map—Healthy Interactions, Inc.
4. *Diabetes Health Professional*: Yearly Product Reference Guide—January issue
5. Diabetes Mall Catalog: www.Diabetesnet.com
6. International Diabetes Center: www.parknicollet.com/Healthinnovations
7. Milner Fenwick: Patient Education Media Catalog: www.milner-fenwick.com
8. National Institute of Diabetes and Digestive and Kidney Diseases: Information Clearinghouses Publications

Formulas
For Insulin sensitivity (IS): 1700 Rule
1700 divided by total daily dose of insulin, e.g., 1700/50 Units = 34 mg/dL or one unit of insulin decreases BS 34 mg/dL

For insulin resistance:
Insulin sensitivity factor divided into gms of CHO = 2 Units/gm CHO

Insulin sensitivity factor Correction factor:
Present BS subtracted by Ideal BS divided by Insulin sensitivity factor, e.g., 235 mg/dL – 100/34 mg/dL = 3.9 units needed to bring BS to desired level

CHO points
Divide the number of CHO grams by 15 and round – to equal the number of CHO points, 150 gms/15 gms CHO per point = 10 CHO points

Insulin to Calorie Point Ratio (per meal):
Total Daily Dose of insulin divided by Calorie points of food, e.g., 15 Units/5 points for breakfast = 3 Units for every calorie point

Insulin to CHO Ratio:
500 (or 450) divided by the total daily insulin dose (50) = the number of CHO grams covered by 1 Unit of insulin, e.g., 150 gms CHO divided by 15 = 1 Unit of insulin to 10 gms CHO

Web Sites

AIM resources	www.americansinmotion.org
Alternative and Complementary Diabetes Information	www.alternativediabetes.com
American Association of Diabetes Educators	www.diabeteseducator.org
American Diabetes Association	www.diabetes.org

American Family Physician	www.aafp.org
American Family Physician – Family Health Info	www.familydoctor.org
Canadian Diabetes Association	www.diabetes.ca
Centers for Disease Control Diabetes Home Page	www.cde.gov.nccdphp.ddt.ddthome.html
Children With Diabetes	www.childrenwithdiabetes.com
Diabetes	www.nd.edu/~hhowisen/diabetes.html
Diabetes Bookstore	www.merchant.diabetes.org
Diabetes.com	www.diabetes.com
Diabetes Disaster Preparedness	www.state.nj.us/health/fhs/documents diabetes_disaster_guidelines.pdf
Diabetes Education & Camping Association	www.diabetescamp.org
Diabetes Forecast	www.diabetes.org/DiabetesForecast
Diabetes Guide to the Internet	www.pslgroup.com/DIABETES.html
Diabetes in America	www.diabetes-in-America.s3.com/default.html
Diabetes in Control	www.diabetesincontrol.com
Diabetes Information	www.mediconsult.com/diabetes
Diabetes Monitor	www.mdcc.com
Diabetes One Stop	www.diabetesonestop.com
Diabetes Self-Management	www.diabetes-self-mgmt.com
Diabetes World	www.diabetesworld.com
Growth Charts	www.cdc.gov/growthcharts
Health Literacy	www.hrsa.gov/quality/healthlit.htm
Juvenile Diabetes Foundation	www.jdfcure.com
Kids and Family-Friendly Web Site	www.kidnetic.com
Max's Magical Delivery: Fit for Kids	www.ahrg.gov/child/dvdobesity.htm
National Association of School Nurses	www.nasn.org
National Diabetes Education Program (DNEP)	www.ndep.nih.gov
National Institutes of Diabetes	www.niddk.nih.gov/NIDDK
North American Association for Study of Obesity	www.obesityonline.org
Online Diabetes	www.OnlineDiabetes.com
Steps to a Healthier You	www.mypyramid.gov
U.S. Department of Agriculture (USDA)–Nutrition	www.nutrition.gov
Wisdom (for kids)	www.diabetes.org/wisdom
Diana Guthrie	www.dguthrie@kumc.edu
Richard Guthrie	www.RAG33@hotmail.com

Index